AF511579

Second Edition

Pathology Practicals

with OSPE

As per the latest NMC Guidelines |
Competency Based Medical Education (CBME) Curriculum
under Graduate Medical Education Regulation

Second Edition

Pathology Practicals

with OSPE

As per the latest NMC Guidelines |
Competency Based Medical Education (CBME) Curriculum
under Graduate Medical Education Regulation

Santosh Kumar Mondal MBBS MD
Professor and Head
Department of Pathology
AIIMS (All India Institute of Medical Sciences)
Kalyani, West Bengal
Ex-Professor, Department of Pathology
BS Medical College, Bankura, West Bengal
Ex-Associate Professor, Department of Pathology
Medical College, Kolkata, West Bengal

CBSPD

CBS Publishers & Distributors Pvt Ltd

New Delhi • Bengaluru • Chennai • Kochi • Kolkata • Lucknow • Mumbai
Gujarat • Hyderabad • Jharkhand • Nagpur • Patna • Pune • Uttarakhand

Disclaimer

Science and technology are constantly changing fields. New research and experience broaden the scope of information and knowledge. The author has tried his best in giving information available to him while preparing the material for this book. Although all efforts have been made to ensure optimum accuracy of the material, yet it is quite possible some errors might have been left uncorrected. The publisher, the printer and the author will not be held responsible for any inadvertent errors or inaccuracies.

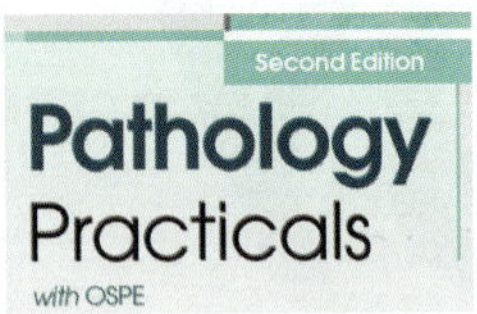

ISBN: 978-93-5466-742-8

Copyright © Author and Publisher

Second Edition: 2024
Reprint: 2026
First Edition: 2019
Reprint: 2020

All rights reserved. No part of this book may be reproduced or transmitted in any form or by any means, electronic or mechanical, including photocopying, recording, or any information storage and retrieval system without permission, in writing, from the author and the publisher.

Published by Satish Kumar Jain and produced by Varun Jain for

CBS Publishers & Distributors Pvt Ltd
4819/XI Prahlad Street, 24 Ansari Road, Daryaganj, New Delhi 110 002, India
Ph: 011-23289259, 23266838 Website: www.cbspd.com
e-mail: delhi@cbspd.com

Corporate Office: 204 FIE, Industrial Area, Patparganj, Delhi 110 092, India
Ph: 011-4934 4934 Fax: 011-4934 4935 e-mail: publishing@cbspd.com; publicity@cbspd.com

Branches

- **Bengaluru:** Seema House 2975, 17th Cross, K.R. Road, Banasankari 2nd Stage, Bengaluru 560 070, Karnataka, India
  Ph: +91-80-26771678/79 Fax: +91-80-26771680 e-mail: bangalore@cbspd.com
- **Chennai:** 18/8B, Subbarayan Street, Shenoy Nagar, Chennai 600 030, Tamil Nadu, India
  Ph: +91-44-26680620, 26681266 Fax: +91-44-42032115 e-mail: chennai@cbspd.com
- **Kochi:** 42/1325, 1326, Power House Road, Opp KSEB, Power House, Ernakulam, Kochi, 682 018, Kerala, India
  Ph: +91-484-4059061-65,67 Fax: +91-484-4059065 e-mail: kochi@cbspd.com
- **Kolkata:** 147, Hind Ceramics Compound, 1st Floor, Nilgunj Road, Belghoria, Kolkata 700 056, West Bengal, India
  Ph: +91-33-25633055/56 e-mail: kolkata@cbspd.com
- **Lucknow:** Basement, Khushnuma Complex, 7-Meerabai Marg (behind Jawahar Bhawan), Lucknow 226 001, UP, India
  Ph: +91-522-4000032 e-mail: tiwari.lucknow@cbspd.com
- **Mumbai:** PWD Shed, Gala no. 25/26, Ramchandra Bhatt Marg, Next to JJ Hospital Gate no. 2, Opp. Union Bank of India, Noorbaug, Mumbai 400 009, Maharashtra, India
  Ph: +91-22-66661880/89 e-mail: mumbai@cbspd.com

Representatives

- **Gujarat** 0-9879558667
- **Hyderabad** 0-9885175004
- **Jharkhand** 0-9811541605
- **Nagpur** 0-8692091830
- **Patna** 0-9334159340
- **Pune** 0-9664372571
- **Uttarakhand** 0-9716462459

Printed at: HT Media Ltd, Greater Noida, UP, India

to

All my beloved Students:
Past, Present and Future

Preface to the Second Edition

It gives me immense pleasure to bring the second edition of *Pathology Practicals*. Considering the rapid progress in the medical education and an overwhelming response to the first edition warranted emergence of the second edition. This edition incorporates CBME (Competency Based Medical Education) and OSPE (Objective Structured Practical Examination) as suggested by NMC/MCI. As per the latest CBME guidelines, the following have been incorporated:

- OSPE (Objective Structured Practical Examination)
- DOPS (Direct Observation of Procedural Skills).

Also, separate chapters on Hemoparasites and Blood Transfusion, have been included. In the chapter OSPE, 100 cases have been discussed. Separate museum specimens OSPE are now part of this second edition.

Hand-drawn schematic diagrams of microscopic slides, included in this book, will be very useful for students. Students will be able to draw these figures on their exercise books as part of their assignments given by teachers. A new chapter on definitions and Other important aspects related to General Pathology will be of great help during viva-voce examination.

Previous year questions (2023 and 2022) are also included in this edition. Like first edition, many colour and black and white pictures, diagrams, flowcharts have been added for easy understanding. In the viva-voce section (end of each chapter), many new questions have been added which are thought provoking and useful during practical/viva examination.

So, there is a sea change in this second edition, which is completely revised, updated, and better illustrated. I thank my parents, wife, and son for their constant support to bring out this edition. Special thanks to Dr Deepika Pandey who was SR of our department. I also thank Dr Tummidi Santosh, Associate Professor, Department of Pathology who lend a helping hand from time to time. Hope, this practical book will be practically a students' companion and will enable them to score high marks.

A humble submission, i.e. suggestions, positive criticism from the faculties as well as students are solicited, which will inspire me in improvisation of the subsequent edition.

Santosh Kumar Mondal
E-mail: santosh.path@aiimskalyani.edu.in

Preface to the First Edition

Francis Bacon once said "Some books to be tasted, others swallowed and some few to be chewed and digested". But books like friends should be a few and well chosen.

Clarifying concepts and inculcating the fundamental tenets in pathology practicals are daunting tasks for any medical teacher. Pathology is a rapidly expanding field of medicine with new techniques. In modern era, tremendous growth is in progress in diagnostic pathology.

In this book, five sections (Haematology, Clinical Pathology, Histopathology and Cytopathology, Museum Techniques and Mounted Surgical Specimens and Problem Cards and Discussion) with a total of 16 chapters have been included. All these chapters are related to pathology practicals. Not only the practical aspect of a test or technique has been described but also the theoretical concept with regard to that particular test has been explained. At the end of every chapter, viva voce questions related to that particular topic have been included that will help the medical students face the examiner during pathology practical examinations.

Real mounted surgical specimens and their gross/macroscopic features will enhance the students' understanding. The problem cards will help to build logical thinking among the medical students. For easy understanding, many colour as well as black and white pictures/ microphotographs, flow charts, diagrams, and tables have been included.

I thank my parents, my wife Shampa and son Soumyadeep for their constant support to complete this work. I thank Dr Debashis Chakrabarty, Associate Professor, Department of Pathology, SSKM Hospital, Kolkata, West Bengal, for helping me during preparation of this book. I also thank my postgraduate students Dr Bidhan Chandra Nayak and Dr Saptarshi Bhattacharya of Bankura Sammilani Medical College for their great help.

Despite our best efforts, some mistakes might creep in. I request all the readers to kindly bring to my notice if there is any mistake or typing error. Your positive criticism, appreciations and suggestions are valuable to us and are most welcome.

Santosh Kumar Mondal

E-mail: dr_santoshkumar@hotmail.com

Contents

Section V: Problem Cards and Discussion

Section VI: OSPE (Objective Structured Practical Examination)

Section VII: Schematic Diagrams (HP Slides) and Definitions of General Pathology

MBBS Curriculum in Pathology and Question Papers

Appendices

Section I

Haematology

1. Blood Collection and Anticoagulants
2. Blood and Bone Marrow Smear Preparation and Staining Methods
3. Marrow Puncture Needle and Examination of Bone Marrow
4. Total Count of WBC, RBC and Platelets
5. Erythrocyte Sedimentation Rate (ESR) and Packed Cell Volume (PCV)
6. Haemoglobin Estimation
7. Bleeding Time (BT), Clotting Time (CT), Prothrombin Time (PT) and APTT
8. Blood Grouping and Rh Typing
9. Haemoparasites
10. Blood Transfusion/Transfusion Medicine

Chapter

1

Blood Collection and Anticoagulants

Blood is the most frequent body fluid used for analytical purpose. Blood is a mesenchymal tissue consisting of a liquid portion called plasma and particulate or formed elements (RBCs, WBCs, platelets) which are suspended in plasma.

Plasma

Blood plasma is a straw-coloured fluid component of blood which normally holds the blood cells in suspension. So, plasma can be called extracellular matrix of blood cells. It makes near about 55% of the total blood value. It is composed mostly of water (up to 95% by volume) and dissolved proteins (6–8%). These proteins are albumin (4.5 g%), globulins (2.5 g%) and fibrinogens (0.3 g%). Apart from proteins, glucose, clotting factors, electrolytes (Na^+, Mg^{2+}, Ca^{2+}, Cl^-, HCO_3^-, etc.). Hormones, carbon dioxide and oxygen are present in the plasma.

Serum

When blood is collected in the test tube or vial without addition of anticoagulants, then blood is clotted. The clot is formed by using blood cells, clotting factor like fibrinogen. The fluid is separated from clot. So, this fluid contains proteins and other elements but lacks fibrinogen (used in the formation of clot).

So, serum is plasma minus fibrinogen.

BLOOD COLLECTION AND PROCESSING

Three general procedures for obtaining blood are (Fig. 1.1A and B):

1. Venipuncture for venous blood
2. Arterial puncture for arterial blood
3. Skin puncture for capillary (peripheral) blood

Venous blood is preferred for most haematological examinations.

Venipuncture or Venous Puncture

Venous blood is best withdrawn from an antecubital vein by means of a dry glass syringe or disposable plastic syringe. The steps are:

i. Position the patient properly, depending on whether the patient is sitting or prone (ambulatory or non-ambulatory). This is to make sure for easy access to the antecubital fossa.

ii. The patient is asked to make a fist, so that veins become more prominent and more palpable.

iii. Select a suitable vein for venipuncture. For veins of the antecubital fossa, the median cubital and cephalic veins may be used alternatively. In case, the patient has an intravenous line, draw venous blood from other arm.

iv. Cleanse the venipuncture site with 70% alcohol (isopropanol) or 1% iodine-

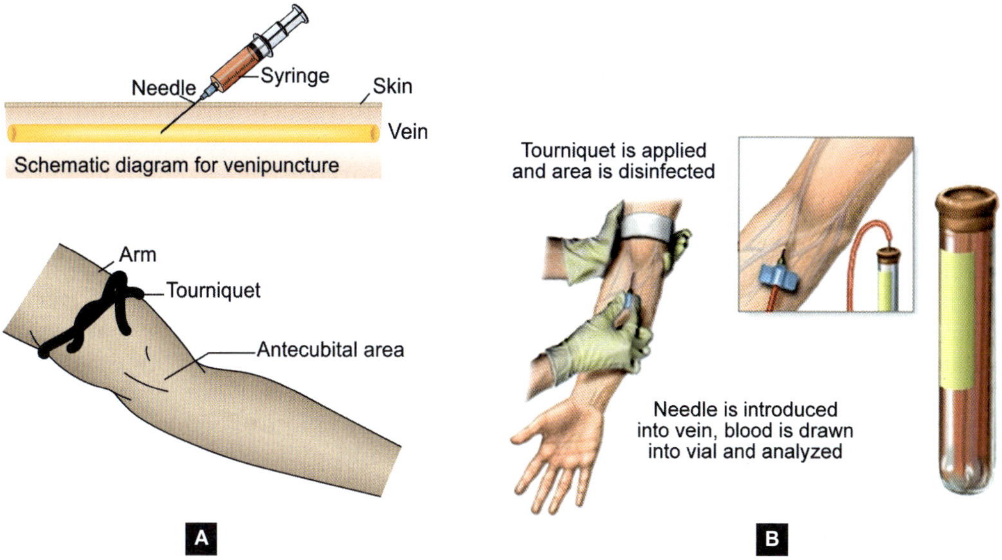

Fig. 1.1A and B: Blood collection procedure

saturated swab stick. Allow the area to dry.

v. Apply a tourniquet few inches above the puncture site. But remember, do not keep the tourniquet for more than one minute.

vi. Hold the vein firmly, both above and below the puncture site. For this, use either thumb and middle finger or thumb and index finger.

vii. Perform the venipuncture. Enter the syringe needle (19 or 20 gauge) at approximately 15° angle to the arm. If using the evacuated system or vacuotainer as soon as the needle is inserted in the vein, ease the collection tube forward in the holder as far as possible, firmly securing the needle holder in place.

viii. Release the tourniquet when blood begins to flow.

ix. After blood collection, place a clean cotton ball or gauze lightly over the site. Withdraw the needle, then apply pressure to site.

x. Now apply an adhesive bandage strip over the cotton ball or gauze to stop bleeding or formation of haematoma.

Note

i. The needles should not be too fine or too long, those of 19 or 20 SWG British standard, American standard 19 SWG = 18 (1.016 mm), 20 SWG = 19 (0.914 mm) are suitable.

ii. If the veins are very small then 23 SWG (= 22 or 0.610) to be used to collect at least 2 ml venous blood.

iii. If veins are selected from dorsum of the hand, it tends to bleed easily. So, care must be taken.

iv. Beware of haemolysis of blood during collection. It can be avoided or minimized by using clean apparatus, withdrawing the blood slowly, not using too fine needle, delivering the blood slowly into the receiver and avoiding frothing during the withdrawal of the blood and subsequent mixing with the anticoagulant.

Arterial Puncture

Arterial blood is used rarely. It is used to measure oxygen and carbon dioxide tension, as well as pH (arterial blood gases or ABGs). These blood gas measurements are critical in the assessment of oxygenation problems encountered in patients with pneumonia, pneumonitis and pulmonary embolism. Also critically ill cardiovascular patients and patients who are undergoing cardiac or pulmonary surgery are monitored for hypoxaemia.

Arterial puncture is technically more difficult than venous puncture. Increased pressure of the flowing blood, makes it more difficult to stop bleeding with the undesired development of a haematoma. The arteries selected for arterial punctures are radial, brachial and femoral arteries in order of choice. Unsuitable sites are oedematous, irritated, near a wound, or in an area of an arteriovenous (AV) shunt or fistula. Although venous blood yields adequate pH values if properly collected but venous blood yields incorrect values for arterial oxygen saturation and alveolar pCO_2.

Skin Puncture (Capillary Blood)

Skin puncture is the method of choice in paediatric patients especially infants. The large amount of blood collected from repeated venipuncture may cause anaemia (iatrogenic), especially in premature infants. Skin puncture is also preferred in geriatric patients because of thinness of skin and loss of skin elasticity which cause venipuncture difficult.

In the neonates and infants, the heel is often used for skin puncture. A deep heel prick is made at the distal edge of the calcaneal protuberance following 5–10 minutes prior exposure to prewarmed water. In the older paediatric population, and in geriatric patients, earlobes or fingers are preferred.

This capillary blood collected by skin puncture is good for making blood smear or for a single routine haematological test. A blood smear prepared from capillary blood without anticoagulant gives better information about blood cell morphology and differential count. But the total count is not very accurate. This is because of dilution by the tissue fluid and sometimes also due to lack of free flow of capillary blood. But if free flow capillary blood is received, then it is as satisfactory as venous blood.

Capillary blood obtained from heel puncture is not good for pCO_2 and pO_2 determination in the first day of life, probably owing to vasoconstriction and poor perfusion of the extremities. In infants with respiratory distress syndrome, heel blood deviates significantly from arterial blood in all parameters except standard bicarbonate and base excess.

The discrepancies between peripheral (capillary) and venous blood are more pronounced if earlobe than finger is chosen for skin puncture. However, if the ear is rubbed well with a piece of cotton or lint until ear is warm and pink, then a good spontaneous flow of blood can be obtained using sterile lancets as prickers. In this case, RBC count, leucocyte count and haemoglobin content almost close to venous blood.

Heel Puncture Method (Fig. 1.2)

A deep puncture in the heel is made after heel is really warm (5–10 minutes prior

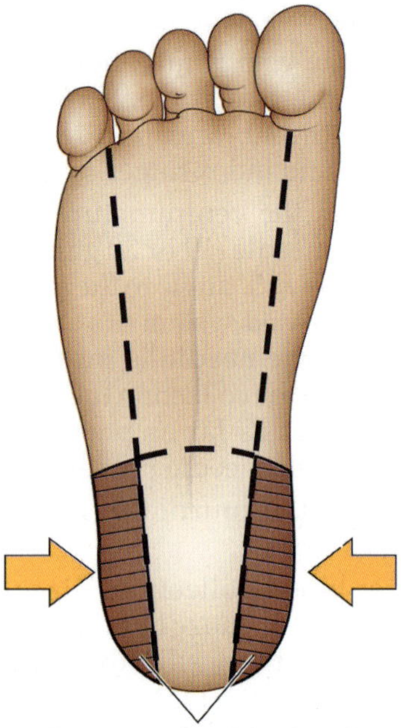

Fig. 1.2: Heel puncture method

exposure to prewarmed water) by using a steel lancet. Ideal sites are the medial or lateral parts of the plantar surface of the heel. Remember, the central plantar area and posterior curvature are not chosen in infants because of risk of injury to the underlying tarsal bones.

Earlobe Puncture Method

Rub the ear until it becomes warm and pink. Then with a sterile lancet prick the earlobe (as it has no bone or cartilage) to a depth of 2–3 mm by a single stab. Wipe and discard first few drops of blood. Collect the blood sample when it flows spontaneously (usually in about 30 seconds). Always use different lancet for different patients.

Finger Prick (Stick) Procedure (Fig. 1.3)

The best locations for finger sticks are the 3rd (middle) and 4th (ring) fingers of the non-dominated hand. Do not select tip of the finger or the centre of the finger. The second (index) finger tends to have thicker and calloused skin, so not preferred. The fifth finger (little finger) tends to have less soft tissue overlying the bone.

1. After selection of site of the finger, put on gloves and cleanse the puncture site with 70% alcohol (isopropanol).
2. Massage the finger toward the selected site prior to puncture.
3. Then with a sterile safety lancet make a skin puncture just off the finger pad.
4. Wipe away the first drop of blood which contains excess tissue fluid/plasma. Take subsequent blood drop into collection tube/device by gentle pressure on the finger; or put the blood drop onto a glass slide.
5. Cap, rotate and invert the collection device/tube.
6. Label it.

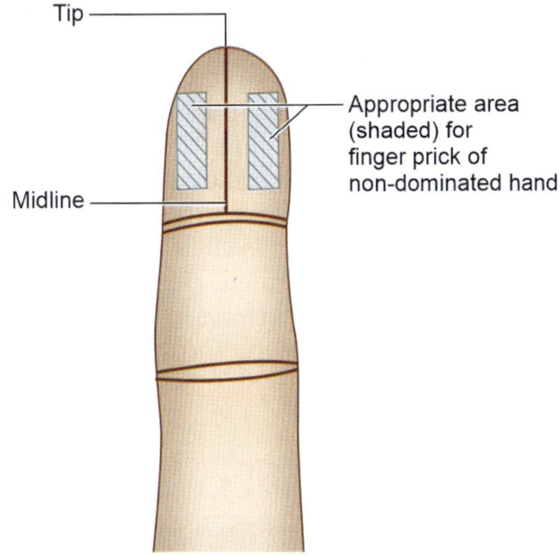

Fig. 1.3: Finger prick (stick) procedure

Differences between Venous and Peripheral (Capillary) Blood

- The platelet count is usually higher in venous than in peripheral blood (average 9% higher, but may go up to 32%). This is probably due to adhesion of platelets to the skin puncture site resulting in lower platelet count in peripheral blood.
- Venous blood and peripheral blood are not same, even though capillary blood is free-flowing which comes from arterioles after skin puncture.
- The RBC count, haemoglobin content and packed cell volume (PCV) are slightly higher in peripheral blood than venous blood. The total leucocyte count (TLC) and neutrophil counts are also higher about 8%, and monocyte count by 12% in peripheral blood. In children, it may be up to 100% higher, both for heel and earlobe punctured capillary blood.
- But the monocytes and neutrophils tend to accumulate in the earlobe if the blood is not free-flowing.

ANTICOAGULANTS

The anticoagulants prevent blood from clotting and as a result, plasma is formed (Table 1.1). Most anticoagulants bind with calcium ions (Ca^{2+}) and remove it by calcium chelating. Calcium is a factor in the coagulation cascade. As the calcium is chelated it cannot work. So, clot is not formed. Heparin, on the other hand, directly interferes in the coagulation process by destroying thrombin as well as thromboplastin.

Platelets + clotting factors + calcium → thrombin which converts fibrinogen → fibrin clot.

1. EDTA (Ethylenediaminetetra-acetic Acid)

It is also called sequestrene and probably the best anticoagulant for routine haematological investigations.

Mechanism of action: It is a powerful calcium chelating or binding agent and acts by binding the calcium in blood. So, active

Table 1.1: Some blood anticoagulants and their use

Name of anticoagulants (requirement per ml of blood)	Mechanism of action	Diagnostic use
1. No anticoagulant for serum in plain vial/tube	No anticoagulant; blood is clotted	Serum: Liver function test (protein, bilirubin, SGOT/AST, SGPT/ALT, alkaline phosphatase γGT, etc.), lipid profile (chole-(sterol, triglyceride, HDL, LDL, VLDL), urea, creatinine, etc.
2. EDTA (1–1.5 mg/ml)	Binds Ca^{2+} and chelates it	Haemoglobin estimation, PCV, TLC, DLC, platelet count, parasite detection (microfilaria, malaria)
3. Trisodium citrate (3.2% aqueous solution; blood to anticoagulant ratio of 9:1 or 4:1 for coagulation studies and ESR respectively)	Binds Ca^{2+} and precipitates it as double salt (calcium sodium salt)	Coagulation studies, prothrombin time, ESR
4. Heparin (0.1–0.2 mg/ml)	Inhibits thrombin in the presence of antithrombin III. Also, it inhibits thromboplastin formation	• Osmotic fragility test • Plasma iron estimation • Demonstration of LE cells • Lymphocyte culture for karyotyping/genetic studies • Lymphoma/leukaemia panel for flow cytometry/ immunophenotyping
5. Sodium or potassium oxalate (2 mg/ml)	Binds Ca^{2+} and chelates it	Blood urea and creatinine
6. Double oxalate (ammonium and potassium oxalate, 2 mg/ml)	Binds Ca^{2+} and chelates it	Hb, TLC, PCV, specific gravity
7. Sodium fluoride (6 mg powder/ml of blood)	• Blocks RBC enzymes for glycolytic inhibition of glucose • Also, chelates calcium	Blood glucose (sugar) estimation

calcium ions are not available for coagulation process.

Concentration of EDTA: A concentration of 1.2 mg of anhydrous salt per ml of blood is required. For dipotassium salt, a concentration of 1.5 ± 0.25 mg/ml of blood is recommended as per International Council for Standardization in Haematology (ICSH). The dipotassium salt is very soluble and is preferred over disodium salt which is less soluble.

Advantages of EDTA

i. Very good anticoagulant for routine haematological investigations. EDTA has the advantage over oxalate anticoagulant because it prevents clumping of platelets *in vitro*. So, platelet count can also be performed on venous blood.

ii. The dilithium salt of EDTA has the advantage that same blood sample can be used for chemical investigations apart from haematological investigations. But dilithium salt is less soluble compared to dipotassium salt and is less preferred.

Disadvantages of EDTA: Excess of EDTA (>2 mg/ml), irrespective of its salts, cause shrinkage and degenerative changes in RBCs and WBCs. Also, excess salt causes significant decrease in PCV and increase in MCHC (mean corpuscular haemoglobin concentration). Excess EDTA causes platelets to swell and then disintegrate, resulting in spuriously high platelet count as the swollen platelet fragments are large enough to be counted as normal platelets.

2. Trisodium Citrate

A 3.2% aqueous solution of trisodium citrate ($Na_3 C_6H_5O_7, 2H_2O$) is the anticoagulant of choice **for coagulation studies**. It is also most widely used anticoagulant **for ESR** (erythrocyte sedimentation rate) also. But for coagulation studies (prothrombin time) 9:1 blood to anticoagulant is used, whereas in ESR determination 4:1 venous blood to anticoagulant is used.

Mechanism of action: Coagulation is prevented by precipitation of blood calcium in the form of a double salt (calcium sodium salt) which is very weakly dissociated.

3. Heparin

Heparin powder or liquid is used in a concentration of 10–20 IU (0.1–0.2 mg) per ml of blood.

Mechanism of action: It acts by inhibiting thromboplastin formation. Also it has antithrombin activity, i.e. inhibiting the action of thrombin on fibrinogen in the presence of plasma of co-factor antithrombin III.

Uses

i. Osmotic fragility test

ii. Chemical investigation like plasma iron estimation

iii. Demonstration of LE cell in SLE patients

iv. Lymphocyte culture for karyotyping/genetic study

v. Lymphoma/leukaemia panel for flow cytometry or immunophenotyping

vi. Nitro blue tetrazolium (NBT) test to assess phagocytic activity of phagocytes.

Advantages: It is an effective anticoagulant and does not alter the size of RBCs. It minimizes chances of haemolysis. Some consider heparin in the form of lithium salt is the ideal universal anticoagulant for blood.

Disadvantages

i. It is expensive

ii. It is inferior to EDTA as anticoagulant

iii. Heparinized blood should not be used for making blood films as it gives a faint blue colouration to the background when blood smears are stained with Romanowsky stains. Also, it causes leucocytes to clump, so TLC and DLC will be erroneous.

4. Oxalate

Potassium, sodium and ammonium oxalates act as calcium chelating agent like EDTA and trisodium citrate. They interact with blood calcium and form calcium oxalate after chelation.

i. Potassium and sodium oxalate: Used mainly for chemical analysis. Concentration of anticoagulant 2 mg/ml of blood.

ii. Double oxalate (Wintrobe's mixture): It is a mixture of two types of oxalates (ammonium oxalate and potassium oxalate in a ratio of 3:2). It is used in a concentration of 2 mg/ml of blood. Preparation of double oxalate mixture is as follows:

- Ammonium oxalate: 1.2 g
- Potassium oxalate: 0.8 g
- Distilled water: 100 ml

This solution contains 20 mg of oxalates (both ammonium and potassium oxalate)/ ml solution. So, 0.2 ml of this solution containing 4 mg of oxalates is sufficient for 2 ml of blood (up to 5 ml blood) as anticoagulants.

Uses

i. Determination of haematocrit value or PCV.
ii. Determination of haemoglobin and total leucocyte count (TLC)
iii. Determination of specific gravity of whole blood or plasma.
iv. Single powder in the form of sodium or potassium oxalate can be used for blood urea and creatinine estimation.

5. Sodium Fluoride

It is used in the concentration of 30 mg powder/5 ml of blood or 6 mg powder/ml of blood. **Mechanism of action:** (i) It chelates calcium and forms calcium fluoride, (ii) it prevents glycolysis by blocking acid phosphorylase enzymes in RBCs but increases amylase activity.

Uses: It is anticoagulant of choice for blood sugar estimation.

For glucose estimation, fluoride may be added to heparin also.

Note

Fluoride inhibits glycolysis of blood cells (RBCs) which may otherwise destroy glucose at the rate of about 5%/hour.

BLOOD COLLECTION TUBES/VIALS AND COLOUR CODE (Figs 1.4 and 1.5)

1. **Red or gold top clot tube:** Contains no anticoagulant. Blood will clot and serum will be formed.
2. **Purple top tube:** Contains EDTA anticoagulant.
3. **Blue top tube:** Contains 3.2% buffered sodium citrate anticoagulant for coagulation studies.
4. **Black top tube:** Contains 3.2% sodium citrate for ESR only.
5. **Light green top tube:** Contains lithium heparin anticoagulant.
6. **Dark green top tube:** Contains sodium heparin anticoagulant used for amino acid and cytogenetic studies.
7. **Gray top tube:** Contains glycolytic inhibitor or sodium fluoride for glucose estimation.
8. **Yellow tube:** Contains acid citrate dextrose (used in blood banking).

SOURCES OF BLOOD COLLECTION ERROR

1. Wrong patient identification or labelling error.
2. Haemoconcentration: Prolonged tourniquet time (>1 minute) restricts blood flow causing false high results, e.g. cell counts.
3. Haemodilution: If blood is collected from an arm with an IV (intravenous), the blood can be diluted and/or contaminated causing false low cell counts.
4. Haemolysis: Caused by traumatic blood drawing technique, vigorous shaking of the blood tube or forcing the blood

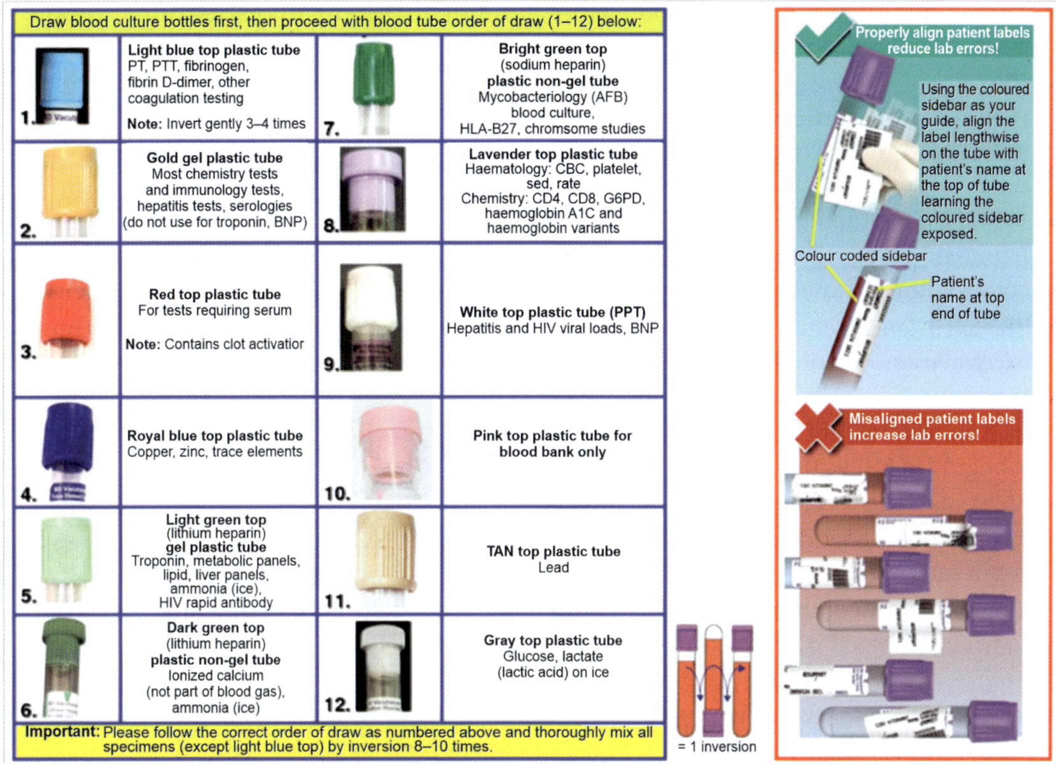

Fig. 1.4: Colour code of top of blood tube/vial and their significance

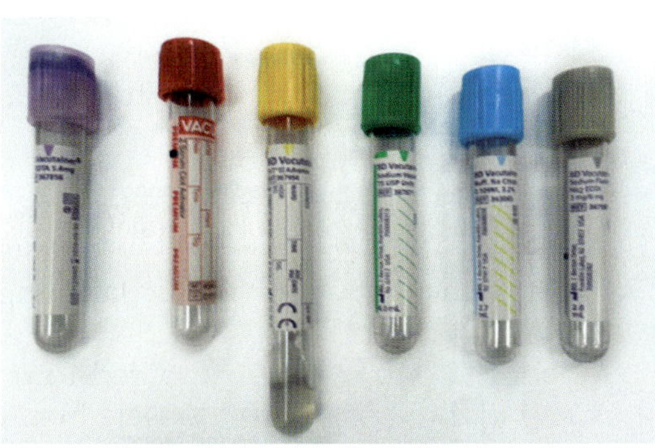

Fig. 1.5: Different blood collection tubes/vials with colour code

through syringe needle into the tube. Rupture of blood cells causes release of cell constituents like potassium, tissue factors and responsible for low RBC counts.

5. Use of wrong anticoagulant/tube: As for example, heparin causes platelet clumping. Hence, unsuitable for platelet counts.
6. Partially clotted blood draws improper mixing of anticoagulant containing tubes or blood obtained using poor blood drawing technique (e.g. too slow) may clot. Cells are trapped in the fibrin clot causing falsely low cell counts.
7. Insufficient fill: All tubes should have minimum draw amounts to maintain the proper anticoagulant concentration to blood volume. As for example, blue top tubes for coagulation test must be full.
8. Proper instruction for the said test not followed, e.g. certain tests have time limits for testing.

EFFECT OF STORAGE OF BLOOD

- When blood is kept in room temperature (18–25°C) for prolonged time, certain changes take place regardless of the anticoagulant use.

- This is obvious in EDTA blood (tripotassium salt > dipotassium salt).
- RBCs begin to swell; as a result, MCV increases, osmotic fragility and prothrombin time increase slowly and ESR decreases.
- The TLC and platelet count gradually fall. It is best to perform TLC and platelet count within 2 hours.
- The fall in leucocyte count is more if there is excessive amount of EDTA (>4.5 mg/ml).
- Reticulocyte count is unchanged for 24 hours at 4°C but at room temperature, it begins to fall within 6 hours.
- Nucleated RBCs (normoblasts) disappear from stored blood within 1–2 days at room temperature.
- Haemoglobin content is relatively stable for days unless it is infected.

For different investigations, blood is collected in tubes with or without anticoagulants. If there is anticoagulant, after mixing the blood cells of whole blood can be analyzed. Centrifugation of whole blood separates the cells from fluid plasma. In the bottom there will be RBCs. Above, there will be plasma containing fibrinogen. In between these two layers, there will be a **buffy coat** containing WBCs and platelets.

If there is no anticoagulant, fibrinogen will be used up to form fibrin strands which entrap blood cells. Centrifugation of this blood will separate the clot from the fluid serum. Serum lacks fibrinogen.

Serum and plasma can be obtained on standing also and they can be taken out by micropipette without disturbing fibrin clot or blood cells respectively. But, centrifugation will give better quality serum or plasma (Fig. 1.6).

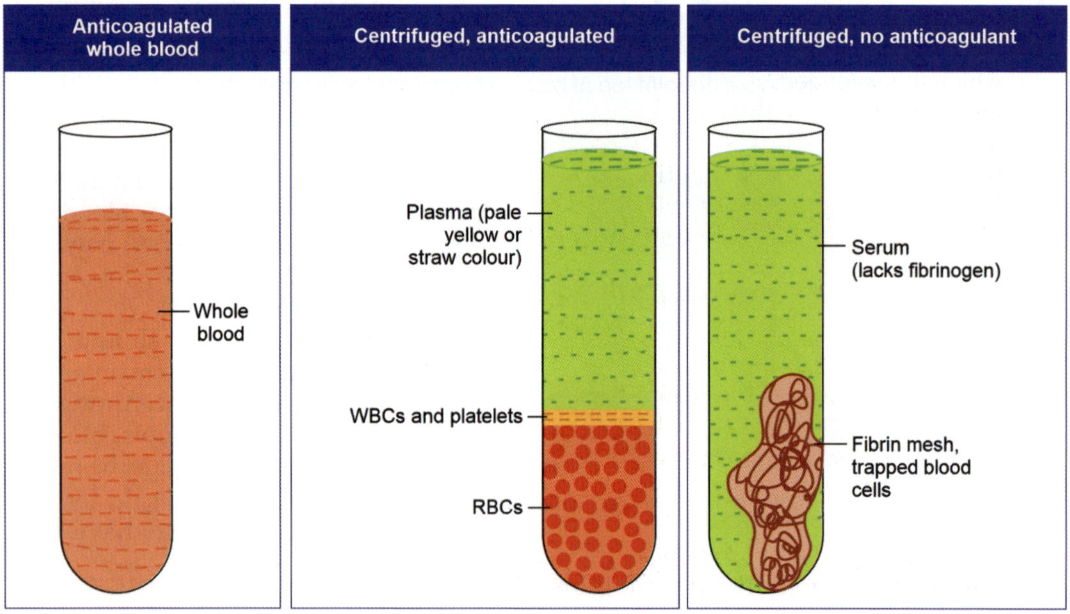

Fig. 1.6: Left tube contains anticoagulated whole blood, middle tube showing plasma and last tube showing serum

VIVA VOCE

Q1. What are differences between serum and plasma?

Ans:

Serum	Plasma
1. Serum is formed as supernatant when blood undergoes clotting	1. Plasma is obtained by centrifugation of anti-coagulant mixed blood. Anticoagulant mixed blood after standing may also give plasma but of poor quality compared to plasma after centrifugation.
2. Serum does not contain fibrinogen, prothrombin and other clotting factors like V, VII, VIII, IX, X, XI and XII which have been used in clotting.	2. It contains all the clotting factors including fibrinogen. But calcium ion is absent.
3. It is used to estimate different biochemical parameters and serum enzymes like uric acid, electrolytes, urea, creatinine, SGOT, SGPT, alkaline phosphatase, etc.	3. It is used mainly for coagulation studies like PT, APTT, TT, etc. Also used for detection of plasma glucose, plasma calcium, plasma ammonia, etc.
4. Serum is clear fluid.	4. Plasma is yellowish or straw coloured.

Q2. What is the ideal gauge needle (bore size) for collection of venous blood?

Ans: If the needle is too large for the vein for which it is intended, it will tear the vein and cause bleeding (haematoma). If the needle, is too small, it will damage the blood cells especially RBCs. So, laboratory tests which require whole blood cells or haemoglobin or plasma will give inaccurate results.

The gauge refers to the inner measurement or opening of the needle. Usually needle gauge of 21G to 23G is preferred for venous blood collection. Small bore needles of 25G or less cannot be recommended and reserved only for problematic venous accesses and newborns. Usually 25G or lesser size may cause haemolysis and inaccurate results of electrolytes especially potassium. Nonetheless, 21G needles are most commonly used for routine tests.

Q3. Why is middle or ring finger preferred for capillary blood collection?

Ans: The best locations for finger sticks are the 3rd (middle) and 4th (ring) fingers of the non-dominated hand. Do not select tip of the finger or the centre of the finger. The second (index) finger tends to have thicker and calloused skin, so not preferred. The fifth finger (little finger) tends to have less soft tissue overlying the bone. Ulnar side of the tip of ring finger is comparatively less innervated. So, needle prick is less painful to the patients.

Q4. Why too much pressure is not given during blood collection from finger prick?

Ans: Needle prick should be deep enough so that free flow blood comes out. Gentle pressure may be applied to start the blood. But too much pressure to finger tip should not be given as tissue fluid will come out which will dilute the blood. So, haematological values will be lowered.

Q5. Why double oxalate is preferred over single oxalate as an anticoagulant?

Ans: Ammonium salt (ammonium oxalate) causes swelling of RBCs while potassium salt (potassium oxalate) causes shrinkage of RBCs. Hence, mixture of these two salts or double oxalate will cause neither RBC swelling nor RBC shrinkage. Normal shape and size of RBCs are maintained. Potassium oxalate: Ammonium oxalate = 2:3.

But oxalates are not preferred as anticoagulant for Hb/TLC/platelet count as they induce morphologic alterations in WBCs and RBCs. So, smear morphology cannot be studied.

Q6. Why excess EDTA is bad as anticoagulant?

Ans: Excess of EDTA (>2 mg/ml), irrespective of its salts, cause shrinkage and degenerative changes in RBCs and WBCs. Also, excess salts cause significant decrease in PCV and increase in MCHC (mean corpuscular haemoglobin concentration). Excess EDTA causes platelets to swell and then disintegrate, resulting in spuriously high platelet count as the swollen platelet fragments are large enough to be counted as normal platelets.

Q7. What is a vacutainer?

Ans: **Vacutainer:** This is a blood collection tube which is sterile glass or plastic tube with a coloured rubber stopper creating a vaccum seal inside of the tube facilitating the drawing of a predetermined volume of blood/liquid. Vacutainer tubes may contain anticoagulant/additives to stabilize and preserve the blood/liquid specimen prior to analytical testing. Tubes containing gel can be easily handled and transported after centrifugation without the blood cells and serum mixing.

Vacutainer tubes were invented by Joseph Kleiner and Becton Dickinson in 1949.

Q8. What are different vacutainers used in haematology?

Anticoagulant/additives	Colour	Blood volume	Uses
1. Plain	Red	6 ml	Most biochemistry including drug levels, serological tests, which uses serum, cross-matching.
2. EDTA-K2	Purple/ Lavender	3 ml	Most haematological tests, HbA1C, molecular genetic tests using blood DNA, blood grouping, crossmatch.
3. Lithium heparin	Green	4 ml	Cytogenetic tests using blood DNA, osmotic fragility test, STAT biochemistry like electrolytes, renal screen, ammonia, etc. After blood is drawn inside by vacuum, it should be inverted gently at least 6 times to prevent clotting.
4. Sodium citrate	Blue	2.7 ml	Coagulation studies. This tube should be inverted at least 3–4 times.
5. Sodium fluoride/ potassium oxalate	Grey	6 ml	Glucose test. It should be inverted gently at least 6 times.
6. SST II, clot activator and serum gel separator, plain	Yellow	5 ml	All tests requiring serum except those few that need red cells as well

Chapter

2

Blood and Bone Marrow Smear Preparation and Staining Methods

Examination of blood and bone marrow smear/film are important haematologic evaluation and to diagnose a haematologic disease. Blood or bone marrow smears should be prepared immediately as delay can cause spurious results.

Here, three methods of making blood smears/films are described

1. Wedge method
2. Spinner or spin method
3. Cover glass method

WEDGE METHOD

This is perhaps the most common method to prepare a blood film (Fig. 2.1A to D). Place a small drop of blood (2–3 mm in diameter) about 1–2 cm from the end of a clean, dust-free slide which is on flat surface. Then without any delay, a spreader (second slide) is hold between thumb and forefinger of the right hand against the surface of the first slide at an angle of 30–45° and move it back to make contact with the blood drop to spread it. Then push the spreader slide at a moderate speed forward until all the blood has been spreaded over the first slide forming a moderately thin film. Ideally, the spreader slide should be clean, dry and slightly narrower than the first slide so that blood does not cross the edge of the first slide and edges of blood film can be examined under the microscope.

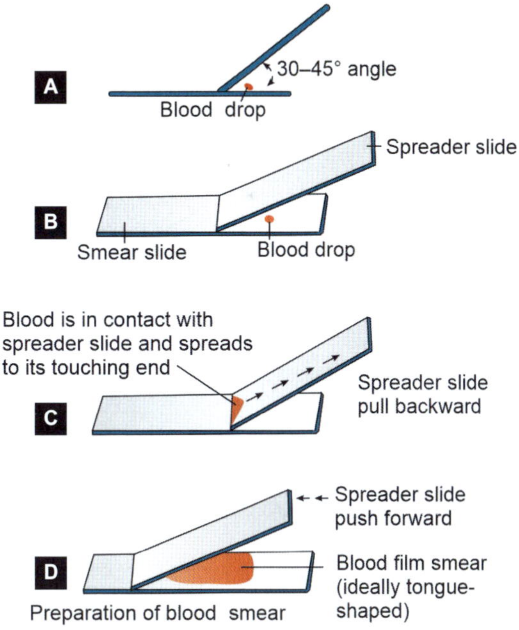

Fig. 2.1A to D: Preparation of blood smears. (A) Small blood drop from 1 to 2 cm from one end of glass slide; (B) Place the spreader slide at an angle of 30° to 45° over the smear slide; (C) Pull back the spreader slide so that it touches the blood drop and spreads throughout the edge of the spreader slide; (D) Push forward to make blood/smear

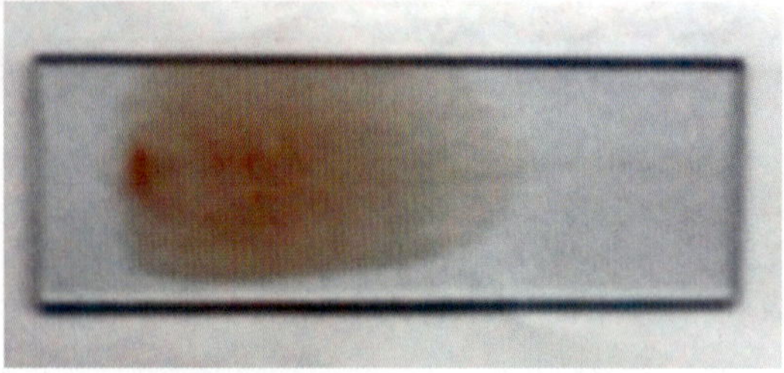

Fig. 2.2: Ideal thin blood smear

Note

a. The blood drop should be such that it can produce the blood film 3–4 cm in length.
b. The ideal thickness of blood film should be such that there will be some overlap of RBC (red blood cells) throughout much of the blood film's length. But the RBCs are separated at the tail end of the film.
c. The film should not cover the entire surface of glass slide.
d. Ideally, there will be a thick portion and a thin portion in a good film and there will be gradual transition from one to the other (Fig. 2.2).
e. The blood film should have an even, smooth appearance and should be free ridges, waves or holes.
f. The edge of spreader slide must be very smooth. Roughed edges will produce ragged tails containing many leucocytes (WBCs).
g. The thickness of blood film can be adjusted by changing the speed of spreading or by changing the angle of the spreader slide or by using a larger or smaller blood drop (Figs 2.3 and 2.4).
h. At a given angle, increasing the speed of spreader slide will cause increase in the thickness of the film.
i. At a given speed, increasing the angle of spreader slide will also cause increase in the thickness of the film.
j. The faster the blood film is air dried, the better the spreading of the individual cells on glass slide. Slow drying of film (as in humid weather) may cause contraction artifacts of the cells.
k. There may be disproportionate monocytes at the tip of the feather (tail) edge or neutrophils just in from the feather edge and both at the lateral edges of the film.

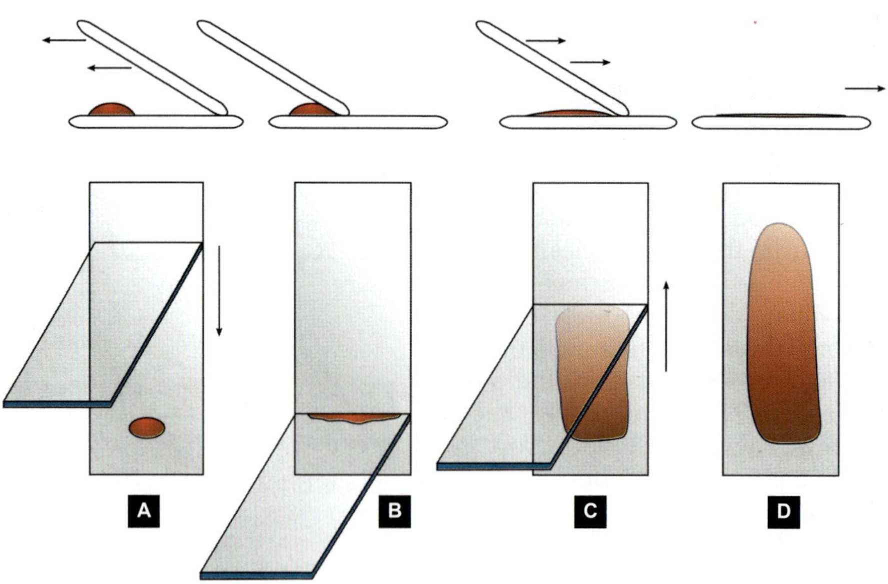

Fig. 2.3A to D: Upper row showing side view of different steps of making a thin blood film. Lower row showing front view of different steps of making a thin blood film

Thin film

- Good preparation—feathered end of the film should be centrally located on the slide with free margins on both sides, when properly prepared, it will be only one cell layer thick at this end.
- Badly prepared smears can cause presence of streaks—as a result of chipped spreader.
- Holes in the film indicate faulty preparation and dirty or greasy slides, respectively.

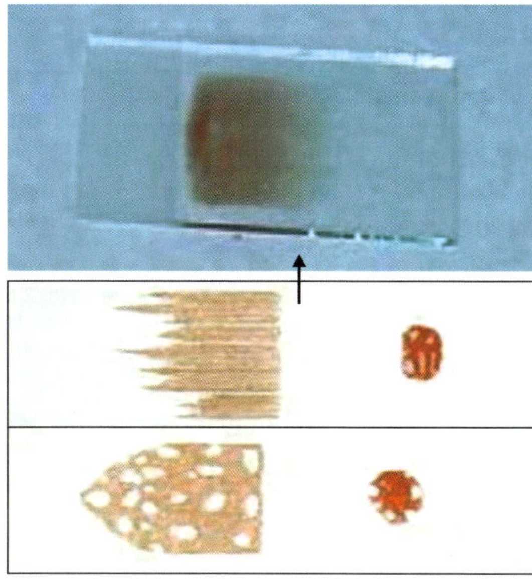

Fig. 2.4: Good and badly prepared thin blood film

SPINNER OR SPIN METHOD

Spinner or spin method is an automated method in which 1–2 drops of blood drops are placed in the centre of a glass slide. Then it is spun at a high speed in a spherical centrifuge (e.g. cytospin) for a short period. The blood drops are spreaded on the glass slide in a monolayer. With this method leucocytes and platelets are distributed uniformly without any distortion.

Note

1. The RBCs may be distorted.To overcome this problem, mix one volume of 9 g/L NaCl (sodium chloride) to 2 volumes of blood for diluting the blood and then put the diluted blood on the glass slide.
2. White blood cells (WBCs) can be easily examined on any spot in the film made by spinner method.
3. Unlike wedge method, it does not produce disproportionate monocytes and/or neutrophils at the tail or lateral edges.

COVER GLASS METHOD

For this, 22 mm square (number one or one and a half cover glasses) are recommended. Touch a cover glass to the top of a small blood drop without touching the skin. Now place it, blood side down crosswise onto another cover glass, so that the corners appear as an eight point star. The small blood drop will spread out quickly and evenly in a thin layer between the two surfaces. Prepare blood film by pulling the cover glasses quickly and firmly apart on a plane parallel to their surfaces. After that, cover glasses are placed on clean paper (film side up) and are air dried.

Blood film from venous blood may be prepared likewise by placing a blood drop on a coverslip and follow the above mentioned steps.

THICK SMEAR AND ITS PREPARATION

While the blood film mentioned above, is suitable for studies of cellular morphology, sometimes thick smears are prepared to detect microfilariae and malarial parasites (Figs 2.5 to 2.7). Thick smears are very useful when parasites (malaria and microfilaria) are scanty but identification of the parasites is less than thin films. Mixed infection (both *Plasmodium vivax* and *falciparum*) may also be missed. Thick smear is also useful when there is severe leucopenia. It helps to perform differential count or at least the proportion of polymorphonuclear to mononuclear cells.

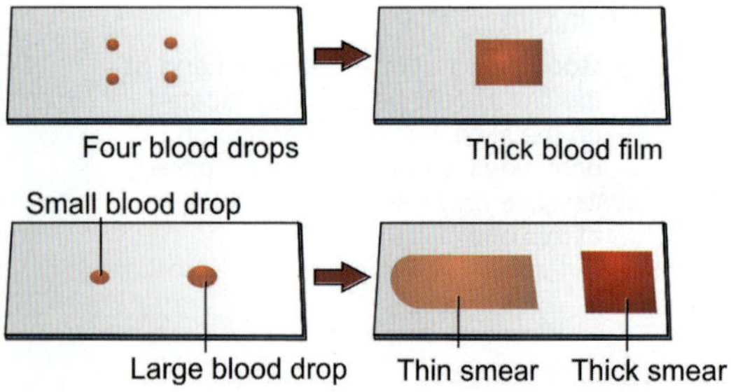

Fig. 2.5: Preparation of thick and thin blood films in the upper panel. Preparation of both thin and thick blood films on the same slide.

Preparation of Thick Film

A drop of blood is placed in the centre of a glass slide and is spreaded out with a corner of another slide to cover an area about four times its original area. The film may be air-dried or dried at 37°C for 30 minutes in an incubator. If the film is satisfactory, then printed matter (small print of newspaper) is just visible.

Alternatively, four small blood drops may be taken in the mid-portion of a glass slide. They are joined together to form a blood film (square shaped) in the mid-portion of the slide.

Sinton proposed to make thin and thick smears onto same glass slide. For this, a large blood drop is taken near one end to make thick smear and one small blood drop is taken in the centre of the slide. Thick smear is prepared from the large blood drop (square shaped) while thin smear is prepared from the small blood drop (tongue shaped) in the same manner as previously described.

Fixation of Blood Films

Blood films need to be fixed before staining to prevent haemolysis when they come in contact with water during water-based (aqueous) stains or water is poured during staining. For this, blood films are coated with acetone-free methyl alcohol for 1–2 minutes. This alcohol (methyl alcohol) denatures the proteins present in the blood and hardens

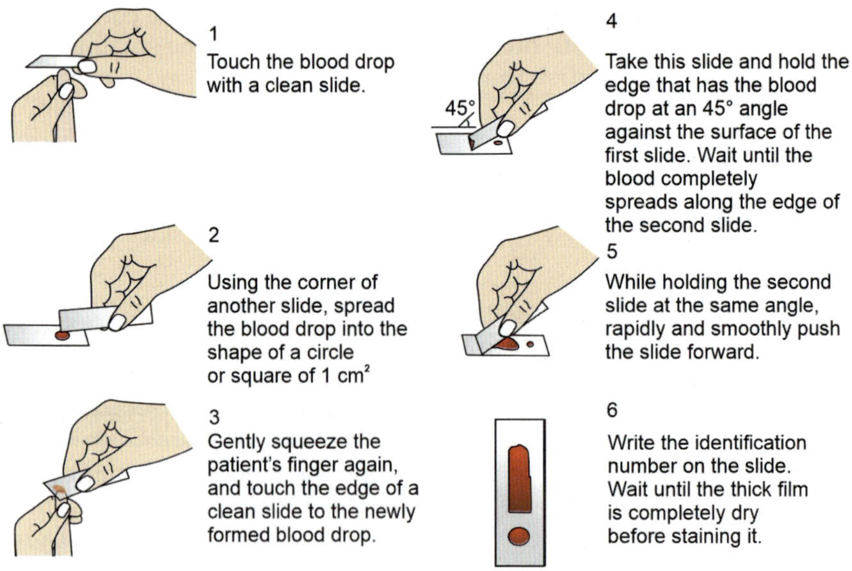

Fig. 2.6: Preparation of a thin and a thick blood film on the same slide

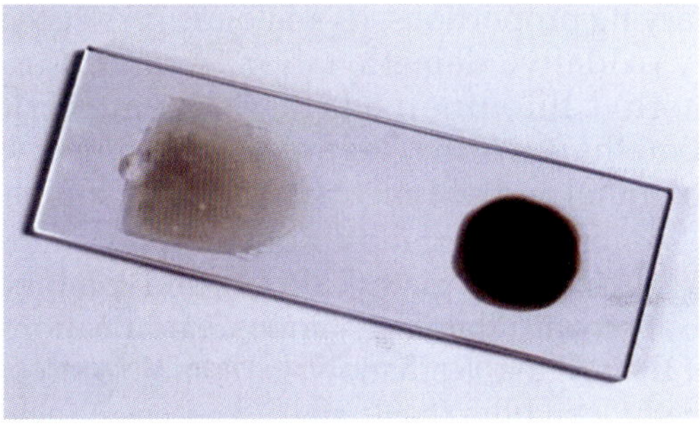

Fig. 2.7: Thin and thick blood films on the same slide. Thin blood film is typically tongue-shaped while thick blood film is circular or square-shaped

the blood cells. As Leishman's stain and Wright's stain contain acetone-free methyl alcohol in the staining solution, the blood films do not require prefixation with alcohol. But Giemsa staining needs prefixation with alcohol as the ready to use staining solution contains only 5% alcohol (suboptimal for fixation).

BONE MARROW ASPIRATE FOR EXAMINATION

1. **Bone marrow films:** Put one drop of aspirate onto slides about 1 cm from one end. Then quickly suck off most of blood present in the aspirate with the help of a fine Pasteur pipette applied to the edge of each drop. Alternatively, keep the glass slides on a slope (to tilt them) for draining away of the blood.

   While the blood is removed, the irregularly shaped marrow fragments adhere to the slide. After that make bone marrow films which will be 3–5 cm in length by using a smooth edged glass spreader of less than 2 cm width. The marrow fragments are dragged behind the spreader and place the marrow cells trailing behind the spreader (trail of cells). The differential count should be made in these cellular trails, starting from the marrow fragment and working back towards the head of the film.

   Fix the bone marrow films and stain them with Romanowsky dyes as for peripheral blood films. But for high quality, a longer fixation time is needed (>20 minutes in methanol).

   Some advocate to add the aspirated marrow material to an anticoagulant like EDTA in a tube and to prepare a marrow films on returning to the laboratory. But there may be a possibility of using excess anticoagulant (only 0.2–0.3 ml of marrow aspirate compared to 2–5 ml of blood). The stained marrow film may show pink-staining amorphous material and some of the erythroblasts and reticulocytes may clump together due to excess anticoagulants.
2. **Bone marrow imprints:** Bone marrow fragments/particles of imprints may also be used for preparation of imprints. One or more visible particles are picked up with a capillary pipette, a toothpick or the broken end of a wooden applicator. The bone marrow particle(s) are transferred immediately to a slide and made to adhere to it by a gentle smearing motion. The slide is air dried rapidly by waving it and then is stained.
3. **Crush preparations:** A small drop aspirate containing a slide near one end. Another slide is placed over the first slide. Slight pressure is given to crush the bone marrow and the slides are separated by pulling them apart in a direction parallel to their surfaces.

   All bone marrow films should be dried quickly by moving them in the air (air dried) or by exposing them to a fan.

   As the bone marrow aspirate is being spreaded, the fat appears as irregular holes and make it sure that the marrow, material not only the blood has been aspirated.

POOR BLOOD SMEARS AND ITS COMMON CAUSES

1. The glass slides should be very clean as dirty slides do not give an even smear.

2. Put an appropriate size of blood drop onto glass slide and make the smear immediately. Delay will cause uneven distribution of WBCs.
3. The spreader slide should be moved steadily and confidently. Jerky movement or loss of contact between spreader slide and smear slide will give poor smears.
4. Angle between the spreader slide and smear slide should be 30° to 45°. Increasing the angle may result in a thick smear, whereas decreasing the result in a thin smear.

FIXING AND STAINING OF BLOOD SMEAR

The smears should be stained immediately after the preparation. Methanol (acetone-free) present in the common Romanowsky stains fix the smear slides in the staining procedure. If staining is delayed then smears must be fixed with methanol for 2–3 minutes. Fixation of smears will prevent distortion of blood cells and smears can be stored for future staining.

In the blood cells, some structural components are acidic while others are basic. Acidic substances stain with basic stain like methylene blue, azure B, etc. and are called basophilic. Examples of basophilic substances are nuclei and nucleic acids. Some basic structures like haemoglobin are stained with acid stains like eosin and are called acidophilic or eosinophilic. Other structures stained by combination of the two are called neutrophilic.

Stains which are composed of both acid and basic dyes are known as "Romanowsky" stains. These stains have the ability to make subtle distinctions during staining of cell and can stain the granules differentially. Neutrophilic granules are weakly stained by azure complexes, whereas eosinophilic granules get stained by acidic component of the dye and basophilic granules which contain acid heparin are stained by basic component of the dye.

The thiazine's basic component consists of methylene blue (tetramethyl thionine) and in varying proportions, its analogues produced by oxidative demethylation: Azure B (trimethyl thionine); azure A (asymmetric dimethylthionine), azure C (monomethyl thionine) and symmetric dimethyl thionine.

As already said most Romanowsky stains are dissolved in methyl alcohol and combine fixation with staining. Various modifications of the original Romanowsky combination of methylene blue (basic stain) and eosin (acid stain) are now used. Usually combination of azure B and eosin Y is used as Romanowsky stain. Common Romanowsky stains are:

1. Leishman's stain
2. Wright's stain
3. Giemsa stain
4. May-Grünwald-Giemsa (MGG) stain
5. Field's stain
6. Jenner's stain
7. MacNeal stain.

Leishman's stain is mostly used in the routine staining of blood film though Wright's stain and Giemsa stain are also very popular (Table 2.1). Giemsa stain is ideal for staining and detecting malarial parasites and other protozoa. Field's stain is used for staining thick film to detect malarial parasites and it offers rapid staining and screening of blood smears. MGG stains are used not only for blood/bone marrow films but also for cytology/FNAC smears.

Leishman's Stain

Reagents

1. Leishman powder (eosin-methylene blue powder): 0.15 g
2. Methyl alcohol (acetone-free): 100 ml

The Leishman powder is placed in a conical flask to which methyl alcohol is added. Then the mixture is warmed to 50°C for 10–15 minutes. It is then filtered. The dye is ripened by keeping the filtrate in sunlight for 3–4 days or in an incubator at 37°C for 7 days.

Method: Dry the film in the air and flood the slide with the stain. After 2 minutes, add double the volume of water and stain the

Table 2.1: Common causes of faulty staining and their corrections

Faulty staining pattern	Causes	Corrections
1. Excessive blue stain	Thick films, prolonged staining time, inadequate washing or too high alkaline pH of stain or diluent.	Staining for less time or using less stain and more diluent. The pH of the buffer should be lowered.
2. Excessive pink stain	Insufficient staining, prolonged washing time, mounting the coverslips before they are dry, too high acidity (very low pH) of the diluents buffer or stain.	Staining time or washing time as advocated pH of buffer and stain should be adjusted.
3. Precipitates on the film	Drying during period of staining, inadequate washing of slide after staining, inadequate filtration of the stain, dust particles on smear or slide and use of unclean slides.	Act as per the cause

film for 7–10 minutes. Then wash the smear in a stream of buffered water until it has acquired a pinkish tinge (up to 2 minutes). After the back of the slide has been wiped clean, set it up right to dry.

Wright's Stain

Reagents

1. Wright's stain powder: 0.2 g
2. Methyl alcohol (acetone-free): 100 ml

The solution is kept at 37°C for a few days before use.

Method: Almost same as in Leishman's staining. When the stain is ripe, a scum of film is formed over the surface of the stain.

Giemsa Stain

Reagents

- Giemsa powder: 0.6 g
- Glycerol: 50 ml
- Acetone-free methyl alcohol: 50 ml

Giemsa powder (0.6 g) is placed in a conical flask. Then 50 ml of glycerol is added. This mixture is warmed at 50°C for 15 minutes with occasional shaking and then 50 ml methanol is added to the mixture. It is now filtered and filtrate is ready for use. But before use the stain should be diluted 1:10 (1 part stain + 9 parts distilled water).

Method: Unlike Leishman or Wright stain, here the blood films should be fixed with methyl alcohol (acetone-free) separately for 3–5 minutes and then dried. Because after 1:10 dilution acetone-free methyl alcohol becomes 5% only (from 50% in original), which is suboptimal for fixation of blood cells. Diluted Giemsa stain (1:10) is poured on the fixed smear and kept for 20–30 minutes. Wash the smear with neutral/distilled water and dry.

May-Grünwald-Giemsa Stain

Reagents

1. May-Grünwald powder: 0.3 g
2. Acetone-free methyl alcohol: 100 ml

Dissolve the 0.3 g powder (dye) in 100 ml methyl alcohol and warm it at 50°C for 10 minutes. During warming shake it from time to time, filter after 24 hours.

Method: Fixed the smear in methyl alcohol for 3–5 minutes. Then stain the film with diluted (1:10) May-Grünwald stain for 5 minutes. Then stain the film with diluted (1:10) Giemsa stain for 15–20 minutes. Wash with buffered water and dry in the air.

Field's Stain

Reagents

1. **Stain A (polychromed methylene blue)**
   a. Methylene blue: 0.26 g
   b. Azure B (optional): 0.1 g
   c. Disodium hydrogen phosphate: 2.5 g
   d. Potassium dihydrogen phosphate: 1.25 g
   e. Water: 100 ml

Dissolve the phosphates in warm freshly boiled water. Then mix the azure B with phosphate solution and dissolve it well. Lastly the dyes (methylene blue) are added and mix well. Filter it.

2. **Stain B (eosin)**
   a. Eosin Y (yellow eosin, water soluble): 0.26 g
   b. Disodium hydrogen phosphate: 2.5 g
   c. Potassium dihydrogen phosphate: 1.25 g
   d. Water: 100 ml

Dissolve the phosphates in warm freshly boiled water. Then mix the dye (eosin Y) with phosphate solution and dissolve it well, filter it.

Staining Method

1. Fix the film for 10–15 seconds in methanol.
2. Pour off the methanol and put 12 drops of diluted stain B (1:4 dilution in water)
3. Immediately add 12 drops of stain A.
4. Agitate the slides to mix the stains.
5. After 1 minute, rinse the slide in water.
6. Differentiate the slide in phosphate buffer for 5–10 seconds at pH 6.6.
7. Wash the slide in water.
8. Place it on end to drain and then dry.

> **Note**
>
> i. A pH to the alkaline side of neutrality accentuates the azure component of Romanowsky stain at the expenses of the eosin and vice versa.
> ii. A pH of 6.8 is usually recommended for general or routine use.
> iii. To look, malarial parasites a pH of 7.2 is recommended in order to detect Schuffner's dots of *Plasmodium vivax, ovale* and *malariae*. (Remember Maurer's dots in *P. falciparum* and Ziemann's dots in *P. malariae*).

Chemical Theory of Romanowsky Staining

The mechanism by which certain components or structure of a cell stain with particular dye, depends on complex differences between the different dyes. As for example, azure B in dimer form is bound to anionic molecules, e.g. phosphate groups of DNA, whereas eosin Y is bound as a monomer to cationic sites of proteins.

As early as the dyes are bound to particular structure of the cell, either electron interaction occurs with dye-dye aggregation or the eosin Y molecule is inserted between the azure B molecules and the complex is held together by charge effect.

So, the acidic groupings of the nucleic acids and proteins of the cell nuclei and primitive cytoplasm determine their uptake of the basic dyes (like azure B). On the other hand, the presence of basic groupings on the haemoglobin molecules determines its affinity for acidic dyes and its staining with eosin (acid dye).

Examination of Romanowsky Stained Blood Smear

At first, examine the stained blood smear under low power for screening. Note the background colour and distribution of WBCs. In an ideal stained smear, three zones can be identified visually. The starting area or the "head" of the smear (where blood drop was originally placed), following which is the "body" and the thin end of the smear known as "tail" (Fig. 2.8).

At the tail end, RBCs lie singly and the neutrophils and monocytes predominate. In the body, RBCs overlap each other to a certain extent and lymphocytes predominate. The ideal area is in-between these "body" and "tail" of the smear where blood

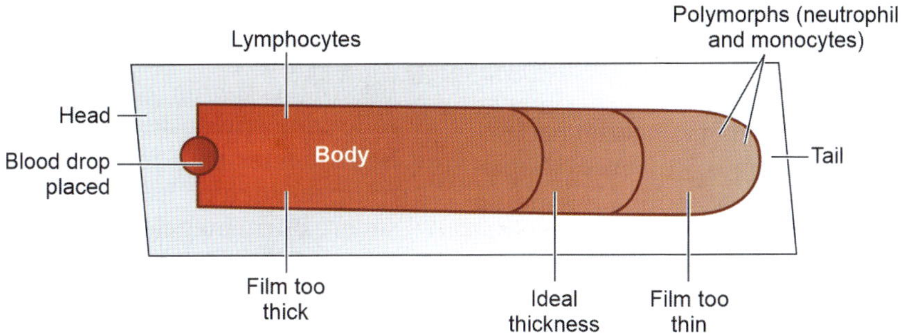

Fig. 2.8: Three zones in stained smears. The head, body and tail

cells are uniformly distributed. Here, the RBCs do not overlap and touch each other slightly.

For differential count of WBCs (Figs 2.9 and 2.10), two methods can be adopted:

1. The original drop of blood spreaded out between spreader and slide (C-C1). The film is made in such a way that representative strips of film like A-A1 and B-B1 are formed from point of application A and B respectively. In order to make an accurate differential count, all leucocytes in one or more strips (like A-A1, B-B1, etc.) should be inspected and classified.

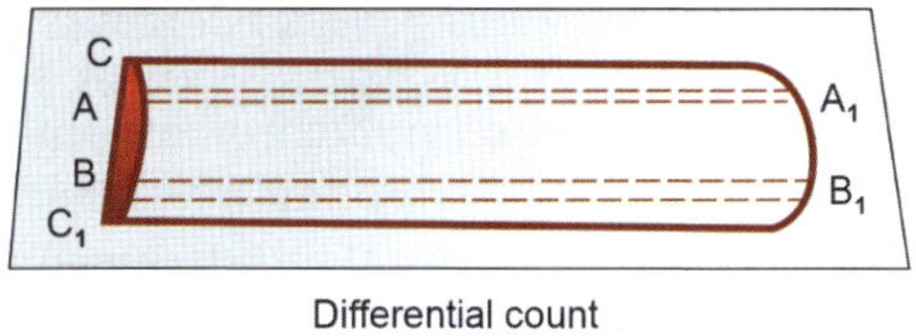

Fig. 2.9: Linear or straight line method of differential count of WBC

2. Choose the ideal thickness of the stained smear. Then inspect and classify all the leucocytes in a serpentine counting pattern (shown diagrammatically) (Fig. 2.10).

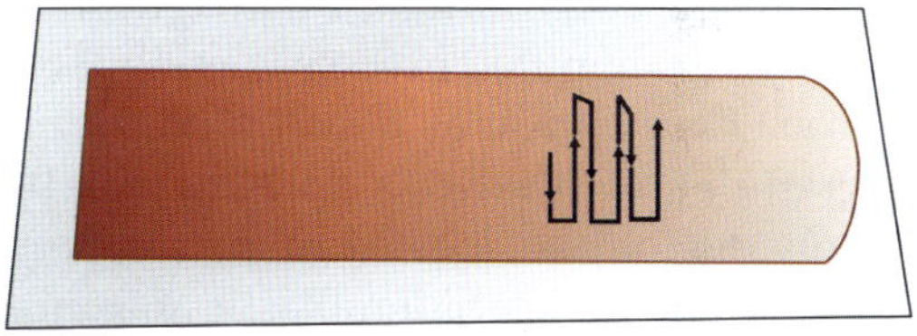

Fig. 2.10: Serpentine counting pattern (area is in between body and tail end of smear)

EXAMINATION OF STAINED BLOOD FILMS

Erythrocytes

The erythrocytes when not crowded together, appear as circular, homogenous discs of nearly uniform size, ranging from 6–8.5 mm in diameter. As for haemoglobinization, normally a small area of central pallor is seen (central 1/3rd) in RBCs.

Colour

1. **Normochromia: Normal RBC** appears pinkish brown due to presence of haemoglobin. Peripheral part looks deep brown while the central part (1/3rd) is pale because of biconcave shape of RBC.
2. **Hypochromia:** When RBC contains less haemoglobin, the central pale area becomes larger and paler. The MCHCs are also decreased.

   Example: **Iron deficiency anaemia.**
3. **Hyperchromia:** The RBCs become thicker and larger and they stain deeply and less central pallor because of increased haemoglobin content (MCH), but the haemoglobin concentration (MCHC) is normal.

   Example: **Megaloblastic anaemia.**
4. **Polychromasia:** Theoretically means many colours but practically RBCs appear bluish grey. This is due to presence of residual RNA in RBC (normally absent in mature RBC). So, young red cell shows polychromasia and larger than mature red cell and may lack central pallor. These

young red cells are called reticulocytes. It is most marked in **haemolysis and blood loss.**

4. **Anisochromia:** It means unequal haemoglobin content due to different populations of RBCs. Hence, different staining patterns of individual RBC. Example: **Iron deficiency anaemia treated with blood transfusion**.

Size

1. Normocytes: **Normal RBC** (6–8 µm in diameter; average 7–7.5 µm)
2. Microcytes: Decrease in size of RBC which may result from fragmentation of normally sized red cells (normocytes) or larger red cells (macrocytes). It occurs in many types of abnormal erythropoiesis, **e.g. iron deficiency anaemia and thalassaemia**.
3. Macrocytes: They are large RBCs having a diameter more than 8 micro mm, a MCV (mean corpuscular volume) more than 95 fl and higher than normal Hb concentration (MCHC). Example: **Megaloblastic anaemia, chronic liver diseases.**
4. Anisocytosis: This is a general term which describes any variation in size of RBC. Example: **Anaemias, thalassaemias**.

Shape

i. **Poikilocytosis:** This is a general term which describes any variation in the shape of RBC.

ii. **Spherocytes:** They are nearly spherical RBC in contrast to normal biconcave disc. Their diameter is smaller than normal and thickness is greater than normal. Tiny bits of membrane (in excess of Hb) are removed from adult RBC resulting the cell with a decreased surface/volume ratio. Example: Hereditary spherocytosis and in some cases of autoimmune haemolytic anaemia.

iii. **Target cells (leptocytes):** These refers to leptocytes (unusually thin red cells), and when stained show a peripheral ring of Hb with a dark, central, Hb containing area. Example: Haemoglobinopathies like thalassaemia, chronic liver disease, following splenectomy, HbC disease.

iv. **Schistocytes (cell fragment)**: It indicates the presence of haemolysis as seen in severe burn, megaloblastic anaemia or in microangiopathic haemolytic anaemia.

v. **Acanthocytes**: These are irregularly spiculated RBCs in which ends of spicules are bulbous and rounded. Examples: Abetalipoproteinaemia, certain liver diseases.

vi. **Burr cells (echinocytes):** These are small cells or cell fragments bearing one or few spines or spicules with regular distribution (unlike acanthocytes where spicules are seen all over RBC surface). Examples: Microangiopathic haemolytic anaemia, severe burns.

Structure or Content

i. **Basophilic stippling (punctate basophilia):** It is characterized by presence within erythrocytes of irregular basophilic granules which vary from fine to coarse. Fine stippling is seen when there is increased red cell production and therefore increased polychromatophilia. Coarse basophilic stippling may be seen in lead poisoning, megaloblastic anaemia or pyrimidine-5-nucleotidase deficiency. This is attributed to an abnormal instability of the RNA in the young red cell.

ii. **Pappenheimer bodies:** These are abnormal granules of iron found inside RBCs and stained by Wright stain and/or Giemsa stain. These bodies are a type of inclusion body formed by phagosomes that have engulfed excessive amounts of iron. They appear as dense, blue-purple granules within RBCs and are usually only one or two, located in the cell periphery. Examples: Sideroblastic anaemia, haemolytic anaemia, and sickle cell disease.

iii. **Cabot rings:** These are ring shaped, figure of eight or loop-shaped structures. These rings are probably microtubules remaining from a mitotic spindle (due to defective erythropoiesis). Examples: Pernicious anaemia, lead poisoning

iv. **Howell-Jolly bodies:** These are smooth, round remnants of nuclear chromatin. Single Howell-Jolly bodies may be seen in haemolytic anaemia, megaloblastic anaemia and after splenectomy. Multiple Howell-Jolly bodies in a single RBC usually indicate megaloblastic anaemia or defective erythropoiesis.

v. **Rouleaux formation:** Rouleaux formation is the alignment of RBCs on one another so that they resemble stack of coins. Examples: Multiple myeloma, other paraproteinaemia (monoclonal gammopathy) and macroglobulinaemia.

White Blood Cells (WBCs)

Differential leucocyte count (DLC) (Fig. 2.11): The DLC is done on the basis of size, cytoplasm with or without granules and type of nucleus of WBCs. The WBC may be divided into:

- **Granulocytes** (WBC with cytoplasmic granules): Neutrophils, eosinophils and basophils.
- **Agranulocytes** (WBC without granules): Lymphocytes and monocytes.

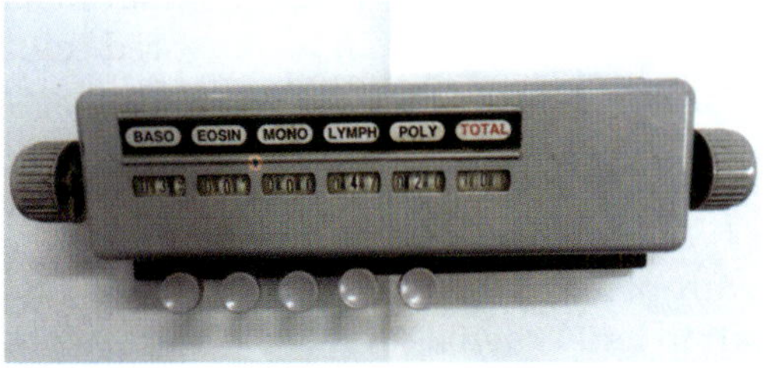

Fig. 2.11: DLC counter (manual) for differential leucocyte count (DLC)

Total leucocyte count (TLC): Normal total leucocyte count in adult person is 4000–11000/mm^3. Leukocytosis refers to TLC more than 11000/mm^3. Leucopenia less than 4000/mm^3.

Neutrophils (Polymorphs) (Fig. 2.12)

This leucocyte averages 12 mm in diameter, they are smaller than monocytes and eosinophils and slightly larger than basophils. **Segmented neutrophil** has at least two of its lobes separated by a filament. **Band neutrophil** has either a U-shaped nucleus of uniform thickness or a strand of nuclear material thicker than a filament connecting the lobes (appearance of "telephonic receiver").

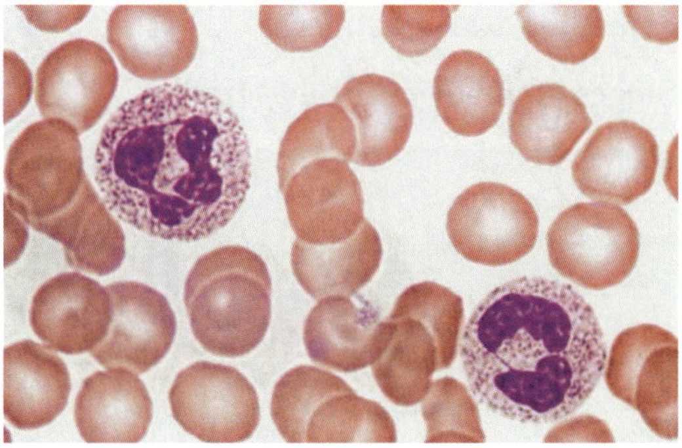

Fig. 2.12: Neutrophils

- The cytoplasm is filled up with tiny granules (0.2–0.3 mm) which stain tan to pink or orange with Romanowsky stains.
- Normal segmented neutrophils: 56% of leucocytes (DLC).
- Normal band neutrophils: 03% of leucocytes (up to 8% may be seen).
- Two lobes neutrophils: 10–30% of neutrophils.
- Three lobes neutrophils: 40–50% of neutrophils.
- Four lobes neutrophils: 10–20% of neutrophils.
- Five lobes neutrophils: ≤5% of neutrophils.
- In women, 2–3% of circulating neutrophils show an appendage at a terminal nuclear segment. This 'drumstick' is connected to the nucleus by a short stalk

and is about 1.5 mm in diameter. It indicates the inactive X chromosome and corresponds to **Barr body**.

Hypersegmented neutrophils (Fig. 2.13): If the peripheral smear shows ≥5% of neutrophils having 5 lobes or ≥1% of neutrophils having 6 lobes, then the neutrophils are called hypersegmented.

Causes

1. Megaloblastic anaemia
2. Uraemia
3. Hydroxyurea treatment
4. Cytotoxic treatment especially with methotrexate treatment.

Stages of neutrophilic maturation

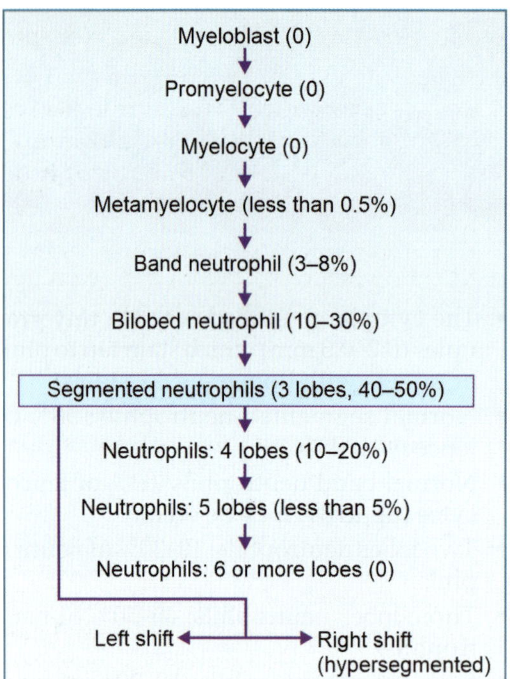

Segmentation of the nucleus of the neutrophil is a normal separation process. With the three-lobed neutrophil as a marker, shift to the left (less nature) or to the right (hypermature) can be understood. A left shift with band neutrophils, metamyelocytes and occasional myelocytes is common in sepsis and usually neutrophils contain toxic granules in cytoplasm. If myeloblast and promyelocytes are seen in peripheral blood, the causes may be leukaemia or leukoerythroblastic anaemia. Sometimes in pregnancy, a significant number of band forms is seen.

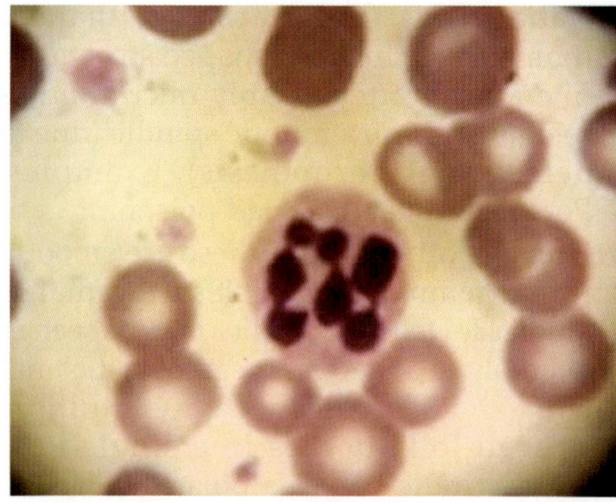

Fig. 2.13: Hypersegmented neutrophils (7 lobes) in megaloblastic anaemia

Arneth count: Neutrophils are divided in five groups according to number of lobe(s), it possesses:

1. Group I : One lobe
2. Group II: Two Lobes
3. Group III: Three lobes
4. Group IV: Four lobes
5. Group V: Five lobes.

One hundred neutrophils are counted in peripheral smear and number of each group of neutrophil is expressed as a percentage.

If there is increase in the group I and II neutrophils (as seen in sepsis) then there is a shift to left. Whereas, if there is more hypersegmented neutrophils (as seen in megaloblastic anaemia), then there is shift to right.

Arneth index: Percentage of neutrophils in groups I, II and ½ of group III is about 60 (normal range 51–65).

Schilling count: In this count, all the granular leucocytes are divided into four groups and the number of each group is expressed as a percentage of the WBCs. The four groups are:

1. Myelocytes
2. Metamyelocytes
3. Band neutrophils
4. Segmented neutrophils

A dividing line is drawn (usually segmented neutrophils' number). A shift to left happens when the number in percent increases, to the left of the dividing line.

Morphologic alterations in neutrophils

Toxic granules: These are dark blue to purple cytoplasmic granules seen in neutrophils (also in metamyelocytes and band forms). Toxic granules are seen in severe bacterial infections and in other causes of inflammation or toxic conditions. These are myeloperoxidase positive and may be numerous or few in number. Toxic granules are azurophil granules that have retained their basophilic staining reaction by lack of maturation or have developed increased basophilia in mature neutrophils. Toxic granules like azurophilic granules seen in neutrophils with prolonged staining time or decreased pH of staining reaction.

Döhle bodies: Döhle inclusion bodies are small, round or oval pale blue-gray structure, usually found at the peripheral cytoplasm of neutrophil. They consist of decomposed ribosomes and endoplasmic reticulum. Originally they were described in scarlet fever, but they are seen in any other infections, in aplastic anaemia, following administration of toxic agents and in burns.

Cytoplasmic vacuoles: It usually indicates severe sepsis, when toxic granules are also present. Cytoplasmic vacuoles will develop as an artifacts with prolonged standing of the blood before smears are made.

May-Hegglin anomaly: Autosomal dominant disease in which pale blue inclusions resembling Döhle bodies are seen. But the inclusions are larger and more prominent than Döhle bodies. Also, they are found in all leucocytes except lymphocytes.

Pelger-Huet anomaly: It is a benign inherited condition in which neutrophil nuclei fail to segment properly. Most of the neutrophils nuclei have two discrete equal-sized lobes connecting by a thin chromatin bridge. The chromatin is coarsely granular and cytoplasmic granular content is normal.

A similar type acquired morphological anomaly, known as pseudo-Pelger cells may be seen in acute myeloid leukaemia (AML). Here, the neutrophils are hypogranular and have irregular nuclear pattern.

Neutrophilia

Definition: When absolute neutrophil count 7500/mm^3 or 72% of DLC.

Relative neutrophilia: It can be divided into primary (clonal) and secondary.

Primary neutrophilia: Myeloproliferative neoplasms (chronic myeloid leukaemia, acute myeloid leukaemia), neutrophilic leukaemia, hereditary neutrophilia.

Secondary neutrophilia: Localized acute infections (pneumonia, tonsillitis, meningitis, acute otitis media), systemic infection (e.g. septicemia), acute rheumatic fever, vasculitis, acute myocardial infarction, burns, leukoerythroblastic reaction.

Leukoerythroblastic reaction: The presence of normoblasts, tear drop cells and immature cells of neutrophilic series (promyelocytes, myelocytes, metamyelocytes, band forms) along with neutrophilia in the blood is known as leukoerythroblastic reaction. It often indicates space-occupying disturbances of the bone marrow such as myelofibrosis with myeloid metaplasia, metastatic carcinoma, leukaemias, multiple myelomas, Gaucher's disease, TB and other granulomatous diseases.

Neutropenia

Definition: When neutrophil count is <43% of leucocytes or an absolute neutrophil and band from <1500/mm^3.

Causes of neutropenia

1. Decreased bone marrow production of neutrophils: Myelodysplastic syndromes, chemotherapy, acute leukaemia, aplastic anaemia.
2. Increased bone marrow production but decreased survival of neutrophils: Hypersplenism, SLE, rheumatoid arthritis, autoimmune and isoimmune neutropenia.
3. Viral infections: Measles, influenza, infectious mononucleosis, HIV infection, hepatitis.
4. Bacterial infection: Miliary TB, overwhelming sepsis, typhoid and paratyphoid, brucellosis, tularaemia.
5. Drugs: Antibiotics (chloramphenicol, cephalosporin, vancomycin), sulfa drugs, antimalarials (chloroquine, quinine), antifungal agents (amphotericin B, flucytosine).

Agranulocytosis

Definition: It theoretically means total absence of granulocytes in the peripheral blood.

But severe granulocytopenia (neutrophils and bands <500/mm^3) also referred as agranulocytosis casually.

Causes: Peripheral destruction of polymorphs or neutrophils (often drugs related).

i. Severe bone marrow failure.

   A neutrophil and band count <500/mm^3 is high risk factor for sepsis, whereas a count <200/mm^3 leads to overwhelming bacterial infections.

Lymphocytes (Fig. 2.14)

At birth, in normal individuals, the absolute numbers of lymphocytes and T cells are highest and may represent 90% of all leucocytes. Thereafter, B cells begin to rise and T cell decreases. In adolescence and adulthood B cells (15%) and T cells (85%) stabilized and lymphocytes constitute 20–40% of all leucocytes. Normally, majority of circulating lymphocytes are small and ≤10% are large.

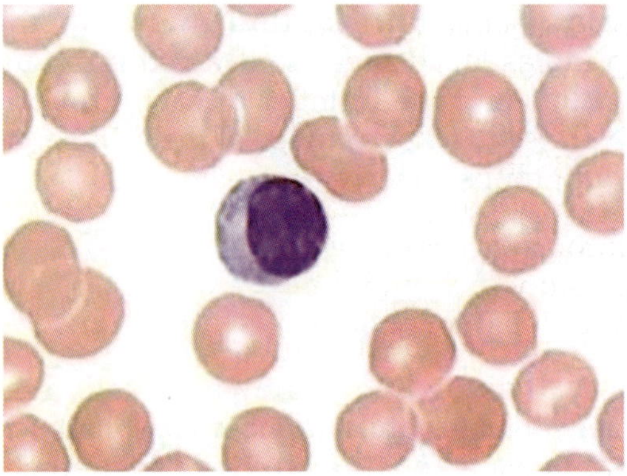

Fig. 2.14: Lymphocyte

The small lymphocytes have a thin rim cytoplasm occasionally containing scanty azurophilic granules. Nuclei are uniform in size (9 μm in diameter) which provides a useful guide for estimating red cell size (average 7–8 μm in diameter). The large lymphocytes (9–15 μm in diameter) have abundant pale blue cytoplasm containing azurophil granules. Because of this, these are known as large granular lymphocytes (LGL) (Fig. 2.15) and basically they are activated B lymphocytes or NK (natural killer) cells. The nuclei of lymphocytes have homogeneous chromatin with some clumping at the periphery.

Türk cells: In bacterial and viral infections, transforming lymphocytes are present. These Türk cells are immunoblasts (10 m in diameter) with a round nucleus and abundant deeply basophilic cytoplasm. Ultimately these cells will transform into

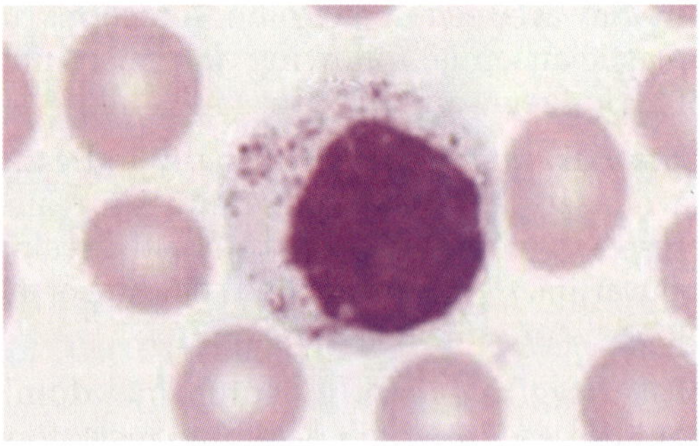

Fig. 2.15: Large granular lymphocyte

plasmacytoid lymphocytes or plasma cells. Occasionally, they may be seen in PBS.

Activated lymphocytes: These cells are seen in PBS in virals infections. These cells have slightly larger nuclei and more open chromatin (less dense) and abundant cytoplasm which may be irregular. Example: Infectious mononucleosis or glandular fever.

Lymphocytosis

Definition: It is defined as an absolute lymphocyte count >4000/mm^3 (or >43%) in adults, >7200/mm^3 in adolescents and >9000/mm^3 in young children and infants.

Spurious lymphocytosis: When there is neutropenia with relative lymphocytosis, but normal absolute lymphocyte count (e.g. typhoid fever, thyrotoxicosis, agranulocytosis).

Causes of lymphocytosis

i. *Viral causes:* Influenza, infectious hepatic viral infection, in various exanthemata like measles, mumps, chickenpox, rubella and infectious mononucleosis.
ii. *Bacterial causes:* Enteric or typhoid fever, tuberculosis, pertusis (whooping cough), secondary syphilis, brucellosis.
iii. *Protozoal causes:* Toxoplasmosis.
iv. *Malignancy:* Chronic lymphocytic leukaemia (CLL), acute lymphoblastic leukaemia (ALL), prolymphocytic leukaemia, hairy cell leukaemia, large granular lymphocytic leukaemia, leukaemic phase of follicular, mantle cell and splenic marginal zone of lymphoma.
v. *Miscellaneous:* Thyrotoxicosis, myasthenia gravis, hypopituitarism, hypersensitivity reaction, stress and drugs (efalizumab).

Lymphocytopenia

Definition: When lymphocyte count is <1500/mm^3 (<18%) in adults, and <3000/mm^3 in children.

Causes: Corticosteroid therapy, Cushing syndrome, sarcoidosis, chemotherapy and radiotherapy, neoplastic conditions especially Hodgkin lymphoma, epinephrine injection, few infections (e.g. acute and chronic retroviral infections of HIV, TB).

Monocytes (Fig. 2.16)

Monocytes are the largest of the circulating leucocytes; 15–18 μm in diameter and constitute 2–10% of leucocytes in PBS.

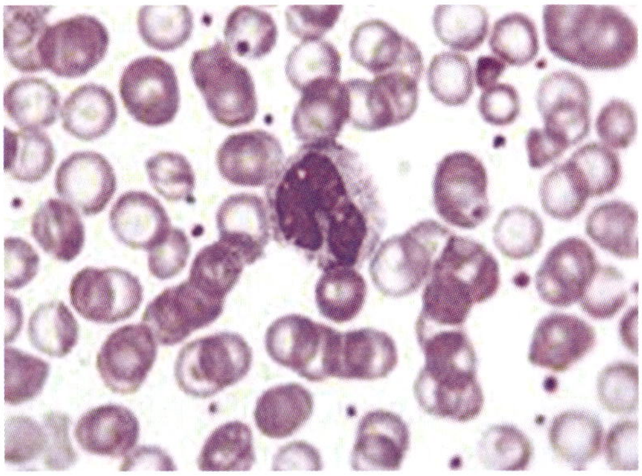

Fig. 2.16: Monocyte

Monocytes are characterized by a large, eccentrically placed nucleus which is stained less intensely than that of other leucocytes. Nuclear shape is variable but there is often a deep indentation giving a horseshoe or even bilobed appearance. The chromatin is finer and more evenly distributed compared to neutrophils. The abundant cytoplasm stains pale grayish-blue with Romanowsky stains. The cytoplasm contains numerous small pink-purple stained lysosomal granules and cytoplasmic vacuoles which may confer "frosted-glass" appearance. Monocytes are highly motile and phagocytic cells which are the precursors of macrophages or histiocytes (found in different tissues). Examples: Kupffer cells in liver, Langerhans cells of skin, osteoclast in bone and microglia in CNS.

Monocytosis

Definition: Absolute monocyte count is >500/mm^3 or >12% of DLC.

Causes

i. Bacterial infections: TB, syphilis, brucellosis, bacterial endocarditis.
ii. Protozoan infections: Malaria, kala-azar, trypanosomiasis.
iii. Rickettsial infections: Typhus, Rocky Mountain spotted fever.
iv. Malignancy: Acute monocytic or myelomonocytic leukaemia, chronic myelomonocytic leukaemia, myeloproliferative neoplasms, Hodgkin and non-Hodgkin lymphoma, multiple myeloma.
v. Carcinomas: Ovary, breast, stomach.
vi. Miscellaneous: Ulcerative colitis, Crohn's disease, sprue, sarcoidosis.

Eosinophils (Fig. 2.17)

Eosinophils are a little larger than neutrophils; 12–17 µm in diameter (average 13 mm). They usually have two lobes in the nuclei bit may have three or four lobes also. The cytoplasm is packed with distinctive spherical gold/orange (eosinophilic) granules. They average 3% of the leucocytes in adults.

The most characteristic ultrastructural features of eosinophils are presence of large, ovoid, specific granules each containing an elongated crystalloid in the cytoplasm.

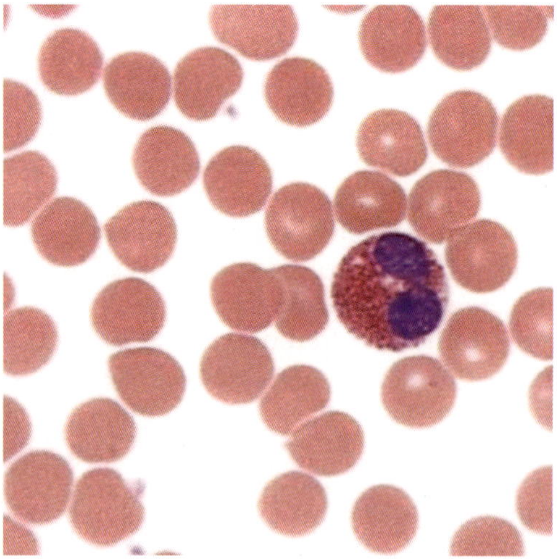

Fig. 2.17: Eosinophil

These specific granules are membrane bound and of uniform size and the matrix contains a variety of hydrolytic enzymes including histaminase. These crystalloids have a cubic lattice structure and consist of an extremely alkaline or basic protein, known as **major basic protein.**

In comparison to neutrophils, eosinophils are easily differentiated by the colour and size of the cytoplasmic granules. Eosinophilic granules are bright red with eosin and a more brick-red with Romanowsky stains. The cytoplasm is colourless. The nucleus stains less deeply compared to neutrophils and most eosinophils have two lobes or segments, rarely more than three.

Eosinophils are phagocytic cells but compared to neutrophils, they have greater oxidative capacity via the hexose monophosphate shunt. Eosinophils have particular phagocytic activity for antigen–antibody complexes.

Eosinophilia

Definition: Absolute eosinophil count >600/mm^3 or >8% of DLC (some use a cut-off value of >>450/mm^3).

Causes

i. Allergic diseases: Bronchial asthma, seasonal rhinitis (hay fever).
ii. Skin disorders: Atopic dermatitis, eczema, pemphigus eosinophilia.
iii. Parasitic infestations: Trichinosis, tapeworm, cysticercosis, visceral larva migrans (due to roundworm) creeping eruption (due to hookworm), Löeffler's syndrome, pulmonary eosinophilia (due to roundworm), tropical pulmonary eosinophilia (due to hyperimmune reaction caused by microfilariae).
iv. Infections: Scarlet fever, Echinococcus infection, early phase of *Pneumococcus pneumoniae*, fungal infections.
v. Neoplastic disorders: Chronic eosinophilic leukaemia, myelomonocytic leukaemia with inversion, mastocytosis, T cell lymphoma, Hodgkin lymphoma.

vi. Drugs: Pilocarpine, digitalis, physostigmine, sulfonamide, etc.

Basophils (Fig. 2.18)

Basophils are the rarest (<1%) of the circulating leucocytes. The basophils are intermediate in a size between neutrophils and eosinophils. Like the eosinophils, basophil has a bilobed nucleus but this is usually obscured by numerous large, densely basophilic (deep blue) specific granules which are larger, but fewer in number than those of eosinophils. In few basophils, most of these granules may be missed as these granules are highly soluble in water and tend to be dissolved away during common blood smear preparation. When basophils are stained with the basic dye, like to toluidine blue, the granules bind the basic dye and the dye changes colour to red. This phenomenon is called **metachromasia** and the granules are called metachromatic granules. The cytoplasmic granules of basophils and mast cells contain proteoglycans consisting of sulphated glycosaminoglycans linked to protein core, this accounts for their metachromatic staining characteristic.

Major function of basophils and mast cells is probably immunological response to certain parasites and allergens. Release of histamine and other vasoactive mediators are responsible for the so-called immediate hypersensitivity (anaphylactoid) reaction, which is characteristic of allergic rhinitis (hay fever), urticaria, some forms of asthma and anaphylactic shock.

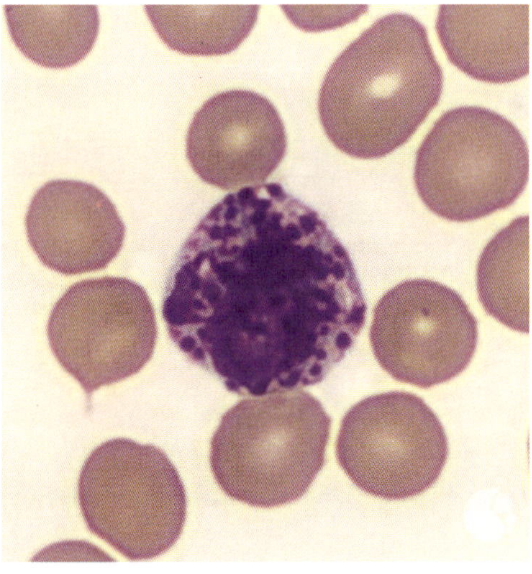

Fig. 2.18: Basophil

Basophilia

Definition: Basophil count is >200/mm^3 or >2% of DLC.

Causes

i. Neoplastic conditions: Myeloproliferative syndromes (chronic myeloid leukaemia, myeloid metaplasia, polycythemia vera), acute basophilic leukaemia, Hodgkin lymphoma.
ii. Infections: Chickenpox, small pox
iii. Hypersensitivity states: Drugs, food, foreign protein injection
iv. Others: Hypothyroidism, nephrotic syndrome, chronic haemolytic anaemia following splenectomy, chronic sinusitis and transient basophilia following irradiation.

Leukaemoid Reactions (Fig. 2.19)

Definition: A leucocyte count of >50,000/mm^3 in non-leukaemic condition.

The PBS (peripheral blood smear) shows an increase in and shift to the left of myeloid cells (band neutrophils, metamyelocytes, myelocytes, some promyelocytes and mye-

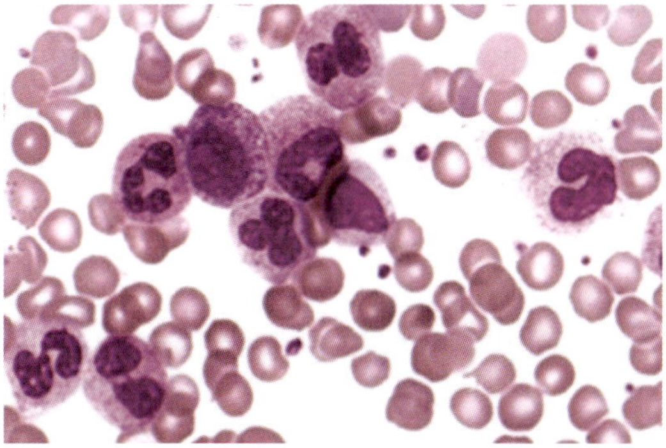

Fig. 2.19: Leukaemoid reactions (neutrophilic)

loblasts); and similar quantitative and quantitative changes in lymphocytes, or eosinophils or monocytes. Depending on the predominant cell, leukaemoid reactions may be neutrophilic (most common), lymphocytic, eosinophilic or monocytic.

Neutrophilic leukaemoid reactions: Excessive neutrophilia along with left shift of myeloid cells. It may occur in many situations like haemolysis, haemorrhage, Hodgkin lymphoma, myelofibrosis, malignancy with bone marrow involvement, severe burns, eclampsia, certain intoxications, and infections (especially tuberculosis).

Examination of PBS is more helpful than bone marrow examination. Increased primary granules (azurophilic granules) in the myeloid cells known as toxic granules, Döhle bodies and cytoplasmic vacuolization may be seen.

Lymphocytic leukaemoid reactions: Very high count of normal-appearing or mature lmphocytes may occur in measles, chickenpox, CMV, pertusis and in infectious mononucleosis. When atypical lymphocytes are many or immature lymphocytes (which may be seen in infectious mononucleosis) then the distinction from lymphocytic leukaemia may be difficult. In tuberculosis, normal-appearing or atypical lymphocytes may be found.

Examination of bone marrow is often helpful, because lymphocytes are minimally increased if at all in marrow, in contrast to PBS. If lymphocytes are increased in both PBS and marrow, then it is lymphocytic leukaemia (when fulfill other criteria).

Eosinophilic leukaemoid reactions: Blood cells as immature as eosinophilic myelocytes rarely appear in PBS in reactive eosinophilia, in which the TLC may exceed $50 \times 10^3/\text{mm}^3$. Eosinophilic leukaemoid reactions usually occur in children usually caused by parasitic infections. In adults, the idiopathic hypereosinophilic syndrome may be a cause.

Leukaemoid reaction is differentiated from leukaemia by

i. Absence of hepatosplenomegaly, lymphadenopathy and haemorrhage.
ii. Presence of blasts/immature cells <5% (in acute leukaemia, blasts ≥20%)
iii. Presence of toxic granules and Döhle bodies in neutrophils (in leukaemia Döhle bodies are absent).
iv. Presence of increased LAP (leucocyte alkaline phosphatase) score but in leukaemia LAP score is decreased.

Platelets (Thrombocytes) (Fig. 2.20)

Platelets (thrombocytes) are small, non-nucleated cells formed in the bone marrow from the cytoplasm of very large cells called megakaryocytes. In blood films from EDTA to blood and stained with Romanowsky stains, platelets are round to oval 2–4 mm in diameter. They are irregular in outline with fine red granules which may be scattered or centralized in the cell. A small number of larger platelets, up to 5 mm in diameter may be seen in normal persons.

Their number in circulating blood range from 150,000 to 400,000/mm^3. If the platelet count is normal, then on the average, one platelet is found per 10–30 RBCs. At 1000X or in oil immersion, this is equivalent to 7–20 platelets per oil immersion field.

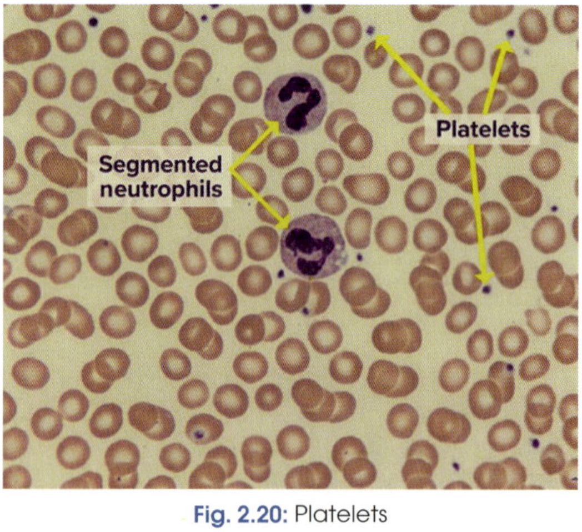

Fig. 2.20: Platelets

Platelet Functions

i. They from plugs to occlude sites of vascular damage by adhering to collagenous tissue at the margin of the wound. Later the platelet plug is replaced by fibrin.

ii. They promote clot formation by providing a surface for the assembly of coagulation protein complexes which are responsible for thrombin formation.

iii. They secrete factors which are involved in vascular repair.

Thrombocytopenia

Thrombocytopenia refers to decrease in the number of platelets in peripheral blood below normal (1.5 lacs/mm^3). But practically a count below 1 lac/mm^3 is considered thrombocytopenia.

Causes

1. *Increased destruction of platelets*
   a. Immune causes: Idiopathic thrombocytopenic purpura (ITP), infections (HIV, dengue, malaria), systemic lupus erythematosus, neonatal alloimmune purpura, post-transfusion purpura.
   b. Nonimmune causes: Thrombotic thrombocytopenic purpura (TTP), disseminated intravascular coagulation (DIC).
2. *Decreased production of platelets*
   a. Hereditary: Wiskott-Aldrich syndrome, Fanconi's anaemia.
   b. Acquired: Megaloblastic anaemia, aplastic anaemia, bone marrow infiltration (leukaemias, lymphomas, metastatic carcinomas), drugs (cytotoxic drugs, ethanol), radiation.
3. **Increased sequestration:** Hypersplenism
4. **Dilutional thrombocytopenia:** Massive blood transfusion.

Thrombocytosis (Thrombophilia)

It refers to increase in the platelet count above normal (4 lacs/mm^3). Thrombocytosis may be primary or reactive (secondary). Primary thrombocytosis due to myeloproliferative disorders can be distinguished from reactive (secondary) thrombocytosis by the presence of leukocytosis, immature WBCs and nucleated RBCs in peripheral blood, defective platelet function (epinephrine-induced platelet aggregation) and splenomegaly in cases of primary thrombocytosis.

Causes of thrombocytosis

i. Primary thrombocytosis: Polycythemia vera, chronic myeloid leukaemia, essential thrombocythaemia, idiopathic myelofibrosis.

ii. Secondary thrombocytosis: Infections, chronic inflammatory diseases, trauma, haemorrhage, iron deficiency, splenectomy, malignancy.

VIVA VOCE

Q1. What are the characteristics of an ideal peripheral blood smear?

Ans:
- The smear should not be too thick or too thin.
- It should occupy about central 2/3rds of the glass slide.
- The smear should be tongue shaped and it should have straight lateral borders.

Q2. What is thick smear and when is it used?

Ans: Thick smear is prepared by spreading a large drop of blood on the slide approximately 2 cm in diameter and dry it. The dried smear is dipped (2–4 times) in tap water to dehaemoglobinize the RBCs and red-coloured solution comes out. The smear is fixed with methanol and stained with Romanowsky stain.

Thick smear is used for quick detection of malarial parasites and for screening of malaria.

Q3. What is fixation of smear and how is it done?

Ans: Fixation means fixation of blood cells and other things of smear to be fixed onto the slide.

So that, during subsequent staining and washing the smear do not wash off.

Usually acetone-free methyl alcohol is used for fixation. Acetone if present, it will wash away the nuclear stain and nuclear stain will be of poor quality. So, acetone-free methyl alcohol is used.

Q4. Why buffered water is used during blood smear staining? What is the ideal pH of buffered water?

Ans: Buffered water is used to maintain optimal pH during staining. If the pH of stain is acidic, it will cause poor nuclear stain and very reddish cytoplasm. On the other hand, if the pH of stain is alkaline, the stained smear will be blue due to improper staining of cytoplasm.

The ideal pH for routing blood smear is 6.8 and for malarial detection is 7 to 7.2. At pH 6.8 (with the use of diluted phosphate buffer), the stained smear imparts a reddish hue to red cells and differential staining pattern of the granules present in granulocytes. To look, malarial parasites, a pH of 7.2 is recommended in order to detect Schuffner's dots of *Plasmodium vivax, ovale* and *malariae*. (Remember Maurer's dots in *P. falciparum* and Ziemann's dots in *P. malariae*.)

Q5. How platelet adequacy and platelet count are made on peripheral blood smear?

Ans: In normal healthy person, platelets are present in clumps as well as discretely. If there are platelet clumps (each clump containing ≥6 platelets), then platelet count is adequate. Usually 3–5 platelets are present per 100 RBCs. If there is <3 platelet/100 RBCs, then platelet count is low and patient is probably suffering from thrombocytopenia.

As per **Henry's clinical diagnosis and management by laboratory's methods**, in stained film from EDTA to blood, there are 7–20 platelets/oil immersion field (1000X) or one platelet per 10–30 RBCs.

For rough estimation of platelet count, take average platelet count in 10 oil immersion field on a blood film, then multiply it by 15,000 which will give reasonably good platelet count (reference WHO laboratory book).

Some advocated that under oil immersion, normal person will have 10–25 platelets per oil field (average 20). Take average platelet count under oil immersion, then multiply by 20,000 if the average is <10, multiply by 15,000 if the average is ≥10.

As per Gradwohl's clinical laboratory methods, the diagnosis is:

No. of platelets/oil immersion field	Estimated total platelet count
• Less than 1 platelet	• Decreased in number
• Several platelets with occasional clumps	• Adequate in number
• Over 25 platelets	• Increased in number

The number of platelets in 10 oil immersion fields multiplied by 2000 closely approximates the platelet count.

There are differences in opinion, but for practical reasons, take average platelet count in 10 oil immersion field on a blood film, then multiply it by 15,000 which will give reasonably good platelet count (reference WHO laboratory book).

Q6. What is platelet satellitism?

Ans: Platelet satellitism is phenomena in which platelets encircle neutrophils. It is usually seen when blood is collected in excess EDTA (though may be seen with other anticoagulants). It is caused by IgG or IgM antibodies that bind the CD16 antigen. CD16 is a low affinity Fc receptor, found on the surface of neutrophils, also present on NK cells, monocytes and macrophages. Satellitism around other leucocytes may be seen and some platelets may even be phagocytosed by neutrophils/WBCs.

Q7. What is "platelet dust"?

Ans: This was first described by Peter Wolf in 1967 which are basically microparticles and are not simply inert products of cellular debris. These microparticles are submicron vesicles shed from a variety of cells. These microparticles have roles in coagulation, cellular signaling, vascular injury and homeostasis. To date, the cell types reported to release microparticles either constitutively or when stimulated that include platelets, blood cells, endothelium, epithelium and many cancer cells.

Q8. What parasites can be identified in peripheral blood smear (PBS)?

Ans:
i. Malaria: Most common parasite found in PBS.
ii. Microfilaria of *Wuchereria bancrofti*
iii. *Leishmania donovani* or LD bodies of kala-azar: Found free or inside monocytes.
iv. *Trypanosoma cruzi*
v. Others: Babesia, Brugia, Mansonella, etc. rarely.

Q9. What is the advantage of Leishman staining compared to Giemsa staining?

Ans: No separate fixation is needed as it contains methanol solvent within Leishman stain itself which will fix the smear. So, Leishman stain fixes and stains the smear simultaneously. Also, shorter time is required compared to Giemsa staining.

Leishman stain is a good alternative to Giemsa for malarial parasite detection. Leishman stain is superior for visualization of RBC and WBC morphology, which can be an advantage for the diagnosis of diseases involving RBCs and WBCs.

Q10. What is the advantage of Giemsa stain?

Ans: Giemsa stain is most complex Romanowsky stain and it contains maximum number of azo compounds. So, Giemsa stain provides maximum intermediate shades and better toning effect. Hence, it is good for microphotography. Also, Giemsa stain is best for malarial parasite detection.

Q11. What is the use of Field's stain and modified Field's stain?

Ans: Field stain was originally used to detect malarial parasite on thick smear. But it can also detect *H. pylori* on thin sections of stomach (paraffin section, 2–4 mm thickness). Also, it can be used as a quick Romanowsky stain for thin blood film and marrow smears. Modified Field's stain is recommended for rapid staining of protozoans, such as *Acanthamoeba* and *Trichomonas* species.

Q12. How would you identify a well stained and good smear microscopically?

Ans: Ideally, the smear should be tongue shaped and after staining, a well stained blood smear will have pinkish tint at the stained portion and no staining on other portion of the slide.

Microscopically well stained smear should show following features:

- Red cells will have pinkish orange colour.
- Nuclei of white cells will be purplish blue.
- Neutrophilic granules should be violet pinkish or pale pink (neutral stain).
- Eosinophilic granules should be orange red (eosinophilic).
- Basophilic granules should be deep purple or buish black (basophilic) and granules should overlap the nuclei.
- The nuclei of the lymphocytes are dark with condensed chromatin.
- The platelets are small, round, membrane bound, pinkish granular structures.

Q13. Why peripheral blood smear does not show schizonts of *P. falciparum*?

Ans: *Plasmodium falciparum* is associated with infected red cells expressing PfEMP (***Plasmodium falciparum*** **erythrocyte membrane protein)** leading to their attachment to the endothelial cells lining small blood vessels. PfEMP forms knobs on the RBC surface and binds to ligands on endothelial cells, including CD36, thrombospondin, VCAM-1, ICAM-1 and E-selectin. It also causes infected red cells to clump together (formation of rosette). All these block blood flow and sequestration of infected RBCs in the capillaries. So, schizonts of *P. falciparum* do not appear in PBS.

Chapter 3

Marrow Puncture Needle and Examination of Bone Marrow

Bone marrow examination is an indispensable adjunct to the study of haematological diseases and sometimes the only way for a correct diagnosis. Apart from haematological disease, many other disorders can be diagnosed by bone marrow examination. It is estimated that in adults, weight of the marrow is 1300–1500 g.

Bone marrow or marrow can be obtained by needle aspiration, percutaneous trephine biopsy or surgical biopsy. Bone marrow aspiration (also called aspiration biopsy) is simple, safe and relatively painless. Aspiration can be performed on outdoor patients. On the contrary, trephine biopsy or surgical biopsy is not simple but can be performed on outdoor patients too.

The advantage of marrow aspiration is that, individual cells are perfectly preserved in the well-prepared marrow films and after staining subtle differences between cells can be recognized easily compared to trephine biopsy/surgical biopsy. But the disadvantage of aspiration is that the arrangement of the cells in the marrow and the relationship between different cells are more or less destroyed during aspiration. Also, in fibrosis (myelofibrosis) or in hypoplastic/aplastic anaemia, no marrow material except blood is aspirated **(called dry tap)**.

The great advantage of trephine biopsy is that it can provide a perfect view of the structure of relatively large pieces of bone marrow (perfect alignment of different cells in marrow biopsy). Also, morphological features of individual cells can be identified by making an imprint or a smear from the marrow tissue obtained.

HISTORY OF BONE MARROW EXAMINATION

- In 1905, the Italian physician Pianese reported bone marrow (BM) infiltration by the parasite Leishmania.
- In 1927, Anirkin, a Russian physician obtained BM from the sternum using a lumbar puncture needle.
- In 1931, Arjeff, introduced needles with a guard.
- In 1935, Klima and Rosegger developed BM needles with guards.
- In 1945, Vandenberghe and Blitstein were the first to use the iliac crest to obtain BM.
- In 1952, Bierman used the posterior iliac crest as the site for bone marrow aspiration and claimed to be very safe site.
- In 1958, McFarland and Dameshek described a trephination technique using the Vim-Silverman biopsy needle.

BONE MARROW ASPIRATION

The various sites for bone marrow aspiration are:

In children

- Tibia → superior medial surface of tibia, inferior to the medial to the tibial tuberosity. This site is favoured for newborn, infants and children <2 years of age.
- Posterior iliac crest and spine
- Calcaneum

In adults

- Iliac crest
- Anterior and posterior superior iliac spine

  (Most favoured site nowadays)
- Spinous processes of lumbar vertebra
- Sternum: It is no longer favoured though was popular in the past.

The sternum should never be attempted in children. The preferred site for children of all ages are posterior superior iliac spine or iliac crest. Upper end of tibia is also a favourite site <2 years of age but caution should be taken as the weak tibia in children is vulnerable to fractures and lacerated injury to major blood vessels may occur in inexperienced hands.

Sternum though very popular site of aspiration in the past, but now is becoming obsolete. Unless the needle is correctly inserted, there is a risk of perforating the inner cortical layer and damaging the underlying large blood vessels and right atrium leading to medical emergencies.

Aspiration from iliac spine or iliac crest has the advantage that a large amount of marrow material can be aspirated and risk of injuring major blood vessels or organs is minimal compared to sternum. Also, unlike sternum, the patient cannot see what is happening or the medical procedure as the patient is lying on his/her side or lying prone. Multiple attempts can be made if necessary without making patient worried.

For aspiration, different needles used are:

1. **Salah bone marrow aspiration needle (Fig. 3.1):** It has three parts:

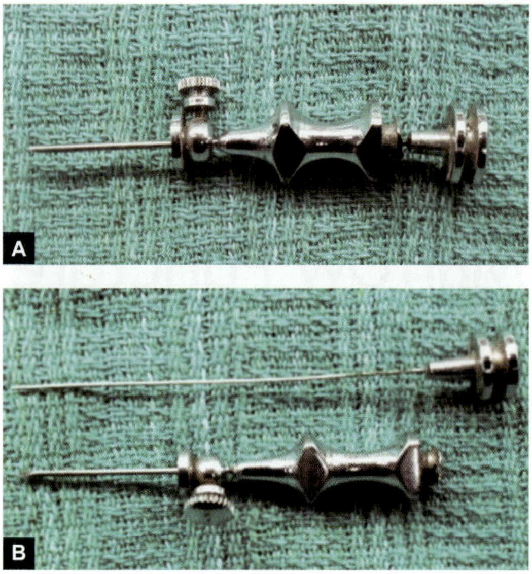

Fig. 3.1A and B: Salah bone marrow needle

   a. Trocar
   b. Cannula or stylet
   c. Adjustable side guard and screw
2. **Klima bone marrow aspiration needle (Fig. 3.2):** Here, there is no screw but there is a guard. But other two parts (trocar and the stylet) are there. Klima needle has the advantage as the guard has no chance of getting slipped and injuring underlying structures.

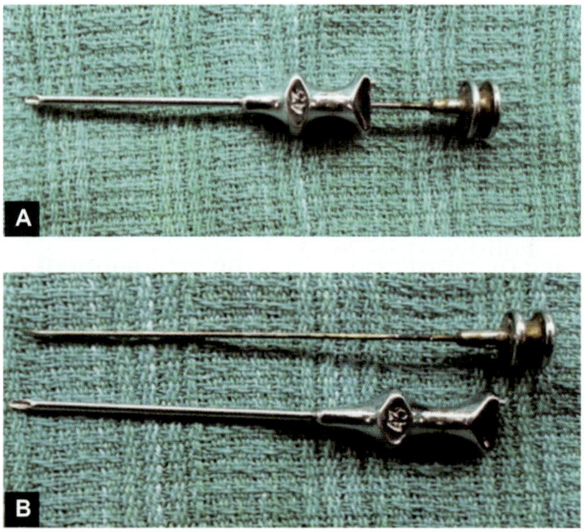

Fig. 3.2A and B: Klima bone marrow needle

3. **Islam's bone marrow aspiration needle**: Here dome-shaped handle and T bar are intended to provide stability and control during aspiration.

Ideal bone marrow needle

- Should be stout
- 7–8 cm in length
- Adjustable guard
- Well-fitted stylet
- Edges well sharpened

Indications of Bone Marrow Aspiration

A. Diagnostic indications

1. Red cell disorders—megaloblastic anaemia, pure red cell aplasia
2. WBC disorders—leukaemia (acute and chronic), subleukaemic leukaemia
3. Platelet disorders—idiopathic thrombocytopenic purpura (ITP)
4. Myeloproliferative disorders and myelodysplastic syndromes
5. Storage disorders—Gaucher's disease, Neimann-Pick disorders
6. Assessment of iron stares (Perls' Prussian blue stain)
7. In evaluation of fever or pyrexia or pyrexia of unknown origin (PUO)
8. Detection of parasites—microfilaria, LD bodies of kala-azar (*Leishmania donovani*), malaria
9. Detection of LE cell in SLE patients
10. Metastatic deposits—different carcinomas
11. Staging of lymphoma (Hodgkin and non-Hodgkin)
12. Follow-up—therapy for leukaemia and lymphoma
13. Plasma cell dyscrasia—multiple myeloma
14. Bone marrow aspirated material as a source of culture to detect infective pathogens like TB, fungus, etc.
15. Granulomas in bone marrow: TB, histoplasmosis, sarcoidosis, lymphoma
16. Cytogenetic studies, molecular genetic studies, cytochemistry and flow cytometry.

B. Therapeutic indications: Bone marrow transplant.

BONE MARROW TREPHINE BIOPSY

Three types of needles are used:

1. Jamshidi trephine needle (Fig. 3.3A): Most popular and most commonly used
2. Islam's trephine needle (Fig. 3.3A)
3. Sacker-Nordin's bone marrow trephine biopsy.

Indications of Bone Marrow Biopsy

- Diagnosis of leukaemia and lymphoma
- Staging of different lymphomas
- Evaluating iron stores, fibrosis, granulomas, abscesses, metastases and vascular lesions
- Detection of metastatic deposit (carcinoma)

Contraindications of Bone Marrow Examination

- Bleeding disorders or diathesis
- Haemophilia
- Infection at site of puncture.

Bone Marrow Aspiration Technique (Fig. 3.4)

Puncture of Ilium (Superior Iliac Spine and Iliac Crest)

The usual site for bone marrow aspiration or puncture is iliac crest in adults. Only needles designed for bone marrow aspiration should be used (Salah's needle or Klima's needle). They should be stout, about 7–8 cm in length with a well-fitted stylet and preferably with a guard (Klima's needle) (Fig. 3.5). The point of the needle and edge of the bevel must be sharp so that it can pierce bone easily. The skin of the chosen site should be cleaned with 70% alcohol (e.g. ethanol) or 0.5% chlorhexidine. Now follow the below mentioned steps:

1. Clean the area with 70% alcohol or 0.5% chlorhexidine as stated above.

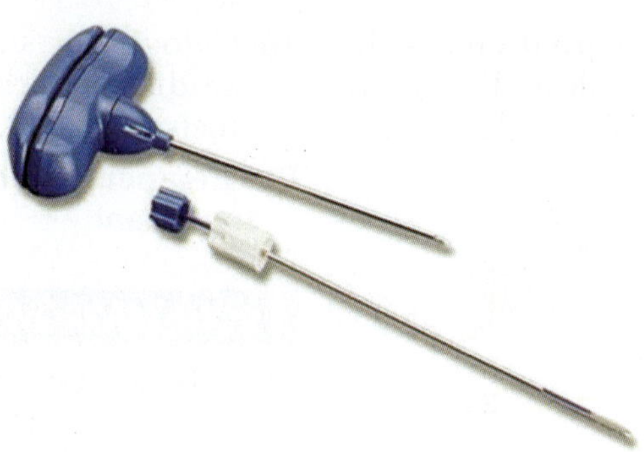

A

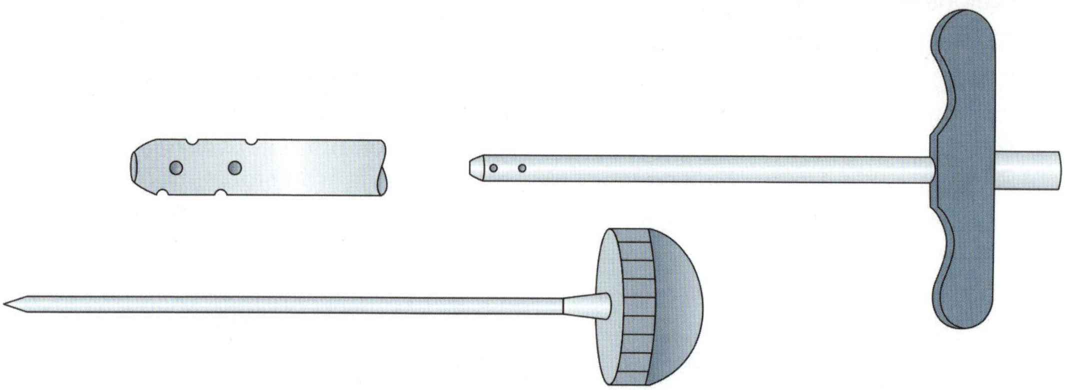

A modified Western of the Islam needle has multiple holes in the distal portion of the shaft in addition to the opening at the tip to overcome sampling error when the marrow is not uniformly involved in a pathological lesion.

B

Fig. 3.3A and B: Jamshidi and Islam trephine needles

2. The skin, subcutaneous and periosteum overlying the site are infiltrated with a local anaesthetic (2% lignocaine) by a 2 ml syringe. Wait for 3–5 minutes.
3. With a boring movement (rotating clockwise and anticlockwise with some pressure but not full rotation). The needle is inserted to the bone. The bone is touched after passing through soft tissue (sensation of hard material as perceived by the person doing the technique). Further insertion as will give sudden release of resistance as if the needle has entered into an empty space.
4. Now the needle has entered into bone marrow space.
5. Take out the stylet.
6. With a well-fitted 2–5 ml syringe, take out 0.2–0.3 ml of marrow material.
7. Take out the needle and seal the puncture site.
8. Immediately prepare marrow films from the aspirated marrow materials.

Puncture of the Sternum

Usual site in sternum is manubrium sterni or the first or second pieces of the body of sternum.

If the manubrium sterni is chosen, the puncture site should be about 1 cm above the sternomandibular angle and slightly lateral to the midline.

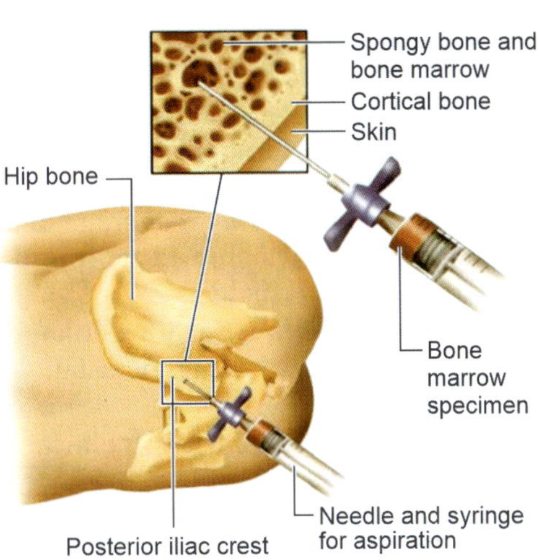

Fig. 3.4: Bone marrow aspiration

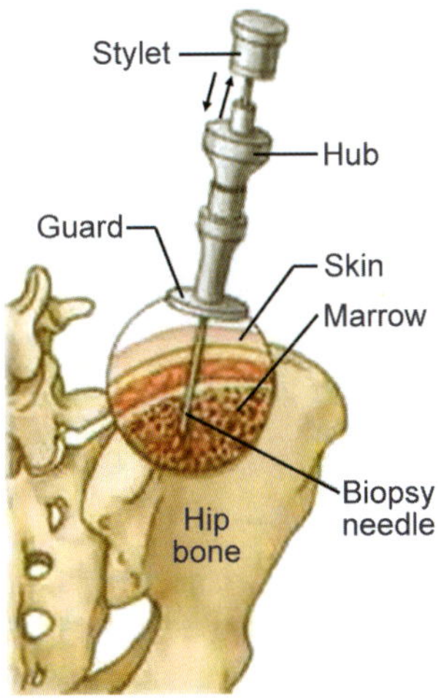

Fig. 3.5: Bone marrow aspiration by Klima's needle

If the body of sternum is chosen, the puncture site should be opposite, the second and third intercostal space slightly lateral to midline.

In case of sternal puncture, it is essential to use the guard. Clean the area as stated in puncture of ilium. Infiltrate lignocaine as stated previously. Now insert the needle with boring movement. After piercing the skin and subcutaneous tissues, when the needle touches the periosteum, adjust the guard on the needle so that the needle can be allowed to penetrate for about 5 mm further (not more than that to avoid risk of injury of blood vessels and organs). Then aspiration is done as stated in puncture of ilium.

Preparation of Marrow Films

Transfer the aspirated material without delay, as it tends to clot quickly. One drop of marrow material is delivered onto each glass slide 1 cm from one end. Get rid of extra blood by quickly sucking off with a fine Pasteur pipette leaving the greyish marrow particles behind. Some advised to tilt the slide or place the slide on a slope so that the lighter blood come down over the slide and then remove it. After removing extra blood, marrow films are prepared by pushing a spreader (glass side) or by a coverslip. The marrow particles/fragments are dragged behind the spreader and leaves a trail behind them. The marrow film should be 3–5 cm length and not more than 2 cm in width.

Bone marrow imprints: One or more visible marrow particles/fragments are picked up with a capillary pipette, or by a toothpick and immediately transferred onto a slide and made to stick to it by a gentle smearing motion. The slide is air-dried rapidly by waving it.

Crush preparations: Marrow particles in a small drop of aspirate may be placed onto a slide near one end. Another slide is carefully placed over the first slide. Now crush the bone marrow particles by giving some pressure and prepared the smear of crushed marrow particles by pulling the slides apart in a direction parallel to their surface.

Confirmation of presence of bone marrow not only blood: Presence of sand like marrow particles and irregular holes of fat in the films give assurance of marrow and not just blood has been aspirated.

Fixation of marrow films and staining: Fix the marrow films and stain them with Romanowsky stain as for peripheral blood (refer to previous chapter).

- Leishman stain is used routinely
- Prussian blue staining may be done to demonstrate iron in haemosiderin deposit or in ferritin and assessment of iron status in body. Iron in haemoglobin is not stained.
- Few slides may be stained with PAS (periodic acid–Schiff) stain or May-Grünwald stain.

Reporting of Bone Marrow Films (Myelogram)

At least 300–1000 bone marrow cells (average 500 cells) should be examined. A myelogram report should include:

i. **General cellularity of marrow:** Whether this is hypercellular or hypocellular or normocellular. As a rough guide cellularity (haemopoietic cells) occupying <25% of the particle is considered hypocellular, whereas cellularity >75–80% is hypercellular. Some follow the simple formula as regards to age → cellularity% = (100 – age)%. So, physiologically children have highest cellularity and elderly lowest cellularity.

ii. **Myeloid–erythroid ratio (M:E ratio):** Leukocytes of all types and stages of maturation are counted together. Likewise, erythroblasts and normoblasts are counted together. A ratio is made. Normal M:E ratio is 1.2:1 to 5:1 (average 3:1). An increased M:E ratio (e.g. 6:1) may be found in erythroid hypoplasia, patients with infection or myeloproliferative disorders like CML. A decreased M:E ratio (<1.2:1) may be seen in normoblastic hyperplasia or in decreased leukopoiesis.

iii. **Type of erythropoiesis:** Whether normoblastic, megaloblastic or dyserythropoietic.

iv. **Type of leukopoiesis:** Myeloblast, promyelocyte, myelocyte, metamyelocyte, band neutrophil and mature neutrophils are present or not (Fig. 3.6). Also seen up to what stage of maturation is present.

v. Number of lymphocytes, plasma cells, monocytes, etc.

vi. **Megakaryocytes:** Number of megakaryocytes is estimated better in tissue sections than in marrow films. Under low power or 100X, an average of 1–3 megakaryocytes should be found in each low power field.

vii. **Abnormal cells (if any):** Leukaemic cells, lymphoma cells or metastatic carcinoma.

viii. **Parasites:** Microfilariae, malaria, LD bodies (kala-azar)

ix. **Iron status:** Done by Perls'-Prussian blue stain. It is reported as negative or 1 + to 5+, storage iron is seen in macrophages (haemosiderin or ferritin). In normal adults it is 2+, whereas 3+ is slightly increased, 4+ is moderately increased and 5+ is markedly increased.

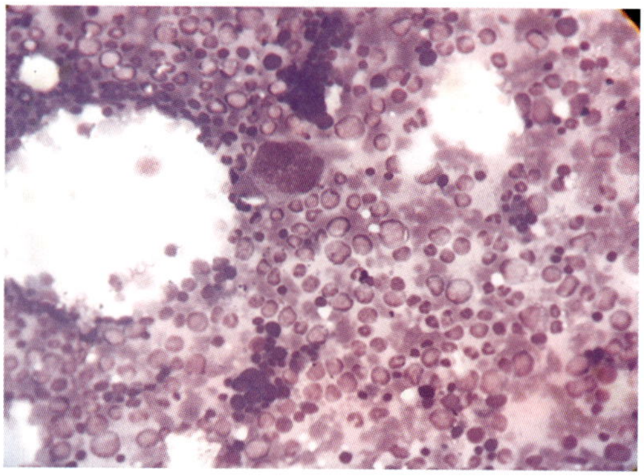

Fig. 3.6: Normal bone marrow shows trilineage haemopoietic cells (oil immersion, Leishman's stain, 1000X)

Summary of Bone Marrow Report

The report (myelogram) should include an estimate of cellularity, M:E ratio, statements about any cytological or maturation abnormalities, an estimate of the number of megakaryocytes, an estimate of the storage iron and proportion of sideroblasts and statement about any abnormal cell or other abnormal findings.

Remember, every bone marrow report (myelogram) (Table 3.1) should be interpreted

Table 3.1: Normal ranges of differential counts in bone marrow in adults (myelogram) in aspirated material

Type of cell	Range (%)
• Reticulum	0.1–2
• Myeloblasts	0.1–3.5
• Promyelocytes	0.5–5
• Myelocytes:	
– Neutrophilic	5–20
– Eosinophilic	0.1– 3
– Basophilic	0–0.5
• Metamyelocytes	10–30
• Neutrophils including bonds	7–25
• Eosinophil	0.2–3
• Basophil	0–0.5
• Monocytes	0–0.2
• Lymphocytes	5–20
• Megakaryocytes	0.1–0.5
• Plasma cells	0.1–3.5
• Proerythroblasts	0.5–5
• Early and intermediate normoblasts (basophilic and polychromatic)	2–20
• Late normoblast (pyknotic or orthochromatic)*	2–10

* The term pyknotic is preferred to orthochromatic as a description of most mature normoblasts or late normoblasts. But cells with fully haemoglobinized or mature cytoplasm (i.e. orthochromatic) is rarely seen in normal bone marrow.

along with a blood smear examination of the same patient. For bone marrow at least 500 cells and for blood smear at least 200 cells should be examined as differential count.

1. Jamshidi Needle (Fig. 3.7)

This needle has the advantages than Turkel and Bethel needles or needles of Vim-Silverman type (sometimes the specimen is crushed and its architecture altered). The Jamshidi needle should be inserted by to and fro rotation through approximately 90°. It should not be continuously rotated because this tends to distort and twist the core of marrow tissue, but once the needle is inserted up to desired length, the needle is rotated clockwise (few rotations) and anticlockwise (few rotations) without any downward pressure. This is done to cut the core tissue and put the tissue within needle.

2. Islam's Needle

This needle has the advantage over other needles, as it can provide long uniform core of marrow-containing bone spicules and there is no distortion of bone marrow architecture. These needles are usually performed

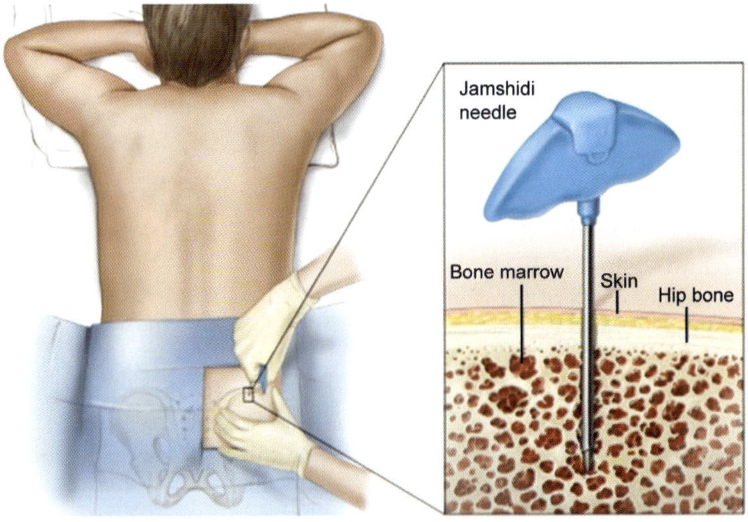

Fig. 3.7: Trephine biopsy by Jamshidi needle

at the anterior or posterior superior iliac spine. The posterior superior iliac spine provides core tissue which is longer and larger than other sites. A large trephine is sometimes of value as it provides sufficient bone marrow material for accurate diagnosis (Table 3.2).

Other trephine biopsy needles

The other trephine biopsy needles are: Westerman Jensen, drills and disposable needles.

Bore Size of Trephine Needles

Trephines have been developed with bore size of 4–5 mm and they can be safely inserted in iliac crest (but a small skin incision and local anaesthesia is required). Bore size of 2–3 mm is also good and provides good material.

Trephine Biopsy/Histological Sections

The needle biopsy and the clotted marrow particles or fragments are fixed in Zenker's acetic solution (5% glacial acetic acid; 95% Zenker) for 6–18 hours or in B-5 fixative for 1–2 hours. Prolonged time in fixation in either fixative will make the tissue brittle. The tissue is processed routinely for embedding in paraffin, cut at 4 mm and stained routinely with haematoxylin and eosin. Giemsa and PAS stains are also frequently used. But sometimes thinner sections are needed (1–3 mm). For this, plastic or resin embeddium medium (not paraffin) is required which enables to cut sections at 1–3 mm thickness.

Examination of Stained Sections

- Haematoxylin and eosin (H&E) stain (Fig. 3.8A and B): This is excellent for demonstrating the cellularity and pattern of the marrow and for revealing pathologic changes such as fibrosis or presence of granuloma or carcinoma.
- Romanowsky stain: Haemopoietic cells are better identified with this stain.
- Reticulin stain (silver impregnation stain): The bone marrow always contains a small amount of glycoprotein matrix which is actually collagen and make supporting network. This collagen or connective tissue is known as reticulin or reticulin fibres. This reticulin can be stained by reticulin stain or silver impregnation stain (Flowchart 3.1).
- PAS stain: To demonstrate any parasite (intracellular or extracellular), myeloblast, lymphoblast, glycogen, etc.
- Myelofibrosis and myelosclerosis: Myelofibrosis refers to an increase in coarse fibres, whereas myelosclerosis refers to an increase in fine fibres. Both fibres are stained by reticulin stain. Coarse fibres predominate in myelofibrosis (chronic or idiopathic).

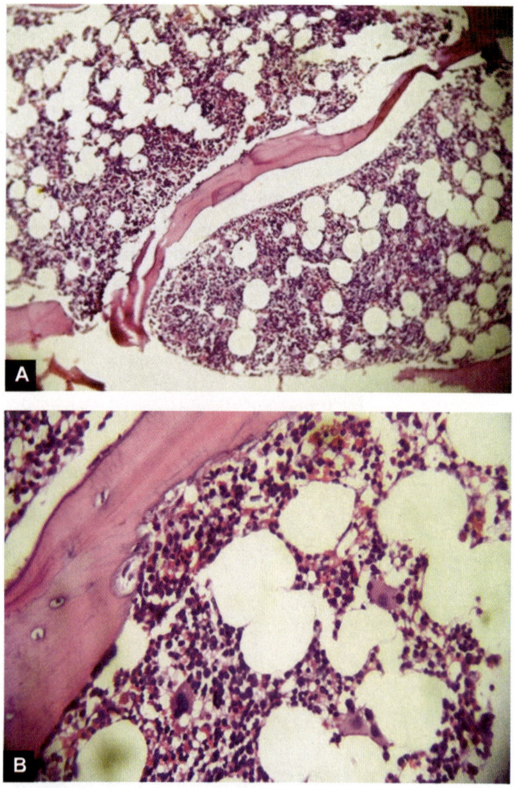

Fig. 3.8A and B: (A) Low power view of trephine biopsy shows marrow tissue, fat spaces and bony trabeculae; (B) High power view shows trilineage (erythroid, myeloid and megakaryocytic/thrombocytic cells) haematopoiesis including megakaryocytes

Table 3.2: Comparison of bone marrow aspiration and bone marrow biopsy

Parameter	Bone marrow aspiration	Bone marrow biopsy
1. Site	Illiac spine, sternum, tibia, spinous process of vertebra	Posterior superior iliac spine
2. Main indications	Suspected haematologic malignancies, unexplained cytopenias	Repeated dry tap, aplastic anaemia, myelofibrosis, lymphoma staging, focal lesions, hairy cell leukaemia
3. Needle used	Salah, Klima	Jamshidi
4. Information obtained	Morphology, cytochemistry, iron stain, flow cytometry (immunophenotyping), culture	Cellularity, architecture, fibrosis, focal lesions
5. Stains and special tests	Romanowsky stain, iron stain, cytochemistry, molecular genetics, flow cytometry (immunophenotyping), culture	H&E stain, reticulin stain, IHC (immunohistochemistry)
6. Reporting time	Same day	Up to 7 days

Flowchart 3.1: Pluripotent marrow stem cell and formation of haemopoietic cells

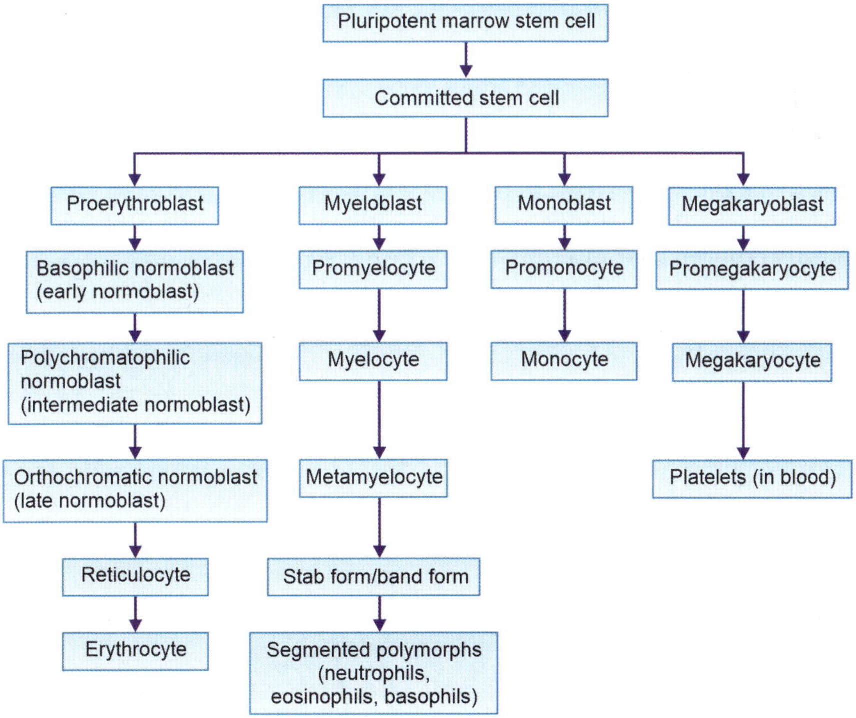

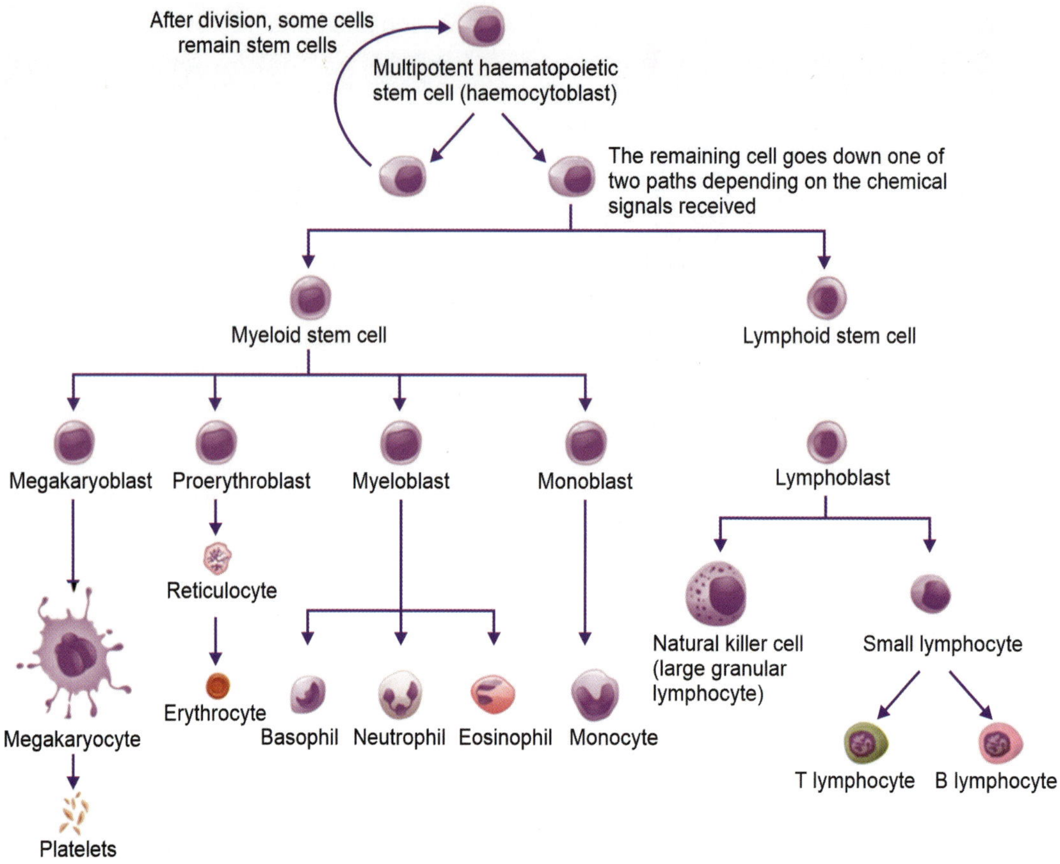

Fig. 3.9: Haematopoiesis of different blood cells in the bone marrow

- Increased reticulin fibres also occur in secondary carcinoma (metastatic deposit), osseous disorders like Paget's disease and hyperparathyroidism, in inflammatory reactions and in other myeloproliferative disorders (particulary lymphoproliferative disorders and proliferation of megakaryocytes) (Fig. 3.9).

VIVA VOCE

Q1. What are the parts of bone marrow needle and how to identify?

Ans: A stout wide bore needle and guard. A stillete is there within the needle which prevents blockage of the needle when it penetrates the skin, soft tissue and bone chips. The guard allows penetration of the needle up to desired length and prevents damage to the underlying tissues/organs.

Q2. What are the differences between Salah's needle and Klima's needle? Which one is better?

Ans: Salah's needle it does not has side screw and guard is fixed to the body of needle itself by a spiral thread.

Q3. Which is the best site and why?

Ans: Posterior superior iliac spine is the preferred site because:

- Patient lies prone and cannot see the procedure (patient can see sternal puncture). So, patient is less apprehensive.
- The procedure is very safe as there is no underlying important structure (like substernal aorta) and risk of damaging vital organs is minimal.

Q4. What are the absolute indications for bone marrow aspiration examination?

Ans:
- Hypoplastic/aplastic anaemia
- Sideroblastic anaemia
- Megaloblastic anaemia
- Aleukaemic/subleukaemic leukaemia
- Assessment of remission during chemotherapy of acute leukaemia
- Kala-azar (acute)
- ITP (Idiopathic thrombocytopenic purpura)
- Multiple myeloma

Q5. What are the relative indications for bone marrow aspiration?

Ans:
- Chronic kala-azar
- Before starting chemotherapy for acute leukaemia
- Staging of lymphoma (Hodgkin and non-Hodgkin lymphoma).

Q6. What is dry tap and what are the causes?

Ans: When only blood and no marrow material is aspirated then it is called 'dry tap'. Common causes are aplastic anaemia, myelofibrosis, and faulty technique.

Q7. How would you confirm that marrow has been aspirated?

Ans: i. Macroscopically, by looking at the granularily. When bone marrow smear is touched the surface is irregular and sand-like feeling due to presence of marrow particles. Marrow particles look glistening.

ii. Microscopically, by looking at the megakaryocytes and fat spaces (in-between marrow cells) under microscope. Marrow particles are dragged during smear preparation, and trail of cells is left behind.

Q8. What are the indications of trephine or bone marrow biopsy?

Ans: All the indications of bone marrow aspiration and 'dry tap' during aspirations (myelofibrosis, myelosclerosis and aplastic anaemia).

Bone marrow biopsy removes a core of bone to evaluate both bone and surrounding tissue (marrow tissue). Also associated cells, protein deposits or inflammatory processes can be assessed. It shows the relationship of the cells to each other or to the bone or the cells' precise location in relation to the bone. Bone marrow infiltration by tumour cells or cancer cells can also be examined which helps in staging in many tumours like Hodgkin and non-Hodgkin lymphomas.

Q9. What are the contraindications of bone marrow aspiration?

Ans: Haemophilia A, haemophilia B, bleeding diathesis and infection at the site of puncture.

Q10. What are the routine stains and special stains for bone marrow smear examination?

Ans: Routine stains: Leishman's stain, Giemsa stain and MGG.

Special stains

i. Perls'-Prussian blue stain: To detect iron status. Absent in iron deficiency anaemia, increased in haemochromatosis, haemosiderosis, refractory sideroblastic anaemia and decreased in aplastic anaemia and pernicious anaemia.

ii. Reticulin stain for myelofibrosis, polycythaemia vera and myeloproliferative disorders (increased in all).

iii. PAS stain, myeloperoxidase stain and Sudan black stain: Differentiate between ALL (acute lymphoblastic leukaemia) and AML (acute myeloblastic leukaemia).

Chapter

4

Total Count of WBC, RBC and Platelets

For total count of blood cells (RBCs, WBCs and platelets) and haemocytometers are used. There are a number of different haemocytometers in the market and each of them has a different grid (device containing horizontal and perpendicular lines) as well as different recommended uses. Different haemocytometers are:

- Neubauer/improved or modified Neubauer chamber
- Louis-Charles Malassez device: French histologist and anatomist (1842–1909) who first invented haemocytometer.
- Burker chamber
- Thoma chamber (Fig. 4.1)
- Fuchs-Rosenthal counting chamber: Used mainly for total eosinophil count.

But most popular and most frequently used haemocytometer nowadays is **improved or modified Neubauer chamber**. Most haemocytometers are manufactured from crystal glass and generally measured 30 × 70 mm with a thickness of 4 mm. Two vertical lines are ground from the glass to define the cell counting area and the double cell counting chambers have a ground out 'H' shape.

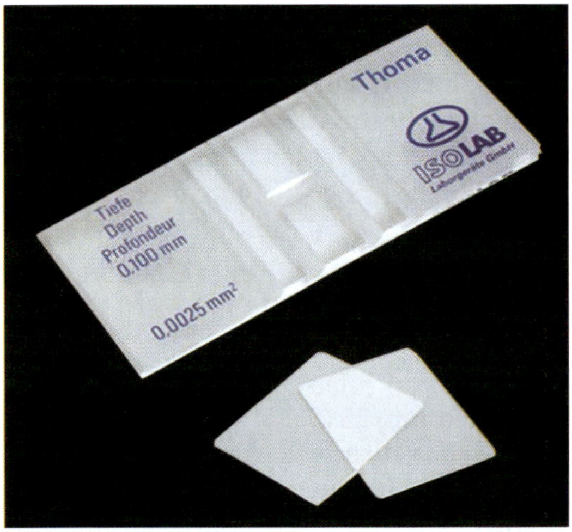

Fig. 4.1: Thoma counting chamber

OLD *VS.* IMPROVED NEUBAUER CHAMBER

- In the old chamber, in the central area, there are 16 large squares each having 16 small squares. But in the improved chamber there are 25 large squares, each containing 16 small squares.
- The triple lines, dividing the central area is not very close in old chamber. But in improved chamber, the triple lines are very close.
- The space occupied by the triple lines in old Neubauer chamber being used to produce extra large space.
- In old chamber, the gap between triple lines was wide and the rectangular space between them looks as similar as the

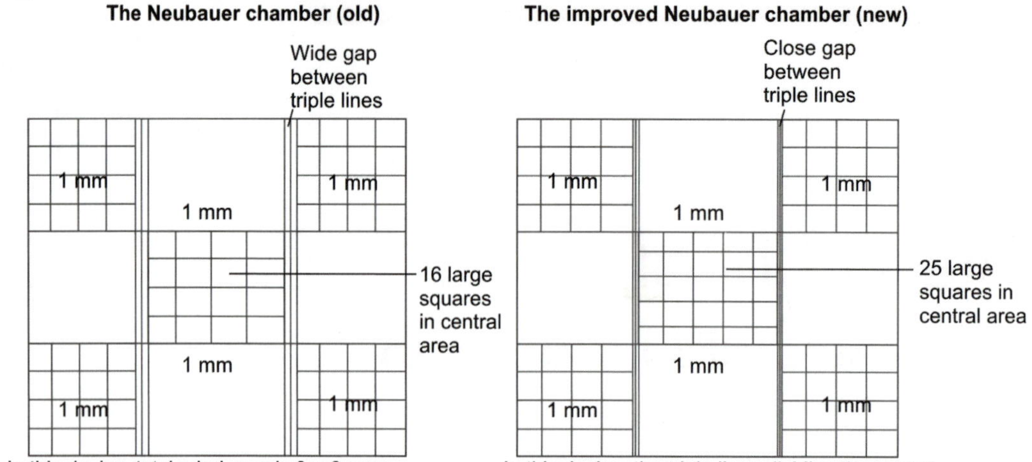

In this device, total ruled area is 3 × 3 mm; the central ruled area is 1 × 1 mm. In the central area 16 groups of 16 small squares separated by triple rulings. The four corner squares are subdivided into 16 squares, and chamber depth is 0.1 mm

In this device, the triple lines dividing the central large square are very much closer to each other. The central ruled area is divided into 25 large squares. Each of these squares is divided to form 16 small squares. The four corner squares are subdivided into 16 squares, and chamber depth is also same (0.1 mm)

Fig. 4.2: Old and improved Neubauer chamber

squares in which the cells are to be counted. So, it makes the count very difficult and chances of error was very high.

- In old Neubauer chamber, the separating lines were very dull and some time it was very difficult to recognize them. But in the improved chamber, the separating lines are vivid and clear (Fig. 4.2).
- By dividing, central space in 25 large squares, the RBC and platelet count have become easier.

Parts of Haemocytometer (Improved Neubauer's Chamber)

(Figs 4.3, 4.4 and 4.6)

i. A counting chamber
ii. A WBC pipette
iii. A RBC pipette
iv. A thick coverslip.

Counting Chamber (Fig. 4.5)

The improved Neubauer's chamber has two ruled stages separated by a small gutter (a shallow trough/channel beneath the edge of a roof). The two ruled stages again are separated from two ridges by gutters, one on each side. The surface of these two ruled stages is 0.1 mm above the surface of the stage. So, when cover glass is kept on the platform of this counting chamber, the space between the bottom of the coverslip and the base of the grooved area becomes 0.1 mm in depth.

There are two chamber stages, one above and one below, which is separated by gutter. Each stage has a ruled area measuring 3 × 3 mm which is divided into 9 squares. This squares measuring 1 × 1 mm each. The four corner squares are divided into 16 small squares (1/4 × 1/4 mm each). The four corner areas (A, B, C and D are used in Fig. 4.6 for counting WBCs.

The central ruled square area (1 × 1 mm) is divided into 25 (5 × 5) small squres in the improved Neubauer's chamber. Each small square is again subdivided into 16 (4 × 4) smaller squares. Area of each small square is 1/5 × 1/5 mm or 1/25 mm^2. For counting

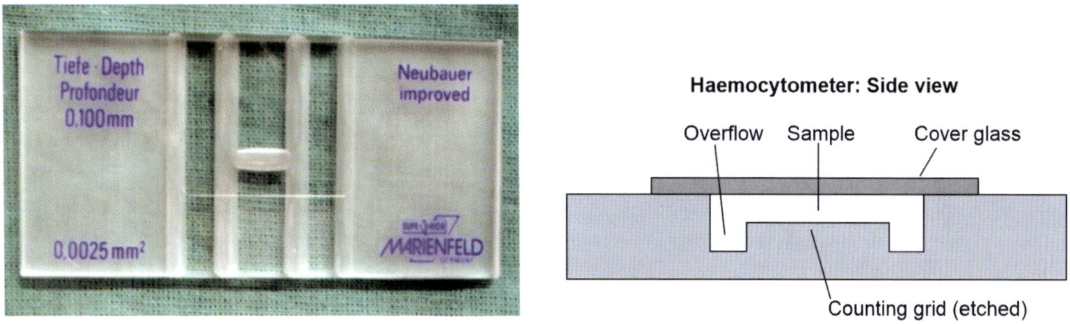

Fig. 4.3: Improved Neubauer's chamber

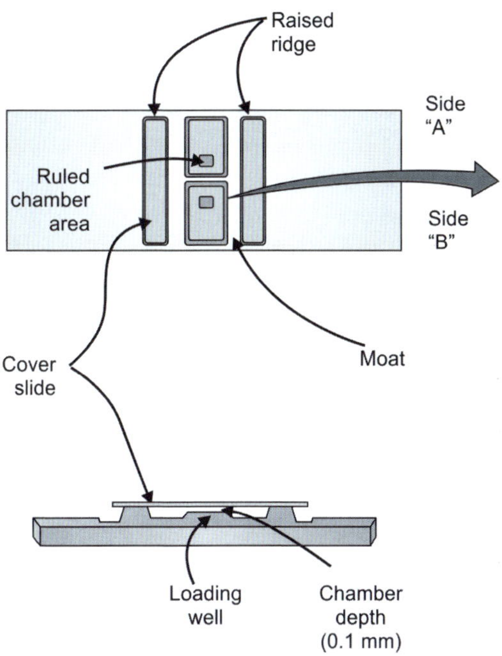

Fig. 4.4: Schematic diagram of using improved Neubauer's chamber

RBCs, this central ruled area is used. Usually four corners and one central square ruled area (blackened in picture) are used total RBC count. This area is also used for platelet count and sperm count from seminal fluid.

WBC Pipette (Fig. 4.7)

The pipette is marked 0.5, 1 below the bulb and 11 above the bulb. There is a white-coloured bead inside the bulb.

Uses

i. Total WBC count of blood (TLC).
ii. Total cell count from different body fluids like pleural fluid, CSF (cerebrospinal fluid, peritoneal fluid).
iii. Total platelet count, if the platelet count is very low.
iv. Total sperm count if the sperm count is low.

Blood or body fluid or seminal fluid is taken by WBC pipette and four corners of the haemocytometer are changed for cell counting.

RBC Pipette (Fig. 4.8)

The pipette is marked 0.5, 1 below the bulb and 101 above the bulb. There is a red-coloured bead inside the bulb.

Uses

i. Total RBC count of blood
ii. Total platelet count of blood
iii. Total sperm count from seminal fluid
iv. Total WBC count in case of leukaemias when there is very high WBC count and counting in the four corners may be problematic.

Blood or body fluid or seminal fluid is taken by RBC pipette and central ruled area of the haemocytometer is charged for cell counting.

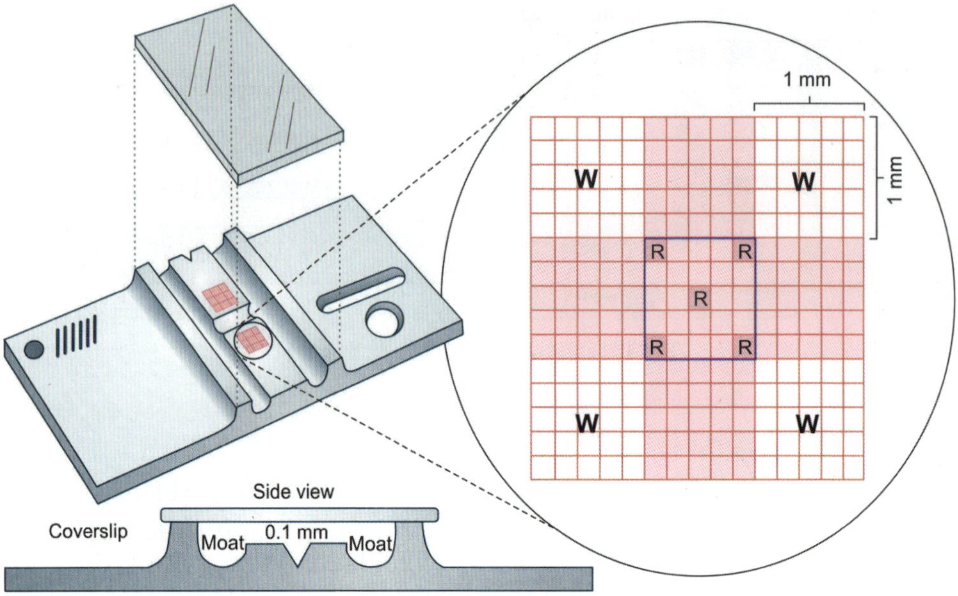

A

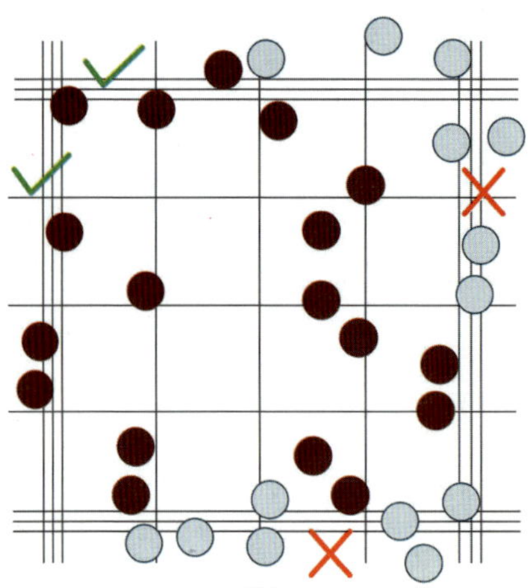

B

Fig. 4.5A and B: (A) Counting of WBC and RBC in the chamber; (B) Right way of counting cells. Cells on the upper and left triple lines are counted (black-coloured circles) while on right and lower triple lines are not counted (white-coloured circles)

Thick Coverslip (Fig. 4.9)

A specially made coverslip which has very smooth surface and even thickness of 0.3 mm or 0.4 mm or 0.5 mm is used. Commonly, coverslip with a thickness of 0.4 mm is used. Two sizes of coverslip are available in the market. One is 16 × 22 mm coverslip which is used for single ruled haemocytometer. The other coverslip is 22 × 23 mm which is used for double-ruled counting chamber.

Differences between RBC pipette and WBC pipette are given in Table 4.1.

White Blood Cell Count (Manual Method)

Blood is collected up to mark 0.5 of WBC pipette, either from EDTA or oxalate mixed

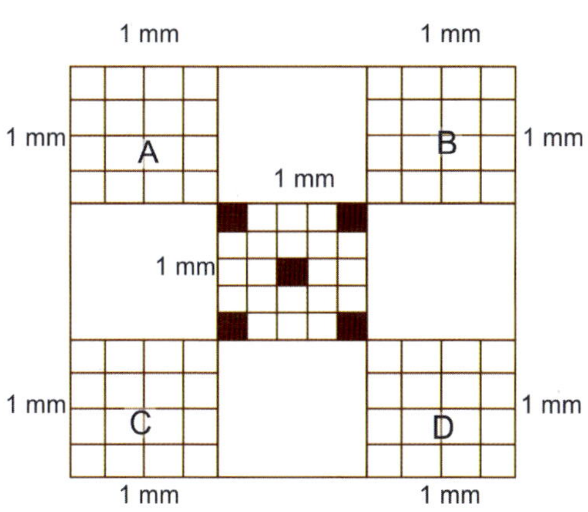

Fig. 4.6: Counting chamber in improved Neubauer's chamber

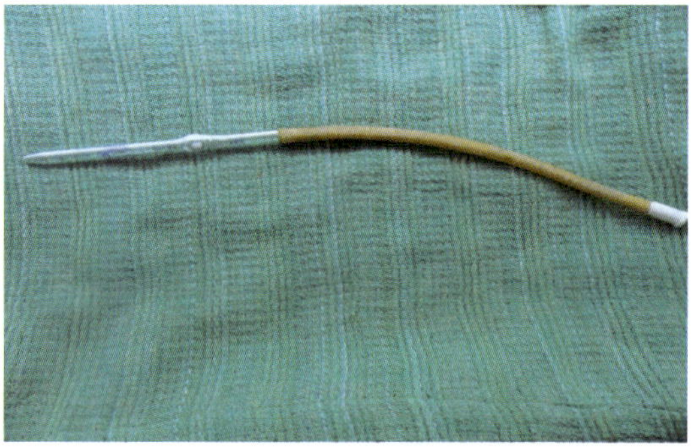

Fig. 4.7: WBC pipette

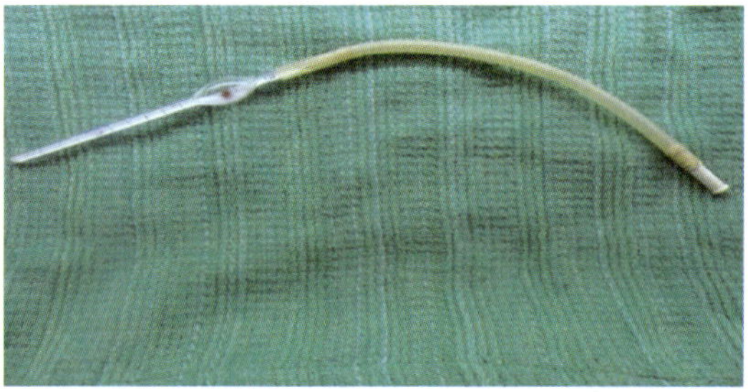

Fig. 4.8: RBC pipette

(anticoagulated) venous blood or after finger prick (fresh blood without anticoagulant). WBC diluting fluid is then sucked up to the mark 11 above in the WBC pipette. Well mixed the blood and WBC fluid in the

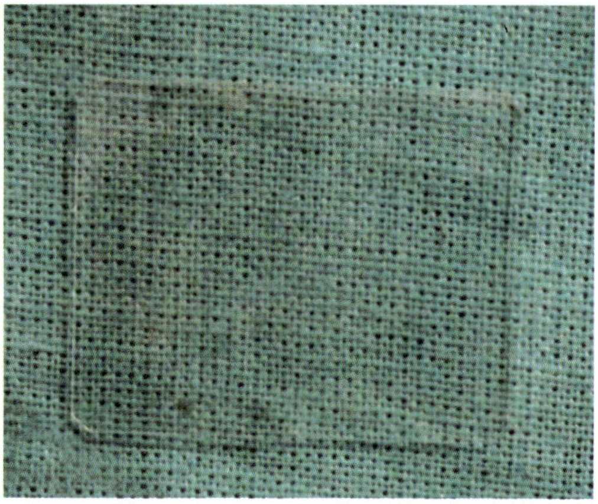

Fig. 4.9: Thick coverslip

Table 4.1: Differences between RBC pipette and WBC pipette

RBC pipette	WBC pipette
1. It has a red bead	1. It has a white bead
2. It has graduations up to mark 101	2. It has graduations up to mark 11
3. Size of bulb is larger	3. Size of bulb is smaller
4. Size of lumen is smaller	4. Size of lumen is larger

pipette by rotating the pipette between fingers by rotation. Then keep it over the table for few minutes (5–10 minutes). The red cells are lysed by the diluting fluid (acetic acid) but the leukocytes remain intact. Nuclei of the WBCs stain deep violet black by methylene blue or gentian violet stains.

Composition of WBC Diluting Fluid

- Glacial acetic acid: 2 ml
- Distilled water: 100 ml
- Aqueous methylene blue
  Solution (0.3%, w/v): 10 drops*
  Or

1% aqueous solution of gentian violet: 1 ml.

* Aqueous methylene blue solution is prepared by dissolving 0.3 gm of methylene blue in 100 ml of distilled water. Filter it before use. Alternatively, gentian violet (1 ml of 1% solution, w/v) can also be used instead of methylene blue (0.3%, w/v).

Dilution of Blood

If the blood is taken up to 0.5 mark, then the dilution is 1 in 20. Because the mark 11 above the bulb is to indicate the total volume of the marked portion of WBC pipette. Firstly, the blood is sucked (up to 0.5 mark), then the WBC fluid is taken. So, blood moves up and is diluted in the bulb and above up to mark 11 (from mark 1 to mark 11), whereas the long bar in the pipette contains only WBC fluid (up to mark 1). So, 10 volumes (11–1 = 10) contain 0.5 ml volume of blood. Hence, the dilution is 1 in 20 or 1:20.

Charging (Filling) the Improved Neubauer's Chamber

- Chamber and coverslip should be clean and dry.
- Hold the WBC pipette slightly inclined and pressure is released slowly with finger so that a small volume of WBC fluid mixed blood is allowed in the chamber under coverslip. This will be accomplished by the capillary action. Blood outside the pipette is wiped with tissue paper or cotton.
- The WBCs are allowed to settle for 2–3 minutes, so that they can be seen in the same plane of focus.

Counting of Leukocytes

WBC count is made under high power (40X) objective; but low power (10X) objective is used to focus them. The WBCs in each of the four large (1 × 1 mm) corner squares (ruled area) are counted, each of this large square has 16 small squares or division. Only WBCs within the squares are counted and cells lying on lines of any two adjacent sides (top and right, or bottom and left) are included in total WBC count.

The volume of each large square = 1 × 1 × 1/10 mm (depth)

So, the volume of four large squares = $1 \times 1 \times 1/10 \times 4$ mm^3 or cu mm = 2/5 mm^3

Let the leukocyte count (WBC) in four large squares is N.

Then, 2/5 mm^3 of volume of blood contains leukocytes = N × dilution factor

Or, 2/5 mm^3 blood contains leukocytes = N × 20

Or 1 mm^3 blood contains leukocytes = $N \times 20 \times 5/2 = N \times 50$.

Note

i. As many leukocytes as possible should be counted; a reasonable and practical figure is to count 100 cells. If 400 cells are counted then chances of error will as low as 5%.

ii. Causes of error: These include mistaking clumped red cell debris or debris or dirt for leukocytes or clumped leukocytes. Clumped leukocytes are usually seen in blood with several hours storage or in heparinized blood (>25 IU/ml of blood).

iii. Filing or charging defects leading to error:
   a. Chamber area incompletely filled
   b. Air bubble anywhere in the chamber area
   c. Any dirt or debris in the chamber (unclean or moist chamber).
   d. Overflow of the counting and ruled area.

iv. Nowadays, bulb pipettes are not recommended because they are easily broken. The volumes of blood used are unnecessarily small and the WBC pipette is difficult to handle. Particularly charging the chamber with pipette is very difficult and needs experience. So, 20 µl micropipette (or Pasteur pipette) is used which is easy to handle.

Red Blood Cell Count (Manual Method)

Blood is collected up to the mark 0.5 in the RBC pipette, either from EDTA or oxalated mixed (anticoagulated) venous blood or after finger prick capillary blood. Wipe tip clean. RBC diluting fluid is then sucked up to the mark 101 in the RBC pipette. Clean the tip of pipette again. It is well mixed and shaken for 2–3 minutes. First few drops are discarded and then counting chamber (central ruled area) is charged. It is then kept in a most chamber or in a Petri dish with wet filter paper and allowed to settle the RBCs for 10–15 minutes; so that they can be seen in the same plane of focus.

Composition of RBC Fluid

- Formalin (40% formaldehyde): 1 ml
- Trisodium citrate: 3.13 g
- Distilled water: 100 ml
- Tinge of eosin (optional)

Formalin acts as a preservative and prevents undesirable growth of microorganism/fungus in the diluting fluid. Eosin tinge is added to distinct the RBCs quickly but not to stain RBCs.

Alternatively, Hayem's fluid may be used (costlier than previous diluting fluid).

Composition of Hayem's Fluid

- Sodium chloride (NaCl): 1 g
- Sodium sulphate: 5 g
- Mercuric chloride: 0.5 g
- Distilled water: 100 ml

Remember the RBC diluting fluid should be isotonic so that RBCs are not lysed. Normal saline can be used if there is no diluting fluid available RBCs and in emergency. But normal saline cause crenation of RBCs and may form rouleax. Hence, not recommended for use.

Counting of RBCs

Red cells are counted in the central ruled are of the improved Neubauer chamber. In the central large square (1 × 1 mm) there are 25 small squares (1/5 × 1/5 mm). Four corners and central small squares are counted for RBCs. Let the RBC count in 5 small squares is N.

Volume of 5 small squares = 1/5 × 1/5 × 1/10 × 5
(depth is 0.1 mm or 1/10 mm)
= 1/50 cu mm or mm^3

So, 1/50 mm^3 blood contains RBCs
= N × dilution factor
= N × 200 (dilution of blood in RBC diluting fluid)

Then, 1 mm^3 blood contains RBCs
= N × 200 × 50/1 = N × 10,000

Note

i. Like WBC pipette, RBC pipettes are also not used nowadays. Instead micropipette or Pasteur pipettes are used.
ii. Error in counting RBC may be due to filing or charging defects (vide WBC count).
iii. Errors may also be due to inaccurate apparatus or due to technical errors (bad technique in collecting blood, insufficient mixing of blood specimen).

Platelet Count (Manual Method)

The diluent consists of 1% ammonium oxalate. Not more than 500 ml should be made at a time. The solution should be filtered through a micropipette filter (0.22 mm) and kept at 4°C.

Method: Use venous blood preferably for platelet counts. Finger pricks may cause clumping of platelets. Fill the blood and diluent as described for RBC count and using RBC pipette. Charge the chamber (central ruled area). Keep the haemocytometer in a moist chamber. Wait for 20–30 minutes to settle down the small platelets.

Using high power (40X) objective with reduced condenser aperture, count the platelets in the same squares as indicated the RBC counting (five small squares). Suppose total platelet count is N. Then as for RBC counting.

So, 1/50 mm^3 blood contains platelets
= N × dilution factor
= N × 200

Then, 1 mm^3 blood contains platelets
= N × 200 × 50/1 = N × 10,000

> **Note**
>
> - If platelet count is low, then WBC pipette may be used (dilution 1:20) and four large corner squares are counted for platelets like WBCs (N × 50).
> - Charged haemocytometer is kept inside a moist chamber or it can be put in a Petri dish with a moistened or wet filter paper. The moist environment does not allow evaporation of platelet fluid. Adequate time (20–30 minutes) is given to settle down the platelets.
> - Platelets under high power objective (light microscope), are small (but not minute) highly refractile particles. Platelets appear bluish and must be distinguished from debris.

ELECTRONIC METHOD FOR BLOOD CELL COUNT

Total WBC count along with other routine haematologic investigations are often done by using electronic instrument like 'Coulter counter' (Fig. 4.10A and B).

The Coulter analyzers utilize the electrical impedance with low-frequency electromagnetic current, high frequency electromagnetic current, laser light scattering, light scattering and absorbance depending on the device used. The compact semiautomated Coulter system provides only the basic WBC count, RBC count, haemoglobin level, haematocrit value. On the other hand, the Coulter MAXM, ONYX, STKR and STKS use positive identification bar code system and close vial sampling. Eighteen to twenty parameters may be assessed, including WBC count, RBC count, platelet count, haemoglobin level, haematocrit value, MCV, MCH, RDW (red cell distribution width) and MPV (mean platelet volume).

Rapid performance, minimal or no technical error, elimination of visual error and biasness, more accurate and precise results are advantages of electronic system over manual or haemocytometer method. In many laboratories, use of manual methods by haemocytometer has become obsolete. Only if the result is very very low or very very high, then it is used (with more dilution for very very high count) as it may be outside the range of the electronic machine.

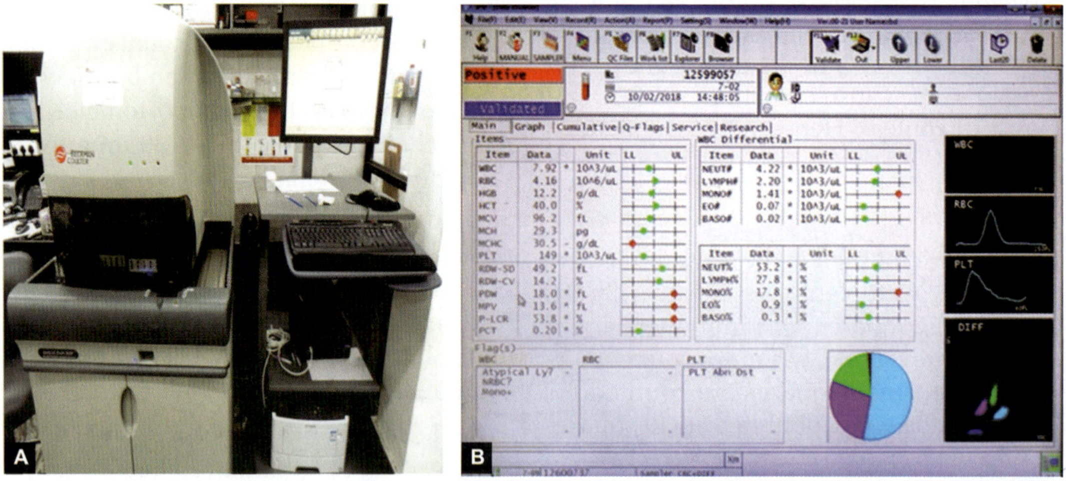

Fig. 4.10A and B: Automated blood cell counters

VIVA VOCE

Q1. How to identify WBC pipette?

Ans: By marks 0.5 and 1 below the bulb and mark 11 above the bulb. Also, a white bead inside the bulb.

Q2. What is the use of WBC pipette?

Ans:
- Used for total WBC count
- Sperm count in semen
- Eosinophil count
- Also may be used to count cells in any fluid where the count is more (>1000/μl), like cell count in CSF, pleural/ascitic fluid.
- RBC count in severe anaemia where RBC count is low.

Q3. How to identify RBC pipette?

Ans: By marks 0.5 and 1 below the bulb and mark 101 above the bulb. Also, a red-coloured bead inside the bulb.

Q4. What is the use of RBC pipette?

Ans:
- Used for total RBC count
- For total platelet count
- For sperm count in semen
- High TLC count

Q5. What is the electronic method for counting WBC? What are the advantages and disadvantages?

Ans: Electronic counter is based on aperture impedance method, or light scattering technology, or both. In this method, particles (WBCs) passing through a chamber in single file scatter the light and convert by a chamber in single file scatter the light and convert by a detector into pulses proportionate to the size of the cells, which are counted electronically. During counting of WBCs, a lysate is used to lyse RBCs.

Advantages
- Easy and rapid method
- High level of precision
- Very large number of cells is counted quickly
- Time saving method

Disadvantages
- The instrument is costly, so beyond the scope of small size laboratory.
- Calibration to be done at regular interval, otherwise there will be error.
- Normoblasts (nucleated RBCs) are counted as leukocytes
- Clumps of platelets are also falsely counted as WBCs.

Q6. What is electronic method of counting platelets? Is it advantageous or disadvantageous?

Ans: The principal is electrical impedance like counting RBCs.

Platelet counting by electronic method is disadvantageous.

Disadvantages
- Debris and fragments of blood cells (small size) are counted as platelets.
- Howell-Jolly bodies and Heinz bodies are also counted as platelets.
- Equipment is costly and calibration error may occur.

Q7. How do you differentiate between platelets and dust particles?

Ans:
- Platelets are refractile
- Platelets are stained light blue when stained by brilliant cresyl blue. Dust particles cannot be stained.
- Platelets have brownian movements but dust particles lack it.

Q8. Which is the best method for absolute eosinophil count (AEC)? What is the composition of diluting fluid for eosinophil count?

Ans: The best method is the automated counter which detects eosiniphil peroxidase during counting. Other methods are Fuchs-Rosenthal counting chamber or hemocytometer or using Dunger's solution. Other dilution fluids are Randolph's diluting fluid, Pilot's stain.

i. Dunger's solution:
   - Acid dye, e.g. eosin or phloxine, 0.1% aqueous solution
   - Water to lyse RBCs and rupture leukocytes

ii. Randolph's fluid:
   - Stock solution A (methylene blue, propylene glycol, distilled water)
   - Stock solution B (phloxine, propylene glycol, distilled water)
   - Working solution is prepared from above stocks 1:1 volume

iii. Pilot's stain:
   - Propylene glycol (50 ml), distilled water 40 ml, phloxine 0.1 aqueous solution, 10 ml; sodium carbonate 1% aqueous solution, 1 ml.

Q9. Why special coverslip not the ordinary one is used while doing various counts by Neubauer chamber?

Ans: Neubauer chamber and its coverslip (thicker than the ordinary coverslip) are so designed that after charging the chamber a fixed/desired amount of fluid is present in-between the ruled chamber and overlying coverslip. And the depth of fluid 0.1 mm (prerequisite for calculation). The ordinary coverslip is thin and light. Fluid depth is not 0.1 mm, so cell counts become erroneous. Moreover, coverslip of Neubauer chamber is uniformly flat while ordinary cover glass is not.

Q10. How do you clean Hb, WBC and RBC pipettes?

Ans: These pipettes are filled with distilled water and cleaned by blowing it out twice. Then, acetone is sucked into the pipette and blown it out. Acetone removes residual water within pipette and dries it completely. When pipette is completely dry, the bead with the bulb moves/rolls freely but if it is wet, bead does not roll freely.

Q11. How sperm count is done in Neubauer chamber?

Ans: Semen diluting fluid (sodium bicarbonate 5 g, neutral formalin 1 ml, and distilled water to make 100 ml). Semen may be diluted in a test tube (0.1 ml semen +1.9 ml diluting fluid) or in a WBC pipette (draw semen to the mark 0.5 and diluting fluid to the mark 11) and mix well. After charging improved Neubauer chamber, wait for 2–3 minutes to settle down the sperms.

Calculation: Count spermatozoa in 2 mm^3 (two large squares at two corners) and multiply by 100,000 or 1 lakh. It gives the number of spermatozoa per ml of semen (unlike in terms of per mm^3 of WBC count).

Normal range: 60–150 million/ml. Count below 20 million/ml is considered abnormal.

Chapter

5

Erythrocyte Sedimentation Rate (ESR) and Packed Cell Volume (PCV)

ERYTHROCYTE SEDIMENTATION RATE

The erythrocyte sedimentation rate (ESR) is the rate at which red blood cells sediment in a period of one hour.

It is also known as sedimentation rate (sed rate).

Brief History of ESR

This test was invented by the Polish pathologist Edmund Biernacki in 1897. In some regions of the world, the test continues to be referred to as Biernacki's reaction. In the year 1918, the Swedish pathologist Robert Sanno Fahraeus along with Alf Vilhelm Albertsson Westergren described the same and is eponymously remembered as Fahraeus-Westergren test. But in the UK, it is usually termed Westergren test which became popular throughout world.

Mechanism of Erythrocyte Sedimentation

The ESR or rate of fall of red cells is governed by the balance between pro-sedimentation factors, mainly fibrinogen and those factors resisting sedimentation, e.g. the negative charge of the erythrocyte (zeta potential). The decreased zeta potential promotes rouleaux formation and hence raised ESR.

ESR depends upon the difference in specific gravity between red cells and plasma. Also, it is greatly influenced by the extent to which RBCs form rouleaux, which sediment stacks of RBCs than single cell. Many other factors are also responsible which include the ratio of RBCs to plasma (i.e. PCV), the plasma viscosity, the bore of the tube, dilution, if any of the blood, the verticality of ESR tube, etc.

The very important factor is rouleaux formation and red cell clumping. This is mainly controlled by the plasma concentration of fibrinogen and other acute phase proteins/reactants, e.g. haptoglobin, ceruloplasmin, α_1-antitrypsin and C reactive protein (CRP). Rouleaux formation is also enhanced by increased concentration of plasma immunoglobulin. On the contrary, it is retarded by higher concentration of albumin and test done with defibrinated blood (≤1 mm/hr), which removes fibrinogen. In anaemia, there may be quantitative deficiency of RBCs, so ratio of RBCs to plasma is altered which results more rouleaux formation and increased ESR.

Methods of ESR Estimation

i. Westergren method
ii. Wintrobe method
iii. Landau method: Not accurate, used in the past in children with limited supply of blood. The method uses capillary blood from heel, toe or fingertip.

iv. Electronic method by automated analyzers.

The first two methods are commonly used methods which are done by manual technique. Of these two, Westergren method is most popular and commonly used method.

Westergren Method using Westergren Pipette (Fig. 5.1)

Though the equipment is sometimes called Westergren tube, it should be called pipette (more scientific term) as it is open at both ends.

Westergren pipette is a slender, thick-walled pipette. It is 300 mm long (i.e. 30 cm or 12 inches) of which lower 200 mm is graduated (markings) and upper 100 mm part is ungraduated. The inner diameter of pipette should not be less than 2.5 mm. The capacity of the tube is about 1 ml.

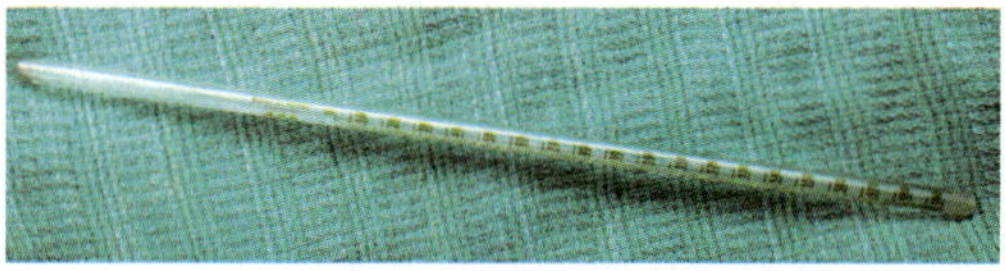

Fig. 5.1: Westergren pipette

Anticoagulant used: 3.2% trisodium citrate solution (no other anticoagulant with this method), 109 mmol/L (32 g/L, $Na_3Ca_6 H_5O_7.2H_2O$). EDTA mixed blood is used in modified Westergren method.

Blood and anticoagulant ratio: For this test 2 ml of venous blood is mixed with 0.5 ml of sodium citrate anticoagulant. So, the blood and anticoagulant ratio is 4:1.

Method or procedure: 0.5 ml of 3.2% sodium citrate solution is taken in a test tube. Then, 2 ml of venous blood (usually from antecubital vein) is mixed with the anticoagulant immediately with the help of a syringe. The sample is well mixed.

The anticoagulated blood is drawn up in to Westergren pipette up to 200 mm mark with the help of a teat or mechanical device (mouth suction is avoided). The pipette is now set exactly vertical in a Westergren stand (Fig. 5.2). A spring clip, pressing on the top and rubber piece at the lower end hold the pipette in the Westergren stand or rack. Now the pipette in the rack which is vertically placed is kept at room temperature without vibration and exposure to sunlight.

Modified Westergren method: It produces the same results but uses EDTA blood rather than citrate as an anticoagulant. In this method, 2 ml of EDTA blood is diluted with 0.5 ml of 0.85% sodium chloride or with 0.5 ml of 3.8% sodium citrate. Precision is poor when EDTA blood is undiluted.

This method has the advantage that same EDTA-mixed blood may be used for other haematologic studies.

Recording result: The RBCs begin to settle down and a clear plasma zone is formed above the settled RBCs. The upper level of the RBC column is read (zero mark is upside and 200 mark is downside) at the end of one hour.

The measurement in mm is ESR (Westergren, 1 hour).

Previously it was thought that mean average ESR per hour (total duration 2 hours) is more accurate.

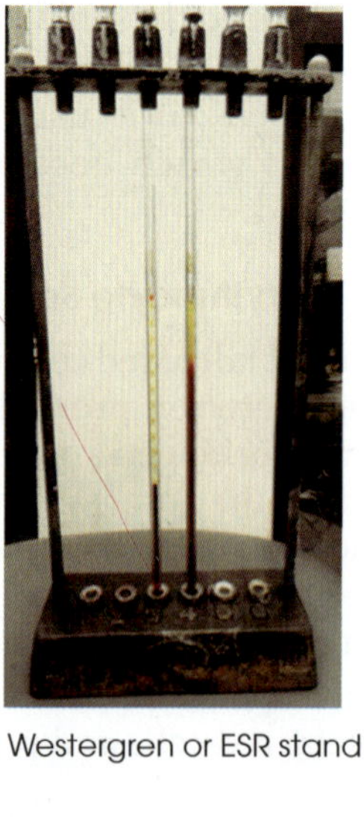

Fig. 5.2: Westergren or ESR stand (rack)

Mean ESR = (1st hour result + ½ of 2 hours result) ÷ 2

But later on, concept of mean ESR disregarded because result after 1 hour gives more accurate result.

Normal range of ESR: The ESR gradually increases with age. Westergren's original upper limit of normal (10 mm/hour for men and 20 mm/hour for women) seems to be low. According to studies by scientists, upper limits of reference values in this method should be as follows:

	Men	Women
i. Below age 50 years	0–15 mm/hr	20 mm/hr
ii. Above age 50 years	0–20 mm/hr	30 mm/hr
iii. Above age 85 years	0–30 mm/hr	42 mm/hr

But in Indian context, acceptable normal range for ESR is

- Men: 4–14 mm/hr
- Women: 6–20 mm/hr
- Newborn: 0–2 mm/hr
- Newborn to puberty: 3–13 mm/hr

Wintrobe's Method

Instrument: Wintrobe's tube is a special, thick-walled glass tube 11 cm long with an internal diameter of 3 mm and the bottom 10 cm are graduated. It has flat inner base. It is calibrated at 1 mm intervals to 100 mm and holds about 1 ml of blood. Graduations are from zero (top) to hundred (bottom) for ESR and zero (bottom) to hundred (top) for PCV.

Anticoagulant: Venous blood is mixed with EDTA (preferred), or double oxalate or heparin.

Methods

1. 2 ml venous blood is collected and mixed with anticoagulant (EDTA) in the vial immediately.
2. Wintrobe tube is filled with this blood till zero mark on top with the help of a Pasteur pipette.
3. The tube is now kept vertically over stand for one hour and is noted by measuring the free plasmatic zone above (descending orders, 0 marks on top and 100 marks on bottom).

Normal range: Men 0–9 mm/hr, women 2–20/hr.

Stages of Sedimentation (ESR)

Stage 1. Rouleaux formation: In this stage (first 15 minutes) red cells form rouleaux and minimum sedimentation occurs.

Stage 2. Formation of fine threads by proteins: During this stage (second 15 minutes) fibrinogen and globulin in plasma form network by forming fine threads. The rouleaux of red cells are trapped within this network and becomes heavier. So, they begin to fall (settling) rapidly.

Stage 3. Rapid fall of protein network: In this phase (third 15 minutes), red cell mass and protein network fall rapidly.

Stage 4. Packing of red cells: In the last 15 minutes, the sedimented red cell mass—protein undergoes packing at the bottom of pipette.

MODIFIED WESTERGREN METHOD

Disposable ESR Pipette (Westergren Method)

A disposable ESR pipette offers a highly accurate, risk free, easy, efficient and safe method for performing *Westergren's ESR determination* directly in a 12 × 75 mm/13 × 75 mm non-vacuum/vacuum blood collection tube (Fig. 5.3A and B).

Disposable ESR pipette is made of clear polystyrene, which gives a clear visibility of the blood for determining ESR. A biodegradable vacuum plug at the bottom,

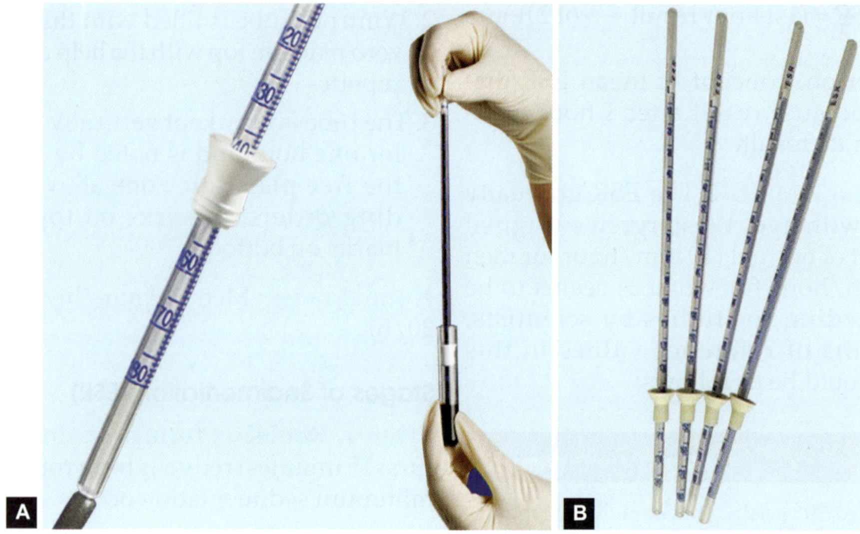

Fig. 5.3A and B: ESR estimation with disposable plastic pipettes (modified Westergren method)

which creates pressure on the blood in the 12 × 75 mm non-vacuum or vacuum blood collection tubes and thus the blood raises up in the pipette till the zero level mark, which acts as a barrier that stops hazardous substances (blood) from escaping through the top of the pipette.

Advantages of a Disposable ESR Pipette

1. A single time use of the pipette.
2. It avoids mouth pipetting and ensures user safety.
3. Can be used with almost all tubes like 12 × 75 mm/13 × 75 mm Non-vacuum/vacuum tubes.
4. Highly accurate, reproducible, risk free, easy, efficient and safe method of conducting an ESR.
5. Fibrous barrier protects user from hazardous aerosols.
6. Speed of application.

Procedure

1. Collect 1.6 ml of whole blood in 0.4 ml of sodium citrate 3.8% solution or take 1.6 ml of EDTA anti-coagulated whole blood in 0.4 ml of saline (use 12 × 75 mm non-vacuum blood collection tubes with 0.4 ml of sodium citrate 3.8% solution).
2. Mix the blood gently.
3. Gently insert the lower end of pipette bearing the vacuum plug in to the blood. Collect ion of tube and using continuous force, push the pipette down to the bottom of the blood collection tube.
4. The blood will automatically rise into the pipette and stop at the "zero" mark.
5. Place the assembly (tube + pipette absolutely vertical on a suitable stand (example rack for ESR pipette). And allow the blood cells to sediment without disturbing it for 60 minutes.
6. At the end of 60 minutes the numerical results are read in millimeters directly from the imprinted scale on the pipette.

Errors Faced while Using a Disposable Pipette

1. If the blood collection tube is cracked
2. If the ESR pipette has not been placed absolutely vertical
3. If the blood collection tube is not gently mixed
4. If the proportion of the blood and sodium citrate/EDTA is improper
5. If the disposable ESR pipette is reused.

VACUETTE® ESR BLOOD COLLECTION TUBES

Instruction for Use

Intended Use

VACUETTE® ESR tubes are used for the collection and transport of venous blood for blood sedimentation rate testing. ESR measurements refer to the Westergren method.

Product Description

VACUETTE® ESR tubes are plastic tubes with a pre-defined vacuum for exact draw volume. They are fitted with colour-coded VACUETTE® Safety Cap (13/75 mm tube) and Brom Butyl Caoutchouc Cap (9/120 mm tube). The tubes, additive concentrations, volume of liquid additives, and their permitted tolerances, as well as the blood-to-additive ratio are in accordance with the requirements and recommendations of the international standard ISO 6710 "Single-use containers for venous blood specimen collection".

The VACUETTE® ESR tubes contain a 3.2 % buffered tri-sodium citrate solution (0.109 mol/L). The mixing ratio is 1 part citrate solution to 4 parts blood. Tube interiors are sterile.

Storage

Store tubes at 4–25°C (40–77°F).

> **Note**
>
> Avoid exposure to direct sunlight. Exceeding the maximum recommended storage temperature may lead to impairment of the tube quality (i.e. vacuum loss, drying out of liquid additives, colouring, etc.)

Handling

Closed VACUETTE® **ESR System** (Fig. 5.4)

Equipment required for ESR measurements:

- A 9/120 mm, graduated, plastic tube with a citrate solution. Draw volume 1.5 ml and 2.75 ml.
- A9/120 mm glass tube with a citrate solution. Draw volumes of 1.6 ml or 2.9 ml are available.
- ESR rack with scale suitable for 1.5 ml/1.6 ml tubes, respectively ESR rack with scale suitable for 2.75 ml/2.9 ml tubes.

Procedures

After blood sampling and also before starting the ESR measurement, gently invert the tube 5–10 times to obtain the correct mixture. Use of a rotating mixer is recommended.

> **Note**
>
> It is recommended to do the determination within the first 4 hours when stored at room temperature. If longer storage is required, keep the specimen at the refrigerator (maximum 24 hours). Note that the sample must be brought to room temperature before use.

1. Place 1.5 ml, 1.6 ml or 2.75 ml, 2.9 ml tube into the corresponding rack vertically. Align the 0 mark at top of scale with the bottom of the meniscus of the blood at the blood-air interface.

   For the 1.5 ml/1.6 ml VACUETTE® ESR tube set timer for 30 minutes. The ESR

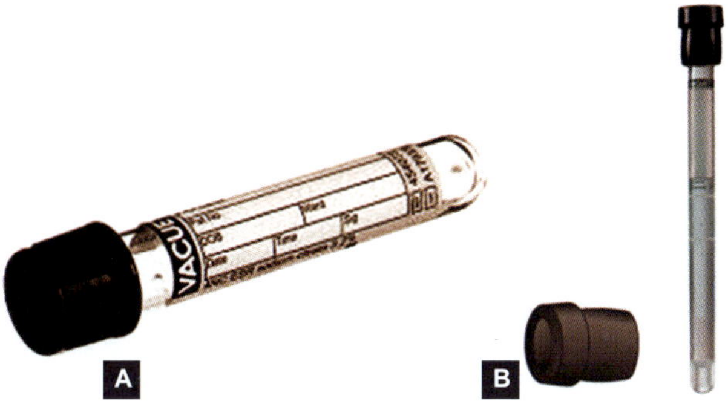

Fig. 5.4A and B: VACUETTE® ESR system

rack suitable for 1.5 ml/1.6 ml tubes delivers only the 1 hour Westergren value after 30 minutes reading time.

For the 2.75 ml or 2.9 ml ESR tube set timer for 60 minutes. The ESR rack for 2.9 ml tubes delivers the 1 hour and if required 2 hour Westergren value after 120 minutes reading time.

2. Discard VACUETTE® ESR tubes without opening.

Note

The conversion scale becomes highly compressed above Westergren values of 100 mm and ESR readings above this level should be repeated using the classic Westergren method if precise values are required.

1.5 ml and 1.6 ml tubes can be used with the following VACUETTE® ESR instruments: SRT 10/II, SRS 20/II, SRS 100/II.

The instrumentation allows for 1 hour Westergren results after 15 minutes or 30 minutes.

(For further information contact Greiner Bio-One or see "VACUETTE® Automated ESR Systems Brochure")

Open VACUETTE® ESR System

The system consists of 3 parts:

1. A 13/75 mm plastic tube with a citrate solution.
2. A graduated pipette with rubber adapter.
3. ESR rack without any scale.

Procedure

After blood sampling and also before starting the ESR measurement gently invert the tube 5–10 times to obtain the correct mixture. Use of a rotating mixer is recommended.

Note

It is recommended to do the determination within the first 4 hours when stored at room temperature. If longer storage is required, keep the specimen at the refrigerator (maximum 24 hours). Note that the sample must be brought to room temperature before use

1. Remove the cap of the tube.
2. Insert the pipette into the opened tube and the blood will fill automatically to the zero-line of the pipette.

Note

If there is a bubble in the column of the pipette, the determination is not valid!

1. Place tube and pipette into the suitable rack. Tube and pipette must be in a vertical position.
2. After 60 and if required 120 minutes, read level between settled erythrocytes and the supernatant plasma from pipette.
3. Afterwards dispose of the tube and pipette together in a suitable biohazard disposal container.

Disposal

1. The general hygiene guidelines and legal regulations for the proper disposal of infectious material should be considered and followed.
2. Disposable gloves prevent the risk of infection.
3. Contaminated or filled blood collection tubes must be disposed of in suitable biohazard disposal containers, which can then be autoclaved and incinerated afterwards.
4. Contaminated ESR pipette and VACUETTE® tubes must be disposed of together in suitable biohazard disposal containers for infectious material.

Disposal should take place in an appropriate incineration facility or through autoclaving (steam sterilisation).

Use of ESR

1. **Diagnosis**
   a. **Marked elevation:** Multiple myeloma, macroglobulinaemia, tuberculosis, hyperfibrinogenemia, myocardial infarction, temporal arthritis, rheumatoid arthritis, chronic kidney disease, SLE, inflammatory bowel disease, polymyalgia rheumatica.

b. **Moderate evaluation:** Chronic infection (chronic osteomyelitis, chronic lung abscess, chronic bronchiectasis), rheumatoid arthritis, neoplasms (Hodgkin lymphoma, carcinomatosis, leukaemia), infective endocarditis, physiological (pregnancy), drugs (oral contraceptives, methyldopa, dextran, vitamin A, theophylline).

2. **Disease severity assessment:** ESR is a component of PCDAI (Paediatric Crohn's Disease Activity Index), an index for assessment of severity of inflammatory bowel disease in children.
3. **Monitoring response to therapy:** ESR has limited role to monitor the response to therapy in certain inflammatory disease such as rheumatoid arthritis, polymyalgia rheumatica and temporal arthritis. In Hodgkin lymphoma, ESR can be used as a crude measure to response. Also, it is used to define one of the several possible adverse prognostic factors in staging of Hodgkin lymphoma.

Causes of Slow or Decreased ESR

- Polycythaemia vera
- Sickle cell anaemia, spherocytosis, poikilocytosis
- Congestive heart failure
- Stages of severe dehydration like cholera, acute gastroenteritis
- Infections: Typhoid and undulant fever, trichinosis, malarial paroxysm, pertusis.
- Allergic states
- Drugs: Aspirin, cortisone, quinine.

In case of sickle cell anaemia, spherocytosis or poikilocytosis, there are abnormal red cells. These abnormalities of RBCs prevent rouleaux formation. Hence, decreased ESR.

Sources of Error and other Interfering Factors

- If the concentration of anticoagulant is higher than recommend the ESR may be elevated.
- Heparin alters the membrane zeta potential of RBCs and cannot be used as an anticoagulant.
- Tilting the pipette accelerates the ESR. The RBCs aggregate along the lower side, whereas the plasma rises along the upper side. Subsequently, the retarding of influence of the rising plasma becomes less effective. An angle of 3° from vertical position, may accelerate the ESR by as much as 30%.
- Plasma factors: An accelerated ESR is seen in elevated levels of fibrinogen and to a lesser extent of globulins. Albumin retards ESR. High rise of plasma viscosity also retards ESR. Cholesterol increases and lecithin decreases ESR.
- The test should be done within two hours. If the blood is stored for more than two hours, ESR will increase.
- If blood is kept in refrigerator, ESR is highly increased. So, refrigerated blood should be allowed to return to normal room temperature before the test started.
- Temperature of the environment: The ideal temperature for the test is 20–25°C. Increase in temperature is directly proportional to increased ESR.
- Bubbles left in the pipette, when the blood is filled, will affect ESR. The cleanliness of pipette is also important.
- Haemolysis may modify ESR.

Different Automated Methods of ESR

(Fig. 5.5A and B)

- Ves-Matic
- ESR STAT-PLUS
- SEDIMAT
- Zeta sedimentation

Advantages of Automated Methods

- Provide more rapid results
- Use small sample volumes
- Save technician time
- Provide increased safety because the need for sample manipulation is decreased.

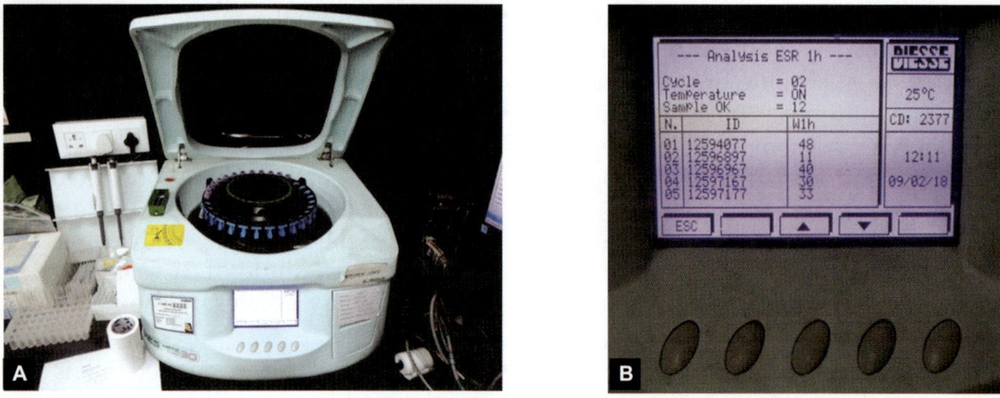

Fig. 5.5A and B: (A) Automated ESR machine; (B) Recording of ESR result

Zeta Sedimentation Rate (ZSR)

EDTA mixed blood (0.2 ml) is filled in a special capillary tube and is centrifuged in special apparatus (zeta fuge, Coulter electronics) for four times, each for 45 seconds. The capillary tube is mechanically rotated at 180° and centrifugation is done in reverse direction at every 45 seconds for four times. The red cell rouleaux develops better and travel down the capillary tube by alternate compaction and dispersion.

Result of ZSR: ZSR is expressed in terms of percentage.

Normal range in adults 40–50%. Rise in ZSR indicates rise in ESR.

Zeta crit: It is the ratio of the height of red cells to the total height of blood column.

Advantages of ZSR

- Requires small amount of blood (0.2 ml)
- No dilution is required.
- Eliminates the effect of anaemia.
- It is more sensitive than Westergren's method of ESR estimation.
- It requires minimum time.

Micro-ESR Method

Barrett (1980) described this micro-ESR method using 0.2 ml of blood to fill a plastic disposable tube 230 mm long with 1 mm inner diameter or internal bore. Both venous and capillary blood are suitable for this method. The tube filled with blood is kept vertically on a stand and the result is read after one hour.

This method has more utility in paediatric patients.

WINTROBE'S HAEMATOCRIT (PACKED CELL VOLUME)

The term 'haematocrit' theoretically means blood separation. Wintrobe haematocrit tube is mainly used for measurement of packed cell volume (PCV).

Definition of PCV

It is defined as the volume of packed red blood cells in a given sample of blood which is expressed as a percentage of the total volume of the blood sample.

Two methods are employed for measurement of PCV.

1. Macro-method using Wintrobe tube.
2. Micro-method using capillary tube.

1. Macro-method—Wintrobe's Tube (Fig. 5.6)

It is a spherical, thick-walled glass tube 11 cm long and has an internal diameter of 2.5 mm with flat inner base. The tube is calibrated at 1–100 mm intervals and holds about 1 ml of blood. The markings on the tube are in

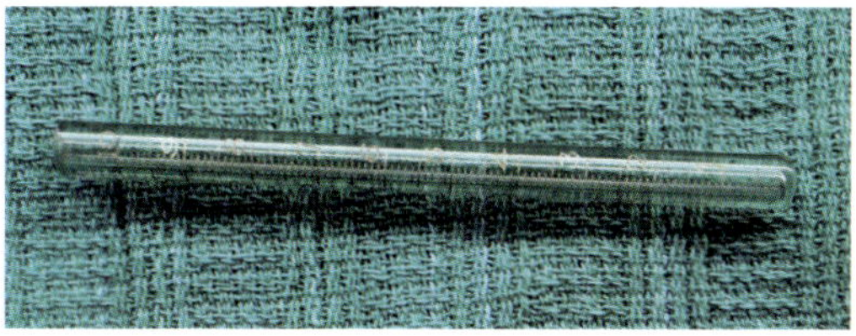

Fig. 5.6: Wintrobe's tube

reversed directions. Ascending marking is used for determination of PCV and descending marking is used for determination of ESR.

Uses

1. Wintrobe's tube is primarily used for determination of packed red cell volume (PCV) of blood.
2. Also it can be used for determination of ESR especially for anaemia correction with the help of correction curve.
3. Buffy coat smear preparation for demonstration of LE cell and staining with Leishman stain in diagnosis of SLE.
4. Abnormal or blast cells in aleukaemic leukaemia.

Blood and anticoagulant: Venous blood anticoagulated with double oxalate powder, EDTA powder or heparin.

Method of PCV Determination (Wintrobe Tube)

1. 2 ml venous blood is taken and immediately mixed with anticoagulant. Mix well by shaking.
2. The Wintrobe tube is filled with anticoagulated blood with the help of a long Pasteur pipette from the bottom up to mark '0' or '10' above.
3. The tube is then centrifuged at 3000 r.p.m. for 30 minutes.
4. The packed cell volume (PCV) is measured by noting the upper level of column of packed red cells by the markings in ascending order. PCV is expressed as percentage of the total volume of blood.

Zones Separated after Centrifugation

1. The layer of packed red cells or PCV is lower most which is usually 45 to 50%.
2. An intermediate thin layer comprises WBCs and platelets. It is above the lower most layer (red cells). The grey-coloured layer is known as buffy coat. Normally, this layer is 2 to 3%. Buffy coat layer is increased in leukaemia and severe degree of leukocytosis.
3. Upper most layer of plasma: This straw-coloured layer is above buffy coat layer and composed of free plasma. This layer may be pink in haemolysis, yellow in jaundice, and colourless in iron deficiency anaemia.

Normal Range of PCV

- Men: 45 ± 5%, i.e. 40 to 50%
- Women: 41± 5%, i.e. 36 to 46%
- At birth: 44 to 62%
- One year infant: 35% (approximate)
- 10 years: 37.5% (approximate)

Increased PCV: Polycythaemia, severe degree of dehydration, cholera, acute gastroenteritis.

Decreased PCV: Anaemia (usually less than 30%)

Sources of Error of PCV

- Inadequate duration and speed of centrifugation.
- Inadequate mixing of blood.
- Excess anticoagulant.
- Irregularity of the bore of Wintrobe tube.
- Trapping of leukocyte—platelet clumps in the tube will result defective red cell packing.

2. Micro-method—Capillary Tube Method for PCV

Nongraduated capillary tube (75 mm in length and about 1 mm internal diameter) is rinsed with heparin solution (1:2000 heparin or 1 in 1000 dilution). Well dry this heparinised capillary tube at 56°C and stored.

When the test is done a capillary tube (haematocrit) is filled up with blood (finger prick or EDTA mixed venous blood) and the empty end is sealed with a micro-burner. The tube is filled up ½ to 2/3 of its length (not the entire length). The tube is then fitted on the micro-haematocrit centrifuge and centrifuged at 12000 r.p.m. for 5 minutes with the sealed end away from the centre.

Calculation of result: Then the capillary tube is taken out and PCB is calculated with the help of a millimetre rule commercially available.

Normal range of PCV (Table 5.1)

- Male: 47 ± 7%
- Female: 43 ± 5%

Advantages of Micro-method

- Time requirement for centrifugation is short.

Table 5.1: Normal levels of packed cell volume (PVC) and haemoglobin

Age and sex	Packed cell volume (PCV)%	Haemo-globin (g/dl)
• Adult male	40–50	13–17
• Adult female (nonpregnant)	38–45	12–15
• Adult female (pregnant)	36–42	11–14
• Children, 6–12 years	37–46	11.5–15.5
• Children, 6 months to 6 years	36–42	11–14
• Infants, 2–6 months	32–42	9.5–14
• Newborns	44–60	13.6–19.6

- Small amount of blood is required to fill the capillary tube.
- Cost effective and easy to work.

Generally, PCV% is three times that of Hb g/dl or Hb%. So, if a person has haemoglobin of 15 g/dl, his PCV will be 15 × 3 = 45% (approx) (Fig. 5.7).

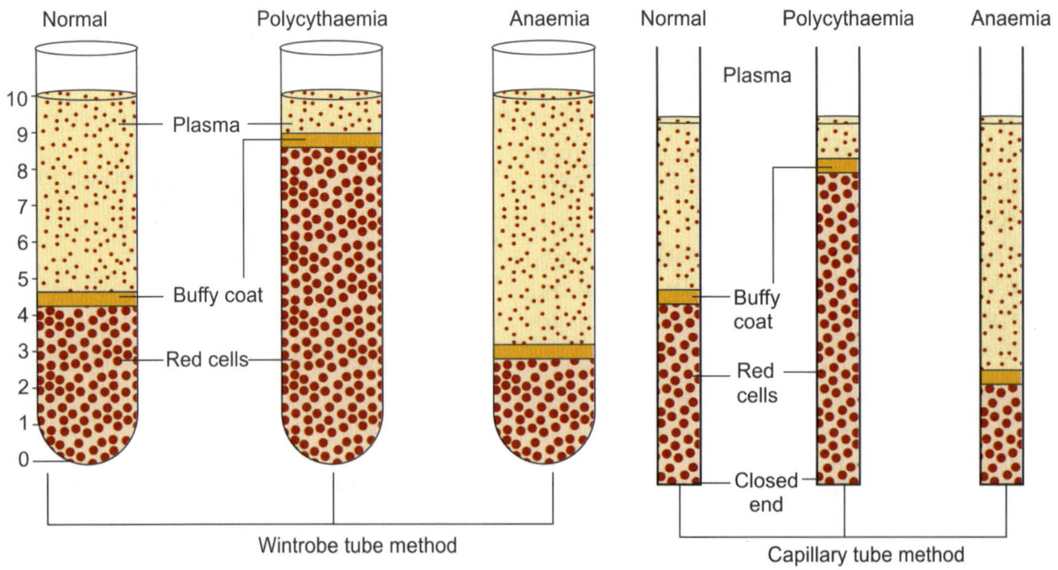

Fig. 5.7: Packed cell volume (PCV) shows comparison of normal, polycythaemia and anaemic blood samples by two different methods (Wintrobe and capillary tube)

VIVA VOCE

Q1. Why ESR is raised in anaemia?

Ans: i. In anaemia there is low erythrocyte mass compared to plasma. This change in the ratio of erythrocyte to plasma favours rouleaux formation and quicker sedimentation.

ii. Microcytes sediment more slowly and macrocytes somewhat more quickly compared to normocytes. The sedimentation of RBCs is directly proportional of RBC aggregates and inversely proportional to the RBC surface area. The microcytes have lower surface area to volume ratio.

Q2. Why ESR is low in sickle cell anaemia and spherocytosis?

Ans: Red cells with abnormal or irregular shape (poikilocytosis) hamper rouleaux formation. In sickle cell anaemia, the RBCs are abnormal in shape (sickle or crescentic in shape). So, ESR becomes low because of slower rouleaux formation.

In spherocytosis, because of the spherical shape (normal biconcave shape) RBCs have more surface area. As ESR is inversely proportional to the RBC surface, this increase in surface area causes decreased ESR.

Q3. How ESR can be used to monitor prognosis of disease?

Ans: ESR can be used to see the response to treatment in some diseases like tuberculosis, rheumatoid arthritis, polymyalgia rheumatica and temporal arteritis. If these diseases respond to treatment, the ESR tends to be lower over time.

In Hodgkin's disease, ESR, of less than 10 mm in first hour indicates good prognosis while ESR of more than 60 mm in first hour indicates poor prognosis.

Q4. Compare Westergren and Wintrobe methods of ESR as far as advantages and disadvantages are concerned.

Ans: Westergren method is more sensitive when ESR is high. Because ESR in this method has three phases with a longer second phase, so sinking of RBCs occurs better in a larger tube add longer second phase gives more accurate result when ESR is high.

But in Wintrobe's tube sinking of RBCs occurs quickly and packing is fast because it has a shorter tube length. So, Wintrobe's method is more sensitive when ESR is low.

Q5. Why Westergren's method is preferred to Wintrobe's method while estimating ESR?

Ans: i. When ESR becomes high Westergren method gives more accurate result.

ii. It is more sensitive because the pipette is longer and there are more markings (graduations).

Q6. What are advantages of Wintrobe's method?

Ans: In this method, ESR is estimated first and then the Wintrobe tube is centrifuged to get PCV. Moreover, the colour of plasma gives clues to certain diseases. Yellow plasma indicates jaundice, red-coloured plasma indicates haemoglobinaemia (intravascular haemolysis) and white in hyperlipidaemia (chyle).

Q7. What is automated ESR method?

Ans: The blood was drawn into special MONOSED vacutainers of Monitor 100® (1.6 ml, 120 mm long, 6 mm diameter) with 1.28 ml of automatic draw containing 0.32 ml of 3.2% sodium citrate. The blood citrate mix reaches up to a maximum length of 60 mm from the bottom of the tube. After proper mixing, the samples were immediately transferred to the analyzer. The ESR reading is taken through a 45 mm high window, 2 mm above the maximum sample level. The Monitor 100® has the advantage of giving the result of 100 samples in 30 minutes (equivalent to 1 hour Westergren reading) and 60 minutes (equivalent to 2 hours Westergren reading). The machine Monitor 100® supplied by Electra Lab, Italy.

Marked discrepancy in the ESR result was noted for high ESR values when compared between manual and automated methods. But it was not seen for normal ESR values. So, a correction factor to be applied when ESR is very high for this automated method.

Q8. What are the length and diameter of Wintrobe's tube? What amount of blood it can hold?

Ans: The tube has length of 110 mm or 11 cm and internal diameter of 3 mm. It is graduated at 1 mm intervals and marked 0 to 100 mm (10 cm) from above downward and also from below upwards.

The tube can hold about 1 ml of blood.

Q9. How PCV is used to determine red cell indices?

Ans: i. Mean corpuscular volume (MCV)

It is the average volume of RBC and is calculated from red cell count and haematocrit volume

MCV = PCV in L/L ÷ RBC count/L (normal value is either 85 ± 8 fl or 77–93 fl)

ii. Mean corpuscular haemoglobin (MCH)

It is the content by weight of haemoglobin of average red cell.

MCH = Hb/L ÷ RBC count/L (normal range is either 29.5 ± 2.5 pg or 27–32 pg)

iii. Mean corpuscular haemoglobin concentration (MCHC)

It is the average of haemoglobin concentration and haematocrit value which is expressed in terms of PCV (0.45 deciliter normally).

MCHC = Hb/dl ÷ PCV in L/L (normal range is either 32.5 ± 2.5 g/dl or 30–35 g/dl).

As MCHC is independent of RBC count and size, it is considered to have greater clinical significance as compared to other red cell indices. It is low in iron deficiency anaemia but usually normal in macrocytic anaemia.

Clinical significance of red cell indices

- In iron deficiency anaemia and thalassaemia, MCV, MCH and MCHC are reduced.
- In anaemia due to acute blood loss and haemolytic anaemias, MCV and MCH are usually within normal limits.
- In megaloblastic anaemia, MCV and MCH are high but MCHC is usually normal. This is because the amount of haemoglobin increases proportionately with the increase in cell size. Hence, MCHC remains normal though MCV and MCH are high.

Q10. What are the values of red cell indices (absolute values) when there is both iron and folate deficiencies?

Ans: Anaemia is macrocytic and hypochromic. So, MCV is high, MCH is low or normal and MCHC is low.

Q11. Why ESR is highly raised in multiple myeloma?

Ans: i. In multiple myeloma, there is increased level of abnormal proteins, known as paraproteins. This abnormal monoclonal antibodies or M proteins can coat red blood cells and interfere with normal electrical charge on the RBC that causes RBC to repel each other. Hence, RBCs stick to one another in linear arrays, a finding referred to as rouleax formation. So, ESR is highly raised.

ii. In multiple myeloma, associated anemia is also present with decreased RBC mass compared to plasma. This change in ratio of RBC to plasma favors stacking of RBC and raised ESR.

Chapter 6

Haemoglobin Estimation

INTRODUCTION

Hemoglobin (American) or haemoglobin (British); abbreviated as Hb or Hgb, is the iron-containing oxygen-transporting **metalloprotein** in the red blood cells of all vertebrate animals as well as the tissue of some invertebrates. It carries oxygen in the blood from respiratory organs (lungs) to other parts of the body or tissues. In the tissues, Hb releases oxygen to permit aerobic respiration which provides energy by metabolic process.

In mammals including humans, the protein component in red blood cell is about 96% by dry weight and approximately 35% when water is included. Hb has an oxygen carrying capacity of 1.34 ml O_2 per gram. The mammalian Hb can bind up to four oxygen molecules. Hb also transports other gases like carbon dioxide (CO_2) in respiratory system, some of which form carbaminohaemoglobin in which CO_2 is bound to globin protein thiol group. It can also bind nitric oxide (NO) to a globin protein thiol group.

Apart from red cells, Hb is also found in the A9 dopaminergic neurons of the substantia nigra, macrophages, alveolar cells and mesangial cells of kidney. In these tissues, haemoglobin does not act as oxygen carrier rather it acts as an anti-oxidant and a regulator of iron-metabolism.

SYNTHESIS OF HAEMOGLOBIN

It is synthesized in a complex series of steps. The heme part is synthesized in mitochondria and in the cytosol of immature RBCs. The globin protein is synthesized by ribosomes in the cytosol of RBC. Production of Hb continues in the cells (RBCs) throughout its early development from the proerythroblast to the reticulocyte in bone marrow. At this stage, the nucleus of mammalian red cells is lost but not in birds and in some other species. Even after losing the nucleus in mammalian RBCs, residual ribosomal RNA allows further synthesis of haemoglobin until the reticulocytes loses its RNA as soon it enters the vasculature. This haemoglobin-synthetic RNA has reticulated appearance and hence it is named **reticulocyte**.

HAEMOGLOBIN DERIVATIVES

Methaemoglobin (Hi)

Methaemoglobin is a derivative of haemoglobin in which the ferrous iron of haemoglobin is oxidized to the ferric state which results in the inability of Hi to combine reversibly with oxygen. The polypeptide chains are not altered.

Up to 1.5% of total haemoglobin may be methaemoglobin in normal person. Increased in the Hi the blood will cause cyanosis and functional anaemia. Cyanosis becomes evident when the methaemoglobin concentration is 1.5 g Hi/dl or 10% of total haemoglobin in blood. Five abnormal haemoglobins have been identified in humans, whose principal consequence is asymptomatic cyanosis as a result of methaemoglobinaemia. These are known as haemoglobin M (HbM) disease.

But most cases of methaemoglobinemia are secondary or acquired mainly due to drugs. These drugs are nitrates, nitrites, quinones, chlorates, sulfonamides, phenacetin, aniline dyes, etc.

Sulfhaemoglobin (SHb)

Sulfhaemoglobin is a mixture of oxidized, partially denatured forms of haemoglobin which is formed during oxidative haemolysis. During oxidation of haemoglobin, sulphur from source is incorporated into the heme rings of haemoglobin. It results in the formation of green-coloured hemochrome, known as sulfhaemoglobin (SHb). Further oxidation of this sulfhaemoglobin will result in the denaturation and precipitation of haemoglobin known as **Heinz bodies**. Unlike methaemoglobin, sulfhaemoglobin cannot be reduced back to haemoglobin (irreversible) and it remains within the cells until they break down.

Sulfhaemoglobin (SHb) has been reported after receiving drugs like sulfonamide, phenacetin, acetanilid, in patients with severe constipation or bacteremia due to *Clostridium perfringens*. Normal person may have <1% sulfhaemoglobin. Sulfhaemoglobinaemia results in cyanosis but is usually asymptomatic.

Carboxyhaemoglobin (HbCO)

Haemoglobin can bind with carbon monoxide (CO) with an affinity 210 times greater than that for oxygen. Carbon monoxide can bind with Hb even its concentration in the air is very low (0.02–0.04%). In this situation, HbCO or carboxyhaemoglobin will be formed.

Endogenous CO is produced during degradation of heme to bilirubin, usually accounts for 0.5% of carboxyhaemoglobin.

Carboxyhaemoglobin cannot bind to and carry oxygen. Also increased concentration of HbCO, shifts the Hb–oxygen dissociation curve towards left resulting in tissue anoxia.

Increased carboxyhaemoglobin is fomed due to acute carbon monoxide posisoning. The chief sources of CO are illuminating gas, gasoline motors, gas heaters and tobacco smoking. Chronic exposure through tobacco/cigarette smoking may lead to chronic increase of HbCO and left shift of oxygen dissociation curve. Hence, smokers tend to have higher haematocrit/PCV (increased red cell mass) and may have polycythaemia too.

NORMAL HAEMOGLOBIN TYPES IN HUMAN

Human haemoglobin is formed of two pairs of globin chains to each of which is attached one molecule of haem (Fig. 6.1). There are six different types of globin chains, designated by the Greek letters α, β, γ, δ, ε, and ζ. The composition of a haemoglobin is specified by a formula such as $\alpha_2 \beta_2$ (adult haemoglobin) which indicates a tetramer containing two α chains (one pair) and two β chains (one pair). The α chain is directed by two α genes, α_1 and α_2 which are present on chromosome 11. The γ chain is directed by two genes like α chains, these are $^{G}\gamma$ and $^{A}\gamma$, which are also present on chromosome 11.

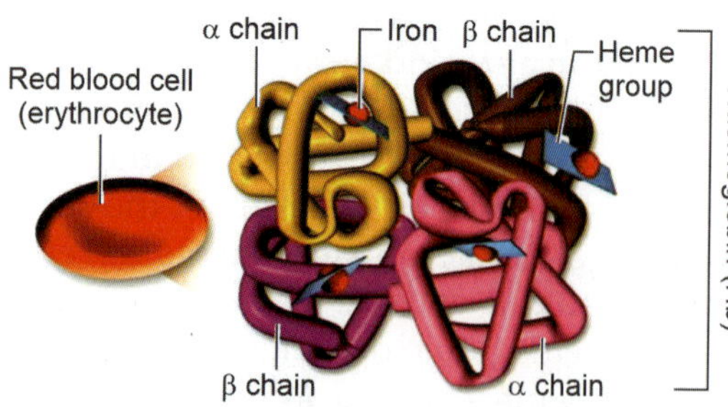

Fig. 6.1: Structure of haemoglobin

In the first three months of embryonic development, when blood cells are produced in the yolk sac, embryonic haemoglobins such as Hb Gower 1 ($\zeta_2 \varepsilon_2$), Hb Gower 2 ($\alpha_2 \varepsilon_2$) and Hb Portland ($\zeta_2 \gamma_2$) are produced. As erythropoiesis shifts to the liver and spleen, the foetal haemogloblin, (HbF) ($\alpha_2 \gamma_2$) appears. When erythropoiesis shifts to the bone marrow during the first year of life, the adult haemoglobins (HbA) ($\alpha_2 \beta_2$) and HbA_2 ($\alpha_2 \delta_2$) begin to be produced.

In the embryo

- Gower 1 ($\zeta_2 \varepsilon_2$)
- Gower 2 ($\alpha_2 \varepsilon_2$)
- Haemoglobin Portland 1 ($\zeta_2 \gamma_2$)
- Haemoglobin Portland 2 ($\zeta_2 \beta_2$)

In the foetus

Haemoglobin F ($\alpha_2 \gamma_2$)

After birth

- **Haemoglobin A ($\alpha_2 \beta_2$),** the most common Hb (95%)
- **Haemoglobin A_2 ($\alpha_2 \delta_2$)**: δ chain synthesis begins late in the third trimester and in adults, it has normal range of 1–3.5%.
- **Haemoglobin F ($\alpha_2 \gamma_2$):** It is present in large amount at birth (65–95%) but in adults, it is trace in amount (<1%).

Hb Variants in Different Diseases

- **Haemoglobin H (β_4):** A variant form of haemoglobin, formed by tetramer of β chains, which may be present in variants of a thalassaemia.
- **Haemoglobin Bart (γ_4):** A variant of haemoglobin, formed by tetramer of γ chains, which may be present in α-thalassaemia.
- **Haemoglobin S ($\alpha_2 \beta_2^S$):** Hb found in sickle cell disease, here glutamine is replaced by valine in β_6 position.
- **Haemoglobin C ($\alpha_2 \beta_2^C$):** Here, there is substitution of glutamic acid by lysine molecule in β_6 position.
- **Haemoglobin SC disease:** A compound heterozygous form with one sickle gene and another encoding haemoglobin C.
- **Haemoglobin AS disease:** A heterozygous form causing sickle cell trait with one adult gene and one sicke cell disease gene.
- **Haemoglobin D-Punjab ($\alpha_2 \beta_2^D$)**: The disease produces mild anaemia.
- **Haemoglobin E ($\alpha_2 \beta_2^E$)**: Another variant due to a variation in the β chain gene. This variant causes a mild chronic haemolytic anaemia.
- **β-Thalassaemia major:** Moderate to high increase of HbF and normal to slight increase of HbA_2.
- **β-Thalassaemia minor:** Moderate to high rise of HbA_2, normal or slight increase in HbF.
- **Hb Bart-hydrops foetalis (α-thalassaemia):** Haemoglobin Bart (γ_4) is 80–90%, some HbH and Hb Portland. Usually HbA, HbA_2 or HbF absent.

DIFFERENT METHODS OF HAEMOGLOBIN ESTIMATION

1. Photocolorimetric method: Cyanomethaemoglobin method or Drabkin's method
2. Acid haematin method or Sahli method
3. Alkaline-haematin method
4. Oxyhaemoglobin (HbO_2) method
5. Tallqvist method
6. Copper sulphate method
7. Lovibond comparator method
8. HemoCue method
9. Chemical (iron content) method
10. Van Slyke's oxygen capacity method or gasometric method
11. Automated analyzer method
12. Spectroscopic method
13. Haemoglobin colour scale method
14. Haldane method.

Of these methods, cyanomethaemoglobin (HiCN) method or Drabkin's method is most widely used and reliable method. Acid haematin method or Sahli's method used in the past mainly in the small laboratories, now become obsolete as it is less accurate. With the invent of automated analyzer, other

Table 6.1: Different methods of haemoglobin estimation and principle of the method

Method	Principle of the method
1. Colorimetric method **A. *Visual colorimetric method*** i. Sahli's method or acid haematin method ii. Alkaline haematin method **B. *Photocolorimetric or photoelectric method*** i. Cyanomethaemoglobin (HiCN) method ii. Automated analyzer iii. Haldane method iv. Oxyhaemoglobin method v. HemoCue method	These methods are based on measuring the colour of haemoglobin of the test compared to standard. This is done either by **naked eye (visually) or by photocolorimetry**. The optical density of a coloured solution is directly proportional to the concentration of the coloured material in the solution
2. Physical method	Specific gravity
3. Gasometric method	Oxygen combining capacity of haemoglobin
4. Chemical method	Iron content of the haemoglobin

methods are being replaced in modern laboratories as it is accurate, reliable and fast (Table 6.1).

Acid Haematin or Sahli's Method (Fig. 6.2)

This method of Hb estimation is not very accurate because different forms of haemoglobins are not converted to acid haematin, and the brown colour which develops is unstable and begins to fade almost immediately after it has its peak. Also, there is subjective biasness of colour matching. It is done in some rural areas where colorimeter is not available.

Principle

Haemoglobin is converted into acid haematin by adding N/10 hydrochloric acid. The acid haematin solution is further diluted with the acid until its colour (brown) matches exactly that of the permanent standard (brown glass reference block) of the comparator block.

But the acid haematin formed in this method is a colloidal suspension and it can not be read in colorimeter which requires optically clear solution.

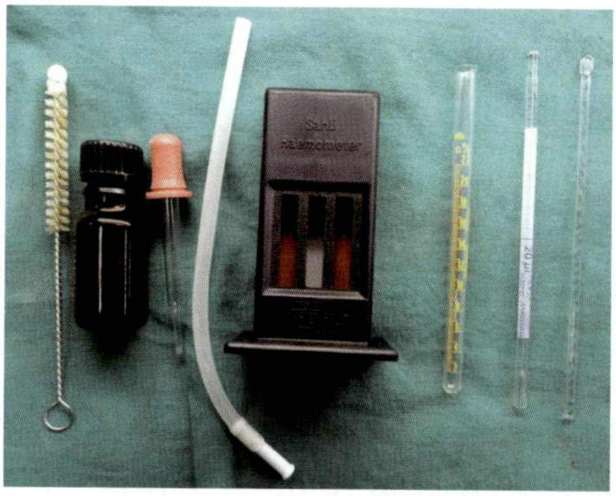

Fig. 6.2: Reagents and equipment for Sahli's method

Reagents and Equipment

1. Hydrochloric acid solution (N/10 or 0.1 N)
2. **Haemoglobinometer pipette or Sahli's pipette:** This is a slender special pipette with a single mark of 0.02 ml or 20 cu mm.
3. **Haemoglobinometer tube (calibrated tube):** This tube has markings on ascending order on both sides. On one side it shows grams per 100 ml (left side) and other side it shows percentage (right side). Presently used Hellige's tubes are square shaped, it has 14.5 g as 100%.
4. **Sahli's haemoglobinometer or comparator box:** It is used to match the colour

of acid haematin formed in the haemoglobinometer tube with that of colour standard in the comparator box.

5. **Glass rod (stirrer):** For mixing the blood in the square/round tube.
6. **Distilled water**

Procedure

The graduated haemoglobinometer tube is filled to the lowest mark, i.e. till 20 mark with N/10 HCl (0.1 N). Now, with the help of haemoglobinometer piptte or Sahli's pipette draw 20 cu mm of blood. This blood can be EDTA or double oxalate mixed or it can be from finger prick (capillary blood). This blood is immediately mixed with the N/10 HCl present in the haemoglobinometer tube. Mix them well by shaking the tube well. The tube is then allowed to stand with in the comparator box and keep it for 10–30 minutes (at least 10 minutes) for full conversion of the haemoglobin into acid haematin (development of brown colour).

Distilled water is then added drop by drop and stirred with a stirrer (glass rod) till the colour matches well with the fixed colour (reference) in the comparator box. The matching or comparison should be done only in natural day light.

Reading: The mark matching with the upper level of diluted acid haematin indicates the level of haemoglobin and is expressed in terms of g/dl.

Note

- After 10 minutes, 95% colour develops (conversion of haemoglobin to acid haematin) and after 20 minutes 98% colour develops.
- This method does not estimate caboxyhaemoglobin, methaemoglobin, foetal haemoglobin and sulfhaemoglobin.
- Non-haemoglobin substances like protein, lipid or cell stroma may affect the colour of blood diluted with N/10 HCl. They may interfere with the converted acid haematin and hence the result.

Advantage of the Method

It is easy, simple and cheap method.

Disadvantages of the Method

i. It is not an accurate method.
ii. It cannot measures all type of haemoglobins like caboxyhaemoglobin, methaemoglobin, foetal haemoglobin and sulfhaemoglobin as it cannot convert these haemoglobins into acid haematin.
iii. As it is a visual method chances of error is high because of subjective variation.

Sources of Errors

i. Improper collection of blood (venipuncture technique, finger prick).
ii. Improper mixing of blood with anticoagulant (EDTA).
iii. Delay in taking results. The brown colour of acid haematin is unstable and the colour fades away with time.

Cyanomethaemoglobin Method (by Colorimetric or Spectrophotometric Method)

As already described, this is the most widely used method of haemoglobin estimation in the world. Also, as a best quality control this method is internationally recommended.

Principle

Blood is mixed with potassium cyanide and potassium ferricyanide mixture. Potassium ferricyanide oxidises haemoglobin to methaemoglobin (Hi). Then potassium cyanide provides cyanide ions (CN^-) to it, and it is converted to cyanomethaemoglobin (HiCN). This cyanomethaemoglobin has a broad absorption, maximum at a wavelength of 540 nm. The absorption of the solution is measured in a photoelectric colorimeter or spectrophotometer using 540 nm wavelength or yellow-green filter with that of a standard HiCN solution.

Remember, in this **method haemoglobin, methaemoglobin and carboxyhaemoglobin can be measured but not the sulfhaemoglobin**

(sulfhaemoglobin can be measured by spectroscopic method or photoelectric method at 620 nm wavelength and alkaline haematin method).

Original Drabkin's solution

- Potassium cyanide (KCN): 50 mg
- Potassium ferricyanide [$K_3Fe\ (CN)_6$]: 200 mg
- Sodium bicarbonate ($NaHCO_3$): 1 g
- Distilled water: 1000 ml.

Modified Drabkin's solution (as recommended by International Committee for Standardization in Haematology or ICSH)

- Potassium cyanide: 50 mg
- Potassium ferricyanide: 200 mg
- Potassium dihydrogen phosphate: 140 mg
- Non-ionic detergent: 1 ml (like Nonidet P40 from Sigma, Triton X-100 or Saponic 218)
- Distilled water: 1000 ml.

The original Drabkin's solution had a pH of 8.6. But the modified Drabkin's solution has a pH of 9.6. This modified solution is less likely to cause turbidity from precipitation of plasma proteins. Also it takes shorter conversion time (3–5 minutes) compared to original Drabkin's solution (15–25 minutes).

Reference solution: It can form to the international specifications and is available commercially. It contains 550–850 mg of haemoglobin/litre and it is dispensed in 10 ml sealed ampoules.

Procedure

20 cu mm (20 µl) of blood is collected (EDTA or oxalate mixed venous blood or capillary blood after finger prick) with the help of haemoglobinometer pipette. This blood is then mixed with 4 ml of Drabkin's solution in a test tube. Invert the test tubes several times for proper mixing. So, dilution of blood is 201 times (dilution factor is 201).

Allow the mixture to stand at room temperature for 15–25 minutes (minimum 15 minutes) for complete development of cyanomethaemoglobin (HiCN). Test solution is compared with the standard and reagent blank in a colorimeter or spectrophotometer.

Calculation

Hb concentration of the test

= optical density of test solution/optical density of standard solution × **concentration standard (mg/100 ml) × dilution factor/1000.**

> **Note**
>
> If 20 cu mm (0.02 ml) of blood is mixed with 4 ml of Drabkin's solution, then dilution factor is 200, whereas if 20 cu mm (0.02 ml) of blood is mixed with 5 ml of Drabkin's solution, then dilution factor is 250.

Advantages

1. The test result is accurate, so, ICSH recommends it.
2. It measures different forms of haemoglobin (except sulfhaemoglobin).
3. The standard solution is commercially available as per international specification (International Committee for Standardization in Hematology or ICSH). So, the test can be easily standardized.
4. Cyanomethaemoglobin reagent (also called Drabkin's solution) is very stable.

Disadvantages

1. The use potassium cyanide (KiCN) in the preparation of Drabkin's solution is a potential health hazard. However, Drabkin's solution contains only 50 mg of KCN/litre, so it is relatively safe. To produce serious health problem/poisoning, someone has to swallow 600–1000 mg of it (12–20 liters of solution).
2. It takes longer time (15–25 minutes) for complete conversion of cyanomethaemoglobin (HiCN). Modified Drabkin's solution takes shorter time (3–5 minutes).
3. If the blood contains carboxyhaemoglobin (HbCO), this rate of conversion is more slower.

Note

- To avoid cyanide (KiCN), lauryl sulphate has been proposed as it has similar properties to HiCN.
- Dilution factor is 200 if 20 μl blood is mixed with 4 ml of Drabkin's solution (i.e. 1:200). But when 20 μl blood is mixed with 5 ml of Drabkin's solution (i.e. 1:250), then dilution factor is 250.

Other Methods of Hb Estimation

1. **Oxyhaemoglobin method:** This is the quickest and simplest method for use with a photoelectric colorimeter. The haemoglobin is converted to oxyhaemoglobin (HbO_2) with the help of liquor ammonia (ammonium hydroxide) solution and is read in 540 nm wavelength or with yellow-green filter. The reliability of this method is not affected by a moderate rise in plasma bilirubin. But the result is not satisfactory in presence of carboxyhaemoglobin, methaemoglobin or sulfhaemoglobin.
2. **Alkaline haematin method:** There are two methods which follows alkaline haematin method: (a) The standard method using Gibson and Harrison's standard, (b) the acid alkali method.

   It is a useful ancillary method under special circumstances as it gives a true estimate of total haemoglobin even if methaemoglobin, carboxyhaemoglobin or sulfhaemoglobin is present. Plasma proteins and lipids have a little effects on the development of colour. Fetal haemoglobin (HbF) and Bart haemoglobin (g_4) cannot be estimated by this method as they are resistant to alkali denaturation normally. But this problem can be overcomed by heating the solution containing HbF or γ_4 in a boiling water for 4–5 minutes.
3. **Spectroscopic method:** For qualitative and quantitative estimation of methaemoglobin and sulfhaemoglobin; spectroscopic examination of blood is very reliable.
4. **Chemical (iron content) method:** Normally iron content of haemoglobin is 0.347%. Hb estimation of blood can be done by estimating total blood iron and dividing it by 3.47. This method is no longer in use.
5. **van Slyke's oxygen capacity method or gasometric method** (Fig. 6.3)**:** It is an indirect method which estimates the amount of haemoglobin from the amount of oxygen it absorbs with the use of van Slyke's apparatus. This method is very complicated.

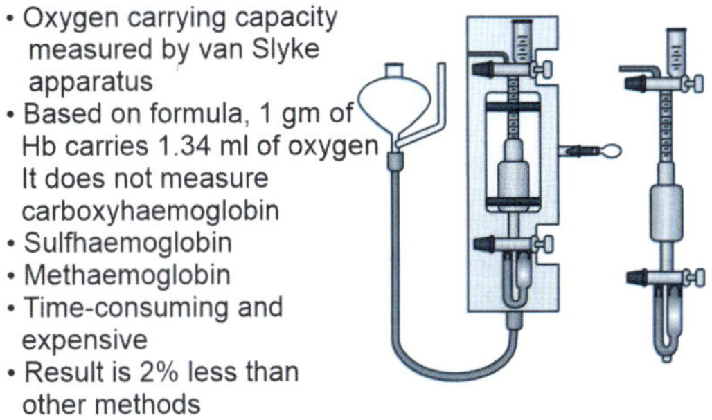

Fig. 6.3: Gasometric method

6. **Specific gravity method:** Normal specific gravity of human average in men is 1.057 and in women is 1.053. By calculating specific gravity of an unknown sample, its haemoglobin content is estimated. This method is very rapid and uncomplicated. It is used to screen the potential blood donors for anaemia.
7. **WHO haemoglobin colour scale method:** The haemoglobin colour scale (HCS) is a simple, rapid and cheap method for Hb estimation with a finger prick sample. It has been developed for use in resource—poor settings when there is no laboratory. The method relies on comparing the colour of a drop of blood sample absorbed onto a filter paper with standard colour on a laminated card, varying from pink to dark red. These colours correspond to haemoglobin levels of 4, 6, 8, 10, 12, and 14 g/dl. Intermediate shades can be identified, allowing haemoglobin levels to be judged to 1 g/dl. This test is used for mass screening of anaemia and has been adopted by World Health Organization (WHO).

8. **HemoCue method:** In this method, the reaction in the microcuvette is a modified azide methaemoglobin reaction. The microcuvette contains three reagents in dried forms (sodium deoxycholate, sodium nitrite, sodium azide) which convert Hb into azide methaemoglobin (HiCN). Single purpose derived photometer (colorimeter) uses double wavelength filters (570 nm and 880 nm) and measures Hb.

It is WHO approved method for Hb estimation among blood donors.

Normal/Reference Range of Haemoglobin

- Adult males: 13–17 g/dl
- Adult females (nonpregnant): 12.0–15.0 g/dl
- Adult females (pregnant): 11.0–14.0 g/dl
- Child: 6 months–12 years: 11.5–15. 5 g/dl
- Chidren: 6 months–6 years: 11.0–14.0 g/dl
- Infants: 2–6 months: 9.5–14.0 g/dl
- Newborns: 13.6–19.6 g/dl

Decreased in Hb concentration: Hb is decreased in all anaemias, in most causes as a consequence of another disease or a deficiency (folate, vit B_{12}, iron).

Increased in Hb concentration

- Hb is increased as a physiologic response to high altitude due to low oxygen tension or in advanced lung or cardiac disease.
- Certain myeloproliferative neoplasms, especially polycythaemia vera (when Hb in men is >16.5 g/dl and in women is 16 g/dl or haematocrit >49% in men and >48% in women).

Limitations of Accurate Hb Estimation

(Table 6.2)

- Errors arise from improper venipuncture or finger prick that may induce haemoconcentration.
- During sample preparation in manual methods, dilution mistakes may occur, or there may be sample turbidity due to improperly lysed RBCs during processing by automated counters which affect the accuracy of the results.
- Hyperlipidaemia, dehydration, marked leukocytosis or high plasma protein result in erroneous result.

Table 6.2: Advantages and disadvantages of different methods of haemoglobin estimation

Name of the method	Advantages	Disadvantages
1. Sahli method	• Simple • Cheap	• Inaccurate results • Inter-observer variability • Colour developed (acid haematin) is unstable • No International Standard
2. Cyanomethaemoglobin method	• Stable compound (HiCN) gives accurate measurement • International Standard available	• Turbidity due to other factors may cause inaccurate results • Time consuming • Reagent cyanide is toxic
3. Tallqvist method	• Simple and rapid • Inexpensive and portable • Reagents and electricity not required	• Results affected by size, thickness of blood spot, temperature, lighting and humidity • Only supplied filter paper can be be used which is limited quantity
4. Copper sulphate method	• Inexpensive • Simple and rapid • Electricity not required	• Inaccurate • Requires fresh solutions • Only ranges of Hb levels are obtained not exact figure • Proper disposal of standard solutions

Contd.

Table 6.2: Advantages and disadvantages of different methods of haemoglobin estimation (Contd.)

Name of the method	Advantages	Disadvantages
5. Haemoglobin colour scale method adapted by WHO	• Simple and portable • Cheap • Electricity not required	• Inter-observer biasness
6. Lovibond comparator method	• Rapid and simple • Useful for routine screening • Electricity not required	• Expensive • Requires precise dilution • Requires large drop of blood • Subjective interpretation
7. HemoCue	• Simple and portable • Rapid and immediate result • Accurate and reliable • Easy to perform • Battery operated	• Expensive as it uses disposable cuvettes
8. Automated analyzer	• Accurate • Reliable	• Expensive • Small laboratories or rural setups cannot afford

Haemoglobin Colour Scale (HCS) Method (Fig. 6.4)

The haemoglobin colour scale is a simple, rapid and cheap method for Hb estimation with a finger prick sample. It has been developed for use in resource-poor settings when there is no laboratory. The method relies on comparing the colour of a drop of blood sample, absorbed onto a filter paper with standard colours on a laminated card, varying from pink to dark red. These colours correspond to haemoglobin levels of 4, 6, 8, 10, 12 and 14 g/dl. Intermediate shades can be identified, allowing haemoglobin levels to be judged to 1 g/dl. This test has been adopted by World Health Organization (WHO).

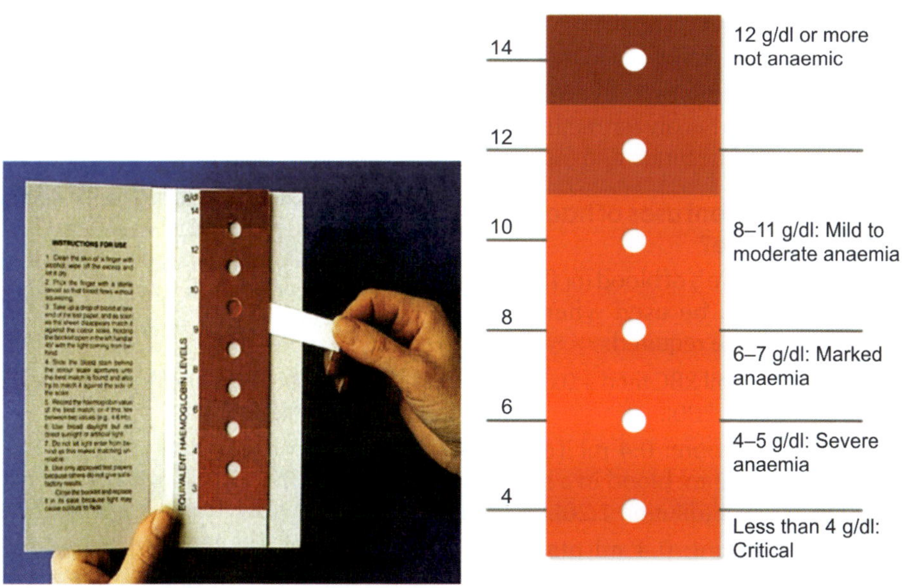

Fig. 6.4: Haemoglobin colour scale (HCS)

VIVA VOCE

Q1. Which is better and practical method for haemoglobin estimation and why?

Ans: In laboratories, where there is no auto-analyzer, cyanomethaemoglobin estimation is most widely used method for haemoglobin estimation. Because it has several advantages over other methods:

i. Cyanomethaemoglobin is a stable compound and colour does not fade easily. But in other methods like Sahli's (acid haematin) method, colour begins to fade after ten minutes. So, in acid haematin method, lower haemoglobin level will be obtained if reading is delayed.

ii. Almost all haemoglobin except sulfhaemoglobin is converted to cyanomethaemoglobin. So, this method can calculate almost all haemoglobins.

iii. This is a colorimetric method, so personal error like matching colour as in Sahli's method is absent.

iv. A stable reference standard is available.

v. The test result is accurate, hence, ICSH (International Committee for Standardization in Haematology) recommends it.

However, automated analyzer method is best as it is reliable, accurate and fastest.

Q2. What are the different uses of haemoglobin (Hb) pipette?

Ans: It uses 0.02 ml (20 mm^3) of blood (or fluid). So, Hb pipette can be used wherever different dilutions are required:

i. For RBC count: 4 ml RBC fluid + 0.02 ml blood (dilution 1:200).

ii. For total WBC count: 0.4 ml Türk's/WBC fluid + 0.02 ml blood in a small test tube to mix it (dilution 1:20).

iii. For platelet count: 0.4 ml platelet count fluid + 0.02 ml blood (dilution 1:20).

iv. For eosinophil count: 0.2 ml of Dunger's fluid + 0.02 ml blood (dilutions 1:20).

v. It can be used for body fluid cell count, sperm count, etc. also.

Q3. Why is N/10 HCl used in Sahli's method, not N/5 or N/15 HCl?

Ans: The Sahli's method (acid haematin method) has been standardized by using N/10 HCl. Brown colour of the comparator glass is equivalent to the colour of acid haematin produced by using N/10 HCl in a standard blood sample which contains 14.8 g% Hb. Test sample is compared against this standard sample.

Q4. In automated cell counter, what chemical regent is used to detect Hb?

Ans: Sodium lauryl sulphate (SLS) is used which converts all Hb into detectable chromogen rapidly.

Q5. What are the physiological variations of Hb concentration?

Ans:

i. Splenic contractions may occur after strenuous exercise which pumps more blood in the circulation as spleen is a reservoir of blood. So, hemoconcentration and falsely raised Hb occurs. Even anticipation of venipuncture (blood) collection may cause splenic contraction as observed by Brown A et al.

ii. Hb raises as increase with altitude.

iii. Hb value highest in the morning and lowest in the evening.

Q6. What are the conditions where Hb is falsely raised?

Ans:

i. When blood is drawn for Hb estimation during intravenous blood transfusion or iron containing drugs.

ii. After burns, acute diarrhoea, severe dehydration due to hemoconcentration.

Q7. In which diseases, Hb level is raised?

Ans:
- Polycythaemia vera
- COPD (chronic obstructive pulmonary disease)
- Emphysema.
- Renal cell carcinoma due to ectopic productions of erythropoietin
- Congenital heart disease in adults
- Smoking for long duration may cause smoker's polycythaemia due to formation of carboxyhaemoglobin.

Q8. What are the conditions where Hb is falsely decreased or spurious/pseudo-anaemia?

Ans:
i. In 3rd trimester of pregnancy, due to increase in plasma volume, Hb concentration falls (1–2 g/dl).
ii. Splenomegaly due to pooling of red cells in spleen.
iii. Congestive heart failure due to fluid retention.
iv. Multiple myeloma/paraproteinaemia.
v. During hypervolaemia (intravenous fluid infusion), Hb level falls.

Q9. Why should the stirrer not taken out of haemoglobin meter tube?

Ans: If stirrer is taken out of tube immediately small amount of acid haematin (formed during reaction) sticking to the stirrer (glass rod) is lost which will give lower Hb result. So, the stirrer should be lifted from the solution in the upper part of the tube when reading is taken.

Q10. In Sahli's method, why are flat comparator glasses and square tube are preferred?

Ans: It is easier to compare flat surface rather curvature or round surfaces. So, square tube containing acid haematin can be easily compared with flat brown surface of comparator box. Error due to curvature can be avoided.

Q11. What is mild, moderate and severe anaemia?

Ans: When Hb value is in between lower limit of normal range to 10.0 g/dl, it is called mild anaemia. When Hb value is 7.0 to 10.0 g/dl, it is called moderate anaemia and when Hb value is <7.0 g/dl, then it is called severe anaemia.

Q12. Which conditions affect Hb estimation /value?

Ans: Hb level is decreased in:

- Anaemia, recumbent position (5–10%), excess squeezing during finger puncture, presence of clots in the sample, inadequate mixing of blood with anticoagulant and "spurious anaemia.
- Causes of "spurious" or "pseudo" anaemia are fluid retention in congestive heart failure (CCF), rise in plasma proteins in paraproteinemias, increased plasma volume in 3rd trimester of pregnancy and pooling of RCBs in splenomegaly.

Hb level is increased in:

- Following strenuous exercise in dehydration (hemoconcentration), at high altitudes, in polycythaemia and prolonged application of tourniquet during venipuncture.

Q13. How Hb is estimated in automated analyzer/cell counter?

Ans:
- First, RBCs are lysed by the lysate and the color is matched against the inbuilt standard color and the Hb value is obtained.
- Then Hb estimation is performed directly by a modification of cyanmethaemoglobin method. Most of the analyzers use a cyanide free biodegradable reagent.
- Hb estimation is accurate, provided these analyzers are frequently standardized. But the standards are expensive.

Chapter

7

Bleeding Time (BT), Clotting Time (CT), Prothrombin Time (PT) and APTT

BLEEDING TIME

Definition: The time required for complete stoppage of free flow blood from a deep puncture wound on the skin is known as bleeding time.

Principle: A standard incision is made on the skin and the total time the incision bleeds (starting of bleeding to end of bleeding) is measured. Cessation of bleeding indicates the formation of hemostatic plugs which are dependent on an adequate number of platelets and on the ability of the platelets to adhere to the subendothelium and to form aggregates.

Standardized Template Method for BT

Materials

- Sphygmomanometer
- Cleansing swabs
- Template bleeding time device (commercially available)
- Filter paper (1 mm thick)
- Stopwatch

Method: Place a sphygmomanometer cuff around the patient's arm above the elbow. Inflate the cuff to 40 mm Hg pressure and keep this pressure throughout the entire test. Clean the ventral (volar) aspect of the forearm with 70% ethanol. Choose an area of forearm skin (cleaned) that is devoid of visible superficial veins. Press a sterile metal template with a linear slit 7–8 mm long firmly against the skin aligned along the long axis of the arm and use a scalpel blade with a guard (the tip of the blade should protrudes 1 mm through the template slit). Then make an incision 6 mm long and 1 mm deep.

Modifications of the template and blade which make two simultaneous cuts with a spring mechanism are also available commercially.

Now, blot off the blood exuding from the cut with filter paper at 15 seconds interval. Do not contact the wound during this procedure. When bleeding has ceased, carefully oppose the edges of the incision and apply an adhesive strip to lessen the rise of keloid formation and an ugly scar.

Normal range: 2.5–9.5 minutes.

Ivy's Method for BT

This test is almost similar to the previous standardized template method. But instead of a standardized incision, two punctures, 5–10 cm apart are made in quick succession using a disposable (or No. 11 surgical blade). The punctures should have cutting depth of 2.5 mm and width of just 1 mm is suitable. When the bleeding has ceased, a sterile adhesive strip is placed on the wounds.

Normal range: 2–7 minutes.

Duke Method for BT

The ear lobule (or heel of an infant) is cleaned with 70% alcohol and allowed to dry. A 3 mm deep stab wound is made with the help of disposable lancet in the margin of ear lobe (or heel). Stopwatch is started when the wound starts to bleed. The flowing blood is soaked by a filter paper lightly and gently at 15 seconds interval. When the wound stops to bleed, the stopwatch is pressed to stop. The time is noted as bleeding time.

Normal range: 2–5 minutes

Interpretation of the Test (BT)

- Bleeding time 1–9 minutes: Normal
- Bleeding time 9–15 minutes: Platelet dysfunction
- Bleeding time >15 minutes: Critical, test must be discontinued and pressure should be applied to the wound to stop bleeding.
- Bleeding time may be prolonged due to low platelet count or thrombocytopenia (<100,000/mm^3). When platelet counts are low, expected bleeding time can be predicted with the following formula:

$$\text{Bleeding time (BT)} = \frac{30.5 \times \text{platelet count/mm}^3}{3850}$$

  A bleeding time longer than that expected calculated time from number of platelet alone (using above formula), may be due to defective platelet function in addition to platelet number.
- The Ivy's method and standardized template method are better to evaluate bleeding time.

Causes of Prolonged Bleeding Time

1. **Thrombocytopenia (platelet count <100,000/mm^3):** It may be primary (essential) or secondary. When the platelet count is <50,000/mm^3, patient may have very long bleeding time and the bleeding may be difficult to arrest. So, bleeding time is contraindicated in this situation.
2. **Defective or qualitative abnormality of platelets:** They may be congenital such as thrombasthenia, storage pool defects or acquired; due to drugs, the presence of paraprotein (multiple myeloma) or platelet abnormalities as in myelodysplastic syndromes (MDS).
3. **von Willebrand's disease:** There is defective platelet adherence to the subendothelium as there is absence/defective von Willebrand factor.
4. **Vascular abnormalities:** As found in Ehlers-Danlos syndrome, or in pseudoxanthoma elasticum.
5. **Deficiency of clotting factors:** Occasionally sever deficiency or factor V or XI or afibrinogenaemia may cause prolonged bleeding time.
6. **Others:** Severe liver disease, leukaemia, DIC, aplastic anaemia.

Interfering Factors

- The normal range may vary if the puncture wound is not of standard depth and width.
- Ingestion of certain drug before the test will cause prolonged BT. Examples: Aspirin, dextran, streptokinase, mithramycin.
- Heavy alcohol consumption may cause prolonged BT.
- Touching the incision, during the test will break of haemostatic plugs or fibrin strands that will lead to prolonged BT.

CLOTTING TIME OR COAGULATION TIME

Definition: Coagulation time is the time required for a whole blood sample to coagulate *in vitro* under standard conditions.

Principle of the test: Coagulation or clotting time (CT) measures all three stages of coagulation (intrinsic pathway, extrinsic pathway and common pathway) (Fig. 7.1) as a whole but it is more sensitive to intrinsic pathway defects. Utmost care should be taken so that thromboplastin (tissue factor) does not enter into the blood sample as a

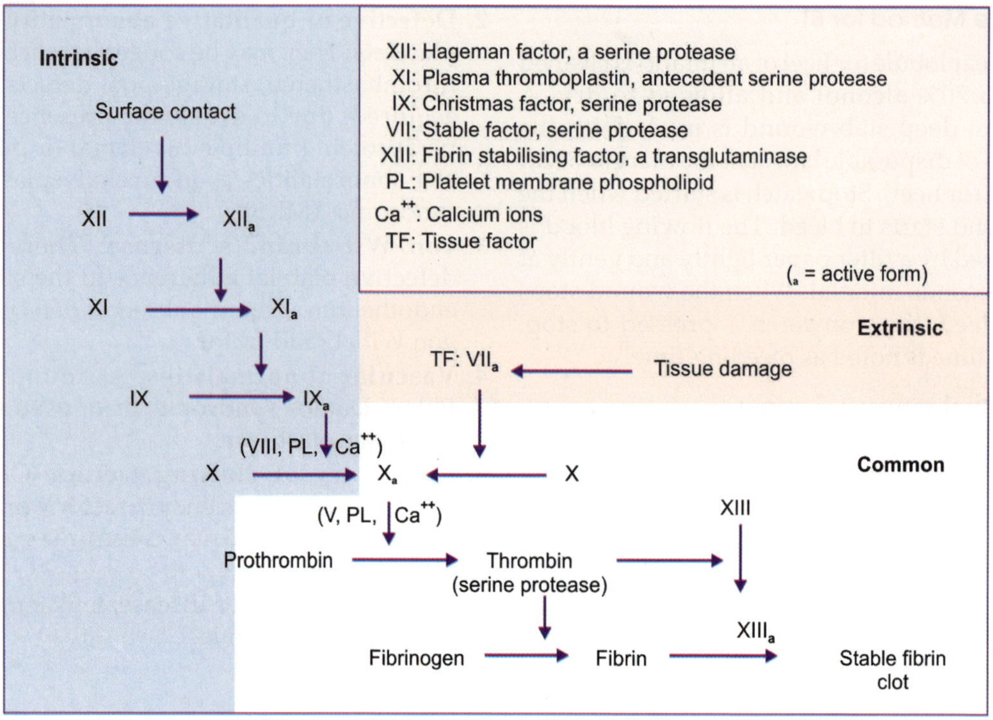

Fig. 7.1: The three pathways that makeup the classical blood coagulation pathway

very small amount will cause shortened CT. It is usually not affected by mild to moderate deficiency of platelets, because for normal coagulation (clotting) only very small number of platelets are required.

Two methods are done for CT

1. Lee and White method
2. Capillary tube method of Wright

Lee and White Method (Fig. 7.2)

Requirements

- Stopwatch
- Equipment for collection of blood
- Clean, dry glass test tubes (10 × 75 mm), three in number
- Water bath (37°C), preferable

Methods

- Make a clear venipuncture with as little trauma to the connective tissue between skin and vein as possible.
- Draw 3–5 ml of blood by a disposable plastic syringe or siliconized dry glass syringe.
- After detaching the needle, deliver 1 ml of blood in each of the three test tubes (10 × 75 mm).
- Place all the 3 test tubes containing blood in a stand so that they remain upright and undisturbed at room temperature. If water bath is available, then place the tubes at 37°C.
- Check the coagulation by tilting the test tubes or by gentle tipping. The first test tube is gently tilted every minute while other test tubes are examined every 30 seconds. When the blood samples are clotted (test tubes can be inverted without blood running down the edge of the tubes).
- The average of the clotting time in three test tubes gives the result.

Normal range: 5–11 minutes at 37°C

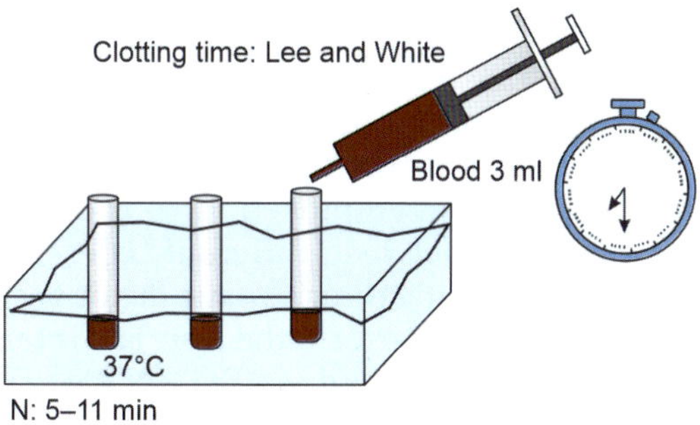

Fig. 7.2: Lee and White method of clotting time

✍ **Note**

i. Rise of temperature will speed up the coagulation process, so the test should be done at a particular temperature.
ii. If the test is done at room temperature (without water bath) then the time will vary with regard to temperature and time of tipping. If someone waits for 10 minutes before starting to tip, then normal CT value may go as high as 20–25 minutes. Whereas if someone waits for 5 minutes before starting to tip, range will be 8–18 minutes.
iii. Vigorous agitation of the test tubes will significantly shorten coagulation time (CT). So, one should tip the tubes very gently to see if the blood has clotted (no movement of blood).

Capillary Tube Methods of Wright

Blood is collected from a clean finger prick (aseptic precautions) in 4–5 fine capillary tubes. The tubes are sealed at both ends by flame (alternatively by chemical plasticine) and the capillary tubes are kept in a water bath at 37°C.

After one minute, one end of the tube is broken gently and the breakage of tube is repeated every 30 seconds until a thin line of unbroken coagulum is stretched between the two broken ends.

Normal range: 6–10 minutes (if test is done in room temperature the CT will be longer; not recommended).

Prolonged Coagulation Time

1. **Haemophilia A** (deficiency of factor VIII. and **haemophilia B** or Christmas disease (deficiency of factor IX).
2. **Anticoagulant therapy** (hyperheparinemia or warfarin therapy).
3. **Hypoprothrombinaemia:** Seen in cirrhosis of liver, obstructive jaundice, vit K deficiency, malignancy of liver.
4. **Fibrinogen deficiency:** When fibrinogen level falls below 50 mg/dl in blood.
5. **von Willebrand's disease**:

PROTHROMBIN TIME (PT)

Definition: Prothrombin time is the time required for clotting of citrated plasma (platelet poor) in a glass test tube after the addition of calcium chloride and thromboplastin (tissue factor) (Fig. 7.3).

Reagents

i. **Patients control plasma samples**: Patients control plasma samples (preferably platelet poor) are prepared from whole blood and citrate anticoagulant in a ratio of 9:1.
   - Sodium citrate (3.2%) solution: 0.5 ml
   - Whole blood: 4.5 ml

   Whole blood and sodium citrate (3.8%) are mixed well gently. Then **platelet-poor plasma (PPP)** is prepared by centrifugation at 2000 g for 15 minutes at 4°C (approximately 4000 r.p.m./minute). It should be kept at room temperature for prothrombin time assay. The test should be done within 2 hours of collection.
ii. **Thromboplastins:** Thromboplastins are tissue extracts obtained from different species and different organs. Majority of thromboplastins now in use are extracts of rabbit brain or lung. It is now commercially available as powder.
iii. **Calcium chloride ($CaCl_2$):** 0.025 mol/litre. The test reagent is prepared fresh before use.

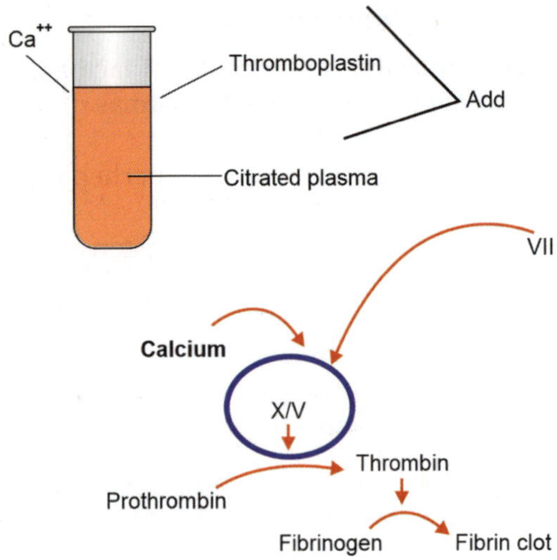

Fig. 7.3: Schematic diagram of prothrombin time (PT)

Points to Remember

- Tissue thromboplastin serves two functions. It activates extrinsic pathway and provides phospholipid surface for certain coagulation reactions.
- Calcium chloride ($CaCl_2$) supplies calcium ions or Ca^{2+} which bind vitamin K dependent factors (II, VII, IX and X) to phospholipid.

Methods (Fig. 7.3)

1. Put 0.1 ml of plasma into a glass test tube placed in a water bath and add 0.1 ml of thromboplastin.
2. Wait for 1–3 minutes to allow the mixture to warm at 37°C.
3. Then add 0.1 ml of warmed $CaCl_2$ (previously kept at water bath in a separate test tube) to that mixture in the glass test tube.

   Mix well the contents and start the stop watch.
4. The test tube is continuously tilted within the water bath and look for clot formation.
5. As soon as the fibrin clot is formed, the watch is stopped and the time is recorded.

Normal values: 11–16 seconds (when rabbit thromboplastin is used)

International Normalized Ratio (INR)

The result of prothrombin time (PT) in seconds which is performed on a normal individual will vary according to the type of analytical system employed. This is due to the variations between different types and batches of manufacturer's tissue factor used in the reagent to perform the test. The **international normalized ratio (INR)** was devised to standardize the test results. Each manufacturer assigns an **ISI (international sensitivity index)** value for any tissue factor they manufacture. The ISI value is usually between 0.94–1.4 for more sensitive and 2.0–3.0 for less sensitive thromboplastins.

The INR is the ratio of a patient's prothrombin time to a normal (control) sample, raised to the power of the ISI value for the analytical system being used.

For example, a ratio of 2.5 (patient's PT to control PT) using a thromboplastin with ISI of 1.4, then INR be calculated using this formula:

INR = $2.5^{(1.4)}$ = 3.61 (normal INR = 1.0 ratio).

Prothrombin index =

$$\frac{\text{PT of control plasma}}{\text{PT of patient's plasma}} \times 100\%$$

Suppose PT of control plasma and patient's plasma are 12 seconds and 16 seconds respectively, then prothrombin index would be $12/16 \times 100\% = 75\%$.

Cause of Prolonged Prothrombin Time (PT)

1. **Oral anticoagulant therapy:** Oral anticoagulants like warfarin interfere with the carboxylation of vitamin K-dependent factors. PT is the standard test for monitoring oral anticoagulant therapy.

   But INR is preferred to monitor patients on anticoagulant therapy. For all other uses, the use of PT is encouraged over INR. The recommended range for INR during most indications for oral anticoagulants is 2–3, or 2.5–3.5 for patients with mechanical heart valves.

2. **Vitamin K deficiency:** PT is useful test to detect vitamin K deficiency. It measures three vitamin K-dependent factors (II, VII and X) out of four (II, VII, IX and X).
3. **Liver disease,** particularly obstructive jaundice, cirrhosis, malignancy of liver.
4. **Inherited deficiency of extrinsic or common pathway coagulation factor(s):** Deficiency of VII, X, V, II or I.
5. **Others:** Post-partum hypofibrinogenaemia, DIC.

ACTIVATED PARTIAL THROMBOPLASTIN TIME (APTT)

Synonym: Partial thromboplastin time with kaolin (PTTK) and kaolin cephalin clotting time (KCCT). Also known as partial thromboplastin time (PTT).

Principle: This test measures the clotting time of plasma after the activation of contact factors but without added tissue thromboplastin, and so it evaluates the overall efficiency of the intrinsic pathway. To standardize the activation of contact factors, the plasma is first pre-incubated with kaolin. A standardized phospholipid is provided to allow the test to be performed on platelet-poor plasma.

Reagents

1. **Platelet-poor plasma:** Both from the patient and control as described in PT.
2. **Kaolin:** 5 g/litre or 0.5 g% in barbitone buffered saline pH is 7.4. A few glass beads are added to aid resuspension. This suspension is stable at room temperature. In place of kaolin, other insoluble surface active substances such as elagic acid or celite can also be used.
3. **Phospholipid:** Commercially available lyophilised reagent and working solution is prepared as per direction. This reagent must be sensitive to detect deficiencies of factors VII, C, IX and XI, at concentration of 20–25 IU/dl.
4. **Calcium chloride ($CaCl_2$):** 0.025 mol/litre.

Methods

1. Mix equal volume of the phospholipid reagent and the kaolin suspension (0.5 ml each) and leave in a glass tube in water bath at 37°C.
2. Place 0.1 ml of control and patient's (test) plasma in two separate glass tubes. Add 0.2 ml of prewarmed kaolin phospholipid solution to these tubes. Mix the contents well and gently. Start the stopwatch immediately.
3. Keep it in the water bath at 37°C and wait for 10 minutes, with occasional shaking.
4. At exactly 10 minutes, add 0.1 ml of prewarmed $CaCl_2$ and start a second stopwatch.
5. The tubes are tilted back and forth in front of a good light source and watch for appearance of fibrin clot. The watch is stopped when the clot forms and the time is recorded. The time taken by the mixture to clot is the APTT (Fig. 7.4).

Normal range: 30–40 seconds.

Causes of Prolonged APTT (Fig. 7.5)

- **Inherited deficiency** of factor VIII and factor IX. Also prolonged in inherited deficiencies of other coagulation factors in intrinsic pathway and common pathway.
- **Circulating inhibitors**: Inhibitors may be of two types—specific and nonspecific.

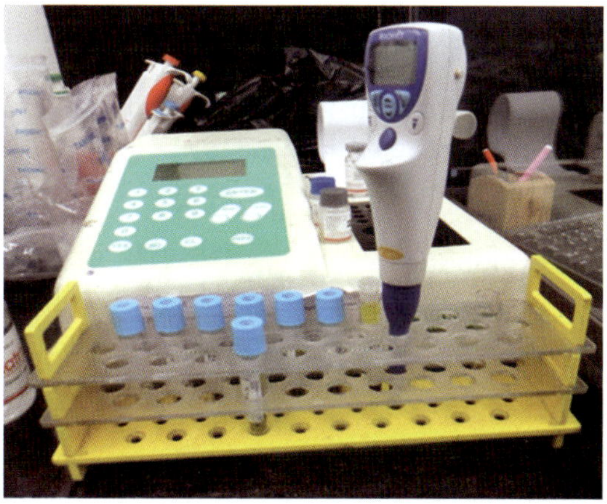

Fig. 7.4: Coagulometer (coagulation analyzer) to determine PT and APTT

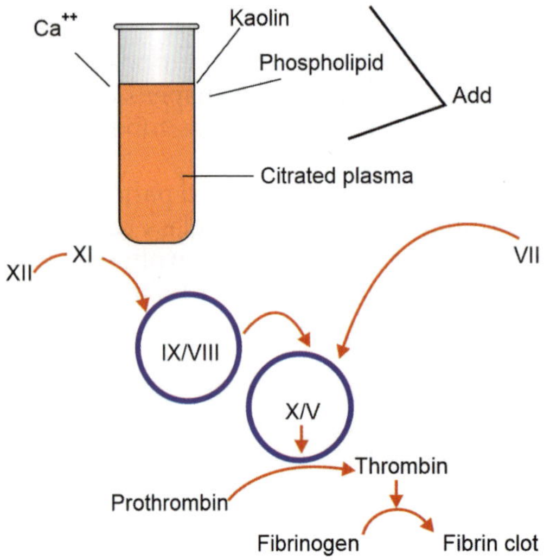

Fig. 7.5: Schematic diagram of activated partial thromboplastin time (APTT)

Specific inhibitors are directed against specific coagulation factors. The most common specific inhibitor is antibody against factor VII. **Non-specific inhibitors** are antibodies that are not directed against specific coagulation factors but block the interaction of clotting factors, e.g. lupus inhibitors.

- Liver disease
- Disseminated intravascular coagulation (DIC)
- Heparin administration: Heparin accelerates the action of antithrombin and inhibits thrombin and factors Xa, XIa and IXa.
- Massive transfusion with stored blood
- A circulating anticoagulant.

Causes of Shortened APTT

- Thrombosis
- Pregnancy

Points to Remember (Fig. 7.6)

- **Bleeding time (BT)**
  - i. It is the time taken for a standard skin puncture to stop bleeding
  - ii. This test examines the ability of blood vessels to constrict and platelets to form a hemostatic plug.
- **Clotting time or coagulation time (CT)**
  - i. It is the time required for a whole blood sample to coagulate *in vitro* under standard conditions.
  - ii. It measures all three stages of coagulation (intrinsic pathway, extrinsic pathway and common pathway).
- **Prothrombin time (PT)**
  - i. It is the time required for clotting of platelet-poor citrated plasma in a glass tube after the addition of thromboplastin (tissue factor) and calcium chloride.
  - ii. The prothrombin time along with its derived measures of prothrombin ratio (PR) and international normalized ratio (INR) are assays evaluating the extrinsic pathway of coagulation.
  - iii. The PT may used along with APTT as the starting points for investigating excessive bleeding or clotting disorders.
- **Activated partial thromboplastin time (APTT)**
  - i. It is used to monitor the functioning of the intrinsic and the common coagulation pathways.
  - ii. A relatively rare cause of prolonged APTT is presence of antibodies against coagulation plasma factors/proteins. These are known as inhibitors. Some of the cause are: Autoimmune diseases, pregnancy, dermatologic conditions, malignancies (prostate cancer, lymphoma), haemophilia A and B, patients receiving clotting factors to control their bleeding disorders.
- Glass syringe should not be used for blood collection in coagulation studies since it activates coagulation.
- Coagulation studies are carried out within 2 hours of collection of blood sample.

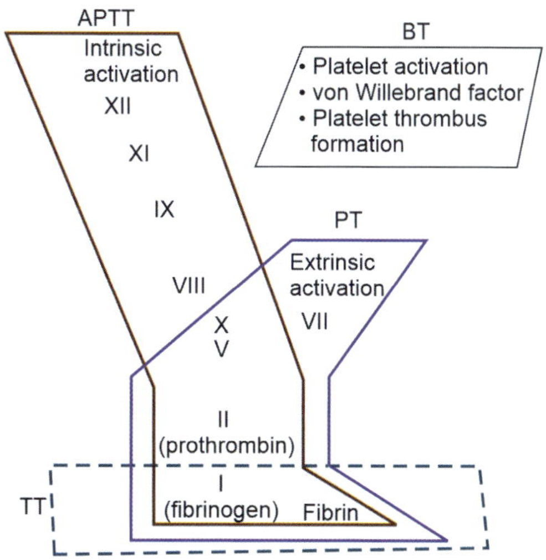

Fig. 7.6: Basic test for haemostasis
BT: Bleeding time, APTT: Activated partial thromboplastin time, PT: Prothrombin time, TT: Thrombin time

VIVA VOCE

Q1. What are intrinsic and extrinsic pathways of coagulation and why are they named so?

Ans: The clotting system can be activated by two pathways—either by intrinsic pathway or by extrinsic pathway. The intrinsic pathway is activated by exposing factor XII to any thrombogenic surface (as for example, glass surfaces or other negatively charged surfaces). On the other hand, extrinsic pathway requires exogenous triggering agent (which was originally provided by tissue extract or tissue thromboplastin prepared from animal tissue rich in tissue factor like rabbit brain). Later on, kaolin or kaolin-cephalin become available commercially which is used nowadays as tissue factor.

But this division is somewhat confusing as intrinsic pathway is relevant *in vitro* (outside body), whereas extrinsic pathway is relevant *in vivo* (within body), after vascular injury/damage.

Q2. Why kaolin and phospholipids are added for doing APTT?

Ans: Kaolin leads to surface contact activation. So, initiating the intrinsic system of coagulation from factor XII onwards. Hence, it is called activated PTT or APTT.

On the other hand, exogenous phospholipids (platelet factor 3) act as alternative to blood platelets and are necessary for coagulation. Within body, platelets are source of phospholipids. This exogenous phospholipid also known as partial thromboplastin. Hence, APTT is also known as partial thromboplastin time.

Q3. Why is incision made parallel to antecubital fossa during template method of bleeding time (BT) estimation?

Ans: Incision is made parallel to antecubital fossa so that no wound is formed as there will be absence of retraction of skin. But if incision is made right angle or obliquely to the antecubital fossa, the skin edges will be retracted and a spindle-shaped wound/scar will be formed.

Q4. What are the effects of circulating anticoagulants in blood?

Ans: Circulating anticoagulants are inhibitors of coagulation like heparin and other anticoagulants present in blood. Presence of circulating anticoagulants cause prolonged PT and APTT.

Q5. If a patient has normal PT but prolonged APTT, then what are the possibilities?

Ans:
i. Defect in intrinsic pathway or congenital deficiency of factors require for intrinsic pathway. As for example, haemophilia A, haemophilia B, deficiency of factor XI, factor XII, prekallikrein and HMWK (high molecular weight kininogen).
ii. Deficiency of von Willebrand's factor (vWF) in von Willebrand's disease (also prolonged bleeding time).
iii. Presence of heparin and other anticoagulants in blood (circulating anticoagulants).

Q6. If a patient has prolonged PT and normal APTT, then what are the possibilities?

Ans:
i. Congenital deficiency of factor VII, which is very rare.
ii. Initiation of oral anticoagulant therapy (warfarin).

Q7. In above scenario (question No. 6), how would you ascertain the exact cause?

Ans: When a patient has prolonged PT and normal APTT, then prothrombin (PT) is repeated with 1:1 mixture of patient's plasma and normal plasma (control) as substrate. If the prolongation is corrected, then the cause is factor VII deficiency.

The normal plasma present in 1:1 mixture supplies factor VII required for normal prothrombin time.

If it is not corrected, then the cause is presence of an inhibitor in blood.

Q8. If a patient has prolongation of both PT and APTT, then what are the possibilities?

Ans: In this case, both tests are repeated with 1:1 mixture of patient's plasma and normal plasma (control) as substrate. If both PT and APTT now become normal, then the patient has deficiency of one or many of these factors; factors I, II, V, and X (common for PT and APPTT).

After that, individual specific assay is done to find out deficiency of particular factor.

Q9. What is thrombin time (TT)? What are the causes of prolonged TT?

Ans: This is time required for testing the conversion of fibrinogen into fibrin. It depends on aqequate fibrinogen levels.

Prolonged thrombin time (TT) is seen in afibrinogenaemia, dysfibrinogenaemia, DIC (disseminated intravascular coagulation) and heparin like inhibitors.

Q10. What is clot retraction study?

Ans: A clot forms at the end of blood coagulation. In normal circumstances, the clot undergoes contraction. When serum is expressed from the clot, the clot becomes denser. The platelets release one substance (called thromboplastin) which is responsible for clot retraction. Normal clot retraction begins within 30 seconds after the blood has clotted, and at 1 hour it is about 30% normally.

Clot retraction test is done when there is suspicion of haemorrhagic disorders related to platelets. Poor clot retraction is seen if platelet count is low (thrombocytopenia) or in poor platelet function with normal platelet count (thrombasthenia).

Q11. Why 3.2% trisodium citrate is used nowadays instead of 3.8%?

Ans: Trisodium citrate 3.8% was used earlier but is no longer recommended as it causes longer PT and APTT results and discrepant INR values. Moreover, INR values based on WHO protocols have been derived using 3.2% and are not validated for 3.8% trisodium citrate.

Q12. How corrections are done in abnormal haematocrit value/polycythemia?

Ans: In polycythemia, volume of plasma is low, whereas haematocrit/ RBC count is high. For this reason, excess of anticoagulant (sodium citrate) remains in test tube. This excess anticoagulant subsequently binds to calcium reagent and cause prolongation of PT and APTT. So, for accurate results volume of anticoagulant should be reduced by using one of these two formulas:

i. Volume of citrate (3.2%) needed

$$= \frac{(100 - \text{Haematocrit}) \times \text{Total tube volume}}{595 - \text{Haematocrit}}$$

ii. Volume of anticoagulant = (Volume of blood in ml) × (100 – Haematocrit) × 0.00185.

Chapter 8

Blood Grouping and Rh Typing

The **term blood group** refers not only to erythrocyte antigen system but also to the immunologic diversity expressed by other blood constituents including leukocytes, platelets and plasma.

International Society of Blood Transfusion (ISBT) Working Party recognizes 35 significant blood group systems though there are about 200 red cell antigens. Landsteiner first discovered **ABO system** in 1901. After that, **MNS system** in 1927, **P system** in 1927, **rhesus** or **Rh system** in 1939, **Lutheran system** in 1945, **Kell system** in 1946, **Lewis system** in 1946, **Duffy system** in 1950, **Kidd system** in 1951 were discovered.

Other significant systems of those 35 systems (recognized by ISBT) are Diego, Yt, Xg, Scianna, Dombrock, Colton, Landsteiner –Wiener, Chido/Rodgers, Hh, Kx, Gerbich, Cromer, Knobs, Indian, Ok, Raph, John Mitton Hagen, I, Globoside, GIL, RHAG.

Most blood group genes (with a few exceptions) are located on the autosomal chromosomes and are inherited following Mendelian rules of inheritance. These blood group genes are expressed equally when inherited in a co-dominant manner (i.e. two allelic forms are expressed equally when inherited in a heterozygous state). The specific alleles at a particular locus of gene in an individual constitute the genotype. Outward expression of this genotype is known as phenotype.

With regard to blood transfusion practice, most important blood group systems are ABO and Rh systems. Because, A, B and Rh D antigens are most immunogenic (they are capable of eliciting a strong antibody response on stimulation) and their alloantibodies can cause destruction of transfused RBCs or they may induce haemolytic diseases of newborn (HDN). ABO antigens are also important for organ transplantation (graft rejection).

Apart from A, B, Rh D antigens other important antigens in transfusion medicine as per their strong immunogenicity are D, K, C, FY^a, c, E, k, e, JK^a, S and s.

Almost always, an individual has the same blood group for life, but very rarely an individual's blood type changes through addition or suppression of an antigen in infections, autoimmune diseases or malignancies. Another rare cause in blood group change is bone marrow transplant.

ANTIBODIES TO RED CELL ANTIGENS

Mainly there are two main types: Naturally occurring and immune or acquired antibodies.

1. **Naturally occurring antibodies:** These antibodies are formed without any antigenic stimulus (RBC antigens). These are present in the serum of persons who lack

that particular antigen(s) in the RBC, e.g. isoagglutinins (antibodies) of ABO blood grouping system. These antibodies are IgM in nature and react to corresponding antigen at a temperature below 37°C. These antibodies very rarely may be seen in other blood group systems.

It is presumed that these antibodies develop due to antigenic stimulus from the similar type of antigens present in the intestinal bacteria or foods consumed by newborns. The infant regards these antigens as foreign and develops antibodies to those foreign antigens which are not present in their own cells/RBCs. Hence, blood group A persons develop anti-B antibodies, blood group B persons develop anti-A antibodies, blood group O persons develop both anti-A and anti-B antibodies while blood group AB persons do not have any antibody.

2. **Immune or acquired antibody:** These antibodies develop when different antigens either in RBC or body fluids are introduced in a person who do not have these antigens. The person consider those antigens foreign and immune or acquired antibodies (agglutinins) are formed. Example: Mismatched blood transfusion or after pregnancy. Most of these antibodies are IgG in nature and react best at 37°C.

ABO SYSTEM

There are four main types of blood groups: A, B, AB and O. Blood group A again can be subdivided into A_1 and A_2. The much rarer A subgroups are A_3, A_x and A_m. But the A_1 and A_2 subgroups are important only. So, ABO system increases to six: A_1, A_2, B, A_1B, A_2B and O. About 80% of blood group A and blood group AB belong to A_1 or A_1B respectively. ABO antigens are found predominantly on erythrocyte membrane protein band 3 and 4.5, membrane glycophorin and structural glycolipids. In addition to red cells, these antigens are also expressed on platelets, white blood cells and various body tissues. As ABO antigens are found on most tissues of the body, they are often referred to as "histo-blood group" antigens. They may be found in soluble form in various body secretions (in secretors).

Although ABO antigens have been detected on erythrocytes in a six-week old foetus but these antigens are poorly expressed at birth. Antigenicity increases gradually and becomes fully expressed around one year of age (some believe full expression needs three years of age).

The blood groups A, B, AB and O are determined by presence or absence of A and B antigens on the red cell membrane (Fig. 8.1, Tables 8.1 and 8.6). There is another antigen called O antigen which remains silent.

Actually, these A, B or O antigens on red cells are controlled by three allelic genes on the long arm of chromosome 9. The A and B genes are co-dominant but the O antigen is amorph or silent (it has no effect on antigenic structure).

The cellular expression of A and B antigens is determined by another gene, called H gene. The H gene (genotype HH or Hh) produces a transferase enzyme, which changes precursor or substance present on RBCs into **H substance**. The A and B genes produce specific transferase enzymes that convert H substance into A and B antigens respectively. But the O gene produces an inactive transferase so that H antigen persists unchanged on red cells.

In the absence of H genes (designated as hh), the precursor substance remains unconverted and H substance is not synthesized. So, A and B genes, if present cannot be expressed and **Bombay blood group (Oh)** type results. Their red cell type is group O. But unlike group O individuals, Bombay blood group persons (Oh) have no H antigen on RBC. As there is no expression of A, B antigens and absence of H antigen, their plasma contain antibodies against all of them, i.e. anti-A, anti-B and anti-H. These antibodies are active at 37°C. Therefore,

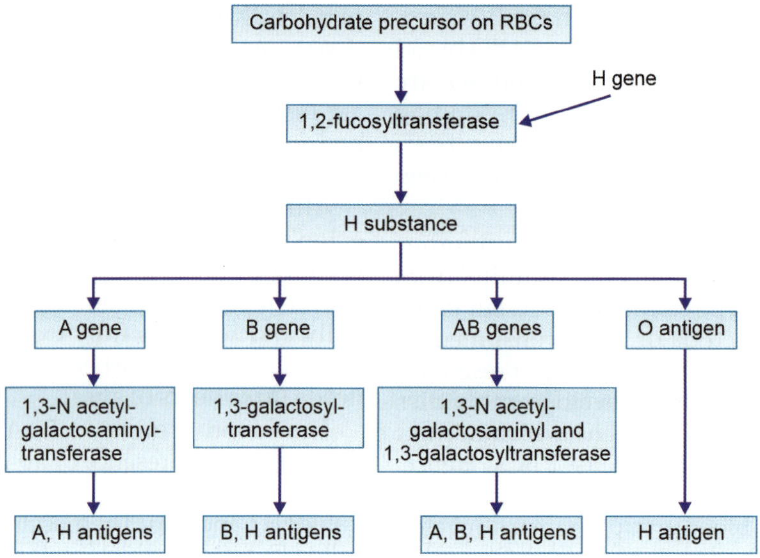

Fig. 8.1: Formation of A, B and H antigens on RBCs

Bombay blood group persons should be transfused only with Oh blood.

Secretors and Nonsecretors

Secretors are persons who secrete A, B, and H antigen (called ABH substances) into body fluids (such as plasma, saliva, sweat, tears, semen, milk, etc.). These ABH substances are secreted in water-soluble form of glycoprotein. The ability of secretion is dependent on presence of a dominant secretor gene (Se). About 80% of Caucasian persons are secretors (genotype Sese or SeSe) and remaining are nonsecretors (sese). Both secretors and nonsecretors express ABO antigens on red cells.

Differences between A_1 and A_2 Subgroups of Blood Group A and AB

Subgroups of A are distinguished by their lack of agglutination with anti-A_1 lectin prepared from *Dolichos biflorus* or with anti-A_1 reagent derived from serum of group O or B persons that has been absorbed with A_2 cells.

In India, frequency of blood group A is 22.88%, blood group B is 32.26%, blood group AB is 7.44% and blood group O is 37.12%.

Features	A_1	A_2
Quantitative differences		
• Reaction with diluted anti-A	+ + + +	+ +
• Antigenic sites:		
a. In adults	1,000,000	250,000
b. In newborns	310,000	140,000
Qualitative differences		
• Reaction with *Dolichos biflorus* (Anti-A_1) lectin	+ + + +	0
• Anti-A_1 in serum	Absent	1–8%
• N-acetylgalactosaminyl-transferase activity	Normal activity (optimal at pH 6)	Decreased activity (optimal at pH 7)

Table 8.1: Antigens, antibodies and other features in ABO blood grouping system

	ABO blood groups			
Antigen (on RBC)	Antigen A 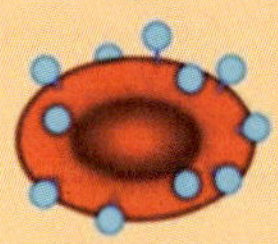	Antigen B 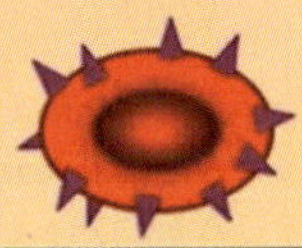	Antigens A + B 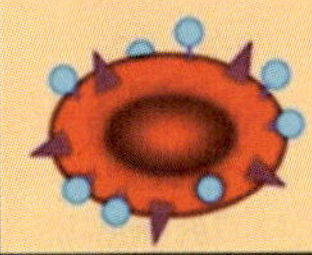	Neither A nor B 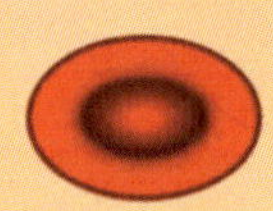
Antibody (in plasma)	Anti-B antibody 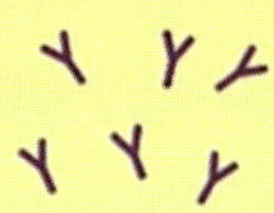	Anti-A antibody 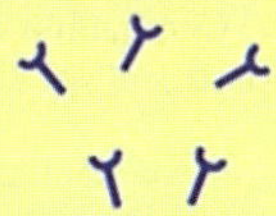	Neither antibody	Both antibodies 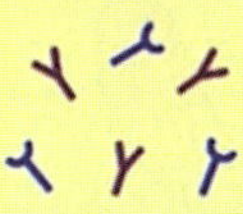
Blood type	**Type A** Cannot have B or AB blood Can have A or O blood	**Type B** Cannot have A or AB blood Can have B or O blood	**Type AB** Can have any type of blood Is the universal recipient?	**Type O** Can only have O blood Is the universal donor?

METHOD OF ABO BLOOD GROUPING

It can be done by slide or tube method or by microplate method. Slide method is satisfactory but not as sensitive as tube method because slide method cannot detect weak anti-A or anti-B reverse serum grouping. Monoclonal anti-A and anti-B reagents are used for blood grouping.

Again, ABO blood grouping can be of two: Forward grouping and reverse grouping.

Forward grouping: Here, one drop of 2–5% red cell suspension is tested with one drop each of commercially prepared anti-A and anti-B.

Reverse grouping: Here, two drops of patient or donor serum are tested against one drop of reagent erythrocytes of known A (usually A_1) and B phenotype. But this is not done in infants under 4 months of age as the corresponding antibodies are normally absent.

Preparing red cell suspension

Depending upon the specific technique employed 2, 5, 10, 20, or 50% red cell suspensions are required. These can be prepared by suspending in saline the packed red cell obtained from citrate or oxalate blood or from a skin puncture into saline.

Preparation of 2% red cell suspension

1. Take 5 ml of normal saline in a test tube. To it, add several drops of anticoagulated or fresh blood.
2. Centrifuge in order to get packed red cells (3000 r.p.m. for 10–20 minutes).
3. Withdraw the supernatant fluid as completely as possible.
4. Add 0.1 ml of this packed red cells to a test tube which contains 4.9 ml of normal saline. Mix them well. This represents 2% red cell suspension (as 0.1 ml of packed red cell in total 5 ml of suspension).

For preparation of 5% red cell suspension, add 0.25 ml of packed red cell to 4.75 ml of saline. For preparation of 10% red cell suspension add 0.5 ml of packed red cells to 4.5 ml of saline in the last step (step 4) of the above procedure.

Slide Method (ABO Grouping)

This method is satisfactory but less preferable compared to tube method. However, in small

Blood group	Antigen + antibody(ies) present		As donor	As recipient
A	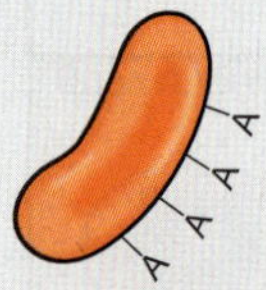 Antigen A	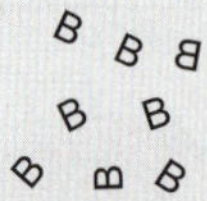 Makes anti-B	Compatible with: A and AB Incompatible with: B and O, because both make anti-A antibodies that will react with A antigens	Compatible with: A and O Incompatible with: B and AB, because type A makes anti-B antibodies that will react with B antigens
B	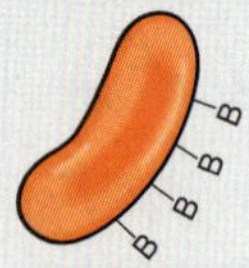 Antigen B	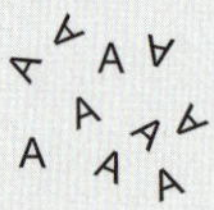 Makes anti-A	Compatible with: B and AB Incompatible with: A and O, because both make anti-B antibodies that will react with B antigens	Compatible with: B and O Incompatible with: A and AB, because type B makes anti-A antibodies that will react with A antigens
AB	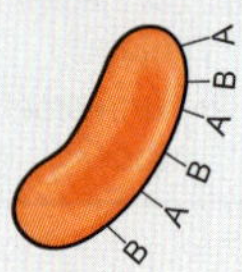 Antigens A and B Antigens A and B	Makes neither anti-A nor anti-B	Compatible with: AB only Incompatible with: A, B and O, because All three make antibodies that will react with AB antigens	Compatible with all groups universal recipient AB makes no antibodies and therefore will not react with any type of donated blood
O	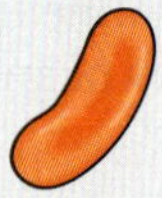 Neither A nor B antigen	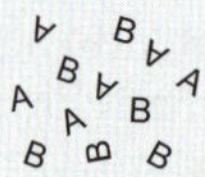 Makes both anti-A and anti-B	Compatible with all groups universal donor O red cells have no antigens, and will therefore not stimulate anti-A or anti-B antibodies	Compatible with: O only Incompatible with: A, AB and B, because type O makes anti-A and anti-B antibodies

Red Blood Cell Compatibility Table

	Donor							
Recipient	O–	O+	A–	A+	B–	B+	AB–	AB+
O–	✓	×	×	×	×	×	×	×
O+	✓	✓	×	×	×	×	×	×
A–	✓	×	✓	×	×	×	×	×
A+	✓	✓	✓	✓	×	×	×	×
B–	✓	×	×	×	✓	×	×	×
B+	✓	✓	×	×	✓	✓	×	×
AB–	✓	×	✓	×	✓	×	✓	×
AB+	✓	✓	✓	✓	✓	✓	✓	✓

laboratories, resource poor set ups, in emergency situations or during mass blood group screening this can be done.

Sample: A 20% red cell suspension is used. Alternatively, fresh blood by finger prick or cells from clotted blood may be used.

Reagent: Monoclonal anti-A and anti-B reagents (commercially available) blue-coloured vial: Anti-A, yellow-coloured vial: Anti-B. Monoclonal anti-AB is also available.

Test procedure (Fig. 8.2A to D and Fig. 8.4)

1. Take a clean glass slide. Mark anti-A on left side corner and anti-B on middle and control on right side corner of that slide.
2. Two drops of blood or 20–40% red cell suspension are placed by a Pasteur pipette at each three demarcated areas.
3. On the left side a drop of anti-serum, on the middle a drop of anti-B serum and on the right a drop of normal saline are added separately.
4. The serum cell suspensions are mixed separately with the help of glass rod or by the corners of another clean slide. Alternatively, wooden swabstick breaking off can also be used.
5. The slide is then tilted with hands gently and carefully for 2–3 minutes.

Test result: Results are read within 2–5 minutes depending on the appearance of agglutination of red cells (positive or negative) as follows:

i. Blood group A: Agglutination with anti-A serum (left corner) but not with anti-B serum (middle).
ii. Blood group B: Agglutination with anti-B (middle) but not with anti-A (left corner).
iii. Blood group AB: Agglutination on both left and middle portions.
iv. Blood group O: No agglutination on left and middle portions.

Control should be negative. If there is agglutination in the control that means either the method or technique is faulty or the reagents are of expired/poor quality.

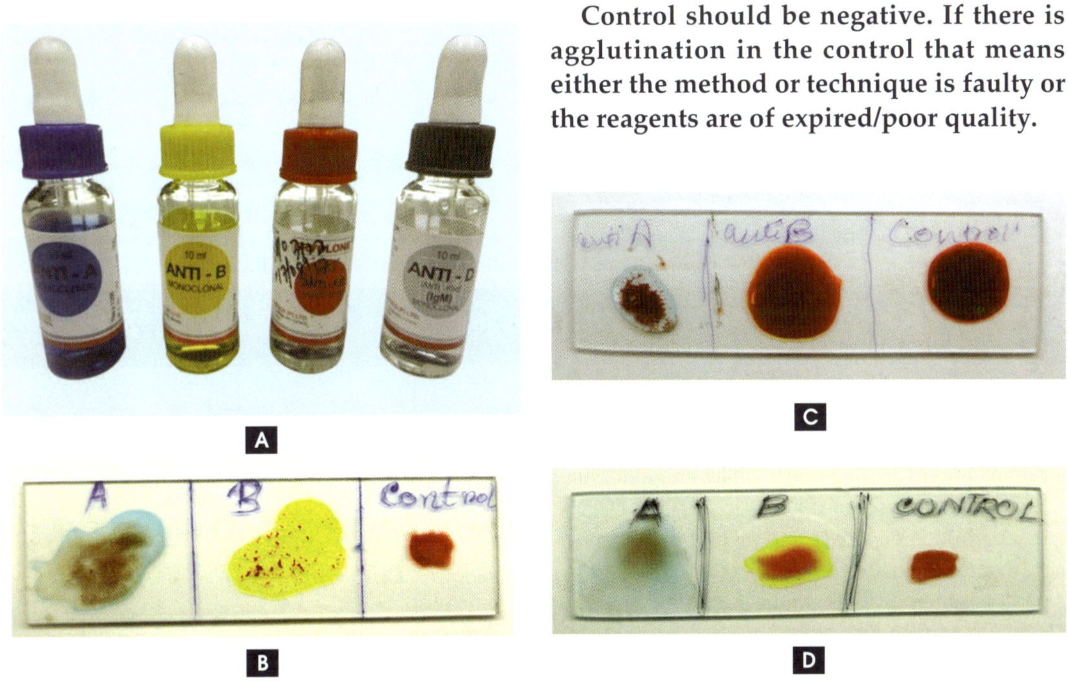

Fig. 8.2A to D: ABO blood grouping. (A) Monoclonal anti-A (green coloured), anti-B (yellow coloured) and anti-AB (colourless) serum. Also anti-D serum (colourless) on rightmost side **(upper left)**; (B) Blood group A **(upper right)**; (C) Blood group B **(lower left)**; (D) Blood group O **(lower right)**

Tube Method (ABO Grouping)

(Fig. 8.3A and B, and Table 8.2)

i. Take 3 glasses or plastic tubes (75 × 12 mm) and add one drop each grouping reagent to 3 tubes to labelled anti-A, anti-B and anti-AB respectively.
ii. Put 1 drop of 2–5% of red cell suspension to each tube.
iii. Mix the suspension by tapping the tubes and leave them undisturbed for 15–30 minutes. Check agglutination.

Test result: Agglutination is judged by the macroscopic appearance of agglutination in round bottom tubes. If positive it will show "graininess", whereas in the absence of agglutination the sedimented cells appear as a smooth round bottom. This agglutination is better visualized under microscope. A scoring system depending upon agglutination pattern can be employed.

For determining the particular blood group following the agglutination pattern in the slide method described early.

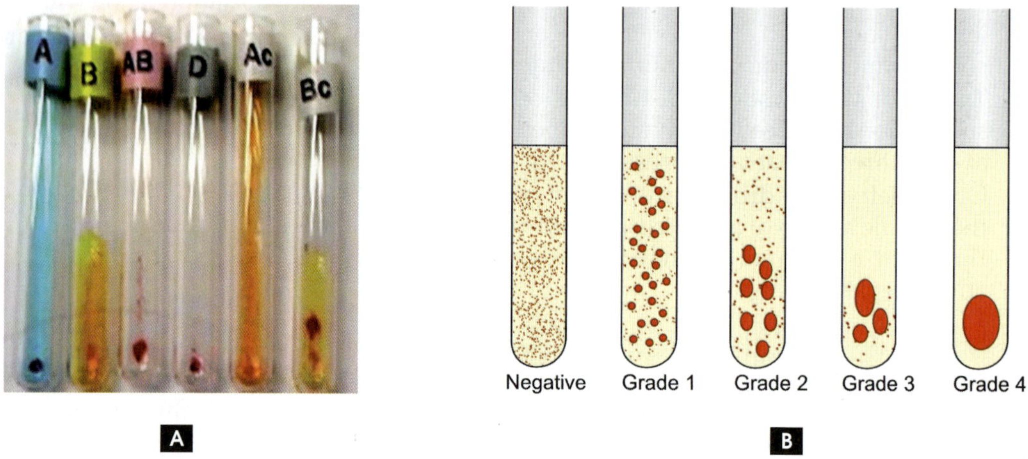

Fig. 8.3A and B: (A) Test tube methods for blood grouping; (B) Scoring system (grades 1 to 4) in test tube method of blood grouping

Table 8.2: Scoring of results in red agglutination tests

Description	Symbol	Agglutination score*
a. Negative result: All cell-free and evenly distributed	–	0
b. Cell button dislodges into fine granules, only visible microscopically	+ or weak (W)	3
c. Cell button dislodges into finely granular clumps, just visible macroscopically	1 +	5
d. Cell button dislodges into many small clumps, macroscopically visible	2 +	8
e. Cell button dislodges into several large clumps, macroscopically visible	3 +	10
f. Cell button remains in one clump, macroscopically visible	4 + or complete (C)	12

***Agglutination score**: Further classification depending upon the number of red cells present in the clump. Hence, clumping of average 12 cells (score 4+), average 10 cells (score 3+), average 5 cells (score 1+).

Serum Grouping (Reverse Grouping)

In the serum grouping or reverse grouping, patient's serum is tested against known red cell antigens on RBCs (Table 8.3). If the patient's serum contains anti-A, anti-B or both it will agglutinate known antigen A, antigen B or both antigens in red cells. Red cells form blood group A contains antigen A, blood group B contains antigen B, blood group AB contains both antigens and blood group O contains no antigen (serves as control) on their red cells. For A antigen, A_1 subtype is commonly used. A_2 cells should be used if there is suspected presence of anti-A_1.

Microplate Method

ABO grouping may be carried out on one U well plate (96 wells) and monoclonal reagents (anti-A, anti-B, anti-AB) are used. Using Pasteur pipette (or commercial reagent dropper) 1 drop of monoclonal reagent or antiserum is added to each well of the U well plate. Then 1 drop of 2–5% patient's red cell suspension is added to these rows. This is done for forward grouping.

For reverse grouping at the same time 1 drop patient's serum or plasma are added to separate wells of the plate. To this known antigens 1 drop (antigen A, antigen B or antigen AB) are added to the serum/plasma. Control may be used.

Now, mix them on a microplate shaker. Leave the microplate at room temperature (20°C) for 15 minutes. Then centrifuge the plate at 700 r.p.m. for 1 minute.

The plate can be read for agglutination by one of the two methods

1. Streaming (microplate set an angle) or agitation.
2. Automated microplate readers.

False Positive Results (ABO Grouping)

- **Rouleaux formation:** Marked rouleaux formation can simulate true agglutination. In reverse grouping the two can be distinguished by repeating the test using serum diluted 1 in 2 or 1 in 1 saline. The rouleaux will disappear but agglutination will persist. If rouleaux are apparent in forward grouping test, then tests should be repeated after washing the patient's red cell thoroughly with normal saline.
- **Cold agglutinins:** Sometimes true agglutination of red cells develops due to cold agglutinins at or below 20°C. If ABO compatibility is ruled out, then the presence of cold agglutinins like anti-P_1 or anti-I antibodies may be the cause of this false positivity. In that case, patient's red cells are washed several times with warm (37°C) saline and blood grouping (ABO)

Table 8.3: Forward and reverse groupings

ABO blood group	Forward grouping		Reverse grouping	
	Anti-A	Anti-B	A_1 antigen on RBC	B antigen on RBC
1. Blood group A	+	–	–	+
2. Blood group B	–	+	+	–
3. Blood group AB	+	+	–	–
4. Blood group O	–	–	+	+

is repeated. There will no chance of false positivity.

- **Warm antibodies:** These antibodies are absorbed to red cell of patient. Agglutinin other than anti-A, anti-B or anti-D (Rh typing) which cause agglutination at 37°C are occasionally seen. Presence of antibodies like anti-Lu, anti-M, anti-K or anti-S antibodies are responsible for this.
- **Bacterial contamination:** Infection of RBCs by bacteria both *in vivo* and *in vitro* may cause polyagglutination in normal sera. Bacterial enzyme expose T receptors on red cell surface. As most human sera contain anti-T antibodies, such infected red cells get agglutinated in normal serum. Hence, blood group O may appear as blood group AB.

False Negative Results (ABO Grouping)

1. Failure of agglutination or weak reactions are usually due to improper sera. If the sera are kept at room temperature for longer time the potency is lost.
2. Failure to add grouping reagent or insufficient volume will cause false negative results.
3. In reverse grouping test, failure to recognize lysis as a positive result may end up in giving false negative reports. To avoid lysis, reagents (anti-A and anti-B) should contain EDTA to prevent complement activation in presence of fresh patient's serum as seen in tile method of grouping.
4. Miscellaneous: Wrong technique, poor quality of red cells, etc.

Rh System

The rhesus (Rh) system was so named because Landsteiner and Wiener (1940) published studies of animal experiments involving the immunization of guinea pigs and rabbits with rhesus monkey erythrocytes. The antiserum produced agglutinated 85% of human erythrocytes, and the antigen defined was called the **Rh factor.**

Using five basic antisera anti-D, anti-C and anti-E, anti-c and anti-e, Wiener identified five different factors or antigens and named them as Rh_o, rh′, rh″hr′, hr″. While Fisher postulated that Rh antigens (C, c, D, d, E, e) are determined by three pairs of closed linked allelomorphic genes which are located on chromosome 1 (Table 8.4). These three pairs are C or c, D or d and E or e. Every human carries one member of these three pairs from each parent. Each gene can control production of a specific antigen. But the antigen controlled by D locus is the strongest immunogen, called the Rh D antigen. The six Rh genes give 8 allelomorphs and 8 antigenic patterns. The nomenclature suggested by Fisher later on accepted by WHO expert by WHO Expert Committee in 1977 (Table 8.5).

Table 8.4: Comparison of Wiener, Fisher and Rosenfield nomenclature

Wiener	Fisher	Rosenfield
Rh_0	D	Rh 1
rh′	C	Rh 2
rh″	E	Rh 3
hr′	c	Rh 4
hr″	e	Rh 5

Table 8.5: The Rh genes and antigens as per Fisher's nomenclature, accepted by WHO (1977)

	Genes	Antigens
Rh positive	CDe	CDe
	cDE	cDE
	cDe	cDe
	CDE	CDE
Rh negative	Cde	Cde
	cdE	cdE
	cde	cde
	CdE	CdE

Rh D is the most strong antigen amongst those 8 antigens and other antigens (which do not have D) are much less antigenic than D and do not have clinical relevance. In clinical practice, therefore, Rh positive or Rh negative depends on the presence of D antigen on surface of red cells which can be detected by adding strong anti-D serum and noting agglutination. Nearly about 95% Indians, 90% Chinese and 85% Caucasians have this Rh D antigen and hence they are Rh positive (Rh+). Only 5–6% Indians do not have Rh D antigens and are Rh negative (Rh–).

During blood transfusion, after ABO compatibility, Rh+ blood can be safely transfused to Rh+ persons. But if the person is Rh– then not only RHD negative blood but also presence of CE antigens should be checked by adding anti-C and anti-E serum. When all these three antigens (CDE) are negative, then only it should be transfused to Rh– persons. This anti-D serum is actually IgG in nature.

There are six antisera corresponding to the Rh antigens. They are anti-C, anti-c, anti-D, anti-d, anti-E and anti-e. But in humans only five of these antisera have been detected and anti-d is absent. This may be probably because d antigen is not immunogenic or amorph to produce antibody against it.

Rh Grouping Method (Fig. 8.4)

Slide Methods

1. Place one drop of anti-D (commercially available) onto a slide.
2. Add two drops of red cell suspension (50%) or whole blood (citrated/oxalated/fresh).
3. Mix well and distribute over a large area of the slide.
4. Tilt it for 2–3 minutes.

Result: Clumping of cells (both macroscopic and microscopic) indicates Rh D positive and no clumps indicate Rh D negative.

Tube Methods

1. Add one drop of anti-D serum in a test tube.
2. Add one drop of 5% red cell suspension and mix well.

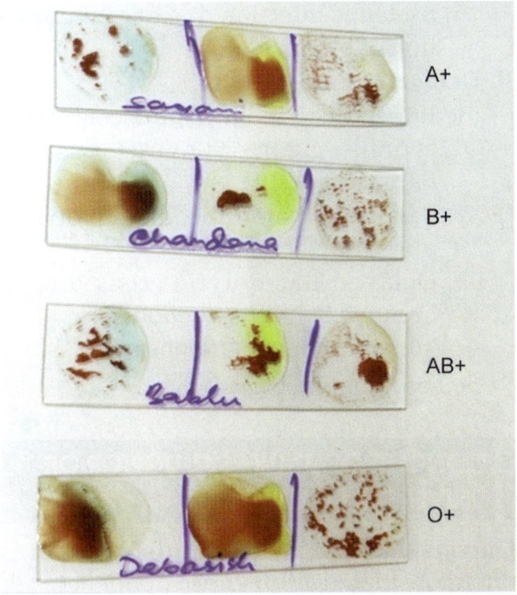

Fig. 8.4: Three compartments. First drop of blood on left side mixed with anti-A serum, middle drop of blood mixed with anti-B serum and last drop of blood on right side mixed with anti-D (Rh) serum. All are Rh group positive with ABO blood grouping of A, B, AB and O respectively

3. Incubate in a water bath at 37°C for 30–60 minutes.
4. Check for agglutination.

Result: Agglutinations or clumps seen under the bottom of the tube indicate Rh D positive and no clumps indicate Rh D negative.

REACTIONS OR COMPLICATIONS FOLLOWING BLOOD TRANSFUSION

A. Immediate complications

1. Rigor followed by pyrexia
2. Allergic urticaria over the body and anaphylaxis
3. Air embolism
4. Haemolytic transfusion reactions leading to haemoglobinuria, haemolytic shock, and renal failure.
5. Cardiac failure due to massive transfusion (volume overload).

6. Systemic infection due to contamination of blood.

B. Delayed complications

1. Infections: Hepatitis, malaria, HIV, syphilis, cytomegalovirus, Epstein-Barr virus (EBV), etc.
2. Past transfusion thrombocytopenic purpura.
3. Delayed haemolytic crisis due to immune body production.
4. Pulmonary microembolism.
5. Thrombophlebitis.

CONCEPT OF UNIVERSAL DONOR OR UNIVERSAL RECIPIENT

Universal donor: Blood group O person is often considered as universal donor because of absence of antigen A or antigen B on red cells. Plasma of blood group O person contains anti-A and anti-B. But these agglutinins or antibodies get diluted when blood is transfused to the recipient (patient) because of large serum in the recipient. So, these antibodies become inactive and no untoward reactions occur.

Universal recipient: Blood group AB person is often considered as universal recipient because of absence of anti-A or anti-B isoantibody in the serum. Any blood group when transfused to these persons, the red cells of donor's blood do not find any antibody to react with. Hence, there is no transfusion reaction.

The above definition is based on ABO grouping system. But when it is combined with Rh typing then persons with blood group O and Rh D negative (Rh–) are called universal donors. Likewise, persons with blood group AB and Rh D positive (Rh+) are universal recipients (Table 8.6).

Table 8.6: Comparison of ABO and Rh blood grouping

Parameter	ABO blood group	Rh blood group
1. Antigenic locus on gene	Chromosome 9	Chromosome 1
2. Antigens	A, B, AB	D (only clinically significant)
3. Distribution of antigens	RBCs, platelets, body fluids, many tissues (called histo blood group)	RBCs only
4. Nature of antibody	Naturally occurring	Immune or acquired
5. Development of antigens	Weak expression at birth (full expression after 1 year of age)	Fully developed at birth
6. Antibody class	IgM	IgG
7. Optimal reaction temperature of antibody	4°C	37°C
8. Whether antibody can fix complement	Yes	No
9. Optimal reaction medium	Saline	Anti-human globulin
10. Haemolysis following mismatched transfusion	Intravascular haemolysis due to complement mediated haemolysis	Extravascular and predominantly in spleen by mononuclear phagocyte (MP) or macrophage system

GEL CARD METHOD (COLUMN AGGLUTINATION OR MICROTYPING SYSTEM)

Microtyping system or column agglutination method is based on gel technology. In this test, gel (dextran acrylamide gel) is held in microtubes contained in a plastic card (hence the name gel card). This sephadex gel presents in each microtube is prepared in a buffer solution. This gel contains group specific antisera/antibody/antiglobulin (for Coombs' test) and sodium azide as preservative. These are incorporated into the gel during manufacture.

Principle of the Test

Cells are poured over the microtube first. As for example, for blood grouping RBC suspension is poured. Then the microtubes are incubated at 37°C followed by centrifugation which pulls the cells downward and react with the antibody incorporated into gel. If antigen over cells are present against particular antibody, haemagglutination will occur (Figs 8.5 and 8.6). Normal RBCs can pass through the gel but the agglutinated RBCs cannot because of their adherence and large size and gel matrix acts as a sieve. The agglutinated RBCs get trapped at various sites within the gel and thus formed a red line (positive test).

If the specific antigen is absent on RBCs, agglutination does not occur and RBCs easily pass through the gel and reach the bottom of the tube. No red line is formed due to absence of agglutination (negative test).

Uses

i. Blood grouping (ABO and Rh typing) and cross-matching
ii. Coombs' antiglobulin test
iii. For diagnosis of sickle cell anaemia, PNH (paroxysmal nocturnal haemoglobinuria)
iv. For diagnosis of different infective organisms (diphtheria, syphilis, measles, parvovirus, etc.)
v. Antibody identification.

Advantages of gel card method

i. This method is easy, accurate, standardized.

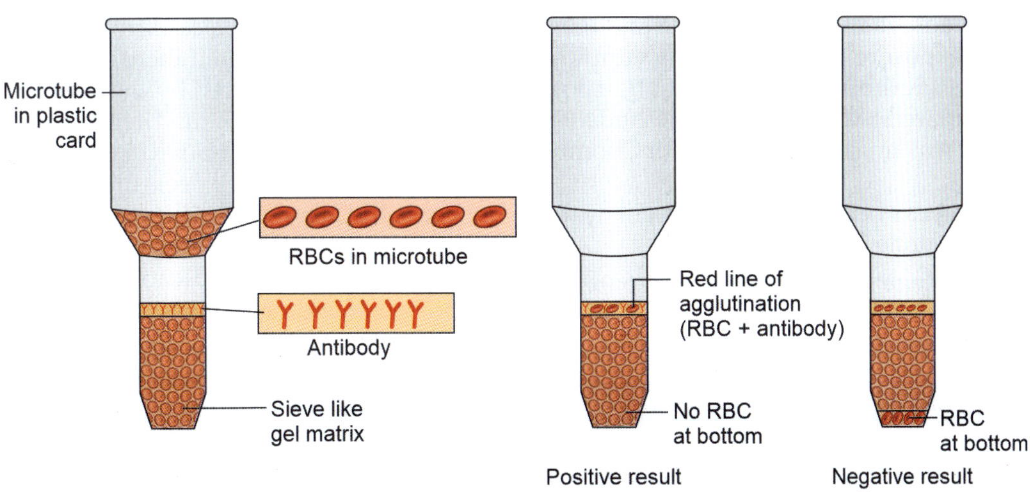

Fig. 8.5: Gel card method of blood grouping (column agglutination or microtyping system)

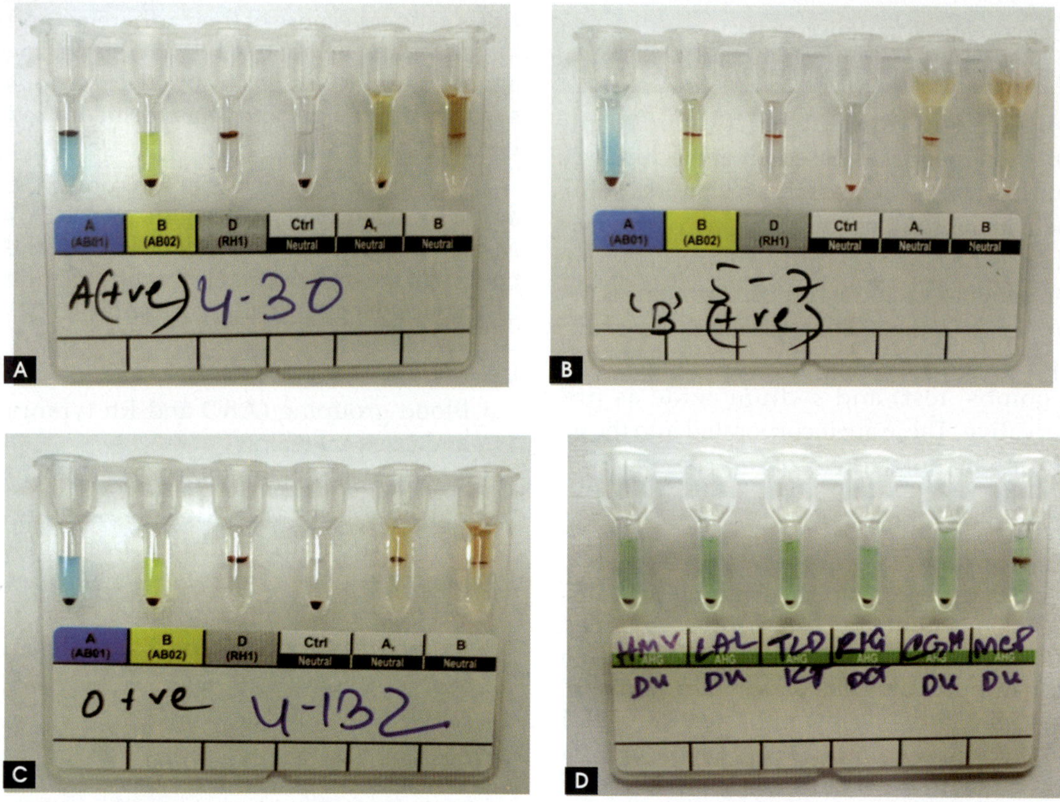

Fig. 8.6A to D: (A to C) showing ABO blood grouping in gel card method. (A) Blood group A+; (B) Blood group B+, (C) Blood group O+. There are six tubes. First one contains anti-A serum, second one contains anti-B serum, third tube contains anti-D serum, fourth tube is control, fifth tube contains antigen A_1, and sixth (last) tube contains antigen B. Particular agglutination is marked by a ring in the middle of that corresponding tube; (D) It shows Du blood grouping system. Among the six cases, only last case is Du positive

ii. It needs small sample volume and reduces exposure to biohazardous samples.
iii. This method has greater sensitivity compared to conventional methods.
iv. Cell washing is not required for Coombs' test.
v. Chances of error is almost absent as this is not done manually.

Disadvantage: It is expensive compared to conventional glass and tube method. Also it needs a special centrifuge.

SOLID PHASE ADHERENCE TECHNOLOGY

This method of cell grouping uses a microplate in which solid phase walls are coated with reagent RBCs or red cell stroma. Serum sample is added to it and if there is antibody in the serum it is captured by the antigen(s) over RBC surface/stroma. Then indicator RBCs (coated with monoclonal IgG) are added and the mixture is centrifuged. This indicator RBCs now attach to the antibody which was captured by coated RBCs. Agglutination occurs and is indicated by diffuse adherence of indicator red cells along the microwell (positive test). If there is no antibody in serum, then there is no agglutination (haemagglutination). This is indicated by RBCs forming a button at the bottom of the microwell (negative test) (Tables 8.7 and 8.8).

Table 8.7: Cause of unexpected results (false-positive or false-negative) during blood grouping

Cell grouping (forward grouping)	
Unexpected negative	**Unexpected positive**
i. ABO subgroup ii. Antisera stored improperly iii. High levels of soluble blood group substances iv. Antigenic suppression seen is leukaemia or cancer	i. Polyagglutinable RBCs ii. Acquired B antigens, seen in gastric or colon cancer, intestinal obstruction iii. Foetomaternal haemorhage iv. Wrong (out-of-group) transfusion v. RBCs coated by Wharton's jelly of umbilical cord vi. Bone marrow transplantation

Table 8.8: Serum grouping (reverse grouping)

Unexpected negative	Unexpected positive
i. ABO subgroup ii. Newborn and elderly persons iii. Immunosuppression iv. Hypogammaglobulinaemia	i. Monoclonal antibodies (immunoglobulins) ii. Transfusion of plasma components iii. Cold-reacting agglutinins

VIVA VOCE

Q1. What is Bombay blood group?

Ans: Both antigens A and B on RBCs are formed from H substance (H antigen). The dominant H gene is located on chromosome 19. This H gene encodes for an enzyme that converts a carbohydrate precursor substance present in red cell into H substance (H antigen). A and B genes encode for specific transferase enzymes that convert H substance into A and B red cell antigens. O gene encodes for inactive transferase enzyme that cannot convert H substance in blood group O red cells.

Rarely, persons do not inherit H gene (very rare HH genotype) and they are unable to produce H substance (H antigen). So, they cannot produce A and B blood group antigens on RBC membrane. This rare blood group is called Bombay blood group or Oh group. It was first discovered in Bombay, Maharashtra, among Marathi speaking people. Hence, it was named Bombay blood group. As, there is absence of blood group antigen A, B and H on RBC membrane, the plasma of Bombay blood group people will contain anti-A, anti-B and anti-H antibodies.

Q2. What are the subtypes of blood group A?

Ans: There are two subtypes—A_1 and A_2 in blood group A. A_1 subgroup is 80% and A_2 subgroup is 20% based on the presence of A_1 antigen or A_2 antigen on RBCs. A_1 has greater number of antigenic site than A_2 (10^6 site vs. 250,000 site). A potent anti-A_1 serum (anti-A_1) can agglutinate A_1 red cells but not A_2 red cells. There is no specific anti-A_2 serum. So, A_2 red cell does not agglutinate and pretends to be blood group O.

However, a saline extract of seeds of *Dolichos biflorus* is now routinely used in subtyping A blood cells (RBCs). It agglutinates A_1 blood cells and A_1B blood cells.

Saline extract of seeds of *Ulex europaeus* is used to agglutinate A_2, A_2B and O cells. It is actually an anti-H lectin.

Q3. Why reverse grouping (serum grouping) is not done before 4 months of age in infants?

Ans: There are no corresponding natural antibodies as regard to antigen(s) present on RBCs in infants below 4 months of age. So, reverse grouping (serum grouping) will give inaccurate result. It will pretend to be blood group AB as serum lacks any natural antibody.

Q4. Which method is better for blood grouping—tube method or slide method and why?

Ans: The tube method is better because the reaction between red cells and anti-serum is enhanced because of centrifugation to make red cell suspension. So, even the weaker antigen like A_2 can be detected apart from other/strong antigen(s). Tube method is recommended for both ABO and Rh blood grouping.

Q5. How would you distinguish agglutination from rouleaux formation?

Ans: When dilution with saline is done, it disperses rouleaux but cannot disperse agglutinated cells. Because agglutinated cells (antigen–antibody bonds) are firmly attached with each other.

Q6. Other than alloagglutination, what are the other causes of agglutination?

Ans: i. Autoagglutination: It is due to presence of cold agglutinin.

ii. Pseudoagglutination: It is aggregates red cells due to nonimmunological cause like excess rouleaux formation as seen in multiple myeloma, or in macroglobulinaemia (due to high level of paraproteins in blood).

iii. Polyagglutination or pan agglutination: If RBCs are contaminated by certain bacteria like *Pseudomonas aeruginosa*, then RBCs may be agglutinated by all blood group sera (antibody) or even by normal human serum. This phenomenon is known as **Thomson-Friedenreich phenomenon**. It is due to unmasking of a particular antigen (T or Tk antigen), which is present on human RBCs. Human serum contains anti-T antibody normally. So, when T antigens on RBCs are unmasked, agglutination occurs in blood groups. This is very rarely observed *in vivo*. *Ex vivo* (*in vitro*), it can be demonstrated by use of an anti-T lectin prepared from peanut.

Q7. What do you mean by one unit of blood?

Ans: Usually one unit of whole blood means 350 ml of whole blood mixed with 49 ml of anticoagulant CPDA-1 (citrate phosphate dextrose adenine 1).

Q8. How blood and blood products are stored?

Ans:
i. Whole blood and packed red cells: At 2 to 6°C in refrigerator for 35 days.
ii. Platelet concentrate: At 20 to 24°C for 3 days with continuous agitation.
iii. Fresh frozen plasma: Below –25°C for one year.
iv. Cryoprecipitate: Below –25°C for one year.

Q9. What is chimerism that can be found unexpectedly during blood grouping?

Ans: Sometimes a blood sample may contain more than one population of red cells. It may result from (i) transfusion of ABO compatible but not ABO-identical blood, (ii) foetomaternal haemorrhage and (iii) bone marrow transplantation (when blood group of donor is different from that of recipient).

Q10. What do you mean by major cross-match and minor cross-match?

Ans: The name 'cross-match' came from the past practice of testing, the recipient's serum against donor's RBCs (major cross-match) and donor's serum against recipient's RBCs (minor cross-match). However, minor cross-match is less important as antibodies in donor blood becomes diluted or neutralized in recipient's plasma (volume is more than donor unit). Minor cross-match is also less important for antibody screening and identification.

Q11. What are the advantages of gel card method for blood grouping?

Ans: In gel card method, the monoclonal antibodies are used (unlike polyclonal antibodies in other methods). So, it is very sensitive and weak antigens can also be detected.

Q12. When blood group of a person can be changed to other blood group?

Ans:
i. Almost always, an individual has the same blood group for life, but very rarely an individual's blood type changes through addition or suspension of an antigen in infections, autoimmune diseases or malignancies.
ii. Another rare cause in blood group change is bone marrow transplantation.
iii. Bacterial contamination: Infection of RBCs by bacteria both *in vivo* and *in vitro* may cause polyagglutination in normal sera. Bacterial enzymes expose T receptors on RBC surface. As most human sera contain anti-T antibodies, such infected red cells get agglutinated in normal serum. Hence, blood group O may appear as blood group AB.

iv. Scientist has discovered a particular enzyme called 98 glycoside hydrolase, extracted from a strain of *Streptococcus pneumoniae*. The enzyme can cut away A or B antigens in blood group A, B or AB to make them more like blood group O. The scientist published their results in *Journal of the American Chemical Society*.

Q13. How different blood groups are associated with disease?

Ans: Persons with blood group A, B or AB will have more chance of heart attacks and heart diseases (due to coronary artery disease) and diabetes compared to blood group O. These people are more likely to develop cognition and memory loss (may be due to high blood pressure and high cholesterol). People with blood group A have been found to have a higher risk of stomach cancer. In blood group O, malaria is less severe. People who are Duffy antigen negative get protection from *P.vivax* infection.

Blood Group A : Heart disease, Stomach cancer.
Blood Group B: Heart disease, pancreatic cancer
Blood Group AB: Thromboembolism (blood clots), dementia
Blood Group O: Skin cancer, renal cancer

Q14. Why blood grouping of partners is done before marriage?

Ans: It is a good idea to know partner's blood group in the event of an emergency (for blood donation). Also knowing blood group is important for pregnancy and Rh factor should be known. If father is Rh +ve and mother is Rh –ve , it may cause Rh incompatibility (usually second and next pregnancies). This Rh incompatibility may cause hemolytic diseases of newborn (HDNB). So, in these cases pregnancies are monitored closely. Also, if needed Rh immunoglobulin (RhoGAM) is given to mother in the 7th month of pregnancy and again within 72 hours after delivery.

Chapter

9

Haemoparasites

HAEMOPARASITES (PARASITES IN PERIPHERAL BLOOD AND BONE MARROW)

Some parasites are found in peripheral blood and bone marrow.

Parasites Found in PBS (Peripheral Blood Smear) and Bone Marrow

- Malaria: Most common parasite found in PBS
- Microfilaria of *Wuchereria bancrofti*
- *Leishmania donovani* or LD bodies of kala-azar: Found free or inside monocytes. Mainly found in the reticuloendothelial cells (macrophages) and megakaryocytes of bone marrow.
- *Trypanosoma cruzi* (causative organism of Chagas' disease)
- Others: Babesia, Brugia, Mansonella, etc. rarely.

Some parasites can be blood-borne. That means

i. The parasite can be found in the blood stream of infected people; and
ii. The parasites may spread to other people through exposure to an infected person's blood (for example, by blood transfusion or by sharing needle or syringes contaminated with blood).

Examples of parasitic diseases which can be blood-borne include African trypanosomiasis (caused by *Trypanosoma brucei*), babesiosis (caused by Babesia, a type of Apicomplexa and also known as Nuttallia), Chagas' disease, leishmaniasis, malaria and toxoplasmosis (caused by *Toxoplasma gondii*). In nature, many blood-borne parasites are spread by insects (vectors) like mosquitoes, sandflies, bugs, ticks, lice, mites, etc. So, they are called vector-borne diseases. But *Toxoplasma gondii* is not transmitted by a vector (by eating infected cooked food which contains cysts).

A parasite is an organism that lives in another organism, called the host, and often harms it. They depend on their host, and often harms it. They depend on their host for survival.

Without a host, a parasite cannot live, grow and multiply. Parasites, unlike predators, are usually much smaller than their host and they reproduce at a faster rate. A parasite either lives within the parts of the body of host or it lives on (outside but in contact) host. Parasites themselves are not diseases but they can spread diseases. The parasite uses hosts resources to fuel its life cycle. It uses host's resources to maintain itself.

Endoparasites: These live inside the host. Examples are tapeworm, hookworm, roundworm, etc. Endoparasites rely on a third organism, known as vector, or carrier.

Epiparasites: These feed on other parasites in a relationship known as hyperparasitism. As for example, a flea may live on a dog, but the flea may have a protozoan in its digestive tract. The protozoan is the hyperparasite.

Types of Parasites

i. **Protozoa:** A protozoa can only multiply or divide within the host. Examples are Plasmodium (malaria), leishmanias, Trypanosoma in blood or bone marrow, *Entamoeba histolytica* (amoebiasis) or Trichomonas in intestine.
ii. **Helminths:** These are worm parasites. Examples are Schistosomiasis, pin-worm, tapeworm, roundworm, etc.
iii. **Ectoparasites:** These live on their hosts (not inside). Examples are lice and fleas.

The important haemoparasites are: (1) Malarial parasites, (2) microfilaria, (3) trypanosomes, (4) leishmaniasis and (5) babesiosis.

Infection with haemoparasites (blood parasites, particularly malaria and filaria may cause enormous human sufferings especially in Indian subcontinent. Malaria and micro-filaria can be diagnosed by careful examination of PBS but bone marrow examination is necessary for diagnosis of Leishmania.

MALARIA

There are four species of Plasmodium (malarial parasites which infect humans: *Plasmodium vivax*, *Plasmodium falciparum*, *Plasmodium malaria* and *Plasmodium ovale*. Among these four species *P. vivax* is the most widely distributed species in the world. In India, incidence is *P. vivax* (70%), *P. falciparurm* (25–30%), mixed infection of *P. vivax* and *P. falciparum* (4–8%) and *P. malariae* (<1%). *P. malariae* has been reported in the Eastern India state of Odisha (Sharna et. al, 2006), while *P. ovale* appears to be extremely rare, if not absent. Odisha has the highest incidence of malaria (40% of all malarial cases in India as per ICMR, 2019).

P. vivax and *P. ovale* both of which cause benign tertian malaria (febrile episodes typically occuring at 48 hours intervals). *P. falciparum*, which is accountable for most deaths due to malaria (malignant malaria and febrile episodes typically occurring at 72 hours intervals). *P. malariae* and *falciparum* may cause nephrotic syndrome (Table 9.1 and Figs 9.1 and 9.2).

Role of Genetic Factors in Malaria

- **Duffy antigen:** People with **Duffy antigen negative** blood group or the Fy (a^-b^-) phenotype in blacks confers protection against *P. vivax* infection. This is due to the fact that *P. vivax* parasite enters RBC at glycophorin receptors present on Duffy antigen site. Black people of West Africa have this immunity towards *P. vivax* as they lack Duffy antigens on red cells. But this protection is available to homozygous people (homozygotes) only.
- **G6PD (Glucose-6-phosphate dehydrogenase) deficiency:** G6PD deficient female heterozygotes get protection against falciparun malaria (*P. falciparum* infection).
- **Sickle cell trait:** Heterozygous patients of sickle cell trait will have comparatively milder form of falciparum malaria. But the homozygotes do not have this advantage.
- **β-Thalassaemia trait:** They also get protection against falciparum malaria.
- HbC and pyruvate kinase deficiency also give protection against malaria.
- **Newborns:** Newborn infants have high level of foetal haemoglobin or HbF (4–6 months of early life) until replaced by adult haemoglobin. HbF is markedly increased in a disease called hereditary persistence of foetal haemoglobin (HPFH) which may be present both in children and in adults. HbF in red cells suppresses the growth of malarial parasite. So, newborns (4–6 months) and patients of HPFH get protection against malaria.

- **HLA subtype:** Certain HLA antigens like class I antigen HLA-BW53 and class II antigen HLA-DRBI 1302 offers some sort immunity against malaria.

WHO Criteria for Severe Malaria

If anyone if these features is present, it is called severe malaria:

- Hyperparasitemia (>5% parasitised RBCs in low endemic area and >10% in hyper-endemic area).
- Renal impairment [serum creatinine (>3.5 mg/dl)]
- Hypoglycaemia (blood glucose <40 mg/dl)
- Unconsciousness or coma
- Prostration (extremely weak or subservient)
- Circulatory collapse or shock
- Multiple convulsions
- Clinical jaundice along with dysfunction of vital organs
- Haemoglobinuria
- Respiratory distress/acidotic breathing
- Metabolic acidosis

Table 9.1: Different features of *P. vivax* and *P. falciparum*

Features	*P. vivax*	*P. falciparum*
Distribution	Tropical countries, subtropics, temperate zones	Tropical countries
Incubation period	8–10 days	8–10 days
RBC infected	Young red cells	All stages of RBCs
Severity of disease	Moderate to severe	Severe
Periodicity of symptoms	48 hours	36–48 hours
Relapse	Yes (due to hepatic hypnozoites)	No
Nephrotic syndrome	Rare	May be
CNS involvement	Rare	Frequent
Microscopic examination		
Form in PBS	Trophozoites (ring form), schizonts and gametocytes	Trophozoites (ring form) and crescents (gametocytes) only. No schizont.
Trophozoite and ring form	Usually single size 2.5 μm; cytoplasm opposite nucleus is thicker. Ring 1/3 diameter of RBC	Single and/ or multiple rings, size of ring smaller 1.25–1.5 μm; cytoplasm regular in outline ring 1/6th diameter of RBC
Nuclei	Single chromatin dots	Single or multiple chromatin dots
Infected RBCs	RBCs are enlarged and pale, Schüffner's dots present	Normal size RBC but crenated, raddish violet colour, Maurer's dot (6–12 in number) in cytoplasm of RBC
Accole' or Applique	Absent	Present. As the parasite attaches itself to the margin or the edge of host cell (RBC), the nucleus and a small part of cytoplasm remains almost outside giving the appearance of 'form applique' or 'accole'.
Schizonts	Size 9–10 μm regular almost completely fill RBC	Size 4–5 μm, fills 2/3 of RBC
Merozoites	12–24 in number, irregularly arranged (grape-like clusters) yellowish brown, fine granules	18–32, arranged like grape-like clusters

Contd.

Table 9.1: Different features of *P. vivax* and *P. falciparum* (Contd.)

Microscopic examination	*P. vivax*	*P. falciparum*
Gametocyte	Spherical or globular much larger than RBC	Crescentic or sickle-shaped larger than a RBC but host cell (RBC) hardly recognisable
Haemozoin	Yellowish-brown, fine granules	Dark brown or blackish
Schüffner's dots or Maurer's dots in cytoplasm	Schüffner's dots	Maurer's dots

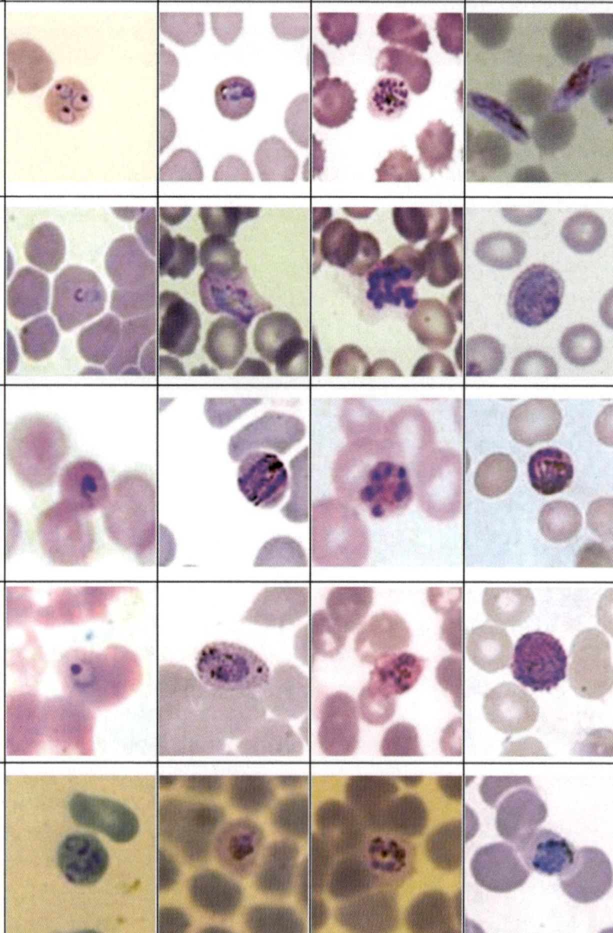

Stages / Species	Ring	Trophozoite	Schizont	Gametocyte	
P. falciparum					• Parasitised red cells (pRBCs) not enlarged. • RBCs containing mature trophozoites sequestered in deep vessels. • Total parasite biomass = circulating parasites + sequestered parasites.
P. vivax					• Parasitised prefer young red cells • pRBCs enlarged. • Trophozoites are amoeboid in shape. • All stages present in peripheral blood.
P. malariae					• Parasitised prefer old red cells. • pRBCs not enlarged. • Trophozoites tend to have a band shape. • All stages present in peripheral blood
P. ovale					• pRBCs slightly enlarged and have an oval shape with tufted ends. • All stages present in peripheral blood
P. knowlesi					• pRBCs not enlarged. • Trophozoites, pigment spreads inside cytoplasm, like *P. malariae*, band form may be seen • Multiple invasion and high parasitaemia can be seen like *P. falciparum* • All stages present in peripheral blood.

Fig. 9.1: Human malaria

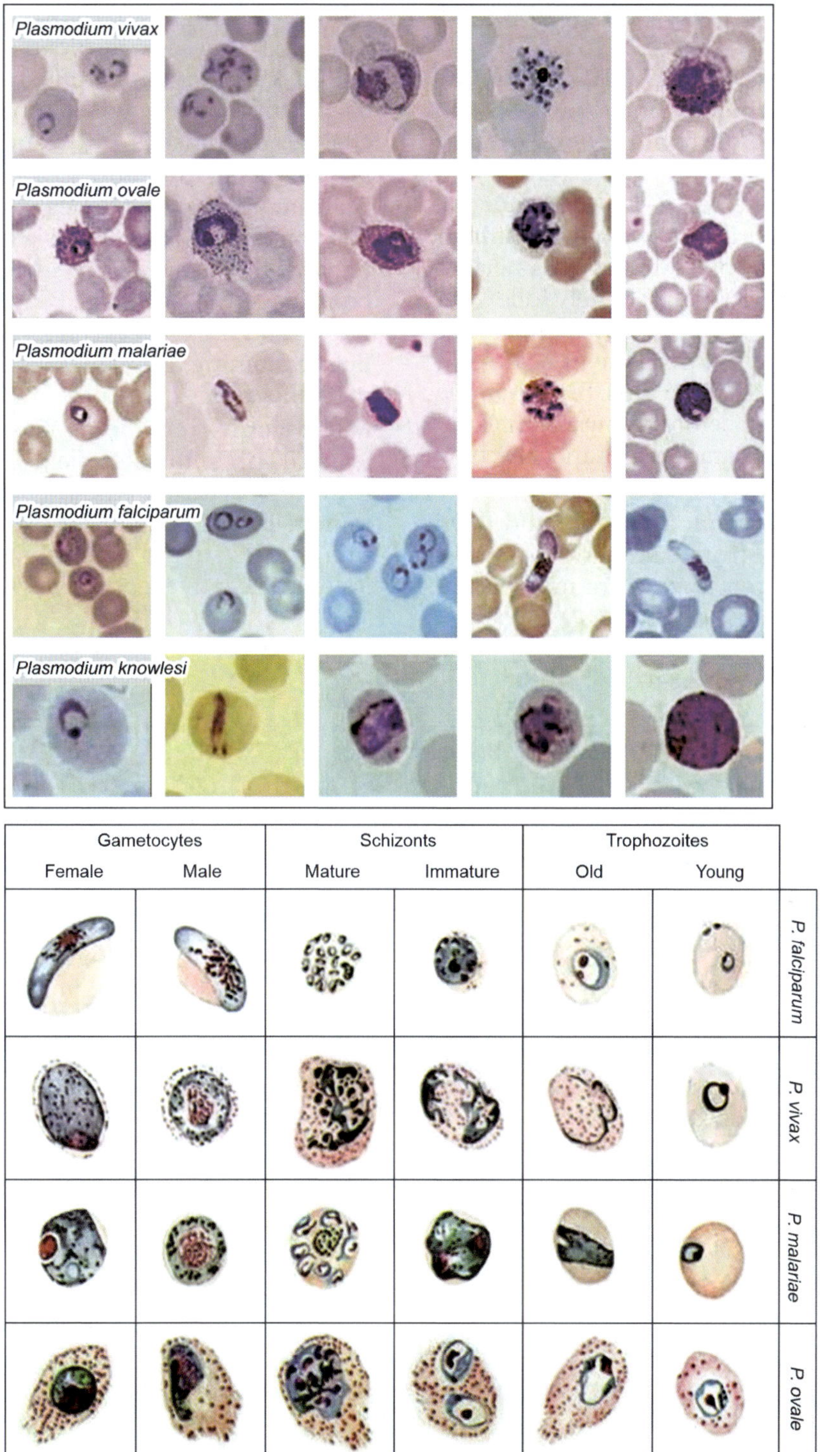

Fig. 9.2: Different species of human malaria

MICROSCOPIC EXAMINATION FOR MALARIA

- **Collection of blood:** Blood smear should be obtained before or at the onset of fever and chills. Some advocate that blood should be collected 2–6 hours after the peak of the febrile paroxysms, as number of parasites is more during this period, collection of blood immediately following a paroxysm of fever usually do not show intraerythrocytic parasites because of lysis of parasitized red cells. Blood sample should be taken before giving antimalarial drugs (if given, parasites to number become less in bloody).
- **Smear preparation:** Both thin, and thick smears made from a finger-prick (skin puncture). Then smears are made immediately. Anticoagulated blood is not preferred. If necessary, blood is collected in EDTA and smears are prepared as early as possible, otherwise, morphologic changes of parasites will occur and diagnosis may be difficult.
- **Staining of smears:** One thick smear and one thin smear are stained with Giemsa on Leishman stain. Thick smear also can be stained by Field's stain. For preparation of thin and trick smear refer to Chapter 2. Before staining, thin smear is fixed with methanol for 1–2 minutes.
- **Microscopic fields to be examined:** At least 100 oil immersion fields (requires 5 minutes) of thick smears and 200 oil immersion fields (requires 15 minutes) of thin smears should be examined 'before issuing a negative report (Figs 9.3 and 9.4).

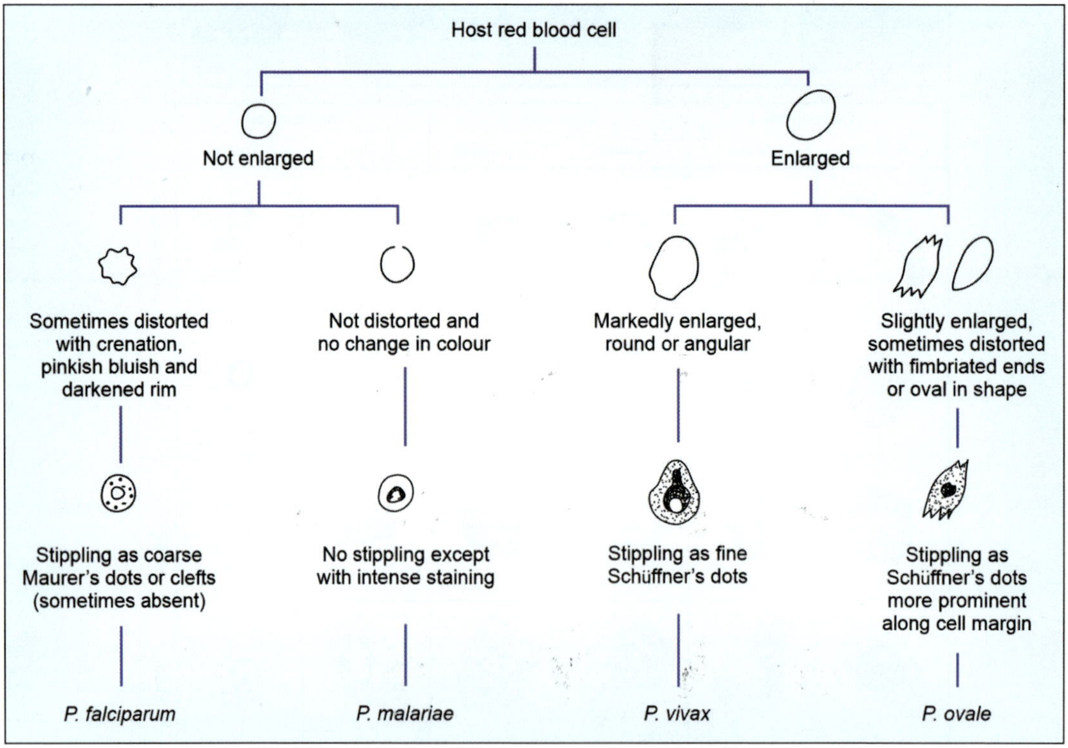

Fig. 9.3: Schematic diagram to diagnose four different species of malaria

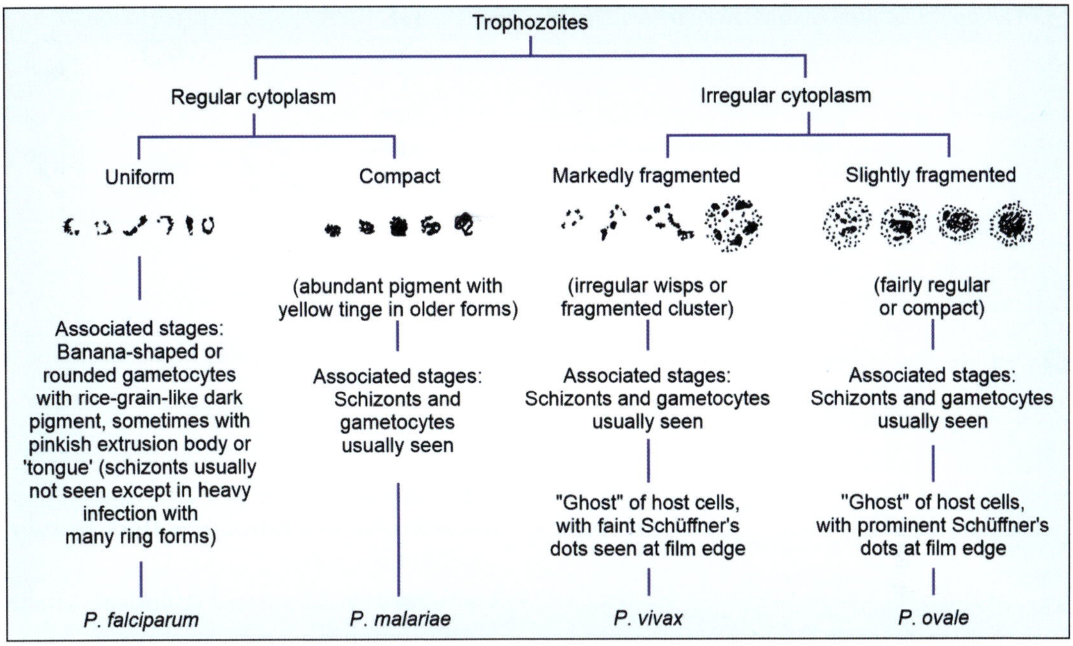

Fig. 9.4: Species differentiation of malarial parasites by cytoplasmic pattern of trophozoites in Giemsa-stained thick blood films

PLASMODIUM FALCIPARUM (*P. FALCIPARUM*)

In the peripheral blood trophozoites, and gametocytes are present. Schizonts are rarely found in PBS.

- **Early trophozoites:** A delicate small uniformly fine cytoplasmic ring with 1–2 small chromatin dots. Ring may be attached (protruding) to the red cell margin (accole form).
- **Late trophozoites:** Compact blue ring with 1–2 red chromatin dots.
- **Schizont:** Very rarely seen except in cerebral malaria. It contains 18–32 merozoites which fill 2/3rds of the RBC.
- **Gametocyte:** Crescentic or sickle or sausage or banana-shaped and larger than RBC (Figs 9.5 and 9.6).

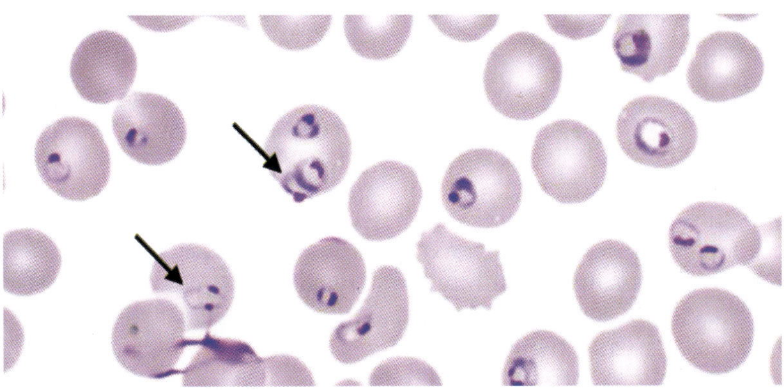

Fig. 9.5: Trophozoites of *P. falciparum*

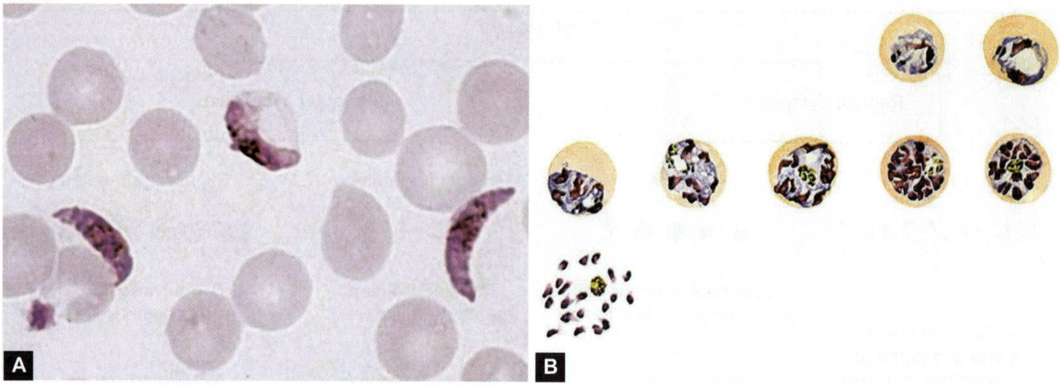

Fig. 9.6: (A) Gametocytes of *P. falciparum;* (B) Schizonts of *P. falciparum*

> **Note**
>
> - **Signet ring form** and **marginal form** usually seen with young or early trophozoites.
> - **Maurer's dots** are seen in the cytoplasm of RBC with early trophozoites. Maurer's dots (also called Maurer's clefts) are red colored granules present in the cytoplasm. They are usually larger and more coarse than Schüffner's dots (found in P. *vivax* and *P. ovale*). Like Schüffner's dots, Maurer's dots appear to play a role in the metabolic pathways of the infected RBCs.
> - In late or mature trophozoites showing haze of pigments may be seen throughout the cytoplasm. Maurer's dots may be found in the cell.
> - Gametocytes may be microgametocyte or macrogametocyte or it may be immature or mature. Remember only mature macrogametocytes are crescentic or banana-shaped. Gametocytes may be male gametocyte (cytoplasm pale blue, nucleus diffuse and larger) or female gametocyte (cytoplasm blue, nucleus small and compact).

Plasmodium vivax (P. vivax) (Fig. 9.7)

Trophozoites, schizonts and gametocytes, i.e. all stages may be found in the peripheral blood (PBS).

- Early trophozoites: Blue cytoplasmic ring, 1/3rd the diameter of RBC. One side of the ring thicker; red chromatin at thinner part of ring.
- Late trophozoites: Irregularly thick cytoplasmic ring (amoeboid form); large red chromatin dot.
- Schizonts: 12–24 merozoites arranged like a rosette with granular yellow-brown pigment in center.
- Gametocytes: Large and spherical. Much larger than RBC.

> **Note**
>
> - Pseudopodia may be found in polychromatophilic erythrocyte
> - Microgametocytes (male): Size: 9–10 μm; cytoplasm: stains light blue; Nucleus: Diffuse large, lies laterally
> - Macrogametocytes (female): Size:10–12 μm, cytoplasm: stains deep blue; Nucleus: Small compact, lies peripherally.
> - Early trophozoite has a cytoplasmic ring (blue), a red nuclear mass (chromatin dot), and an unstained area called **nutrient vacuole**.
> - The trophozoites possess a very active amoeboid movement and constantly thrusts out pseudopodia inside the RBC, giving rise to diverse forms.
> - After a period of about 10 hours, yellowish brown pigment (hemozoin) granules appear in the cytoplasm.
> - Schizont appears after a period of growth of about 36–40 hours and represent full grown (mature) trophozoites. At this stage the parasite becomes rounded in shape and has lost all amoeboid activities. According to the stage, the schizont may be immature, schizont (nucleus not divided) and mature schizont (nucleus divided) (Fig. 9.5).

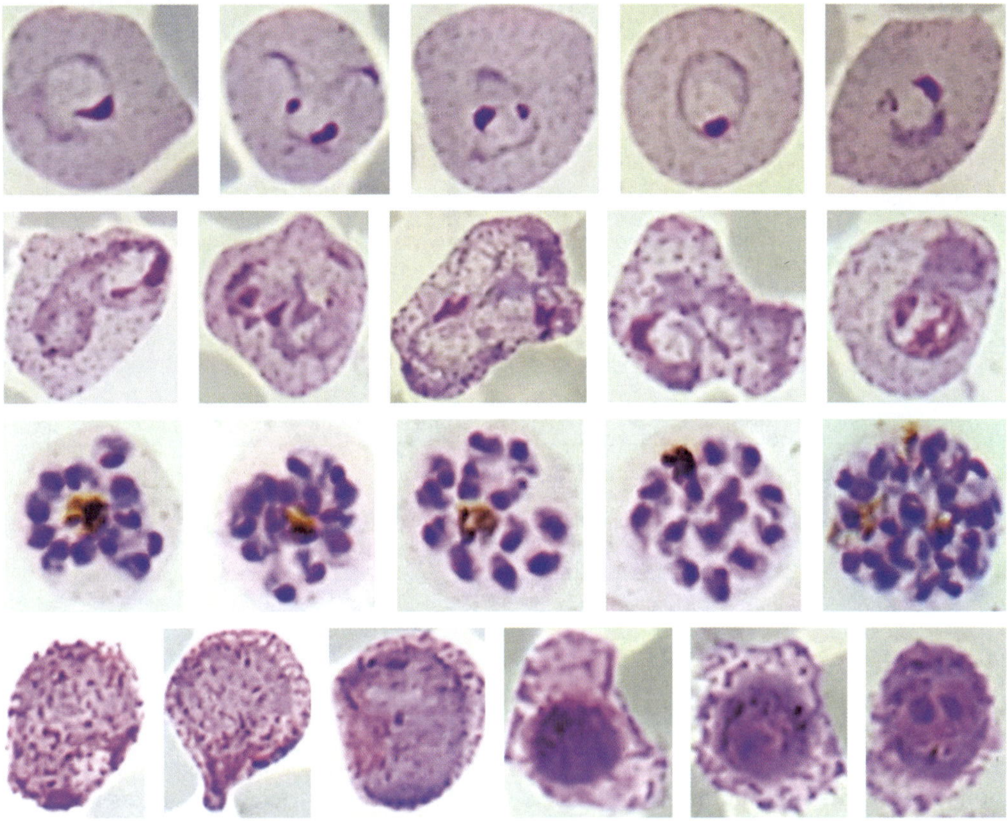

Fig. 9.7: *Plasmodium vivax.* First row: Early trophozoites, Second row: Late trophozoites, Third row: Schizonts, Fourth row: Gametocytes

THICK SMEAR FOR MALARIAL DETECTION

Preparation and straining: Thick smear is prepared by spreading a large drop of blood from center of a glass slide. It is spreaded with the corner of a spreader slide or a stick in such a manner that an evenly spread circular or rectangular smear of size 15 × 15 mm is obtained.

After that smears are air dried. For better results, thick smears can be dried in an incubator at 37°C for 15 minutes. Thick smears are not fixed in methanol (unlike thin smears) as they will be dehaemoglobinised.

The smears are then given a few dips in tap water until red coloured solution comes out (**dehaemoglobinisation of the smear**) Now, the smear is fixed in methanol (after dip in tap water) and stained with Leishman's or Giemsa or Field's stain.

Thick smear is a concentration method for malarial parasites. One microscopic field (oil immersion) of thick smear is equivalent to 40–50 microscopic fields of a thin smear. However, thin smear is essential for morphology and to characterize the type of malarial parasites. Thick smear is of use for quick detection or for mass surveys (Fig. 9.8).

Malarial Pigments

Due to parasitemia of RBCs, physiology of red cell is disturbed, globin part of the haemoglobin is broken down and resynthesized into parasite protein. The unutilized

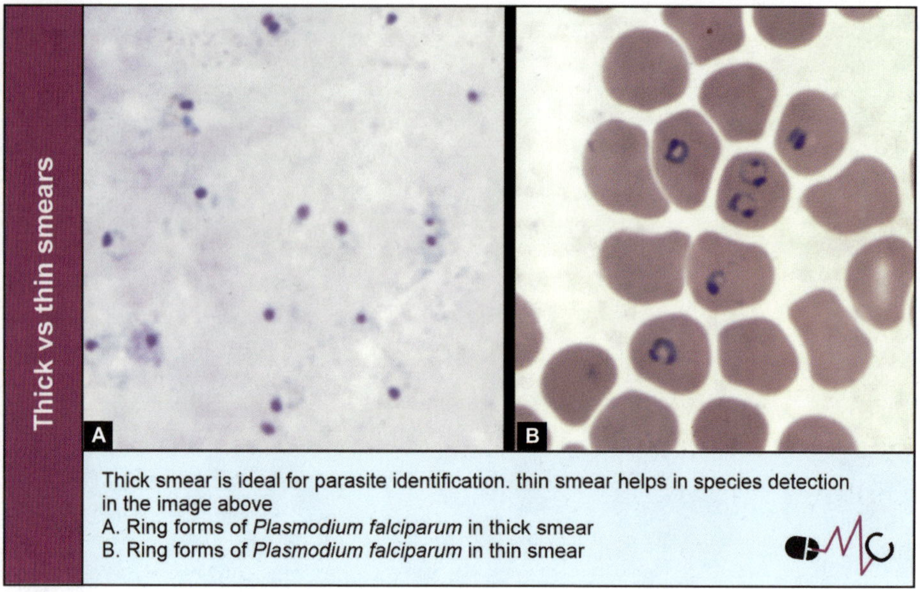

Fig. 9.8: *Plasmodium falciparum*; (A) Thick smear; (B) Thin smear

part of globin is called **haemozoin**—a brown coloured pigment presents in the parasite and known as **malarial pigment**. Haemozoin is responsible for the pigmentation of various organs like liver, spleen, brain, etc. (Fig. 9.9).

Parasite Density (PD)

High density of parasite is associated with a severe disease. The prognosis becomes worse if mature form of parasites (with malarial pigment) predominates in blood. This means prognosis will be better if PBS shows only ring forms (early trophozoites) and >50% of all forms. Prognosis will be bad if PBS shows many mature trophozoites and schizonts (>20% in number).

To calculate parasite density, 200 WBCs are counted on a **thick smear**. Number of parasites present per µl of blood is calculated from this formula:

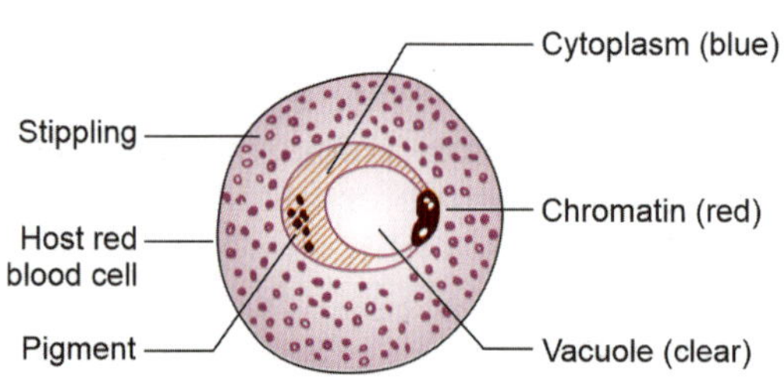

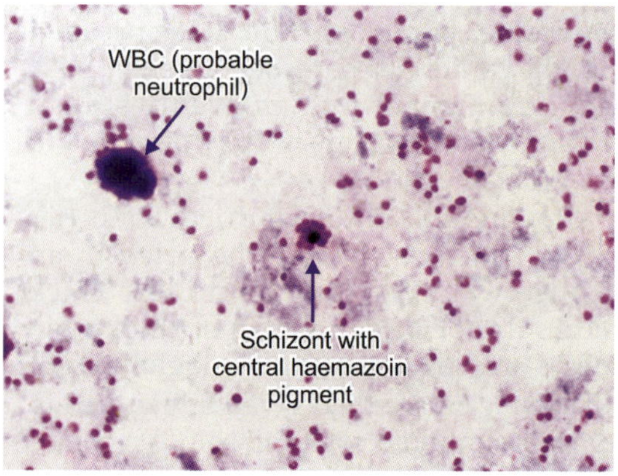

Fig. 9.9: Malarial pigments

Parasite density (PD) on thick smear

$$= \text{Total WBC count}/\mu l \times \frac{\textit{Number of parasites}}{200}$$

that is (total WBC count/µl × Number of parasites) ÷ 200

Assuming a WBC count of 8000/µl, the number of parasites is multiplied by 40 to get PD. However, if accurate WBC count is known, then a better estimate of PD is obtained.

In a **thin smear**, number of parasites amongst 1000 RBCs is counted and reported as a percentage. Number of parasites in 1 µl of blood can be calculated if RBC count in millions/µl is known.

PD on thin smear = Red cell count in millions/µl × Parasite percentage, i.e. number of parasites in 1 µl of blood or PD.

If the RBC count is not known, then it can be arbitrarily taken as 5 millions/µl.

Significance of parasite density (PD)

i. Calculation of PD is of significance in *P. falciparum* infection. PD >10% is an indication for exchange transfusion.

ii. For effective antimalarial treatment (treatment response), percent parasitemia should be calculated (PD) daily till no more parasites (excluding gametocytes) are found.

Parasite Index (PI)

This is calculated by estimating the number of parasitised RBCs among 1000 RBCs. Only asexual forms (ring, trophozoite and schizont) are included for calculating the PI (parasite index). The parasite load is graded on a scale of I–IV corresponding to 0–5%, 6–10%, 11–20% and > 20%. This is calculated on thin smears So,

PI (Parasite index) =

$$\frac{\textit{Number of parasitised RBCs}}{1000\ \textit{RBCs}} \times 100\%$$

Blood Alterations in Malaria

PBS also shows monocytosis with moderate leukopenia. Two-thirds of patients infected with *P. falciparum* infection also show anaemia with to increased reticulocyte count (due to haemolysis) and thrombocytopenia.

Anaemia progressively becomes progressively severe due to hypersplenism.

Reporting of Smear (Result)

In the presence of malarial parasites, blood smear should be reported as follows:

- Smear is positive or negative for malarial parasite
- Name of species (*P. vivax* or *P. falciparum* or mixed, etc.)
- Red cell stages (early trophozoite, ring form, late trophozoite, schizont, gametocyte, accole form, amoeboid form, etc.)
- Parasite density (especially in *P. falciparum*).

RAPID TEST FOR MALARIA: MICROTYPING TEST (GEL CARD)

Recently, simple nonmicroscopic, rapid diagnostic kits are available in the market. These tests detect malarial antigen by immunochromatographic method. The antigens against which commercial test kits presently available are:

- **Parasite, lactate dehydrogenase (pLDH):** This is an enzyme of glycolytic pathway which is present in all four human malarial species. But there are forms of LDH for each species. Level of pLDH correlates with parasite density.
- **Parasite aldolase:** Aldolase based tests are less sensitive for non-falciparum species.
- **Histidine rich protein 2 (HRP-2):** It is synthesized by asexual stages and young gametocytes of *P. falciparum* and expressed on red cell surface.

Of the different antigenic tests, **gel card,** or **microtyping test** for malarial pLDH antigen is very popular. For this test, 10 µl of fresh/frozen/dried whole blood is taken. RBCs are lysed and pLDH from parasitized RBCs is released. Presence of pLDH is detected using monoclonal antibodies against specific epitomes of pLDH (immunochromatographic test: Optimal).

Test based on HRP-2 is useful to detect *P. falciparum* infection. But HRP-2 antigens remain longer in circulation than pLDH. So, more false + ve cases may be reported even after malarial treatment: (immunochromatographic test: Optimal).

Positive test indicates active Plasmodium infection and it can differentiate various species of malarial species. It can also determine strains of Plasmodium resistant to therapy by repeating the test 48 hours after treatment (Fig. 9.10).

Other Methods of Malarial Detection

i. **Fluorescent microscopy:** Nucleic acids of the parasite are stained, with fluorescent dyes and visualized by fluorescent microscopy.
ii. **PCR based test**: These tests are based on the detection of nucleic acid sequence specific to *Plasmodium* species. Primers targeting the *Plasmodium* species 18S rRNA genes are used.

Artifacts Mimicking Malaria on Smears

- The most common artifact in thin smear/films are blood **platelets superimposed on red blood cells**. These platelets should be readily identified because they do not have a true ring form. Platelets do not show differentiation of the chromatin and cytoplasm and do not contain pigments.
- **Clumps bacteria or platelets** may be confused with schizonts.
- At times, masses of fused platelets may resemble gametocytes of *P. falciparum* but do not show the differential staining or the pigment.
- Precipitated stain and contaminating bacteria, fungi, or spores may also be confused with these parasites.

Filaria (*Wuchereria bancrofti*)

Wuchereria bancrofti is confined to tropical and subtropical regions. In India, the disease is confined to the regions along the banks of big rivers, and sea coast. Adult worms localize in the lymphatic vessels and lymph nodes causing lymphatic obstruction to lymph flow resulting in lymphedema and elephantiasis. Embryos of *W. bancrofti* (microfilaria) pass through lymph nodes, lymphatics and enters circulating blood.

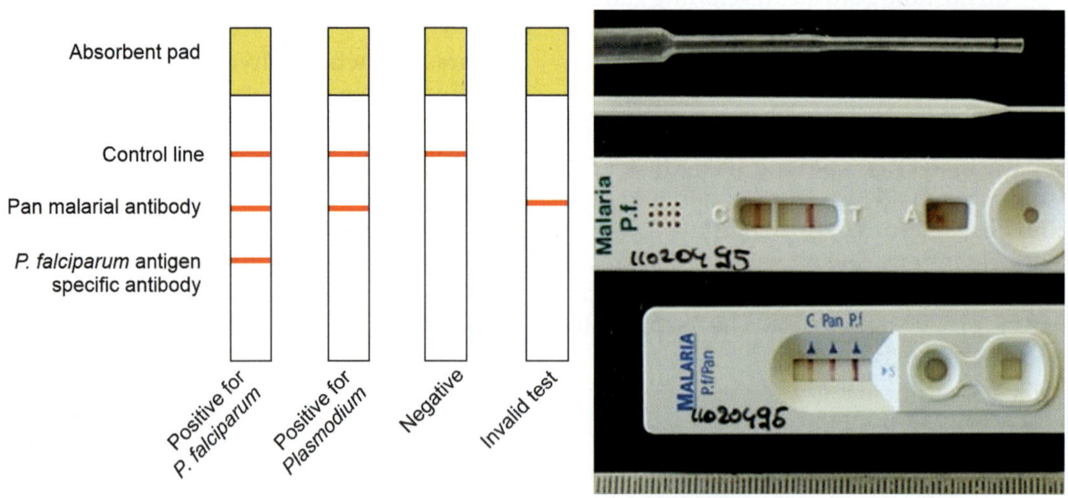

Fig. 9.10: Rapid diagnostic kits for malaria

Demonstration of this microfilaria in PBS is diagnostic clue of filariasis.

Collection of blood: The blood sample should be collected at night between 10 pm and 2 am as microfilariae exhibit nocturnal periodicity. Midnight smears can also be examined.

From blood sample, microfilariae can be demonstrated in

i. Thin blood smear
ii. Thick blood smear
iii. Unstained wet preparation: For this, 2–3 drops of blood are taken in a slide and a coverslip is placed. Microfilariae are recognised by their movements causing agitation of the wet smear and can be confirmed by examining under a low power objective.

  If the smear is to be examined next morning then the coverslip is sealed with Vaseline to prevent drying of blood drop.
iv. Concentration method: Take 5 ml of blood in EDTA vial. Centrifuge at 2500 r.p.m for 5 minutes. Discard the plasma and take buffy coat and sediments of cells. Make 4–6 smears out of it. Air dry, fix in methanol and stain in Romanowsky stain.

Alternatively, 5 ml blood + 10 ml distilled water is taken in a tube and the mixture is shaken vigorously till blood is completely haemolysed. Centrifuge the tube at 2500 r.p.m. for 15 minutes. Deposit after centrifugation is examined under for microfilaria.

Morphology of filaria: Microfilaria measures about 290 µm, in length and 6 µ in breadth. A hyaline sheath engulfs the larval body but hyaline sheath is longer than body. Somatic cells appear as granules and extend from head to terminal tail sheath, which is a distinguishing feature of *W. bancrofti* microfilaria (tail end free).

Bone marrow examination: Sometimes, bone marrow examination also reveals microfilariae of *W. bancrofti* (Fig. 9.11).

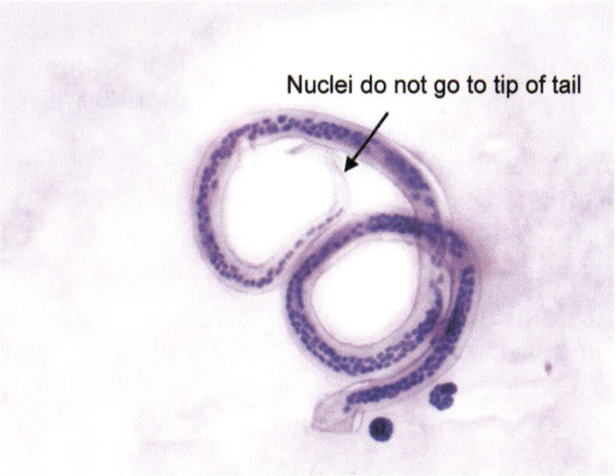

Fig. 9.11: Filaria (*Wuchereria bancrofti*) in blood

Rapid immunochromatographic test: This is a card test, highly sensitive and specific test for diagnosis of active infection caused by *Wuchereria bancrofti*. This card test is available in the market (ICT diagnostics).

This test detects circulating antigens of filaria in a finger prick blood sample. In contrast to microscopic examination, blood sample can be collected at any time of the day. There is no cross-reactivity with other filarial organism like *Brugia malayi*.

Positive result is obtained even microfilariae are not present in blood and adult worms live in lymphatics/lymph nodes. But the test may give positive result for up to 18 months following successful treatment of filariasis.

Leishmaniasis (*Leishmania donovani*)

The parasite *Leishmania donovani* (LD) causes kala-azar or visceral leishmaniasis. In India, it is endemic in the states of Bihar, Odisha, Chennai and Eastern parts of Uttar Pradesh. **Amastigote forms, known as LD bodies** can be found in the reticulum cells of bone marrow and spleen. So, **bone marrow examination and splenic puncture** is done to identify LD bodies **(amastigote form)**.

LD bodies are small, round, 2-4 µm in diameter with a nucleus and a pod-shaped kinetoplast.

Rarely LD bodies are seen free on in monocyte in peripheral blood when parasitemia is very high. So, it may be found from buffy coat preparation of peripheral blood.

PCR (molecular diagnosis): Target regions for PCR analysis are genes encoding r-RNA, repetitive nuclear DNA sequences and kinetoplast DNA. PCR which amplify a 120-bp fragment of kinetoplast DNA has the highest sensitivity (Fig. 9.12).

Trypanosomes/Trypanosoma

Trypanosoma is a unicellular parasitic protozoon. The name is derived from the Greek *trypano* (borer) and *soma* (body) because of their corkscrew-like motion. Most trypanosomes are heterogenous (requiring more than one obligatory host to complete cycle) and most are transmitted via a vector. Trypanosoma is a motile flagellate protozoon. The kinetoplast contains the mitochondrial DNA and the nucleus contains the genomic DNA.

Trypanosomes infect variety of hosts and cause various diseases, including the fatal human diseases like sleeping sickness caused by *Trypanosoma brucei* and Chagas disease caused by *Trypanosoma cruzi* (Fig. 9.13).

The diagnosis can be made by demonstrating **trypomastigote forms (amastigates of trypanosoma)** in PBS or bone marrow.

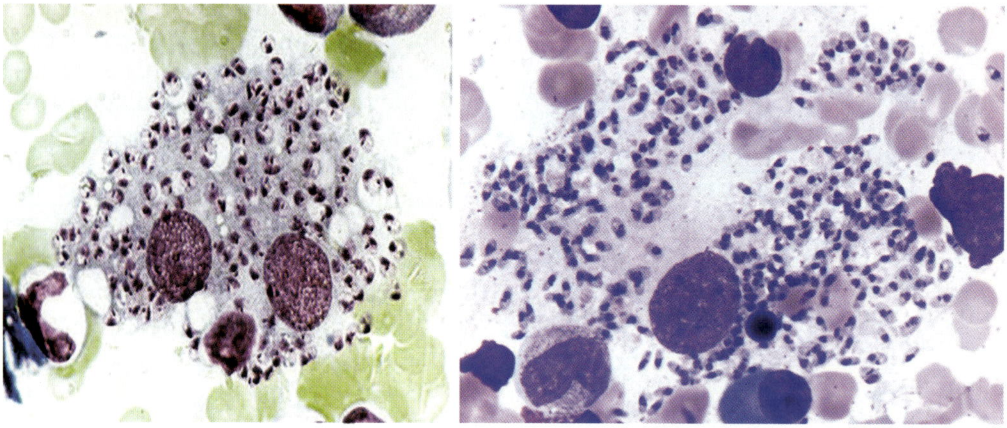

Fig. 9.12: LD bodies in bone marrow

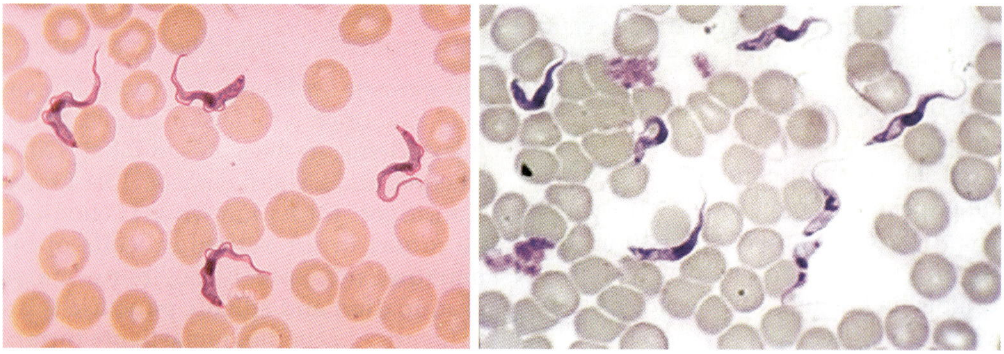

Fig.9.13: *Trypanosoma cruzi* in peripheral blood smear

Babesiosis (Fig. 9.14)

Babesiosis is a malarial-like parasitic disease caused by infection with Babesia. Human babesiosis is transmitted by tick bite.

Diagnosis can be done by demonstrating Babesia parasites in RBCs on PBS. Morphologically it looks like ring form of malarial parasite and can be confused with *Plasmodium* infection (Table 9.2 and Fig. 9.16). Diagnosis can also be done by antibody testing (indirect fluorescent antibody test, IFA). The antibody level (titer) rises in about 2–4 weeks after infection and declines/wanes at 6–12 months (Fig. 9.15).

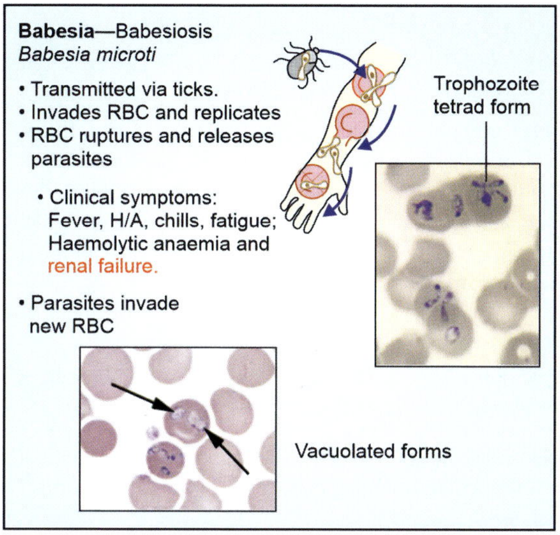

Fig. 9.14: Schematic diagram of babesiosis

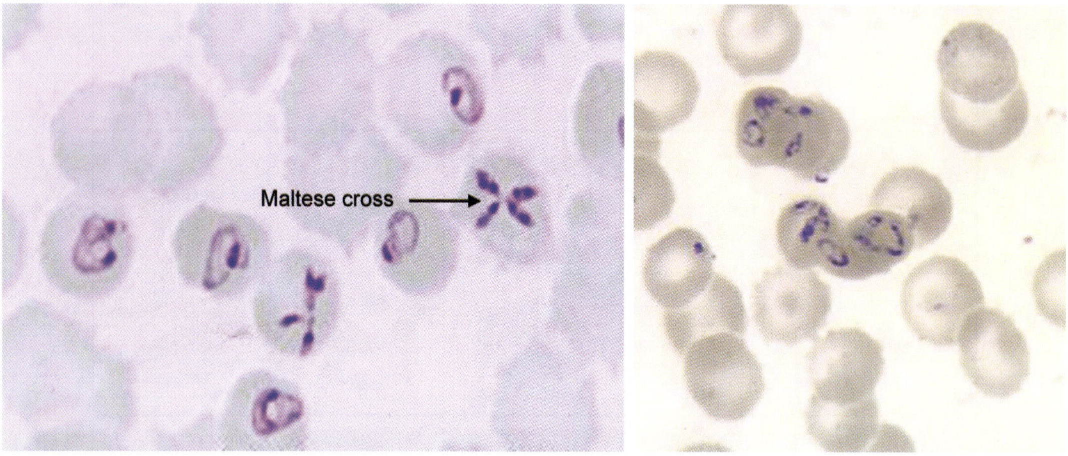

Fig.9.15: Babesiosis on peripheral blood

Table 9.2: Morphological differentiation of malaria parasites (Fig. 9.16)

	P. vivax	*P. falciparum*	*P. ovale*	*P. malariae*
Infected RBC	Enlarged, Schüffner dots	Normal size, Maurer clefts	Enlarged, oval and fimbriated, Schüffner dots	Normal or microcytic, stippling not usually seen
Ring form (early trophozoites)	Large, thick, usually single (occasionally 2) in cell, large chromatin dot	Delicate, frequently 2 or more accole, small chromatin dot	Thick, compact rings	Very small, compact rings
Late trophozoites	Amoeboid, central vacuole, light blue cytoplasm	Compact,vacuolated, somatimes 2 chromatin dots	Smaller than *P. vivax*, slightly amoeboid	Band across cell, deep blue cytoplasm
Gametocytes	Spherical, compact, almost fills cell, single nucleus	Crescent or sausage shaped, diffuse chromatin, single nucleus	Oval, fills three-fourths of cell, smaller than *P. vivax* but similar	Round, fills one-half to two-thirds of cell, similar to *P. vivax* but smaller
Schizonts	12–24 merozoites, irregularly arranged	18–24 merozoites, filling two-thirds of cell	8–12 merozoites filling three-fourths of cell	6–12 merozoites in daisy head around central mass of pigment
Pigments	Fine granular, yellow-brown	Dark to black clumped mass	Coarse light brown	Dark, prominent at all stages

In *P. falciparum* infection, percentage of RBCs infected should be reported. Schüffner dots: Fine stippling; Maurer dots or clefts: Large, irregularly shaped, red-staining dots; Accole forms: Parasite that is marginalized to edge of cell

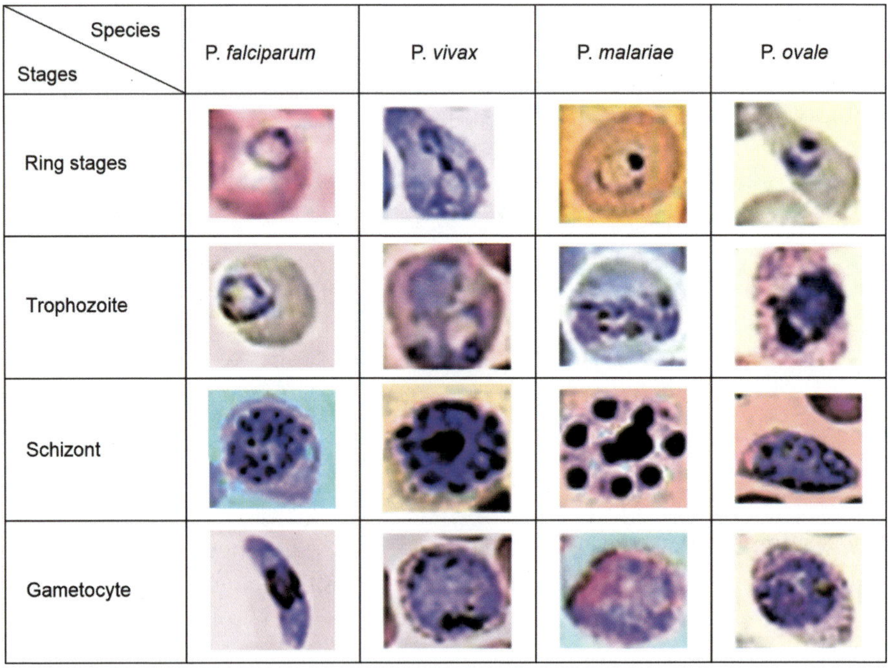

Fig. 9.16: Differentiation of malaria parasite

Chapter 10

Blood Transfusion/ Transfusion Medicine

Transfusion medicine is a multidisciplinary speciality concerned with the proper selection and utilization of blood components as well as the removal of blood or blood components in the treatment of prevention of disease.

The term blood banking is being replaced by the term **transfusion medicine** in order to stress the increasing role of patient care and evaluation of clinical results in this speciality. The blood components—red cells, platelets, granulocytes, fresh frozen plasma and cryoprecipitate—are made directly from a unit of whole blood, using different methods of physical separation (i.e. centrifugation and freezing).

Blood derivatives like albumin, plasma protein fraction, immune serum globulin, coagulation factor concentrates are produced by pharmaceutical companies and are usually made from plasma pools of thousands of donor units, using modifications of the Cohn ethanol fractionation technique. The basic principle of this method is that different proteins can be precipitated from plasma, without denaturation, by adjusting the amount of ethanol added.

Whole blood: One unit of donor blood collected in a suitable anticoagulant—preservative solution and which contains blood cells and plasma.

Blood components: A constituent separated from whole blood, by differential centrifugation of one donor unit of plasma by fractionation.

Blood derivatives: A product obtained from multiple donor units of plasma by fractionation (Fig. 10.1).

BLOOD TRANSFUSION

Blood transfusion is the process of transferring blood/blood products from donor into the blood circulation of recipient within stipulated time.

Types of Blood Transfusions

- **Whole blood donation:** In this one unit (350 ml) of whole blood is collected with a suitable anticoagulant.
- **Autologous donation:** In this type, blood is collected for an individual for subsequent transfusion to the same individual from whom the blood is collected.
- **Apheresis donation:** In this method, whole blood is removed from donor and is separated. Only desired portion is retained and the remaining portion is returned to the donor.
- **Massive blood transfusion:** It is defined in adults as replacement of >1 blood volume, e.g. 100% blood volume in

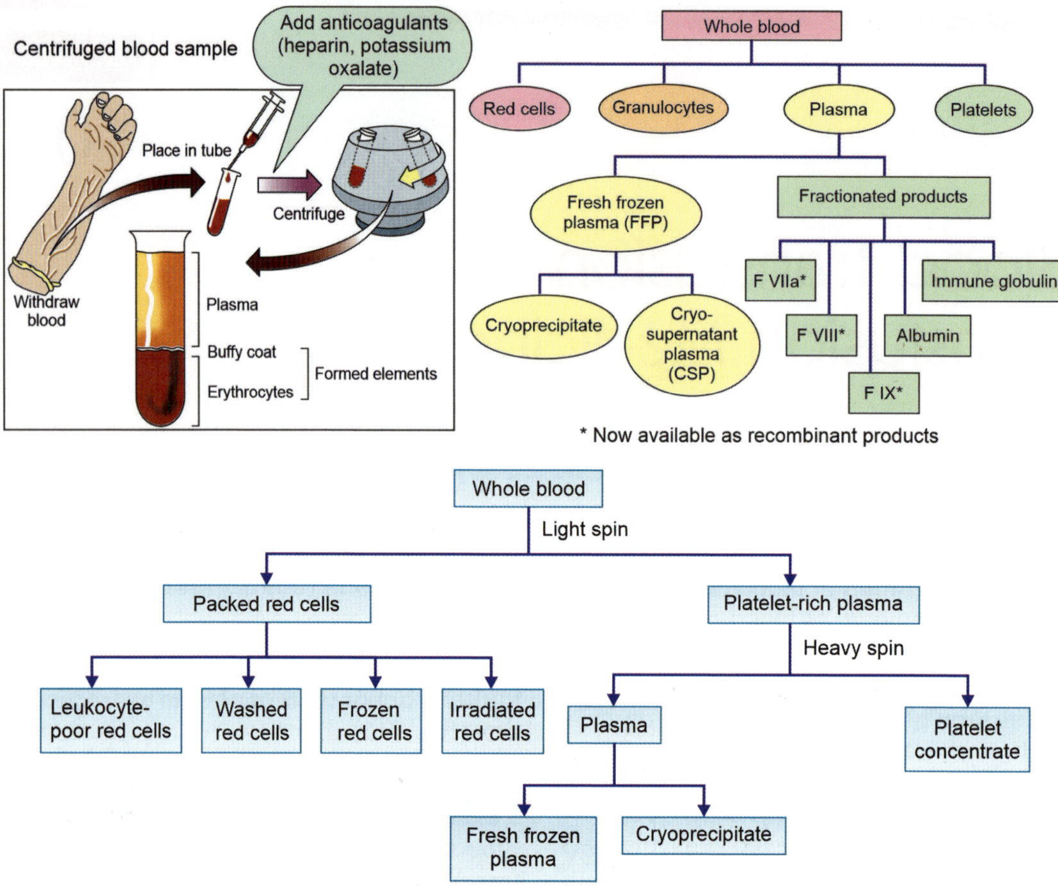

Fig. 10.1: Blood component preparation from whole blood (within 6 hours of collection)

24 hours or >50% of blood volume in 4 hours (adult blood volume is approximately 70 ml/kg). In the past, it was defined as the replacement by transfusion of 10 units of red cells in 24 hours. For children, 100% blood volume in 24 hours or >50% blood volume in 3 hours.

- **Emergency blood transfusion:** If the patient's blood group cannot be determined, then the patient should be transfused with O blood group red cells which are Rh negative with colloids/crystalloids.

Donor Selection for Blood Transfusion

- The donor should be healthy and free from diseases of heart, lung, liver and kidney.
- Donor should not suffer from cancer, diabetes, epilepsy, tuberculosis, bleeding, allergy, malaria, sexually transmitted diseases.
- The donor should be between 18–65 years of age.
- Weight should be >45 kg.
- Time interval between two blood transfusions: 3 months.
- Donor should have eaten something in the last 3 hours.
- Whole blood donation to be deferred for 3 days after platelet/plasmapheresis.
- Blood pressure should be controlled.
- No skin disease at the phlebotomy site.

Preference of Blood Group for Routine Blood Transfusion

- The first choice is the donor blood of the same ABO group as that of the recipient.
- If same ABO blood group is not available, then blood of an alternate but compatible group may be transfused as per mentioned below.

Recipient blood group	Donor blood group	
	first choice	Alternative or second choice
A	A	O
B	B	O
AB	AB	A→ B→ O (in this order)
O	O	Nil

To reduce the risk of haemolysis in a case of non-identical but compatible blood transfusion of ABO group, packed red cells instead of whole blood should be transfused (i.e. most of the plasma which contains anti-A and/or anti-B should be removed.

Salient Features of Blood Transfusion

- Blood should be transfused through a sterile, disposable administration set incorporating a **standard filter (170 μm pore size)**. This filter retains clot or cellular aggregates but permits passage of single cells and microaggregates.
- The usual needle size is 18 or 19 gauge.
- The solution is the blood bag usually contains citrate phosphate dextrose adenine (CPDA)-1. Amount of CPDA-1 is 49 ml for 350 ml of blood or 63 ml for 450 ml of blood.

Function of each component of CPDA is mentioned below

i. **Citrate:** Anticoagulation by binding of calcium in plasma.
ii. **Phosphate:** Acts as a buffer to minimize the effects of decreasing pH in blood.
iii. **Dextrose:** Maintenance of red cell membrane and metabolism. Also needed for ATP generation for viability of red cells.
iv. **Adenine:** Generation of ATP (energy source).

Collection of Blood for Transfusion

- Blood is collected by phlebotomy under aseptic conditions using sterile, plastic bag with anticoagulant. Nowadays, CPDA1 is used as an anticoagulant.
- Mix the blood with anticoagulant gently and periodically during its collection.

Anticoagulants used as preservatives:

- CPD (citrate phosphate dextrose)
- CPDA-1 (citrate phosphate dextrose adenine-1)
- ACD (acid citrate dextrose): Not used nowadays.

Composition of Preservatives

CPD

- Trisodium citrate: 26.30 g
- Sodium dihydrogen phosphate: 2.28 g
- Dextrose: 25.50 g
- Citric acid: 3.27 g
- Distilled water: To make 1 litre.

CPDA-1

- Trisodium citrate: 26.30 g
- Sodium dihydrogen phosphate: 2.22 g
- Dextrose: 31.8 g
- Citric acid: 3.27 g
- Adenine: 0.275 g
- Distilled water to make 1 litre.

Acid Citrate Dextrose (ACD)

- Trisodium citrate: 22.0 g
- Citric acid: 8.0 g
- Dextrose: 24.6 g
- Distilled water to make a final volume of 1 litre.

Storage of blood (*see* Fig. 10.14)

i. Whole blood and packed red cells are stored in a refrigerator at 2–6°C for 35 days.
ii. Platelets are stored at 20–24°C for 3 days.
iii. Fresh frozen plasma and cryoprecipitate are stored at ≤–18°C for one year.

Pre-donation check-up

Donor blood: The following tests are routinely performed

- ABO and Rh blood grouping.
- Screening tests for HBsAg, ant-HCV, anti-HIV-1 and HIV-2 and serum alanine aminotransferase (ALT).
- Screening tests for malaria and syphilis.

Recipient blood: The recipient's ABO and Rh blood grouping.

Compatibility Testing (Pre-transfusion)

Before blood or its components are transfused one must know whether donor blood or components are compatible with recipient's blood.

To check compatibility, following tests are done:

- ABO and Rh typing of the donor and recipient
- Cross-matching: But for transfusion of platelets or fresh frozen plasma, cross-matching is not needed.
- Antibody screening test of donor's and recipient's serum.
- Review of patient's past blood bank history and records if done earlier.

CROSS-MATCHING

Cross-matching is very important before any blood transfusion. It detects any antibody present in the patient's serum which will react with the donor's cells during transfusion.

Importance of Cross-matching

- It detects the presence of any clinically significant, unexpected antibodies in the recipient's serum which may react with donor's red cells. So, cross-match prevents transfusion reaction.
- It is the final check of ABO compatibility between donor and recipient.

Types of Cross-match

It can be divided into two major groups, namely major and minor cross-matching. Major cross-matching consists of mixing donor's red cells with recipient's or patient's serum. On the other hand, minor cross-matching consists of mixing patient's (recipient's) red cells with donor's serum (Tables 10.1 and 10.2).

Table 10.1: Types of cross-match

Cross-match type	Donor's component	Recipient's component
Major cross-match	Red cells	Serum
Minor cross-match	Serum	Red cells

Table 10.2: Different techniques of major cross-match

Types of cross-match	Antibody detection in recipient's serum
• Saline cross-match	IgM
• Antiglobulin test or Coombs test	IgG
• Albumin technique	IgG
• Enzyme technique	IgG mainly and some IgM

Procedure of Major Cross-match

The simplest method is:

- Place one drop of patient's serum in a glass test tube (Fig. 10.2).
- Add one drop of 5% saline suspension of donor's red cells to the above test tube.

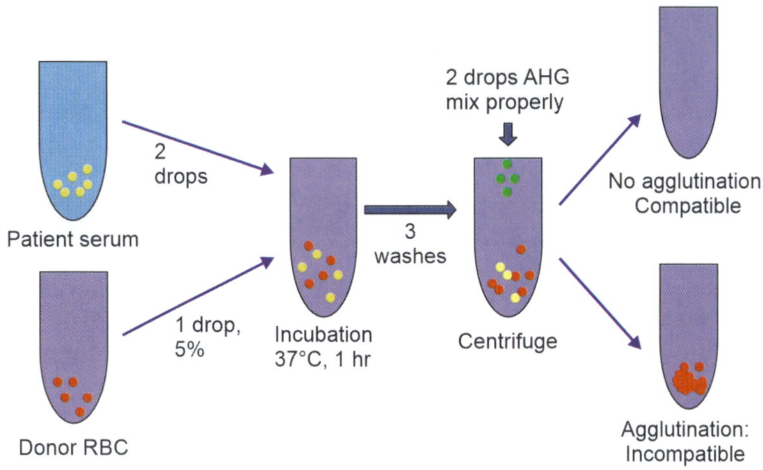

Fig. 10.2: Major cross-match

- Mix them and incubate at 37% for 30 minutes. Centrifuge at 1000 rpm for 1–2 minutes.
- Examine the tube for agglutination or haemolysis. Also check under microscope.

Interpretation of Result

- If there is no agglutination or haemolysis, that mean the donor's blood is compatible with that of patient's blood and can be safely transfused.
- Agglutination or haemolysis indicates mismatching. In this scenario, recipient should not be transfused with the donor's blood or component.

Procedure of Minor Cross-match

- Place one drop of donor's serum in a glass test tube.
- Add one drop of 5% saline suspension of recipient's red cells to the above test tube.
- Mix them and incubate at 39°C for 30 minutes.
- Centrifuge at 3000 rpm for 1 minute.
- Observe for agglutination or haemolysis (Fig. 10.3).

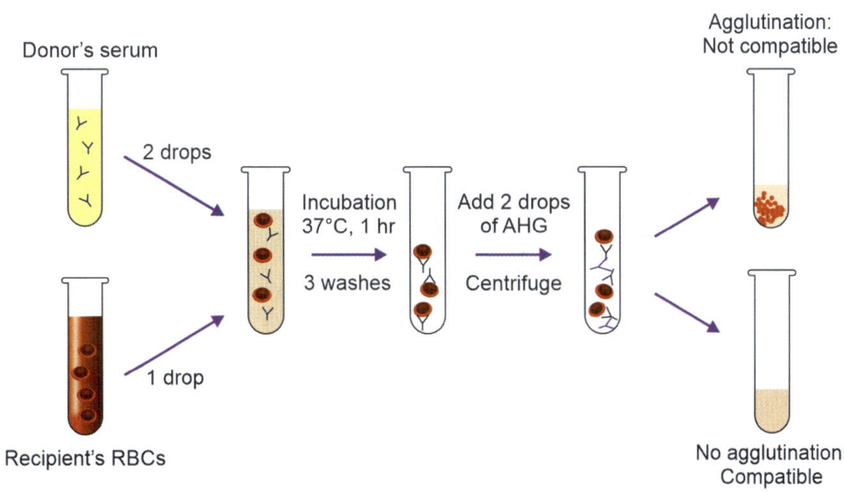

Fig. 10.3: Minor cross-match

INDIRECT COOMBS' TEST (ANTIGLOBULIN TEST)

Saline suspension red cells of donor are incubated with patient's serum. Washed in saline and add antiglobulin agent. Re-centrifuge and examine for agglutination or haemolysis. It will detect any IgG antibodies in patient's (recipient's) serum.

Interpretation of result

- If there is no agglutination or haemolysis, it indicates compatibility of donor unit with patient's (recipient's) serum.
- Agglutination or haemolysis indicates incompatibility and should not be transfused (Fig. 10.4).

Antibody Screening and Identification

Patient (recipient's) serum should be tested for the presence of clinically significant (unexpected or irregular) antibodies. In this procedure, serum of the recipient is tested against a set of blood group O screening cells of known antigenic type. If there is any clinically significant antibody in patient's serum it will be identified. Then the blood unit without the corresponding antigens is selected for compatibility test.

APHERESIS

Definition: Apheresis is an automated blood collection procedure wherein whole blood is removed from a donor or a patient. Then desired component is separated and the remainder of the blood is returned to the donor or patient.

Types of Apheresis

- Donor apheresis
- Therapeutic apheresis: Component of blood contributing to the disease is removed and the remainder is returned back.

Advantage of donor apheresis: Large amounts of a specific component can be collected; minimizes number of donors to which recipient is exposed.

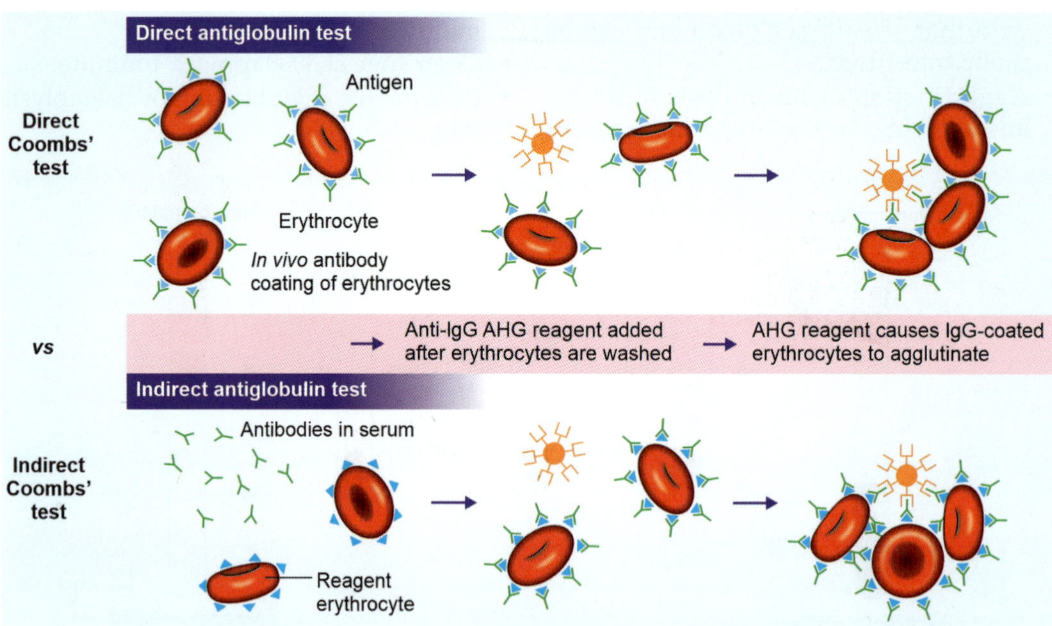

Fig. 10.4: Direct Coombs' test *vs* indirect Coombs' test

Components Collected in Donor Apheresis

- **Red cell apheresis:** 2 units of red cells can be removed if the donor is larger and has higher haematocrit than for single red cell donations. At least 16 weeks interval needed (deferral) if two units of red cells are collected.
- **Plateletpheresis:** Platelet count of the donor should be >1.5 lacs/mm^3 (especially for frequent donor). Donation interval should be at least 2 days. Donor should not have taken aspirin for at least 36 hours before donation. It contains ≥3 × 10^{11} platelets.
- **Leukapheresis:** Not commonly used. For collection of large number of leukocytes; drugs or sedimenting materials need to be administrated to the donor and donor consent for that purpose is needed.
- **Plasmapheresis:** The donor should be larger (≥110 pounds or 50 kg) for infrequent plasmapheresis. Donation interval should be at least 4 weeks.

Therapeutic Apheresis

- **Cytapheresis:** For treatment of sickle cell disease (to reduce HbS and replace with HbA), hyperleukocytosis (to remove excess leukocytes in leukaemia), malaria (to reduce parasite load)
- **Plasmapheresis:** Removal of abnormal plasma proteins (e.g. myasthenia gravis, GB syndrome, TTP, monoclonal gammopathies) (Fig. 10.5).

WHOLE BLOOD (Fig. 10.6)

- One unit of blood is collected in a suitable anticoagulant preservative solution (CPD-1). Its total volume is about 400 ml (350 ml of blood + 49 ml of anticoagulant). Shelf life in CPD-1 is 35 days.
- It consists of cellular elements (red cells, white cells and platelets) and plasma. But it contains no liable coagulation factors (factor V, factor VIII) and no functionally effective platelets.

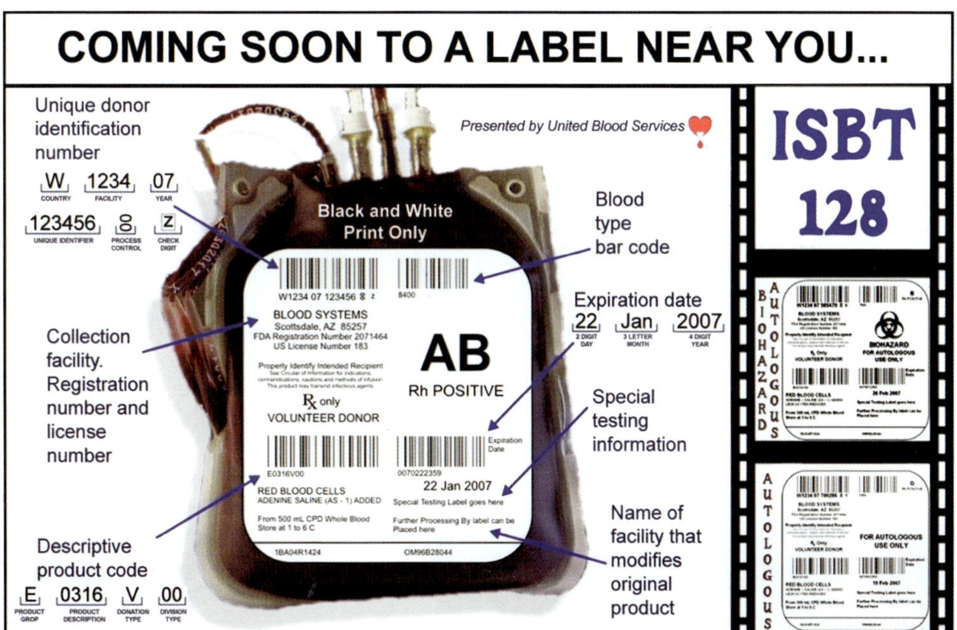

Fig. 10.5: Identification of different points of one unit of blood/blood product

- It is stored at 2–6°C in appropriate blood bank refrigerator.
- Transfusion of whole blood commence within 30 minutes of removal from the refrigerator, and should be complete within 4 hours of starting.
- Transfusion of one unit raises haemoglobin by 1 g/dl or haematocrit by 3%.
- Haematocrit of whole blood 35–45% and haemoglobin 12 g/dl
- Indication: Acute massive blood loss, exchange transfusion, non-availability of packed red cells.
- Risk of volume overload in patients with chronic anaemia and compromised cardiovascular function.
- 450 ml of blood
- 63 ml of anticoagulant solution.
- Hct: 36–44%
- No components have been removed.
- Store at 1–6°C
- Shelf life-
  – Citrate-phophate-dextrose (CPD)
  – CPDA-1 (adenine): 35 days
  – AS-1, AS-3, AS-5–42 days
- Administer through standard blood filter (150–280 microns)
- Infuse within 4 hours of issue.

RED CELL COMPONENTS

1. Packed red cells (red cell concentrate)

- **Preparation:** Whole blood is either allowed to sediment overnight in a refrigerator 2–6°C or it is spun in a refrigerated centrifuge. Supernatant plasma is separated from red cells in a closed system by transferring the plasma to the attached empty bag. Red cells with small amount of plasma are left behind in the primary blood bag.
- Haematocrit 55–75% or haemoglobin 20 g/dl.
- Raises haemoglobin by 1 g% or haematocrit by 3%
- Stored at 2–6°C and shelf life 35 days in CPDA.
- Ideal haematocrit should be 70–75% after preparation from one unit of whole blood. But haematocrit should not cross 80%, otherwise preservative will not be effective for support of red cells.
- Volume: 250 ml.
- Indications: Replacement of red cells in anaemia and in acute/massive blood loss (along with crystalloid or colloid) (Fig. 10.7).

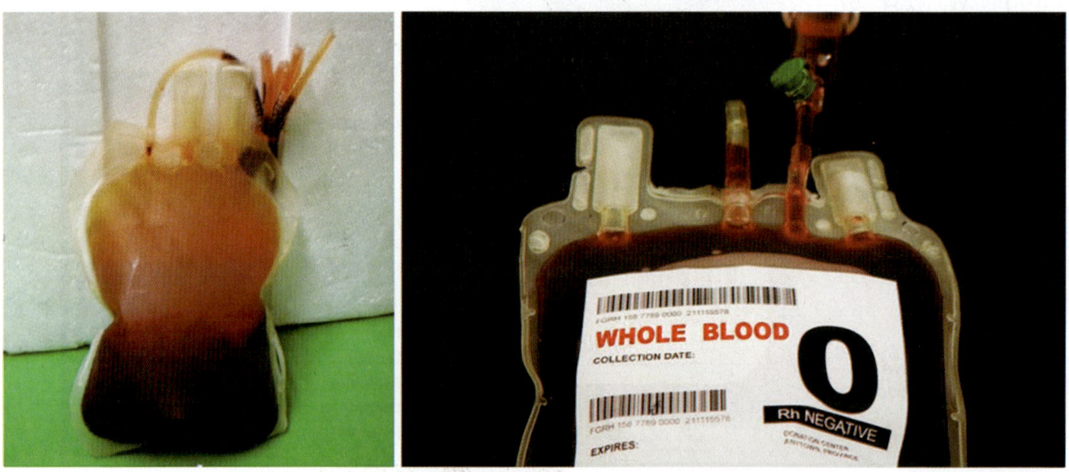

Fig. 10.6: Whole blood

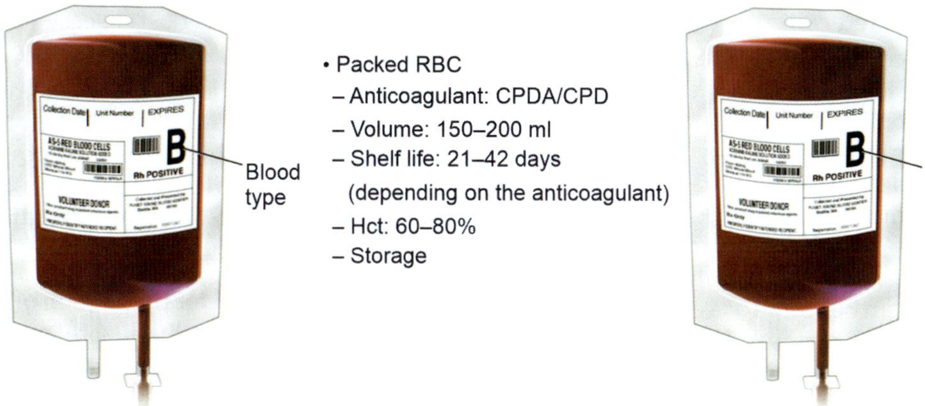

Fig. 10.7: Packed red blood cells

2. Red cells in additive solution (red cell suspension)

These are red cells with minimal residual plasma with an added additive solution. This increases shelf life of red cells (in CPDA) from 35 to 42 days.

Additive solutions like AS -1 AS -3, AS-5 and SAGM (which contains saline, adenine, glucose and mannitol).

Preparation: After collection of whole blood in the primary collection bag (containing CPDA-1), maximum amount of plasma is removed after centrifugation and transferred to a satellite bag (**satellite bag 1**). The additive solution from another satellite bag (**satellite bag 2**) is transferred into the primary collection bag (containing packed red cells) in a closed system within 72 hours of collection.

Advantages of this method are

i. Red cells with improved viability are obtained (shelf-life increases from 35 to 42 days).

ii. Maximum amount of plasma can be removed for preparation of plasma components.

iii. Flow of infusion is improved due to reduction in viscosity.

Indications: Same as for packed red cells.

Contraindication: Red cells in SAGM are contraindicated for exchange transfusion in neonates.

3. Leukocyte-poor red cells

- These are red cells from which most of the white cells have been removed. They are obtained by passing blood through a special leukocyte-depletion filter at the time of transfusion. They can also be prepared in the blood bank.
- By definition, leukocyte-depleted red cells should contain $\leq 5 \times 10^6$ white cells per bag.

  Indications

  i. To avoid febrile transfusion reactions in persons who require repeated transfusions or who have earlier been sensitised to white cell antigens.

  ii. To avoid sensitisation to HLA antigens. As for example, in patients with severe aplastic anaemia, who are likely to receive allogenic bone marrow transplant. But it cannot prevent graft-versus-host disease.

  iii. To reduce the risk of transmission of cytomegalovirus (CMV) in some patients.

4. Frozen red cells

- Red cells can be stored frozen for up to 10 years when stored at or below –65°C. But for this, a cryoprotective agent such as glycerol is added. Glycerol prevents red cell dehydration and formation of ice crystals that causes red cell lysis.
- After deglycerolization (washing with decreasing concentration of saline), red cells can be stored at 4–6°C for 24 hours, if closed system is not used.
- With this method, virtually all plasma, anticoagulant, leukocytes and platelets are removed.
- Indications: i) It is used for storage of red cells with rare blood groups, for further autologous transfusions. ii) It is used for individuals who have repeated febrile nonhaemolytic transfusion reactions. iii) it can be given to IgA deficient patient as it is safe for them.

5. Irradiated red cell

- Viable T lymphocytes in donor blood can induce life-threating transfusion associated graft-versus-host disease (GVH) in at risk patients.
- Gamma-irradiation (250 c Gy) of red cells inactivates T lymphocytes and prevents graft versus host disease. This component can be stored at 4–6°C up to original expiry date or 28 days from irradiation.

Indications

i. It is indicated for prevention of GVHD in susceptible individuals like immunodeficient individuals and patients receiving blood from first degree relatives.

ii. It is used for intrauterine or premature neonate transfusions (Fig. 10.8).

6. Washed red cells

- Red cells can be washed with normal saline to remove plasma proteins, white cells and platelets.
- Shelf-life of red cells after washing is 24 hours at 4–6°C. About 20% of red cells are lost in the process.

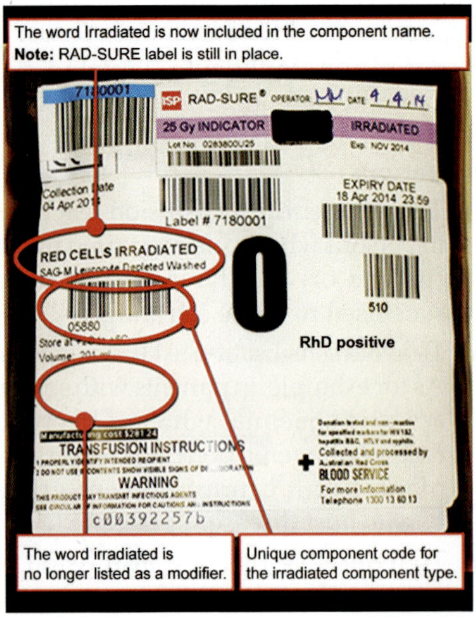

Indications for irradiated blood

- Pre-/post-haematopoietic stem cell transplant
- Hodgkin's disease
- Low birth weight neonate (<1,200 g)
- Neonatal exchange transfusion
- Intrauterine fetal transfusion
- Related donor
- HLA-matched donor or cross-match compatible platelet donor
- Treatment with either fludarabine or 2-CDA

Fig. 10.8: Identification of irradiated blood

- **Indications**
  i. Use of such cells is restricted for IgA-deficient individuals who have developed anti-IgA antibodies as exposure will lead to anaphylaxis.

PLATELET COMPONENTS

1. Platelet Concentrate (Random Donor Platelets)

- Obtained from whole blood and platelets are separated from whole blood within 6 hours of collection. Remember whole blood should be kept at room temperature.
- One unit of whole blood is centrifuged (light spin) to obtain **platelet-rich plasma (PRP)**. PRP is then transferred to the attached satellite bag and spun at high speed to get platelet aggregates (at the bottom) and **plate-poor plasma or PPP** (at the top). Most of the PPP is return back to the primary collection bag or to another satellite bag, leaving behind 50–60 ml of PPP with the platelets.
- Platelets are stored at 20–24°C with continuous agitation (in a storage device called platelet agitator). Maximum storage period 3–5 days.
- One unit of platelet concentrate contains $\geq 45 \times 10^9$ platelets. Transfusions of one unit of platelet concentrate will rise the platelet count in the recipient by about 5000/µl.

  Indications
  i. Bleeding due to thrombocytopenia (immune mediated or secondary), where platelet count is <20,000/mm^3
  ii. In case of abnormal platelet function or platelet function defects
  iii. In DIC (disseminated intravascular coagulation).
- The usual adult dose is 4–6 units of platelet concentrate (or 1 unit/10 kg of body weight). These units (which are from different donors) are pooled into one bag before transfusion. This dose will raise the platelet count by 20,000–40,000/µl.

> **Note**
> - Platelets have ABO antigens on their surface but do not express Rh antigen.
> - It is advisable to transfuse platelets from Rh negative persons to Rh negative patients/persons.

2. Plateletpheresis (Single Donor Platelets)

- In this method, a donor is connected to blood cell separator machine in which whole blood is collected in an anticoagulant solution. Then platelets are separated and retained. Remaining components are returned back to the donor.
- With this method, a large number of platelets can be obtained from a single donor (equivalent to 6 units of platelet concentrate or $\geq 3 \times 10^{11}$) and recipient is not exposed to many donors.
- **Indications**
  i. It is especially suitable if HLA-matched platelets are required (that means if the patient has developed refractoriness to platelet transfusion due to the formation of allo-antibodies against HLA antigens.)

Contraindications
- TTP (thrombotic thrombocytopenic purpura)
- Haemolytic uraemic syndrome.

Corrected count increment (CCI): After transfusion, platelets will survive for only 3–4 days in circulation. Therefore, patients requiring platelet need frequent platelet transfusions. These patients may develop antibodies against platelets and HLA antigens which will reduce the survival of transfused platelets. It is important to know whether the patient has become refractory or unresponsive to such transfusions. This is done by determining whether there will be anticipated increase in platelet counts by calculating corrected count increment or CCI.

CCI = Post-transfusion platelet count =

$$\frac{\text{Pre-transport platelet count} \times \text{BSA}}{\text{Number of platelets transfused (in multiples of } 10^{11})}$$

BSA = Body Surface Area (calculated from a nomogram using height and weight)

CCI >7500/µl at 10–60 minutes following transfusion indicates adequate platelet count increment.

GRANULOCYTE CONCENTRATE

- **Preparation:** Granulocytes for transfusion can be obtained either from a single donor unit by differential centrifugation or by leukapheresis. Leukapheresis is preferred because of better granulocyte yield, which can further be enhanced by administration of corticosteroids to the donor.
- But granulocyte concentrates are seldomly used. The reasons are:
    i. When collected from single donor, it contains a smaller number of granulocytes and is heavily contaminated with red cells.
    ii. Transfusion of granulocyte concentrate often results in complications (e.g. lung infiltration, non-haemolytic transfusion reactions, etc.).
- **Indications**
    i. Patients with severe neutropenia (when granulocyte count <500/mm^3 (agranulocytosis).
    ii. To combat infections, like in neonatal sepsis and granulomatous disease.
    iii. Bone marrow depression.

    But rather than transfusing granulocyte concentrates, many clinicians prefer to administer growth factors for myelopoiesis like G-CSF/GM-CSF.

PLASMA COMPONENTS

Plasma can be obtained either by centrifugation of a unit of whole blood or by plasmapheresis. Various components can be prepared from plasma. The main plasma components are: Fresh frozen plasma, plasma frozen within 24 hours of phlebotomy and cryoprecipitate.

1. Fresh Frozen Plasma (FFP)

- **Preparation**: To prepare the FFP, plasma is separated from whole blood by centrifugation, transferred into the attached satellite bag, and then rapidly frozen at –18°C or at lower temperature. This procedure is carried out within 6 hours of collection because after 6 hours, labile factors (factor V and factor VIII) are lost. FFP contains all coagulation factors.
- **Volume:** 200–250 ml
- **Storage:** It can be stored at below –18°C for 1 year. When required for transmission, FFP is thawed between 30–37°C for about 30–45 minutes. Then it is temporarily stored at 2–6°C and should be used within 24 hours.
- **Indications**
    i. Patients on anticoagulant drug therapy
    ii. Antithrombin deficiency
    iii. Liver disease
    iv. Vitamin K deficiency
    v. TTP
    vi. DIC
    vii. Inherited deficiency of a coagulation factor for which no specific concentrate is available.
- Dosage: 10–20 ml/kg (3–6 units in adults) over a period of 1–2 hours. ABO compatible FFP is preferred to avoid the risk of haemolysis of patient's RBCs by antibodies in donor plasma.

    Fresh grozen plasma contains coagulation factors and other plasma protein (per unit or bag)

Volume	–	200–250 ml
Factor VIII	–	0.6 IU/ml
Fibrinogen	–	250–300 mg/bag
Proteins	–	Albumin, globulin, etc.

1 IU/kg of factor VIII or factor IX (one IU/kg) raises the factor VIII levels in plasma by 2% and factor IX levels by 1% respectively.

Shelf life: One year

Storage tem: –20°C or below

Q.C. requirements: The entire proems of preparation and freezing should be completed with 8 hours after collection.

Volume: 50 to 200 ml

Definite indications for the use of FFP

1. Replacement of single factor deficiencies
2. Immediate reversal of warfarin effect
3. Haemorrhagic disease of newborn
4. DIC with evidence of bleeding
5. Thrombotic thrombocytopenic purpura (TTP)

Conditional uses for the use of FFP

1. Massive transfusion
2. Liver disease
3. Cardiopulmonary bypass surgery
4. Newborn with septicaemia

No justification for the use of FFP

1. Hypovolaemia
2. Plasma exchange procedures except TTP
3. Reversal of prolonged INR in the absence of bleeding.

2. Plasma Frozen within 24 Hours after Phlebotomy

Plasma is separated and is frozen at –18°C between 8 and 24 hours of collection. This contains all coagulation factors, but may have reduced level of factor V and factor VIII in comparison to FFP.

Indications: Similar to FFP.

3. Cryoprecipitate (CRYO)

Cryoprecipitate is prepared from plasma, which has been separated freshly (within 6 hours of collection) by rapidly freezing at a temperature ≤18°C. Then thawed it slowly at 4–6°C. Plasma and a white flocculent precipitate are obtained. This mixture is centrifuged and supernatant plasma is removed leaving behind the whitish cryoprecipitate in 10–20 ml of plasma.

This prepared cryoprecipitate (one unit) is now refrozen at a temperature ≤–18°C and can be stored for 1 year. When required for transfusion, cryoprecipitate was thawed at 30–37°C and can be stored at 2–6°C temporarily for 6 hours. This unit can be transferred to patient. Each unit of cryoprecipitate must contains ≥80 IU of factor VIII and ≥150 mg of fibrinogen. It also contains von Willebrand factor, factor XIII and fibronectin.

Indications: It is mainly used for treatment of fibrinogen deficiency and factor XIII deficiency. Though it can be used for treatment of haemophilia A (factor VIII deficiency) and von Willebrand disease, but nowadays it is not preferred as virus-inactivated factor VIII concentrates and recombinant factor preparations are available (Fig. 10.9).

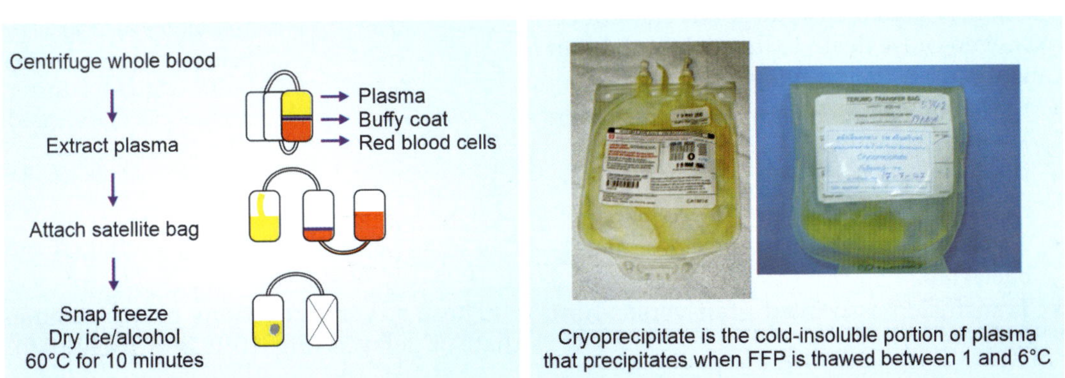

Fig. 10.9: Cryoprecipitate (CRYO)

PLASMA DERIVATIVES

Plasma derivatives are prepared by fractionation of large volumes of pooled human plasma. After fractionation, these derivatives undergo virus-inactivated procedures. Some important plasma derivatives and their uses are listed in Table 10.3.

Recombinant Factor Concentrate

With the advent of recombinant DNA technology, factor VIII, IX and VIIa can be produced by this method. This technique has eliminated the risk of viral transmission. But products produced by this technique are costly. These products are sterile, lyophilized and stable making the administration easier and more scientific compared to blood components.

Indications

i. Factor VIII concentrate for treatment of haemophilia A, von Willebrand disease
ii. Factor IX concentrate for treatment of haemophilia B.
iii. Factor VIIa (rFVII a) for treatment of haemophilia A or B with inhibitors and factor VII deficiency (Table 10.4).

Table 10.3: Important plasma derivatives and their uses

Plasma derivative	Use
• Human albumin solutions	i. It is used as a replacement fluid in therapeutic plasma exchange ii. For treatment of diuretic resistant oedema due to hypoproteinaemia.
• Factor VIII concentrate	i. Treatment of haemophilia A ii. Severe von Willebrand disease.
• Prothrombin complex	i. Treatment of deficiency of factor IX, factor VIII with inhibitors against factor VIII. ii. Inherited deficiency of factors II, VII and X
• **Immunoglobulins**	
a. Nonspecific immunoglobulins	i. Treatment of hypogammaglobulinaemia, ii. Autoimmune thrombocytopenic purpura iii. Neonatal sepsis iv. Passive prophylaxis of viral infections like hepatitis, rubella and measles
b. Specific immunoglobulin	i. Anti-RhD immunoglobulin is used for prevention of sensitisation to RhD antigen in Rh negative women giving birth to a Rh positive baby. ii. Tetanus immunoglobulin, hepatitis B immunoglobulin, varicella-zoster immunoglobulin are used for passive prophylaxis of that particular infection

ADVERSE EFFECTS OF BLOOD TRANSFUSION

Blood transfusion is generally safe and effective. But sometimes adverse effects may be seen. These are called blood transfusion reactions. Occasionally, these adverse effects may even cause death to the recipient. Main causes of transfusion-related deaths are:

- Immediate acute haemolytic transfusion reaction due to ABO incompatibility.
- Pulmonary edema and congestive heart failure due to circulatory overload.
- Complications related to infections (mainly bacterial).
- Transfusion associated graft-versus-host disease.
- Transfusion of physically damaged red cells (e.g. heat, cold).

These adverse reactions may be immediate or delayed (Fig. 10.10 and Table 10.5).

Table 10.4: Storage of different components

Cells	Method of preparation	Storage temperature	Lifespan
Packed red cell	5000 g for 5 minutes	2–6°C	35–42 days
Fresh frozen plasma (FFP)	5000 g for 5 minutes at 22°C	–20°C	1 year if frozen, 24 hours if thawed
Platelet-rich plasma (PRP)	2000 g for 3 minutes at 22°C	20–24°C with constant agitation	5 days
Cryoprecipitate	Derived from FFP after thawing at 4°C	Frozen –18°C	1 year if frozen, 16 hours if thawed
Granulocyte concentrate	5000 g for 5 minutes	24°C	Transfuse within 24 hours of collection
Clotting factor concentrate	Lyophilised preparation	+4°C	Half life is 12 hours
Albumin	Plasma concentrate	Room temperature	Half life is 14 days
Protein C and protein S	Fractionation of plasma	+4°C	Several years
Immunoglobulins	Fractionation of plasma	+4°C	21 days

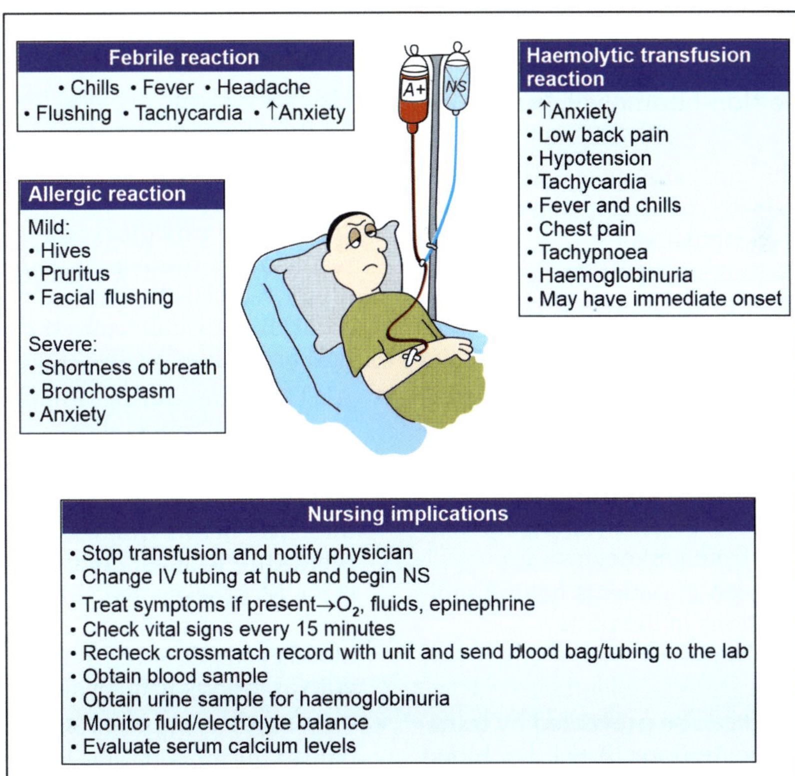

Fig. 10.10: Blood transfusion reaction

Table 10.5: Adverse effects of blood transfusion

Immediate (<24 hours)	Delayed (≥24 hours)
Non-immunological causes • Fever and shock (due to presence of antibodies against WBC or platelet antigens). • Haemolysis (due to physical destruction of blood caused by overheating or freezing) • Congestive heart failure (due to circulatory overload following large volume of blood transfusion)	*Non-immunological causes* • Hepatitis (mostly hepatitis B and C) • AIDS (if donor is HIV positive) • Iron overload (due to multiple transfusion) • Malaria • Syphilis • Viral infections (e.g. CMV)
Immunological causes • Haemolysis (due to ABO incompatibility) • Anaphylaxis (due to IgE antibody) • Urticaria (due to presence of antibody against plasma proteins of donor) • Febrile reactions (due to antibody against leukocyte antigen of donor) • Non cardiac pulmonary oedema (due to antibody against leukocytes of donor or compliment activation)	*Immunological causes* • Haemolysis (due to secondary response of antibody to RBC antigens) • Graft-versus-host disease (due to donor's leukocyte HLA antigens) • Post-transfusion purpura (due to development of antiplatelet antibody)

Some of the common adverse effects will be discussed here.

Fever (Febrile Non-haemolytic Transfusion Reaction)

- Fever is the most common reaction and constitutes >90% of transfusion reactions and 1% of all transfusions.
- It is defined as an unexplained rise of temperature of at least 1°C during or shortly after transfusion (<6 hours).
- This is due to the presence of WBC and platelet antibodies in the recipient's blood as a result of previous transfusion or pregnancies. It is caused by the release of pyrogenic cytokines such as interleukin - 1(IL-1), IL-6, IL-10 and tumor necrosis factor (TNF) from leukocytes.
- Commonly seen in patients having multiple transfusions in the past.
- Signs and symptoms: Fever, chills and tachycardia.
- Prevention: It can be prevented by transfusing leukocyte poor blood, i.e. blood from which buffy coat has been removed.
- Treatment: Antipyretics like paracetamol.

Haemolysis and Acute Haemolytic Transfusion Reaction (AHTR)

- Haemolysis due to blood transfusion can be due to both non-immunologic and immunologic causes.
- **Acute haemolytic transfusion reaction (AHTR)** is a medical emergency which results from intravascular destruction of donor red cells by antibodies in the recipient. It is usually caused by preformed IgM antibodies against donor red cells.
- AHTR occurs during, immediately after or within 24 hours following blood transfusion.
- AHTR usually results from ABO-mismatched blood transfusion to the recipient due to most commonly a clerical error. Most severe reaction occurs if blood group A is transfused to a recipient of blood group O. Severe reaction may occur with as little as 10 ml of blood transfusion.
- Signs and symptoms of AHTR: Fever, pain at the infusion site, loin or back pain, tachycardia, oozing from venipuncture site, hypotension and haemoglobinuria.

- Another cause of haemolytic reaction may be incompatibility of Rh, Kell or Duffy system. Patient gets iso-immunised and antibodies are formed after many weeks or months of transfusion. These are also called **delayed haemolytic transfusion reaction (DHTR).**
- Most of these haemolytic transfusion reactions are due to incorrect labelling, wrong identification of patient, error in blood grouping and failure to detect weak antibodies.
- Laboratory findings:
  i. Haemoglobinaemia (pink coloration of plasma after centrifugation of post-transfusion of blood).
  ii. Haemoglobinuria
  iii. Positive direct Coombs' test
  iv. Raised indirect serum bilirubin
  v. Schistocytes and spherocytes on PBS.

ANAPHYLAXIS

- This rare adverse effect occurs in IgA – deficient recipient who has anti-IgA antibodies (due to previous transfusion) and is now getting blood containing IgA antibodies. This leads to activation of complement and formation of anaphylatoxins (C3a and C5a).
- Signs and symptoms: Nausea, vomiting, flushing, respiratory distress, urticaria, hypotension and shock.

Urticaria

- It occurs due to presence of sensitising antibodies in the recipient which reacts with exogenous antigen, such as milk or egg protein present in the plasma of the donor.
- So, urticaria is common in the patients who suffers from atopic diseases, e.g. asthma, hay fever, etc.

Circulatory Overload

- Transfusion associated circulatory overload (TACO) occurs due to very rapid and excessive administration of blood, plasma or other intravenous blood components.
- It may cause congestive heart failure and pulmonary oedema. This is particularly so in an anaemic patient. Elderly patients, infants and pregnant women in third trimester are more prone to congestive heart failure.
- Signs and symptoms of cardiac failure: Dyspnoea, peripheral oedema, cough, distension of jugular veins and breathlessness.

Graft-versus-host Disease (GVHD)

- GVHD is more common in bone marrow transplant and is rare in blood transfusion. It may occur in patients with immunodeficiency like AIDS, lymphoma, chemotherapy and radiotherapy.
- Though it is rare, but is a lethal complication of transfusion with 90% mortality rate.
- GVHD is mediated by immunocompetent lymphocytes present in blood products which cause immunologic response against the recipient.
- Onset is 3–30 days after transfusion.
- Signs and symptoms: Fever, skin rashes, diarrhoea, infection.
- Patients having risk of GVHD should receive irradiated blood products to prevent immunologic response.

Bacterial Contamination

- The risk is low with plastic closed multipack system compared to glass bottles.
- Transfusion of blood product with platelet concentrates carries more risk as platelets are stored at higher temperature (20–24°C).
- The organisms are commonly cold growing gram-negative bacilli such as pseudomonas and also some coliform organisms.
- Platelets are usually contaminated by gram-positive cocci like Staphylococcus, Bacillus, etc. Red cells (stored at 4–6°C)

are contaminated by *Yersinia enterocolitica, Serratia liquefaciens and Pseudomonas fluorescens*.

- Signs and symptoms: High grade fever, rigors, hypotension and shock.
- Laboratory findings: Inspection of blood bag for discoloration, clots, cloudiness or haemolysis. Gram staining and culture of blood from blood bag and from recipient to detect causative bacteria. Direct Coombs' test is negative.
- Prevention: Blood should be given within 4 hours and prolonged storage of blood at room temperature should be avoided as it causes growth of contaminated bacteria.

Other Infections

- **Hepatitis B virus:** It is a DNA virus and can be transmitted by both cellular and plasma components. Blood and blood components are tested for HBs Ag before transfusion. HBsAg positive donors are excluded from blood donations. Donor screening for HBsAg and anti-HBc is mandatory in some countries. But in India, test for HBsAg is only mandatory.
- **Hepatitis A virus:** It is an RNA virus and is rarely transmitted by transfusion. Donors with hepatitis A or who are in close contact with this virus are deferred for 1 year. Test for hepatitis A antigen or antibody is routinely not done.
- **Hepatitis C virus:** This RNA virus is the **most common cause of transfusion transmitted hepatitis**. This infection is transmitted by both cellular and plasma components. Chronic hepatitis, cirrhosis and hepatocellular carcinoma may occur. Anti-HCV antibody test is done for donor screening.
- **HIV:** This is RNA retrovirus and has two subtypes HIV-1 and HIV-2. HIV can be transmitted by both cellular and plasma components. The test used to detect HIV is anti-HIV-1 and 2 antibodies by **ELISA (screening test)**. **Western blot test is more specific**. To reduce the window period (from 22 days to 10 days), **nucleic acid testing (NAT)** for HIV RNA is recommended.
- **Malaria:** It can be transmitted by transfusion readily. For prevention antimalarial drugs are given in endemic areas. Before transfusion, blood should be checked for malaria (Fig. 10.11).
- **Syphilis** (*Treponema pallidum*): Transmission through transfusion is rare because *T. pallidum* does not survive in refrigerator for storage of blood. It is inactivated at 4°C after 4 days.

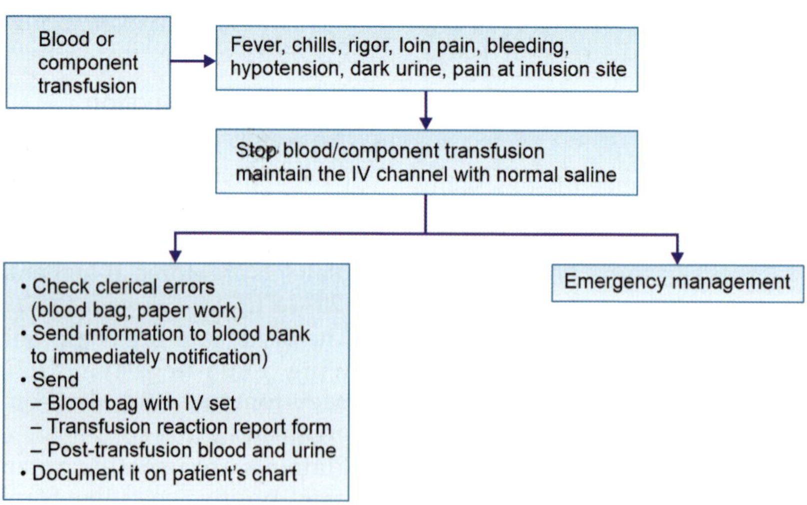

Fig. 10.11: Management protocol after a suspected transfusion reaction

CENTRIFUGATION

Outcome of centrifugation depends on two factors: The relative centrifugal force (RCF) and the duration of centrifugation. The RCF, of g force is the product of $1.118 \times 10^{-5} \times r \times N$ (where r is radius, and N is number of revolutions per minute or r.p.m.). The following speed is useful for preparation of different blood components:

i. 5000 g for 5 minutes for preparation of packed RBC or platelet concentrate,

ii. 5000 g for 7 minutes for preparation of cryoprecipitate or cell free plasma. These combinations are called **"heavy spin"** as opposed to 2000 g for 3 minutes, known as a **"light spin"**, which is used to produce platelet-rich plasma.

For preparation of a platelet concentrate, centrifugation is performed at room temperature (20°C to 24°C). For all other blood components, centrifugation is carried out between 1 and 6°C. Balancing the material in opposite sides of the centrifuge head is important and can be easily done with rubber disks different weights.

Platelets are in high demand. The whole blood unit, with its two attached satellite bags is first centrifuged using a **light spin to get PRP (platelet-rich plasma)** in the upper portion and red blood cells in lower portion. The PRP about 250 ml is expressed into an attached satellite bag, leaving the RBC in the primary bag (Fig. 10.12). The three attached bags are recentrifuged using a **heavy spin** to

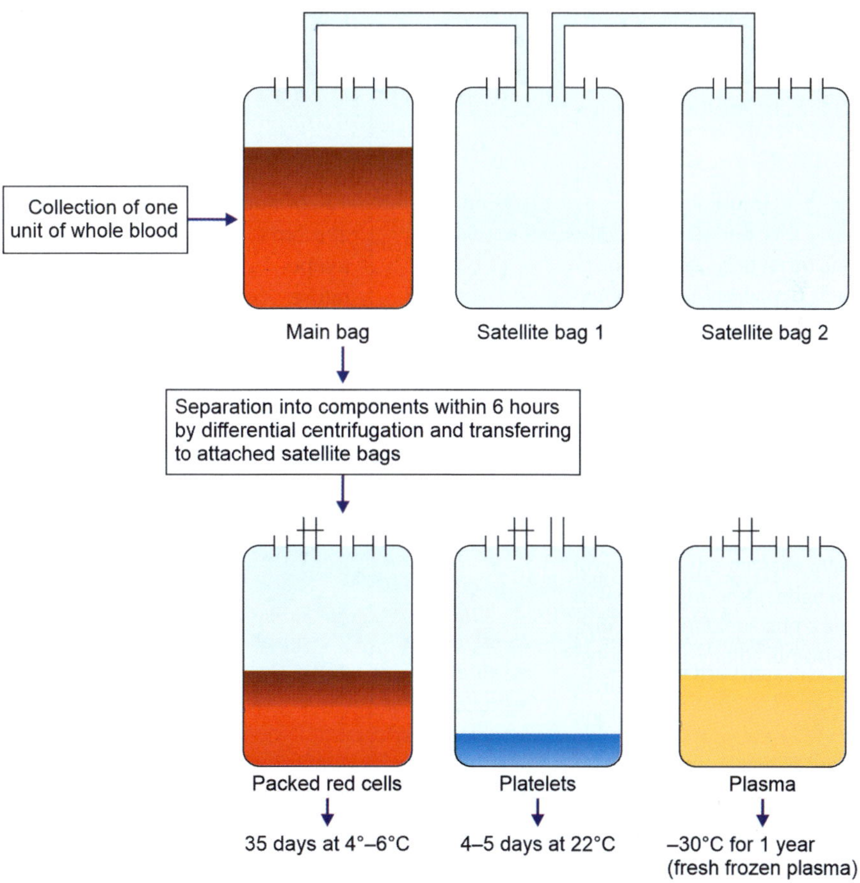

Fig. 10.12: Separation of blood components from whole blood

Table 10.6: Common blood components and derivatives

Blood components and derivatives	Characteristics	Approximate volume	Shelf life	Indications and components
Whole blood	Blood 350 ml, CPD or CPD-1 49 ml	400 ml	ACD or CPD: 21 days. CPD-1:35 days at 1–6°C	Acute massive blood loss, exchange transfusion, non-availability of packed red cells. The flow characteristics are rapid
Packed red cells	Packed RBC with reduced plasma volume. Hct 69%. WBC, platelets and coagulation factors as for whole blood	250 ml	As for whole blood	Replacement of red cells in anaemia. May be used in acute/massive blood loss. Flow characteristic is slow as Hct is high. Can be used with colloids and crystalloid to increase rate of flow.
Random donor platelet concentrate	Platelets (5.5×10^{10}), some WBC (i.e. lymphocyte), 50 ml plasma, few RBC (less than 0.5% haematocrit)	5–60 ml, 4–6 units for adult (1 unit/ 10 kg)	5 days at room temperature (20–24°C)	Used for quantitative and qualitative platelet disorders. May be used when bleeding (slow ooze) due to thrombocytopenia or for prophylaxis. 6–10 units raise platelet count about 50,000/mm^3
Granulocyte concentrate	Granulocyte (1.0×10^{10}) and other WBCs, 250 ml plasma, minimal platelets, RBC about 10% Hct	300 ml	12–24 hours at room temperature	Patients with sepsis, severe neutropenia (neutrophil count <500/mm^3 and bone marrow depression)
Fresh frozen plasma (FFP)	Plasma proteins, all coagulation factors, complement	200–260 ml	1 year at –18°C or colder	Bleeding patient with multiple coagulation deficiency, DIC, liver disease, TTP
Cryoprecipitate	80 units of factor VIII, other plasma proteins, von Willebrand factor, factor XIII, fibrinogen (200 mg), fibronectin	10–15 ml	1 year at ≤–18°C	Most useful for von Willebrand disease, factor XIII deficiency or hypofibrinogenaemia
Factor VIII concentrate	Quantity of factor VIII units are marked on lyophilized bottle	25 ml, as per manufacturer's instructions for reconstitution with diluents	2 years at 2–8°C	Used for haemophilia A (factor VIII deficiency). Lacks high molecular weight von Willebrand factor
Albumin	5 g/100 ml; 25 g/100 ml	250–500 ml; 50–100 ml	3 years at <30°C.	Most useful for hypovolaemic shock or hypoproteinaemia

Contd.

Table 10.6: Common blood components and derivatives (Contd.)

Blood components and derivatives	Characteristics	Approximate volume	Shelf life	Indications and components
Immune serum globulin	Mostly IgG and some IgA and IgM-	10 ml	3 years at <30°C	Treatment or prophylaxis of hypogammaglobulinaemia
Rh immuno-globulin	IgG anti-D (RhO)	1 ml	1½ years at 2–8°C	Prevents haemolytic disease of the newborn in Rh negative mother exposed to Rh positive red cells

produce an aggregated platelet button from PRP. About 200 ml plasma (platelet-poor) removed, leaving 50 ml pf platelet-poor plasma with platelet button. From this 200 ml **platelet-poor plasma FFP** is prepared (Table 10.6).

Transfusion-related Acute Lung Injury (TRALI)

- Pathogenesis: Presence of antibodies in the donor's plasma against recipient's HLA II antigens located on the neutrophils which leads to neutrophilic aggregation in the pulmonary vasculature and endothelial damage there. This leads to clinical symptom there.
- TRALI develops within 6 hours of transfusion.
- It is a cause of non-cardiogenic pulmonary oedema.
- Fresh frozen plasma (FFP) is the commonest blood product to cause TRALI. Mostly seen after sepsis and cardiac surgeries.
- Clinically, it is characterised by acute onset of respiratory disorders associated with oxygen desaturation (hypoxaemia) and bilateral lung infiltrates.
- Infections complications: These are common with platelet preparations. These can be prevented by donor screening (Table 10.7).

TRANSFUSION REACTION INVESTIGATION

Most adverse reaction investigations are conducted to make sure that this is not due to acute intravascular immune haemolysis from an ABO-incompatibility or mismatched transfusion. In the suspected case the intravenous line (IV line) must be kept open with crystalloids if immediate treatment is necessary to treat hypotension. Notify the blood bank immediately.

Table 10.7: ABO and Rh compatibility in blood transfusion

Blood type of recipient	Blood type of donor					
	A	B	AB	O	Rh^+	Rh^-
A	Yes	No	No	S		
B	No	Yes	No	S		
AB	S	S	Yes	S		
O	No	No	No	Yes		
Rh^+					Yes	Yes
Rh^-					E	Yes

S: Substitute as packed red blood cells or wash to eliminate antibodies. E: Only under extreme conditions, especially if the recipient is a young female

Furthermore, the following investigations should be done in case of suspected mismatched blood transfusion.

- Clerical check of the tag (written information) on the blood bag, the blood bag label and the patient identification for discrepancies.
- Investigation of the pre-transfusion clotted blood specimen an EDTA anticoagulated post-transfusion blood specimen and the blood bag.
- Perform a Gram's stain on the blood in the bag and a culture to identify the causative organism/bacteria.
- Repeat the ABO/Rh typing, antibody screen and the cross match to observe if a patient antibody is directed against donor cells. If an antibody is suspected, perform an RBC panel to identify the antibody.
- Examination of post-transfusion urine.
    - i. Look for dark color of urine, if present, test for haemoglobinuria.
    - ii. Test for haemolysis (extravascular and intravascular).
- If DIC is suspected, then perform PT, APTT, platelet count, fibrinogen and fibrin split products on a post-transfusion anticoagulated blood (Table 10.8).

Table 10.8: Investigation of haemolysis due to transfusion reaction

1. Check for incompatibility
• Clerical causes: An identification error will show the type of incompatibility
• Serological causes:
i. Repeat ABO and Rh grouping of the patient (pre-transfusion and post transfusion) as well as donor's blood
ii. Repeat cross-match test with pre- and post-transfusion serum
iii. Direct antiglobulin test (DAT) or direct Coombs' test (pre- and post-transfusion samples.
iv. Screen for red cell antibodies.
2. Check for haemolysis
• Perform tests for patient's plasma and urine for haemoglobin
• Schistocytes and spherocytes may be present on blood smear
3. Check for bacterial contamination/infection
• Gram stain and culture of donor's blood
4. Check for disseminated intravascular coagulation (DIC)
• Coagulation screen
• Measure fibrinogen level and fibrin degradation product (FDP)
• Platelet count
• Blood film (red cell fragmentation)

INTERNAL QUALITY CONTROL IN BLOOD BANK

Internal quality control (IQC) is the backbone of any quality assurance programme. IQC is the set of procedures undertaken by the staff of a laboratory for continuously and concurrently assessing laboratory work and emergent results, to decide whether they are reliable enough to be released.

Drifted trend: Seen when the control value moves progressively in one direction from the mean for a minimum of three days. Suggests that a problem is gradually developing, such as deterioration of a reagent or control.

Dispersion: Increase in random errors and lack of precision. Suggests inconsistency of technique or fluctuations in instrumentation function.

Shift: Abrupt changes observed when a problem develops suddenly. May be due to instrument malfunction or an error in technique (Fig. 10.13 and Table 10.9).

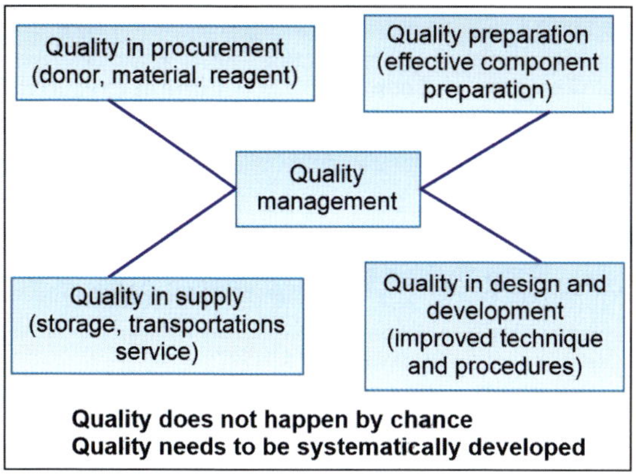

Fig. 10.13: Quality management in blood transfusion

The quality requirements involve

- Quality control and proficiency testing
- Internal and external audits
- Personnel and organization
- Premises, equipment and materials
- Blood pocessing
- Complaints and component recall
- Investigation of errors and accidents

Equipment QC

Equipment	Method of control	Frequency of control	Control executed
Laboratory refrigerator, freezers, water bath	Thermometer, precision thermometer	Daily	Technologist
Blood bag refrigerator, freezer containing transfusates	Graphic recorder plus independent audible and visual alarm for appropriate high and low temperature parameter	Daily	Technologist
Laboratory refrigerator, freezer, water bath	Precision thermometer # For calibration #	Every 6 month	Technologist
Equipment Cell counter	Method of control Calibration, reference samples,	Frequency of control Daily	Control executed by technologist
pH meter	Control solution pH 4–7, 7–10	Each time of use	Technologist
Platelet agitator	Frequency of agitation	Monthly	Technologist
Laminar flow blood	Air pressure	Daily	Microbiologist
Laminar flow blood and sterile area filter	Particle counter	3 times/month	Microbiologist
Cryofuge	Precision RPM meter plus stopwatch to control speed, acceleration and retardation	Twice/month	Technologist

Contd.

Contd.

Equipment	Method of control	Frequency of control	Control executed
Cryofuge	Temperature	Daily	Technologist
Table centrifuge	RPM meter plus stopwatch to control speed, acceleration and retardation	Daily	Technologist
Haemoglobin Spectrophotometer	Calibrate with standard	Daily	Technologist
Haemoglobin Spectrophotometer	Hb-QC sample	Monthly	Technologist
Equipment	Method of control	Frequency of control	Control executed by
Blood mixer	Control weighing and mixing	Twice/month	BM engineer
Blood bag tube sealer	Pressure on bag and tube	Every bag and weld	Technologist
Blood transport container	Temperature control device	Every time on use (on receipt)	Technologist

Table 10.9: List of qualitative (QL) and quantitative (QN) tests done in blood bank

Tests for donor selection	Tests for collected blood product	Tests for final pre-transfusion	Serological test done
• Haemoglobin (QN) • Platelet count (QN) • Serum albumin of donors (QN)	• HIV (QN)/(QL: Card test) • HBsAg (QN)/(QL: Card test) • HCV (QN)/(QL: Card test) • VDRL/RPR (QL) • MP (QL) • Factor VIII (QN) • Fibrinogen (QN) • PTTK (QN), • Pyogenic culture (QN)	• Haemoglobin (QN), • PCV (QN), • Platelet count (QN), • pH (QN) • TRBC (QC) • TLC (QN)	• Blood grouping (QL) • Crossmatching (QL) • Antibody screening/ plasma identification (QL) • Direct Coombs' test (QL) • Indirect Coombs' test (QL)

Equipment/Reagents which are Needed for in-house Checks (IQC)

- ELISA reader/kits
- Blood Grouping equipment/reagents
- Crossmatching cards/antibody screening
- Haematology analyzer/reagents
- pH meter
- Rapid cards/RPR (rapid plasma reagin) or VDRL/MP
- Coagulation analyzer

Selecting controls/calibrators: A calibrator has a known concentration of substance (analyte) being measured. Calibrator is used to adjust instrument, kit, test system in order to standardize the assay. Calibrator is not a control. A control has a known range of analyte. Usually 2 or 3 levels (L1, L2, and L3) of controls are used. Control should be run along with patient sample and is used to validate day-to-day reliability of the test systems (Fig. 10.14).

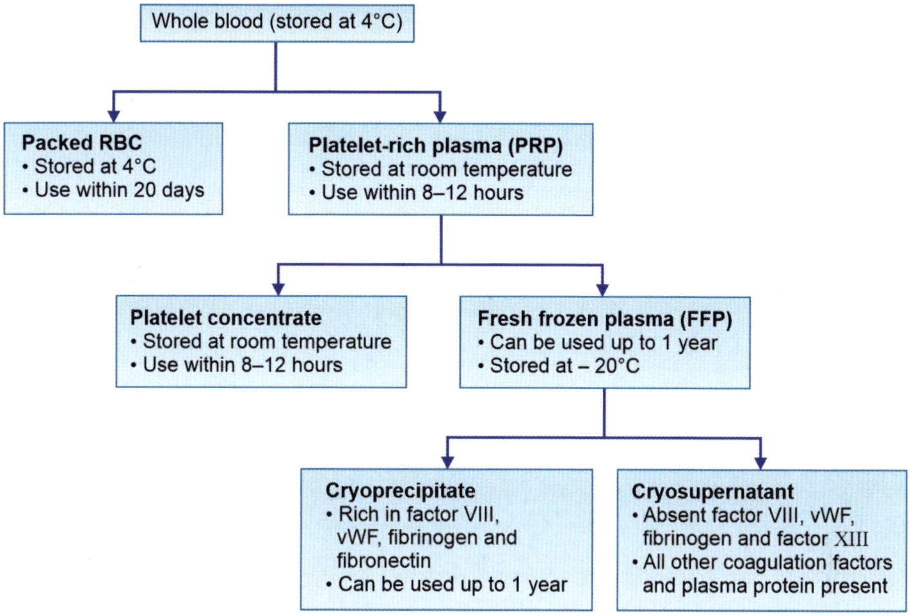

Fig. 10.14: Blood and different components and their use and storage

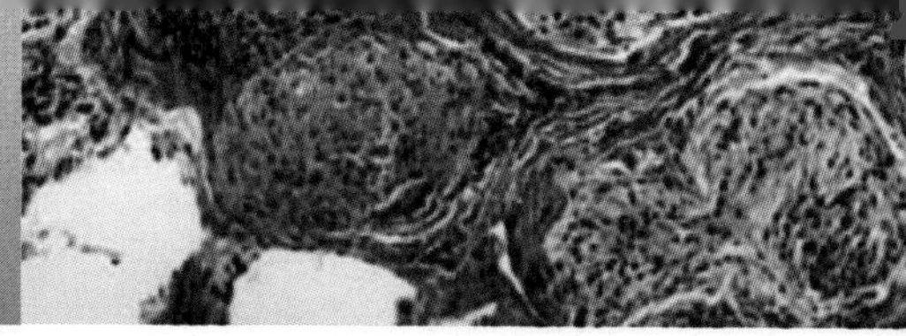

Section II

Clinical Pathology

Chapter

11

Lumbar Puncture Needle, Cerebrospinal Fluid and Body Cavity Fluids

Cerebrospinal fluid (CSF) is produced in the choroid plexuses (70%) and the remainder is formed around the blood vessels and along the ventricular walls. It is produced at a rate of 500 ml/day. It leaves the ventricular system through the medial and lateral foramina, flowing over the brain and spinal cord surface with the subarachnoid space.

The functions of CSF are to collect wastes, circulate nutrients, cushion and lubricate the central nervous system. Resorption of CSF occurs at the arachnoid villi. Total volume of CSF is 90–150 ml in adults and 10–60 ml in neonates.

Blood–brain barrier: When a dye (trypan blue) is injected in living animal/human, it results in staining of all tissues except brain and spinal cord. It was explained by postulation of an existence of a blood–brain barrier. Anatomically, this barrier represents the barrier in the capillary endothelium in contact with astrocyte foot processes. On the other hand, blood CSF barrier is represented by the choroid plexus epithelium and the endothelium of all cerebral capillaries in contact with CSF that accounts for different concentrations of solutes in plasma and CSF. Certain substances in the CSF are tightly regulated by specific transport system (e.g. H^+, K^+, Ca^{++}, Mg^{++}, HCO_3^-), whereas other like glucose, urea and creatinine diffuse freely. Water, chloride, carbon dioxide and oxygen also diffuse rapidly through the barrier easily (Table 11.1).

LUMBAR PUNCTURE (LP) NEEDLE

It is a sterile long slender needle with a stilette. It is about 10 cm long and has a bore of 1–1.5 mm.

Uses

i. Used for lumbar puncture.
ii. Cisternal puncture in case of babies.
iii. Can also be used for aspiration of body fluids from pleural cavity, peritoneal cavity, joint space, etc.
iv. In some cases of guided (CT/USG) FNAC of intra-abdominal or intrathoracic organs.

Lumbar Puncture Method

Evaluation of lumbar puncture (LP) (Fig. 11.1) is essential for the diagnosis of clinically suspected infectious meningitis, subarachnoid haemorrhage, leptomeningeal neoplastic disease and noninfectious meningitis.

Relative contraindication of doing LP: Local skin infection in the lumbar area, suspected spinal cord mass lesion, suspected intracranial mass lesion, any bleeding diathesis.

Haematological work up: A functional platelet count is >50,000/mm^3, and/or INR <1.5 are advisable to perform LP safely.

Table 11.1: Reference values of CSF in adults

Parameter	Conventional units	SI units
i. **Protein**	15–45 mg/dl	0.15–0.45/L
• Prealbumin	2–7%	
• Albumin	56–76%	
• α_1-Globulin	2–7%	
• α_2-Globulin	4–12%	
• β-Globulin	8–18%	
• γ-Globulin	3–12%	
ii. **Electrolytes**		
• Osmolality	280–300 mOsm	280–300 mmol/L
• Sodium	135–150 mEq/L	135–150 mmol/L
• Potassium	2.6–3.0 mEq/L	2.6–3.0 mmol/L
• Chloride	115–130 mEq/L (720–760 mg%)	115–130 mmol/L
iii. **pH**		
• Lumbar fluid	7.28–7.32	
• Cisternal fluid	7.32–7.34	
iv. **Other constituents**		
• Glucose	40–80 mg/dl	2.4–5.6 mmol/L
• Ammonia	10–35 μg/dl	6–20 μmol/L
• Creatinine	0.6–1.2 mg/dl	45–92 μmol/L
v. **pO_2**	40–44 mm Hg	
vi. **pCO_2**		
• Lumbar fluid	44–50 mm Hg	
• Cisternal fluid	40–46 mm Hg	

LP Technique (Fig. 11.2)

Proper position of the patient is important. Two different positions can be used:

i. *Lateral decubitus position:* Most common and routinely performed.
ii. *The sitting position:* Less common, preferable in obese patients.

In both the positions, the patient should be instructed to flex the spine as much as possible. In the lateral decubitus position, the patient is instructed to assume the foetal position with the knee fixed towards the abdomen. In the sitting position, the patient should be blend over a table with his/her head resting on folded arm.

The entry site for a LP is below the level of the conus medullaris, which extends to L1–L2 in most adults. Thus, L3–L4 or L4–S1 interspace can be utilized for entry site. The posterior superior iliac crest should be identified and the spine palpated at this level. It represents the L3–L4 interspace, with the other interspace referred from this landmark. The midpoint of the interspace between the spinous processes represents the entry point for the thoracocentesis needle.

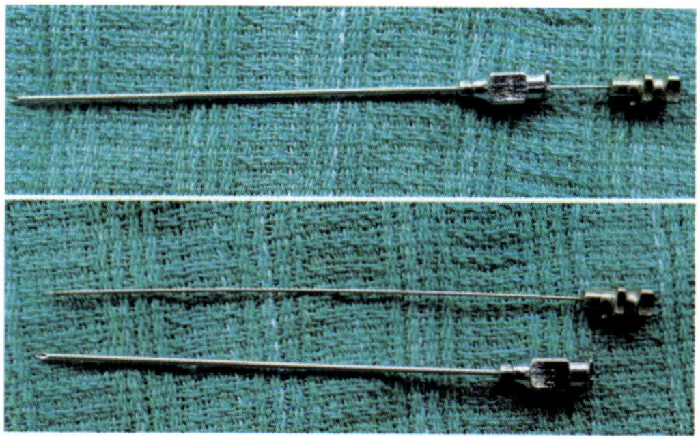

Fig. 11.1: Lumbar puncture (LP) needle

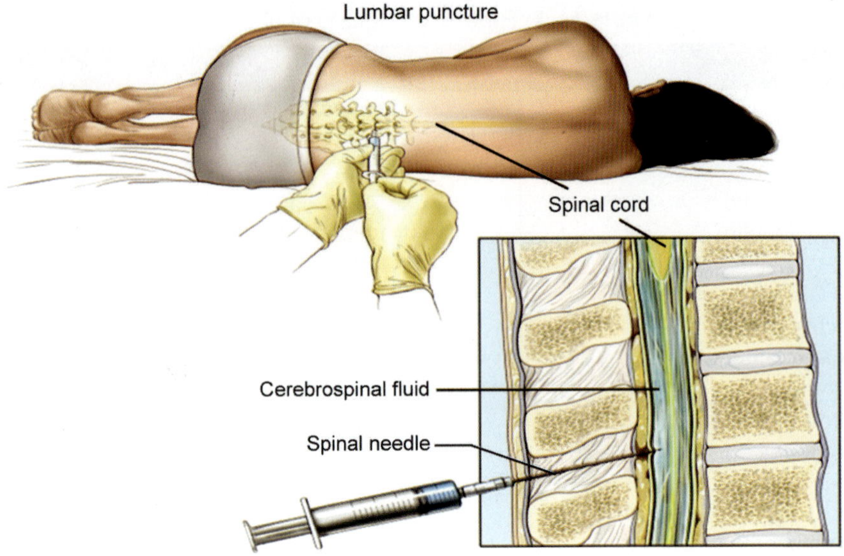

Fig. 11.2: Lumbar puncture technique

Overlying skin is properly cleansed with antiseptics. The skin and fascia of lumbar space selected for puncture are infiltrated with 1–2% lignocaine. Wait for 3–5 minutes.

Properly sterilised LP needle with stilette within it is pushed forward and slightly upward in midline between L3 and L4 vertebrae till a peculiar "give-way" sensation the needle is felt. The stilette is then removed. Pressure of CSF may be measured by fitting the nanometer to the needle or by counting drops (normally 60 drops/minute).

The CSF is then collected (total 10–15 ml) in 3 sterile tubes/vials. First tube is used for biochemical, second tube for microbiological and the third tube for cytological (pathological) examinations.

Ordinarily the CSF specimen is divided into 3 sterile tubes: Tube 1 for biochemistry and immunology studies, tube 2 for microbiological examination, and tube 3 for cell count and differential. An additional tube may be inserted in the No. 3 position for cytology if malignancy is suspected. Avoid glass tubes because cell adhesion to the glass affects the cell count and differential (Table 11.2). Specimens need to be received in the laboratory and processed quickly to minimize cellular degradation, which begins as soon as one hour after collection. Refrigerator is contraindicated for microbiological culture specimens because fastidious organisms like *H. influenzae* and *Neisseria meningitidis* will not survive.

Once, the required amount of CSF is collected, the stilette should be replaced and the LP needle is quickly withdrawn.

Postprocedure: To minimize the chance of a post-LP headache, the patient should be instructed to lie prone for at least 3 hours. If a headache develops then bed rest, hydration, and oral analgesics are often helpful.

NORMAL VALUES OF CSF

- Appearance: Clear and colourless
- Normal opening adult pressure: 90–180 ml of water in an adult in the lateral decubitus position.
- Cell count: Adults: WBC → 0–5 cells/mm^3, RBC → 0/mm^3
  Newborns: WBC → 0–30/mm^3, RBC → 0/mm^{3+}

Table 11.2: Differential cell count

Cell type	Adults (%)	Neonates (%)
• Lymphocytes	62 ± 34	20 ± 18
• Mononuclear cells and monocytes	36 ± 20	72 ± 22
• Neutrophils	2 ± 5	3 ± 5
• Histiocytes	Rare	Rare
• Eosinophils	Rare	Rare
• Ependymal cells	Rare	Rare

Macroscopic Examination

i. **Turbidity** or cloudiness begins to appear with WBC count >200 cell/mm^3 and RBC count >400 cells/mm^3.

ii. **Clot formation** in CSF may be seen in patients with traumatic taps, complete spinal block (Froin's syndrome), suppurative or tuberculous meningitis.

iii. **Xanthochromia:** The CSF is centrifuged, and the supernatant fluid is compared with a tube of distilled water. Xanthochromic CSF is pink, orange or yellow due to RBC lysis and haemoglobin break down. Pale pink, orange xanthochromia is noted after subarachnoid haemorrhage. Yellow xanthochromia is derived from bilirubin. It develops 12 hours after a subarachnoid bleeding, reaches peak at 2–4 days and persists for 2–4 weeks.

CSF xanthochromia may also be due to bilirubin in jaundice patients, artifactual red cell lysis caused by detergent contamination of the needle or tube, carotenoids (orange) in dietary hypercarotenemia, and rifampicin therapy (red-orange).

iv. **Protein coagulum:** Normal CSF does not show protein coagulum. Fibrin clot may form on standing when protein content is very high (>1000 mg%). A fine **cobweb** or **spider web coagulum** is seen in tuberculous meningitis when CSF is allowed to stand overnight. This cobweb coagulum may contain tubercle bacilli which may be seen after staining with ZN stain.

CSF Pressure

It is directly related with the pressure in jugular veins and vertebral veins. So, it is decreased in circulatory collapse and is increased in:

- Congestive cardiac failure (CCF)
- Superior mediastinal syndrome
- Breath holding, physical straining, pressure against abdomen.

CSF pressure is also increased if there is raised intracranial tension, such as

- Meningitis, encephalitis, meningoencephalitis
- Cerebral tumour, cerebral abscess
- Cerebral oedema
- Cerebral haemorrhage.

Indications for Collection of CSF

A. Diagnostic indications

- Meningitis, encephalitis, meningoencephalitis
- Subarachnoid haemorrhage (SAH)
- Central nervous system (CNS), syphilis
- Spinal cord tumour
- Multiple sclerosis
- Intracranial haemorrhage due to injury
- Intracranial space occupying lesion
- Differential diagnosis of cerebral infarction versus intracerebral haemorrhage: Almost in 80% of cases, the latter show blood or xanthochromia.

B. Therapeutic indications

- Relief of intracranial pressure
- Removal of exudate or blood from subarachnoid space
- Introduction of anti-meningococcus or anti-tetanus serum

- Introduction of spinal anaesthesia, radiographic contrast media or drugs.

Contraindications of Performing LP (Lumbar Puncture) Procedure

- Spinal cord tumour
- Brain tumour at cerebropontine angle
- Septicaemias
- Brain abscess (chance of spreading)
- Recent intracranial haemorrhage
- Patient is having convulsions (epilepsy)
- Cardiovascular disease (advanced)

Complications of LP

- Postpuncture persistent headache
- Death due to asphyxiation especially in infants
- Paresis followed by paralysis in cases of spinal cord tumour
- Implantation of skin and subsequent development of implantation dermoid if stylette is not used.
- Development of cerebellar coning followed by sudden death if there is increased intracranial pressure/tension.

Differential Cell Count

A differential performed in a Neubauer's counting chamber is unsatisfactory as low cell numbers have poor precision and identifying the cell type beyond granulocytes and mononuclear cells in a wet preparation. To improve precision and accuracy, different methods have been adopted:

i. **Cytocentrifuge:** It is recommend method for all body fluids including CSF. From 30 to 50 cells can be concentrated from 0.5 ml of normal CSF. This is rapid, and allows Romanowsky staining of air-dried cytospins.

ii. **Filtration method:** It provides excellent cell recovery slightly better preservation than cytocentrifuge but more time-consuming and costly. Romanowsky stain cannot be used. But the advantages are the ability to concentrate large volumes of CSF for cytological examination or culture while retaining the fluid filtrate for additional studies.

iii. **Sedimentation method**: It provides high quality smears, but the yield is not as good as filtration method. These methods are more cumbersome than cytocentrifugation.

Disease Detected by Laboratory Examination of CSF

1. **High sensitivity, high specificity**
   Bacterial, tuberculous and fungal meningitis
2. **High sensitivity, moderate specificity**
   - Subarachnoid haemorrhage
   - Viral meningitis
   - Multiple sclerosis
   - Paraspinal abscess
   - Central nervous system syphilis
3. **Moderate sensitivity, high specificity**
   Meningeal malignancy
4. **Moderate sensitivity, moderate specificity**
   - Viral encephalitis
   - Subdural haematoma
   - Intracranial haemorrhage

BODY CAVITY FLUID

The pleural, peritoneal and pericardial serous cavities usually referred to as body cavities and are lined by single layer of mesothelial cells. These mesothelial cells are made up of flattened or cuboidal epithelium, which is supported by a rich network of capillaries, lymphatics and loose connective tissue. The visceral and parietal surfaces are separated by a potential space which usually contains 10–50 ml fluid (pleural fluid 10–20 ml, peritoneal fluid 10–50 ml and pericardial fluid 10–50 ml). This fluid is pale yellow, clear serous fluid which acts as lubricant.

Normally, serous fluid has a glucose concentration similar to those of blood, a

Table 11.3: CSF findings in some common disorders

	Normal	Subarachnoid haemorrhage	Pyogenic/ bacterial meningitis	Viral meningitis	Tuberculous meningitis	Fungal meningitis
CSF pressure	50–180 mm H_2O		↑↑↑	N/	↑↑	
Colour	Crystal clear or colourless	Blood stained Xanthochromic	Turbid cloudy or opalescent	Clear	Clear/ slightly turbid	Slightly turbid/ clear
Coagulum of protein	Absent	Absent	Big protein clots within few minutes	Absent	Fine, thread-like cobweb or spider coagulum	Present as thread-like
Protein content	15–45 mg/dl		↑↑↑ (100–600 mg%)	(60–80 mg%)	↑↑ (80–140 mg%)	(60–160 mg%)
Glucose	40–80 mg%	Normal	Decreased 10–20 mg%)	Normal/ increased	Decreased (20–50 mg%)	Decreased (20–50 mg%)
Chloride	720–760 mg% (110–125 mEq/L)	Normal/ slightly increased	Decreased	Decreased	Marked decreased	Marked decreased
Total cell count	1–4/ mm^3	Increased RBC	1000–10,000 or more/mm^3	5–300/ mm^3	100–600/ mm^3	40–400/ mm^3
Cell type	Lymphocytes	RBC	Mostly neutrophils (>90%)	Lymphocytes	Mostly lymphocytes (>90%)	Neutrophils and/or lymphocytes; eosinophils in coccidioides
Gram stain	Nil	–	Gram-positive or gram-negative cocci or bacilli found	–	–	–
ZN stain	Nil	–	–	–	Acid-fast bacilli	–
PAS/GMS or fungal stain	Nil	–	–	–	–	Positive, filaments or spores of fungus

Table 11.4: Differences between transudate and exudate

Parameters	Transudate	Exudate
• Colour and appearance	Pale yellow, clear	Cloudy or haemorrhagic opaque
• Cause	Increased hydrostatic pressure or diminished colloidal oncotic pressure of blood	Increase capillary permeability due to various agents
• Specific gravity	<1.015	>1.015 (usually ≥1.018)
• Protein	<1 g%	>2 g%
• Glucose	Normal (15–30 mg%)	Low
• Fibrin	Poor	Rich, may form fibrin clot
• LDH (lactate dehydrogenase)	Normal	Increased
• Fluid/serum protein ratio	<0.5	>0.5
• Fluid/serum LDH ratio	<0.6	>0.6
• Cell count	Few	Many
• Cell type	Few mesothelial cells, occasional lymphocytes	Many inflammatory cells as per cause
• Bacteriological study	Negative	Usually positive if inflammatory causes, negative if neoplastic causes

pH 7.0 and protein concentration of <2 g%. The cellular contents are a few mesothelial cells and occasional lymphocytes.

Accumulation of serous fluid is called effusion, e.g. pleural effusion, peritoneal effusion and pericardial effusion. It can be transudate or exudate.

Laboratory Investigations

Specimen: Specimen (body cavity fluid) should be collected aseptically. The fluid should be collected in 3 sterile containers (test tubes/vials)—one for cytological examination, one for biochemical and other for microbiological examinations.

1. ***Physical examination:*** This includes macroscopic examination, determination of specific gravity and others.
2. ***Microscopic examination:*** Examination for total cell count and differential cell count (stained smear). Look for any neoplastic/malignant cell.
3. ***Chemical examination:*** Usually done for protein and occasionally for glucose, chloride and LDH, mucin or clotting test also reflects the behaviour of certain proteins.
4. ***Laboratory culture:*** To identify the particular infective organism.

Mucin clot test: Addition of 2–3% acetic acid to fluid.

Synovial Fluid

Synovium refers to the tissue lining synovial tendon sheaths, bursae and diarthrodial joints except for the articular surface. Synovium is composed of 1–3 cell layers which form a discontinuous surface overlying fatty, fibrous or periosteal joint space.

Synovial fluid is an imperfect ultrafiltrate of plasma combined with hyaluronic acid produced by the synovial cells. Small ions and molecules like glucose and urea cross easily into the joint space and their concentration is similar to plasma. But large molecules are absent or are present in only trace amounts. Synovial fluid acts as a lubricant and adhesive and provides nutrients for the avascular articular cartilage.

Table 11.5: Causes of pleural, peritoneal and pericardial effusion

Fluid type	Pleural	Peritoneal	Pericardial
1. Transudate	• CCF (congestive heart failure) • Nephrotic syndrome (hypoproteinaemia) • Hepatic cirrhosis	• CCF • Nephrotic syndrome • Hepatic cirrhosis	–
2. Exudate	**Neoplasms** • Bronchogenic carcinoma • Metastatic cancer • Lymphoma • Malignant mesothelioma	**Neoplasms** • Hepatocellular carcinoma • Metastatic cancer • Lymphoma • Malignant mesothelioma	**Neoplasms** • Metastatic cancer • Lymphoma
	Infections • Tubreculosis • Pyogenic pneumonia • Viral pneumonia • Mycoplasmal pneumonia	**Infections** • Tuberculosis • Bacterial peritonitis • Appendicitis (secondary bacterial peritonitis)	**Infections** • Tuberculosis • Bacterial pericarditis • Fungal pericarditis • Viral or mycoplasmal pericarditis
	Others • Trauma • Pulmonary infarct • SLE • Rheumatic disease	**Others** • Trauma • Bile peritonitis • Pancreatitis	**Others** • Trauma • Myocardial infarction • SLE • Rheumatic disease

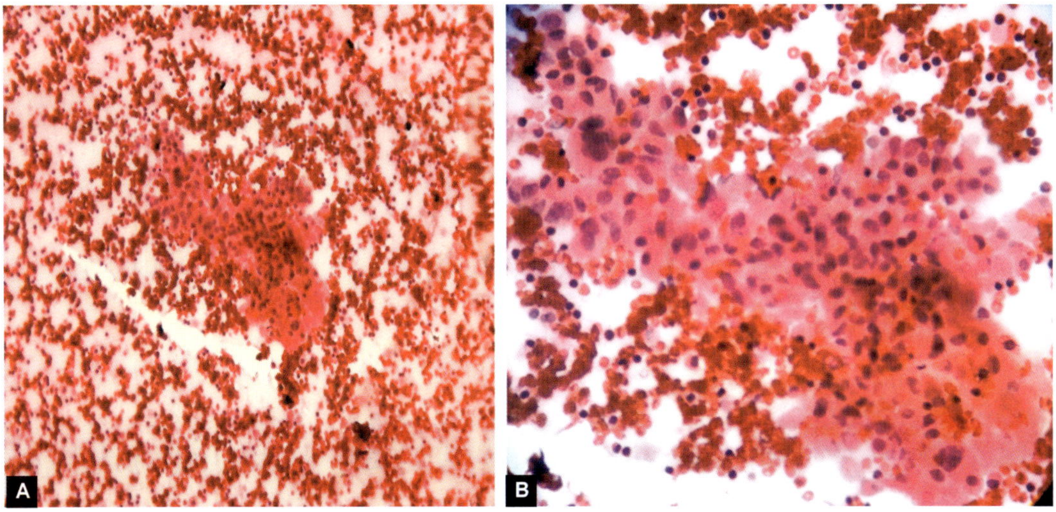

Fig. 11.3A and B: Granuloma in pleural fluid. (A) Low power view; (B) High power view. Granuloma is formed by clusters of epithelioid histiocytes (macrophages)

Normal Synovial Fluid

Volume in a joint: 0.1–2.0 ml

Colour and appearance: Transparent, straw coloured.

Chemical composition

- Protein: 1–3 g/dl (albumin 55–70%, α_1-globulin 6–8%, α_2-globulin 5–7%, β-globulin 8–10%, γ-globulin 10–14%)
- Hyaluronate: 0.3–0.4 g/dl
- Glucose: 70–110 mg/dl
- Uric acid: 2–8 mg/dl
- Lactate: 10–20 mg/dl.

Cytology: Usually 1–2/mm^3 (lymphocytes or histiocytes; a few synovial cells). Maximum range up to 20/mm^3.

Investigations of Synovial Fluid

1. **Inflammatory fluid:** Turbid, and yellow. Cell count 3000–5000/mm^3. Protein content is elevated, viscosity diminished and glucose level normal or low. This may be due to gouty arthritis, other inflammatory arthritis and occasionally septic arthritis.

   A fair number of plasma cells is found in rheumatoid arthritis (>500/mm^3). In septic arthritis, the neutrophil count is high and go up to 50,000/mm^3. The enzyme lactate dehydrogenase (LDH) is elevated in rheumatoid arthritis, gouty arthritis and infectious (septic) arthritis.
2. **Noninflammatory fluid:** It is clear, viscous and amber-coloured. WBC count is <200/mm^3 (mostly mononuclear cells). Protein is low and glucose normal (transudate). Seen in trauma and osteoarthritis.

Mucin Clot Test (Ropes Test) (Fig. 11.4)

Addition of acetic acid to synovial fluid precipitates hyaluronate into a mucin clot, which may be graded as good, fair and poor. Mucin clot reflects the polymerization of synovial fluid hyaluronate.

Mucin

Mucin is a mucopolysaccharide or glycoprotein which is the chief constituent of mucus.

Principle of test: It measures how well-polymerized the hyaluronic acid is?

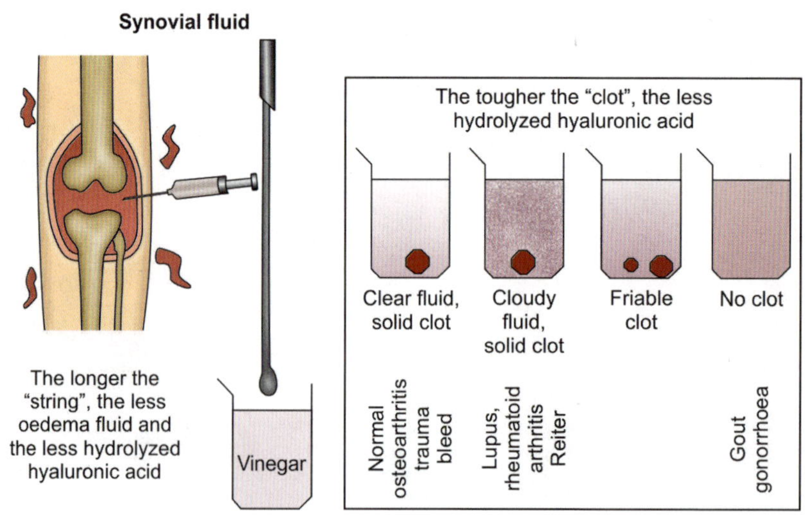

Fig. 11.4: Mucin clot test (Ropes test)

Table 11.6: Synovial fluid in normal and in disease conditions

Finding	Normal	Disease category			
		Group I (noninflammatory)	Group II (inflammatory)	Group III (infections)	Group IV (haemorrhagic)
• Appearance	Clear, straw coloured	Yellow, transparent	Yellow, cloudy, turbid or bloody	Yellow and purulent	Xanthochromic or red-brown
• WBC count	0–150/ml	<3000/ml	3000–75,000/ml	50,000–200,000/ml	50–10,000/ml
• Neutrophil percentage (%)	<25%	<30%	>50%	>90%	<50%
• RBC (if any)	No	No	No	Yes	Yes
• Glucose content	0–10 mg/dl	0–10 mg/dl	0–40 mg/dl	20–100 mg/dl	0–20 mg/dl

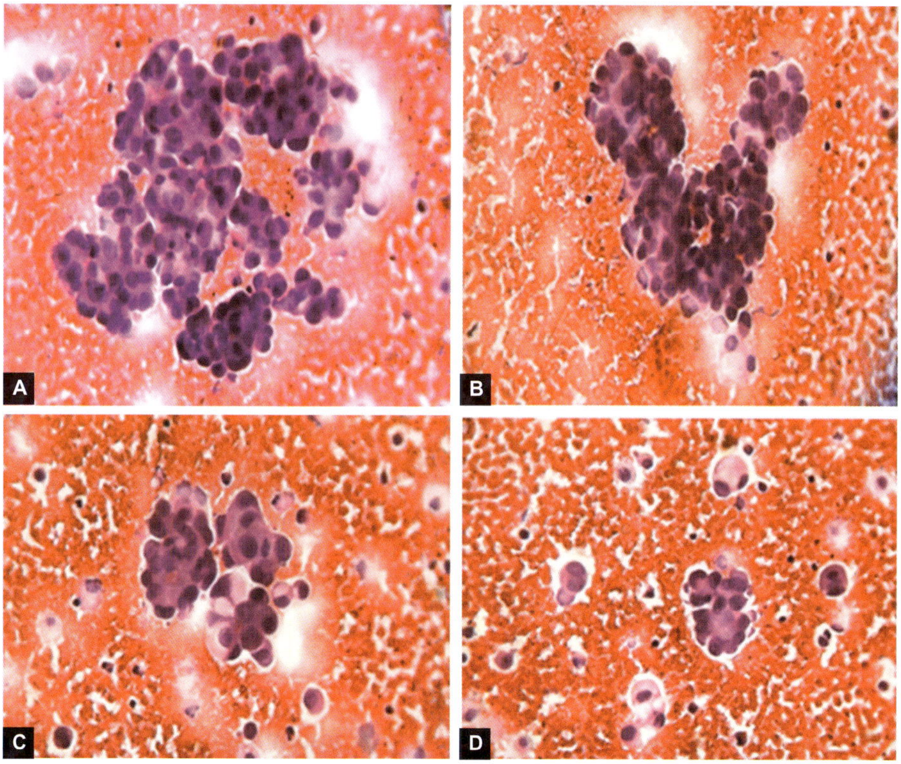

Fig. 11.5A to D: Adenocarcinoma cells in fluid cytology (peritoneal fliud). (A) Low power view showing sheets and papillary pattern of malignant cells (MGG × 100); (B) Low power view showing sheets and papillary pattern of malignant cells (Pap × 100); (C) High power view showing mucin vacuoles among tumour cells (Pap × 400); (D) High power view showing adenoid/pseudoglandular pattern of tumour cells. Few signet ring cells are also seen in the background (Pap × 400)

Table 11.7: Distinguishing feature among reactive mesothelial cells, mesothelioma and adenocarcinoma cells (exfoliated)

Feature	Reactive mesothelium	Mesothelioma (malignant)	Adenocarcinoma
1. Cellularity	Variable	High (often)	Variable
2. Edges of group of cells	Berry like group (<10 cells) with scalloped contour, 'window' present	Berry like groups with scalloped contour, 'window' present	Large clumps (>10 cells), smooth contoured cohesive group with "hard" edges
3. Cell sheets	May be seen but single cell is also seen	Rare	Not found
4. Acinar structures	Not found	May be found	Common
5. Papillary structures	Rare	May be found	May be found
6. Multinucleated cells	Occasional	Frequent	May be found
7. N:C ratio	Low, a little cell to cell variation	Low, a little cell to cell variation	High, cell-to-cell variation
8. Nuclei	Round with smooth contour	Enlarged nuclei with smooth contours	Anisonucleosis, often with irregular contours
9. Nucleoli	May be prominent	Often macronucleoli	Often prominent
10. Cytoplasm	Abundant and dense with peripheral fuzziness	Abundant and dense with peripheral fuzziness	Variable amount, not dense, sharp borders
11. Cytoplasmic vacuolation	May be found	May be found	Often present
12. Cytoplasmic mucin (vacuoles)	Absent	Absent	Often present
13. Cytoplasmic glycogen (vacuoles)	Often found	Often abundant	May be found
14. Cytoplasmic lipid (vacuoles)	Frequent small perinuclear vacuoles	Frequent, small perinuclear vacuoles	Seen in cases of clear cell carcinoma of kidney
15. Electron microscopy (scanning EM or SEM)	Majority show vesicles or blebs covering the surfaces. A few cells are covered by regular microvilli (MV) and show openings of pinocytic vacuoles	Numerous, long, slender microvilli	Short, plump, microvilli

Test method: A few drops of synovial fluid are added to 10 ml of 5% acetic acid in a beaker and swirled for 1–2 minutes. The result is interpreted as:

- **Good mucin clot:** A solid clot in a clear solution
- **Fair mucin clot**: A soft clot in a slightly turbid solution
- **Poor mucin clot**: A friable (crumby) clot in a turbid solution
- **Very poor mucin clot**: No clot, turbid fluid

Inflammation in the joint space damage the hyaluronic polymers, shortening them.

Good mucin clot: Osteoarthritis, trauma, haemophilic arthritis.

Fair mucin clot: Lupus and rheumatoid arthritis.

Poor and very poor mucin clot: Septic and crystalline (gout) arthritis, gonorrhoea.

Polarised Microscopy

Crystals and cellularity are analysed by polarised microscope. Needle-shaped crystals of monosodium urate (usually intracellular) are seen in gouty effusions. Rhomboid-shaped crystals are seen in pseudogout and chondrocalcinosis.

Light's Criteria for Pleural Fluid

There are three parameters:

1. Pleural fluid protein/serum protein ratio >0.5.
2. Pleural fluid LDH/serum LDH ratio >0.6.
3. Pleural fluid LDH greater than two-thirds of the upper limits of normal of the serum LDH.

If at least one of the above three criteria is present, the fluid is virtually always an exudate.

If none is present, the fluid is always a transudate.

VIVA VOCE

Q.1. What are the different uses of lumbar puncture needle?

Ans: i. Most important use is to draw CSF (cerebrospinal fluid)

ii. It may also be used for aspiration from pleural cavity, peritoneal cavity or from joint spaces.

Q.2. Why is L_3–L_4 or L_4–L_5 vertebra chosen for lumbar puncture?

Ans: Spinal cord in humans extends up to L_1 vertebra level. So, if aspiration is done between L_3–L_4 and L_4–L_5 level, there will be no damage to spinal cord and CSF is collected safely. But in small children, conus medullaris extends lower than in adults, so puncture is done L_4–L_5 or lower.

Q.3. When CSF pressure is high, why lumbar puncture is contraindicated?

Ans: It may cause herniation of cerebellum and coning of medulla which may be fatal.

To prevent this, precaution is taken if it is to be done. After introduction of lumbar puncture needle, stylet is partially and slowly withdrawn so that CSF comes drop by drop and not in a jet as CSF pressure is high.

Q.4. How would you differentiate between haemorrhage due to pathological cause and traumatic tap?

Ans:

Parameters	Pathological	Traumatic tap
i. Presence of blood in subsequent collection from 3rd–4th tube onwards	Present in all tubes	Absent
ii. Xanthochromia (yellowish colour) of the supernatant CSF	Present	Absent
iii. Latex agglutination test for cross-linked fibrin derivative D-dimer specific for fibrin degradation	Present	Absent
iv. Haemosiderin laden macrophages and/or erythrophagocytosis under microscope	Present	Absent

Q.5. What is the significance of coagulum in CSF?

Ans: Fibrin clots may be formed on standing when protein content in CSF is very high (>1000 mg/dl, normal 15–45 mg/dl).

In tuberculous meningitis, fine cobweb (thread-like) coagulum is often seen in CSF when it is allowed to stand overnight (prolonged time). This cobweb coagulum may take up tubercle bacilli which may be detected by ZN stain.

Q.6. What is the normal volume of different body cavity fluids and how does it appear?

Ans: Peritoneal cavity contains 10–50 ml, pericardial cavity contains 10–50 ml and pleural cavity contains 10–20 ml of serous fluid. It appears as a pale yellow, clear serum fluid and serves as friction lubricant.

Q.7. What is fibrinous exudate?

Ans: Exudates have higher protein content (>2 mg/dl). When fibrinogen enters body fluid the sample clot after collection and is called fibrinous exudate.

To prevent this, EDTA may be added to the collecting vial/tube.

Q.8. What is the significance of ADA (adenosine deaminase) estimation?

Ans: ADA enzyme is related to purine metabolism and associated with immunodeficiency. Elevate ADA level is seen in tuberculous effusions irrespective of HIV status. There are two isoenzymes of ADA one in ADA I and another is ADA II. The ADA II isoenzyme form is released from activated lymphocytes in tuberculosis. Level >36 U/L in fluid and >54 U/L in serum suggest tuberculosis.

Q.9. What is the significance of high level of hyaluronic acid in serous fluid?

Ans: This is found in effusions caused by malignant mesothelioma (diffuse) and in metastatic deposits of Wilms' tumour over serous surfaces.

Higher level of hyaluronic acid in serous fluid increase the viscosity giving a honey-like consistency.

Q.10. What is globulin test in CSF?

Ans: There are two types of tests done to detect globulins in CSF.

a. **Pandy's test**: In a small test tube, place 1–2 ml of saturated solution of phenol. To it add, 1 drop of CSF. Cloudiness against a black background indicates presence of globulin. It is reported as O (nil), 1+, 2+, 3+ or 4+.

b. **Ross Jones test**: Pour 0.5 ml of clear CSF over 1 ml of saturated solution of ammonium sulphate in a test tube. A thin white ring is formed at the juncture of two fluids. If it disappears on mixing, then it is reported as 1+. Heavy cloudiness persists even after mixing is reported as 4+.

Q11. How CSF fluid is used for different investigations?

Ans: Collected CSF (total 10–15 ml) is divided in 3 sterile tubes/vials. First tube is sent for biochemical, second tube for microbiological and the third tube for cell count and differential count in pathology.

An additional tube may be inserted in the No. 3 position for cytology if malignancy is suspected. Avoid glass tubes because cell adhesion to the glass affects the cell count and differential. Specimens need to be received in the laboratory and processed quickly to minimise cellular degradation, which begins as soon as one hour after collection. Refrigeration is contraindicated for microbiological culture specimens because fastidious organisms like *H. influenzae* and *Neisseria meningitidis* will not survive.

Chapter

12

Urine Examination

Urine examination provides a wide variety of useful information regarding the disease involving the kidney and lower urinary tract. In the evaluation of urine, many tests are done. These tests include: Chemistry, microbiology, routine urine wet analysis, and some other special tests. Some modern techniques like immunocytochemistry, DNA ploidy, cell cycle analysis and molecular genetics (PCR) are also performed on urine specimens.

At present, **three types of urinalysis** are performed. These are:

1. A screening wet urinalysis (routine examination of urine)
2. A reagent strip (dipstick or multistick paper strip)
3. Specialised urinalysis (like cytological examination of malignant cells, PCR, DNA analysis, flow cytometry, etc.).

Composition of Normal Urine

A normal healthy person excretes approximately 1500 ml of urine in 24 hours. Normal urine is clear and pale-yellow in colour which has typical aromatic odour due to presence of volatile organic acids. The yellowish colour of urine is due to presence of urochromes, which comes as breakdown product of urobilinogen. Freshly voided urine is slightly acidic (pH 6.0 to 6.8) which becomes alkaline on standing due to release of ammonia from urea decomposition. This urea decomposition occurs due to role of contaminated bacteria which initiates urease activity that splits urea.

Urine is composed predominantly of water (95%) and other soluble waste products (urea, creatinine, uric acid) and excess electrolytes (sodium, potassium, calcium, chloride, phosphate and others). Most hormones and drugs after their function in the body, are usually excreted through urine. So, urine can be ideal specimen for evaluating hormonal disorders and drug overdose.

Normal urine after standing will often crystallise certain chemicals like urates and phosphates under alkaline conditions and urine becomes turbid now. Epithelial cells, WBC, RBC are occasionally seen in normal urine. Their presence in increased number indicates a pathological condition or disease.

Urine Collection Methods

Urine specimens may be collected in a variety of methods according to type of specimen required the collection type and patient type.

- **Randomly collected specimen (Table 12.1):** It is usually not preferred as urine may be collected soon after patient has consume water/fluid (urine is diluted).

Table 12.1: Benefits of common tests performed with urine specimens

Type of test	Detection	Clinical Screening	Use Diagnostic	Clinical Monitoring	Use Prognostic
1. Wet urinalysis (routine examination)	Glycosuria (diabetes) Proteinuria Haematuria Leukocyturia Infections Crystalluria	++++	++	++	+
2. Reagent strip (dipstick, multistick)	Glycosuria Proteinuria Haematuria Leukocyturia Infections	+++	+/-	+	+
3. Urine microbiology (culture, etc.)	Infections	++	++++	++	+
4. Conventional urinalysis	Glomerular and renal tubular disease Lower urinary tract disorders Non-bacterial infections	+	++++	+++	++
5. Modern diagnostics (PCR, DNA analysis, flow cytometry)	Urothelial cancer	–	+	+++	++

- **First morning specimen:** It is the choice of specimen for urinalysis and microscopic analysis because the urine is generally more concentrated.
- **Midstream clean catch specimen:** This specimen is strongly recommended for microbiological culture and antibiotic susceptibility testing because of reduced incidence of cellular and microbial contamination.
- **Timed collection specimen:** It may be required for quantitative measurement of certain analytes (creatinine, urea, sodium, potassium, calcium, uric acid, catecholamines, metanephrines, vanillylmandelic acid (VMA), etc.).
- **Collection from catheters** (e.g. Foley's catheter): For patients who have difficulties to micturate and are using catheters.
- **Suprapubic aspiration:** It may be necessary when a non-ambulatory patient cannot be catheterised or where there are concerns about obtaining a sterile specimen by conventional methods.
- **Paediatric specimen:** For infants and small children, a special urine collection bag or condom may be attached to the urethral opening.
- **24 hours specimen:** It is of value to quantify 24 hours urinary protein excretion (helpful to diagnose nephritic syndrome and other cause of heavy proteinuria).

Urine Collection Recommendations (the CLSI* Guidelines)

- Primary (routine) specimen containers to have a wide base and a capacity of at least 50 ml.
- Sterile collection containers for all microbiological specimens.
- 24 hours specimen containers to have a capacity of at least 3 litres.
- Specimen containers should have secured closure to prevent specimen loss and to protect the specimen from contaminants.
- Amber-coloured container for specimen required for assay of light sensitive analytes such as urobilinogen and porphyrins.

Preservation of Urine

The urine should be examined within 1–2 hours after voiding. If delay is anticipated, then the specimen is best preserved in a refrigerator (but do not freeze) at an acid pH and without any preservative.

Chemical preservatives prevent decomposition and contamination of bacteria and fungi.

- **Toluene** (2 ml/100 ml urine): It is best all-round preservative. But it interferes with the protein examination by sulphosalicylic method.
- **Thymol** (one crystal): It can preserve urine for a few days. However, it may have false positive reaction for protein.
- **Boric acid** (1% or 1 g/100 ml urine): It is used for many hormones and other substances.
- **Formalin** (1 drop/30 ml urine): It is an excellent preservative for the formed elements (erythrocytes, WBC, casts, etc.).
- **Sodium carbonate:** Rarely used for preservation of urobilinogen.
- **Sodium fluoride**

Physical Examination of Urine (Table 12.2)

Urine Volume

The 24 hours urine discharged by a healthy adult with normal water/fluid intake is about 1500 ml. Because it varies widely with

* Clinical and Laboratories Standards Institute, USA.

Table 12.2: Urine report of a normal adult

Physical examination
• Urine volume: 600–2000 ml/day (24 hours) • Colour: Pale yellow or straw coloured • Appearance: Clear (cloudy if there is phosphate) • Odour: Faint aromatic • Sediment: Nil • Specific gravity: Range 1.003–1.035 (specific gravity of distilled water is 1, also written as 1003–1035, but normal adults with adequate fluid intake specific gravity will be 1.016–1.022)
Chemical examination
• pH (reaction): 4.6–8 (mean 6.1), acidic • Protein (mainly albumin): Scant amount (<150 mg/24 hours urine) • Reducing substance (glucose): Nil or glucose ≤130 mg/day urine • Ketone bodies: Nil • Bile salt and bile pigment: Nil • Bence-Jones protein: Absent • Urobilinogen: 0.5–2.5 mg/24 hours or 0.5–1 mg/dl • Phosphates: Nil or trace • Nitrites: Nil
Microscopical examination
• WBC: 0–5/HPF (usually 0–2, but up to 5/HPF in morning urine)* • RBC: 0–2/HPF • Cast (hyaline casts): 0–2/lpf • Epithelial cells (squamous, cuboidal or transitional ≤15–20/HPF (usually 3–5/HPF) • Crystals: Urates, uric acid, calcium oxalate in acid urine and phosphates, biurates in alkaline urine normally may be present • Bacteria: None • Yeast: None • Parasite (Trichomonas, *Schistosoma haematobium*, microfilaria): None

HPF: High power field, lpf: Low power field, *increased number may be seen in menstruating women.

fluid intake, physiological condition and diet of the human body. Urine discharged during day is about 3–4 times more than that of night. Children (6–12 years) discharge about 800–1200 ml of urine and infant about 500–600 ml of urine in 24 hours.

A urine volume >2000 ml/24 hours is termed **polyuria** and urine <400 ml/24 hours is called **oliguria**. **Anuria** is complete absence of urine formation. **Oligoanuria** when <100 ml/day.

Causes of polyuria

- Diabetes insipidus/diabetes mellitus
- Compulsive water drinking
- Intravenous saline/fluid infusion
- Chronic glomerulonephritis
- Chronic pyelonephritis
- Benign nephrosclerosis
- Hyperparathyroidism
- Addison's disease
- Drug like diuretics

Causes of oliguria

- Severe dehydration (diarrhoea, vomiting, excessive sweating)
- Acute glomerulonephritis (mainly in children)
- Renal ischaemia in a patient of shock
- Obstruction to urinary outflow
- Bilateral hydronephrosis
- Toxic or ischaemic nephrosis
- Blood transfusion reaction or following surgery.

Colour

The yellow colour of normal urine is mainly due to the pigment urochrome and to a small amounts of urobilins and uroerythrin. Urochrome excretion is believed to be proportional to the metabolic rate and it is increased in high fever, thyrotoxicosis and starvation. The uroerythrin (pink pigment) may be deposited in uric acid or urate crystals (black dust deposit) and it should not be confused with blood. Colourless or pale urine in a normal person may be seen after high fluid intake and darker urine (deep yellow or mustard coloured) when fluids are withheld.

Change in urine colour (pathologic and others)

- Red urine: Frank haematuria (gross haematuria), haemoglobinuria or methaemoglobinuria, beets and aniline dye.
- Brown black: Methaemoglobinuria, presence of melanin and homogentisic acid (alkaptonuria)
- Yellow-green: Bilirubin, biliverdin
- Milky white: Presence of chyle in urine (chyluria), plenty of neutrophils (pyuria), emulsified paraffin used in vaginal cream.
- Cloudy: Excess phosphates, carbonates, urates and uric acid in urine, prostatic fluid, radiographic dye.

Specific Gravity

Specific gravity is the density of a substance (weight per unit volume) as compared to that of the density of water which is 1.000 (also written as 1000). Specific gravity of a solution largely depends on the amount of solute present and also on temperature of the solution. It increases with increasing concentration of solute and decreases with increasing temperature as urine volume increases with temperature and density decreases.

Kidney can produce urine with specific gravity which ranges from 1.005 to 1.035. Urine of low specific gravity is called **hyposthenuric** (≤1.007). Urine of fixed specific gravity about 1.010 is known as **isosthenuric**. The specific gravity of the protein-free glomerular filtrate is about 1.010 and its osmolar concentration is about 285 mOsm.

Specific gravity of normal urine is contributed by urea (20%), sodium chloride (25%), sulfate and phosphate mainly. Normal adult with normal diets and normal fluid intake produces urine of specific gravity 1.016–1.022 during a 24-hour period. If there is no fluid intake for 12 hours or 24 hours then specific gravity becomes 1.022 or ≥1.026 respectively.

Causes of high specific gravity

- Concentrated urine: Due to excessive sweating, fever, vomiting.
- Acute nephritis
- Uncontrolled diabetes mellitus (crystalloids not the colloids are responsible)
- All causes of oliguria.

Cause of low specific gravity (<1.010)

- Excessive fluid or water intake
- Diabetes insipidus
- Chronic nephritis
- Hypertension with renal involvement
- All causes of polyuria except diabetes mellitus

Cause of low and fixed specific gravity (1.010–1.012)

- End stage renal disease (chronic nephritis)
- Arteriosclerotic kidney
- ADH deficiency

Measurement of Specific Gravity of Urine

It can be done by following methods:

a. **Urinometer (hydrometer):** The urinometer vessel is filled with three-fourths full with urine (about 70–80 ml, minimum 15 ml urine). The urine should be foamless. The urinometer is inserted with a spinning motion to make sure that the instrument is floating freely without touching the sides or the bottom of the container. Read graduations at the lowest level of the urinary meniscus. If the urine amount is less than dilute the urine to raise the volume till 70–80 ml. Take the reading and multiply by the dilution factor (take last two digits).

   Correction factor for temperature: Add or subtract 0.001 for each 3°C above or below the standardisation temperature (usually 20°C).

   Correction for protein and glucose: Subtract 0.003 for every 1 g/100 ml of protein and 0.004 for every 1 g/100 ml of glucose.

b. **Refractometer:** The refractive index of a solution is related to the content of dissolved solids present. It is the ratio of the velocity of light in air to the velocity of light in a solution. The instrument requires only a few drops of urine (unlike the minimum 15 ml of urine necessary for urinometer).

   In Goldberg refractometer, the specific gravity of urine can be read directly from the calibration. But the specific gravity reading on refractometer is usually slightly lower than a urinometer reading on the same urine by about 0.002.

c. **Reagent strips/dipsticks:** This is basically colorimetric method. The principle of the specific gravity area is based on a pKa change of certain penetrated polyelectrolytes in relation to ionic concentration. The reagent is sensitive to the number of ions in the urine specimen. An indicator changes colour in relation to ionic concentration and is translated to specific gravity values.

Chemical Examination of Urine

pH

The pH (reaction) of urine can be measured by:

- Litmus paper or other pH indicator papers: It can detect broad range of pH 1 to 12. Note the colour change. If red = acidic, orange = normal, yellow = alkaline.
- Reagent strip: Indicators like methyl red and bromothymol blue give a range of orange, green and blue as the pH rises. The test permits differentiation of pH values to half a unit within the range of 5 to 9.
- pH electrode: pH can be measured by pH meter with a closed glass electrode.
- **Titration method:** The pH of the urine is largely dependent on the amount of

mono- and di-basic phosphate present. Titratable acidity is measured by titrating an aliquot of 24-hour urine (collected on ice) with 1/10 (N) NaOH with pH 7.4 as an endpoint.

Causes of acidic urine

- Ketosis: Diabetes, starvation, fever in children.
- Systemic acidosis: Metabolic acidosis, respiratory acidosis.
- Acidification therapy: Acidification therapy when used to treat urinary tract infection.
- Others: Diet containing high protein, some fruits like cranberries.

Causes of alkaline urine

- Alkaline tide: The urine becomes less acid after a meal as a result of secretion of acid into the stomach. On the contrary, at night during the mild respiratory acidosis of sleep, a more acid urine may be formed.
- Systemic alkalosis: Severe vomiting, excess alkali ingestion, hyperventilation.
- Urinary tract infection: Caused by Proteus and Pseudomonas. They split urea to bicarbonate and ammonia.
- Alkalinization therapy: It is used to prevent crystallization of uric acid, oxalate, cystine, streptomycin and sulphonamides.
- Others: Diet high certain fruits and vegetables, especially citrus fruits.

Test for Reducing Substance (Glucose)

Glucose and other reducing substances in urine can be detected by:

a. **Copper reduction test**
   i. Benedict's test
   ii. Fehling's test
   iii. Copper reduction tablet test
b. **Reagent strip method:** Glucostix, clinistix, multistix, chemstrip (glucose oxidase-peroxidase method)
c. **Osazone test:** In this test, glucose osazone crystals are formed which are detected microscopically.

In the past, the two tests which had been most commonly used to show the presence of reducing substances in urine are those of Benedict and Fehling (more commonly Benedict's test). In these two tests alkaline cupric copper solutions are reduced to cuprous oxide.

Benedict's test and Fehling's test are mainly used to detect whether glucose is present in the urine or not. Other reducing substances that give positive results are:

- Other sugars: Pentoses, fructoses, galactose and lactose (but not sucrose)
- Salicylic acid
- Ascorbic acid (vit C)
- Homogentisic acid
- Creatinine
- Uric acid
- Formaldehyde

Benedict's Qualitative (Semiquantitative) Test

Benedict's reagent (qualitative)

- Tri-sodium citrate: 173 g
- Sodium carbonate (anhydrous): 100 g
- Copper sulphate: 17.3 g
- Distilled water, add up to: 1000 ml.

Dissolve tri-sodium citrate and sodium carbonate in 500 ml of distilled water. Dissolve copper sulphate in 500 ml of distilled water with gentle heat in another container. Mix the two solutions.

Principle of the test: All monosaccharides and disaccharides (glucose, galactose, lactose, pentose, levulose) reduce cupric sulphate in alkaline environment into insoluble cuprous oxide of yellow or red colour.

$$\underset{\text{(cupric ion)}}{Cu^{++}} \xrightarrow{\text{hot alkaline solution}} \underset{\text{(cuprous ion)}}{Cu^{+}}$$

$$Cu^{+} + OH \longrightarrow CuOH \text{ (yellow)}$$

$$2\,CuOH \xrightarrow{\text{heat}} Cu_2O \text{ (red)} + H_2O$$

Method: To 5 ml of Benedict's qualitative reagent (blue in colour) add 8 drops of urine (0.5 ml). Boil it over a flame for 3–5 minutes or set in a boiling water bath for 5 minutes. Cool it. Notice the change in colour.

- Negative: No change in colour (blue)
- Trace: Pale green with slight cloudiness
- 1+ (<0.5% glucose): Green or yellow-green deposit
- 2+ (0.5–1% glucose): Yellow deposit
- 3+ (1–2% glucose): Orange or orange-red deposit
- 4+ (>2% glucose): Brick red precipitate

Sensitivity of the test: ≥50 mg%

Fehling's Test

Fehling's reagent

1. *Solution A*
   - Copper sulphate: 34.65 g
   - Distilled water: 500 ml
2. *Solution B*
   - Sodium hydroxide: 125 g
   - Sodium potassium tartarate: 173 g
   - Distilled water: 500 ml

Method: In a test tube take 2.5 ml each of solution A and solution B of Fehling's reagent. Mix well and boil. Add 8 drops (0.5 ml) of urine and boil again for 3–5 minutes. Cool it. Notice the change in colour and get the result (as in Benedict's test).

Benedict's Quantitative Test for Sugar

Quantitative reagents

- Sodium carbonate (anhydrous): 100 g
- Sodium/potassium citrate: 200 g
- Potassium thiocyanate: 125 g
- Copper sulphate: 18 g
- Potassium ferrocyanide (5%): 5 ml
- Distilled water up to: 1000 ml

Method: If the Benedict's qualitative test for urine is positive (Fig. 12.1), then this quantitative test can be done to ascertain exact amount of sugar present in urine. If strongly positive, then urine may be diluted (1:10). In a conical flask, take 25 ml of Benedict's quantitative reagent. To it, add 15 g of crystalline sodium carbonate and boil. When it is boiling then add urine sample drop by drop from a graduated burette until the blue colour completely disappeared and a chalky white colour develops.

At this point, all cupric ion originally in solution is reduced. *It is known that 0.05 g of sugar is needed for complete reduction of this 25 ml of Benedict's quantitative reagent.*

Calculation: Suppose, we have tested 20 ml of diluted urine (1:10 dilution)

So, 20 ml diluted urine contains 0.05 g of sugar

Or, 20 ml undiluted urine (original urine) contains 0.05 g × dilution factor = 0.05 × 10 (here)

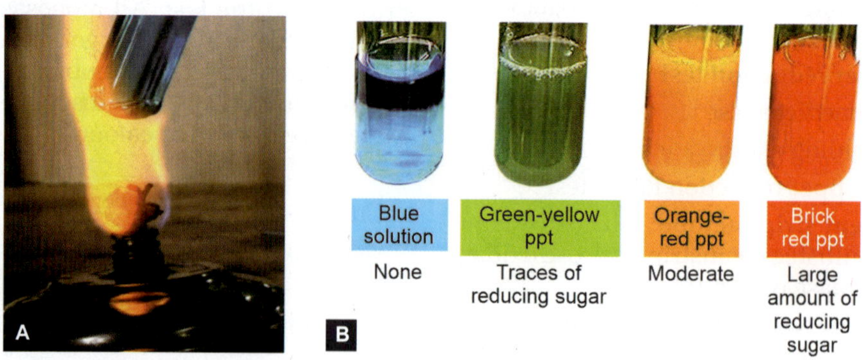

Fig. 12.1A and B: Benedict's qualitative test for urinary glucose

Or, 100 ml undiluted urine contains =

$$0.05 \times 10 \times 100 \div 20 \text{ g}$$
$$= 2.5 \text{ g\% sugar (glucose)}$$

If there is no urinary dilution, the dilution factor is 1.

Reagent Strip Method

This test is based on a specific glucose oxidase and peroxidase method, a double sequential enzyme reaction. Reagent strips differ in the chromogen used. It may be used for semi-quantitative results.

$$\text{Glucose} + O_2 \xrightarrow{\text{glucose oxidase}} \text{gluconic acid} + H_2O_2$$

$$H_2O_2 + \text{chromogen} \xrightarrow{\text{peroxidase}} \text{oxidised chromogen (colour change)} + H_2O$$

The glucose oxidase strip test is specific for glucose. It does not react with lactose, galactose, fructose or reduce metabolites of drugs.

- **Clinistix (*o*-toluidine chromogen)**: Colour changes from pink to purple. It can detect 100 mg/dl of glucose.
- **Multistix (potassium iodide chromogen):** Colour changes from blue to brown within 30 seconds.
- **Chemstrip (aminopropyl-carbazol chromogen):** Colour changes from yellow to orange-brown at 60 seconds.
- **Chemstrip $^{u}G_c$ (tetramethylbenzidine chromogen):** These strips have different sensitivities to urine glucose, range is 60 mg/dl to 5 g/dl. Colour changes at 2–3 minutes.

Note

i. False positive result may be obtained by strongly oxidising cleaning agents in the urine container.

ii. Use of sodium fluoride as a preservative causes false negative results.

iii. High specific gravity of urine decreases colour development.

iv. All reagent strips should be protected from humidity, otherwise it will reduce the reactivity.

v. For optimal result, of this enzymatic reactions, urine should be kept at room temperature.

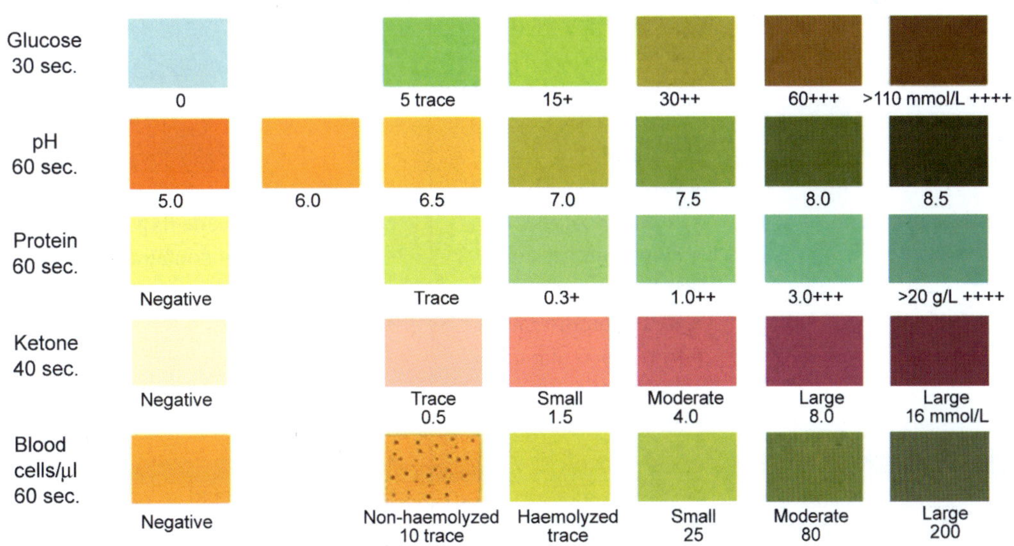

Fig. 12.2: Multistix for chemical examination of urine

Sugar in Urine and its Significance

1. **Glycosuria with hyperglycaemia**
   - Diabetes mellitus
   - Other endocrine disorders: Hyperthyroidism, hyperpituitarism, acromegaly, Cushing's syndrome, phaeochromocytoma.
   - Pancreatic diseases: Haemochromatosis, cystic fibrosis (late stage), carcinoma, severe chronic pancreatitis.
   - CNS dysfunction: Intracranial injury, tumours or haemorrhage (especially in hypothalamus).
   - Drug induced: Thiazides, corticosteroids, ACTH, oral contraceptives.
   - Massive metabolic derangement: Uraemia, sepsis, cardiogenic shock, severe burns, advanced liver disease.
2. **Glycosuria without hyperglycaemia**
   - Renal glycosuria: Normally, sugar does not come into urine unless it is >180 mg/dl in blood. But in case of renal glycosuria renal threshold for urinary sugar is reduced. So, sugar appears in without high blood sugar level.
   - Renal tubular dysfunction: Fanconi's syndrome, galactosaemia, cystinosis, lead poisoning, multiple myeloma.
   - Pregnancy (differentiate it from gestational diabetes)
3. **Non-glucose sugars in urine**
   - *Galactose:* Galactosaemia in newborn due to deficiency of galactose-1-phosphate uridyltransferase or galactokinase.
   - *Lactose:* May appear in urine in late pregnancy or during lactation.
   - *Fructose:* During parenteral feedings with fructose and in association with inherited enzyme deficiencies that cause benign essential fructosuria.
   - *Pentose:* Ingestion of large amounts of fruits, causing the excretion of L-xylose and L-arabinose.

Table 12.3: Comparison between Benedict and reagent strip (glucose oxidase) methods for urinary sugar detection

Test result	Benedict's test	Reagent strip (glucose oxidase) method
1. True positive	• Glucose • Galactose • Lactose • Fructose • Maltose • Pentose	• Glucose
2. False positive	• Ascorbic acid • Homogentisic acid • Salicylates • X-ray contrast media • Anti-tubercular drugs • Levodopa • Stress, excitement	• Hydrogen peroxide (H_2O_2) • Hypochlorite in container • Pregnancy and lactation • Stress excitement
3. False negative		• Ascorbic acid • Homogentisic acid • Large amount of salicylates • Deteriorated reagent strips

- *Sucrose:* After ingestion of very large amounts of sucrose. It gives negative results with glucose oxidase or copper reduction tests. (Sucrose is not a reducing substance.) It can be separated by chromatography.

4. **Tests for protein in urine (proteinuria):** Normal urine contains up to 150 mg/day or 10 mg/dl (1–14 mg/dl) of protein depending on urine volume.

The proteins in urine are derived from plasma and urinary tract. Albumin and small molecular plasma globulins constitute about 2/3rds of the protein, and 1/3rd is the glycoprotein secreted by the thick part of the ascending loop of Henle and possibly the distal tubule. This glycoprotein is known as Tamm-Horsfall protein. It is believed that this protein forms the matrix of all casts. It forms a meshwork of fibrils which may trap cells, cell fragments or granular material. Enzymes and proteins from tubular epithelial cells, immunoglobulin A in secretions of urinary tract, other desquamated cells and leucocytes are other proteins found in very small amount in normal urine.

Plasma proteins with MW < 50,000–60,000 pass through the glomerular membrane and are normally reabsorbed by proximal renal tubular epithelial cells. Albumin which has MW of 69,000 is filtered out only in small amount. Immunoglobulin light chains, retinol binding protein, β_2-microglobulin and lysozyme are excreted in small amounts. Anderson in 1979, demonstrated more than 200 urinary proteins.

Qualitative or Semiquantitative Tests

Heat and Acetic Acid Test

Principle of the test: Urinary proteins are coagulated and denatured by heat and thus rendering the solution turbid (turbidometric method). Acetic acid (3%) is added to the urine to make it slightly acidic. It facilitates the precipitation of protein, and in addition, avoid false positive results due to precipitation of phosphates which are nomal constituents of urine. But excessive amount of acid or alkaline medium should be avoided as it may produce meta-proteins (acid or alkaline) which are not coagulated by heat.

Method (Figs 12.3 and 12.4): Take 10 ml urine in a clean test tube (15 ml capacity) or two-thirds portion of the test tube. Hold the test tube at the bottom with a test tube holder and start heating the upper half-inch or inch of the column of urine (keep the open end of the test tube away from you). If white cloudiness appears, it may due to protein or phosphates. Add 2–3 drops of 3% acetic acid. If the cloudiness disappears it is due to phosphates, but if the cloudiness persists, it is due to protein in urine. If cloudiness appears when heated and disappears when cooled down it is Bence-Jones protein.

Results

- Negative: No cloudiness
- Trace: Hardly visible cloudiness
- 1+: Cloudiness present but no granular flocculation
- 2+: Heavy and granular cloudiness but no flocculation
- 3+: Dense cloud but no marked flocculation
- 4+: Thick, curd-like precipitate and coagulation.

Sulphosalicylic Acid Test

Take 2 ml of centrifuged (clear) urine specimen. Add equal volume of 3–5% sulphosalicyclic acid solution. Invert to mix and wait for 10 minutes. Note the degree of turbidity.

- Negative: No turbidity (<0.005 g%)
- Trace: Faint turbidity (0.01 g%)
- 1+: Distinct turbidity but no granulation (0.01–0.05 g%)
- 2+: Turbidity with granulation but no flocculation (0.05–0.2 g%)
- 3+: Turbidity with granulation and flocculation (0.2–0.5 g%)
- 4+: Clumps of precipitate (>0.5 g%)

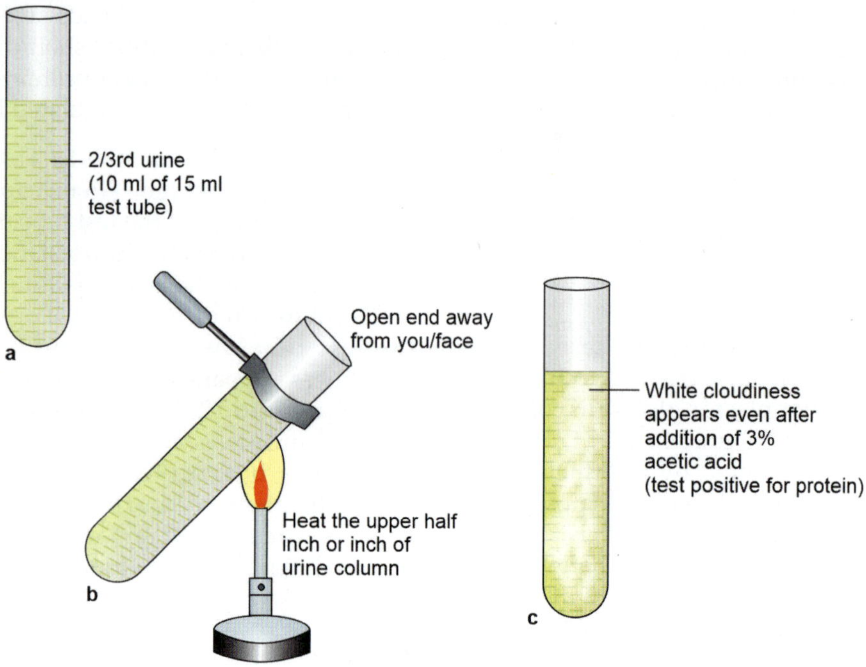

Fig. 12.3: Schematic diagram of different steps (a, b and c) of heat and acetic acid test for urinary protein detection

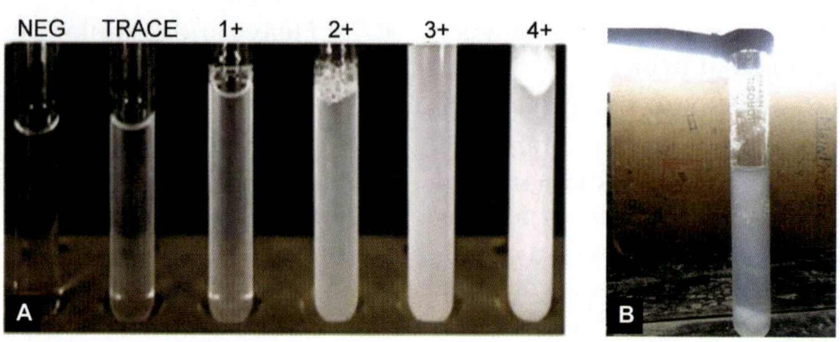

Fig. 12.4A and B: (A) Interpretation of heat test for detection of urinary protein; (B) Showing 2+ positivity

Sulphosalicyclic acid test is more sensitive than heat test. It can detect 5–10 mg/dl of urinary protein.

Heller's Nitric Acid Test

Take 1 ml of concentrated nitric acid (fuming) in a test tube first. Then add 2 ml urine by the side of test tube with the help of a pipette and make a layer on the top of acid. A whitish ring appears at the junction of the two fluids due to formation of metaprotein which appears as precipitates. It is due to presence of albumin in urine (Fig. 12.5).

Reagent Strip Method

This test is based on protein charge and change in pH. As proteins carry a charge at physiologic pH, their presence elicits a pH change. The reagent strip is impregnated with tetrabromophenol blue buffered to an acid pH of 3 or tetrachlorophenol tetrabromosulfophthalein. This area is yellow in

Detection

a. *Heat coagulation test*

5 ml of urine and heat the upper part of the tube—agglutination is formed in the upper part

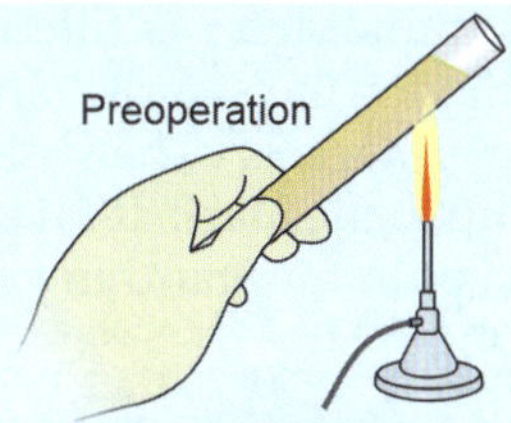

b. *Heller's test*

3 ml conc HNO_3 + 3 ml of urine on side of TT—**white ring** at the junction indicate albumin

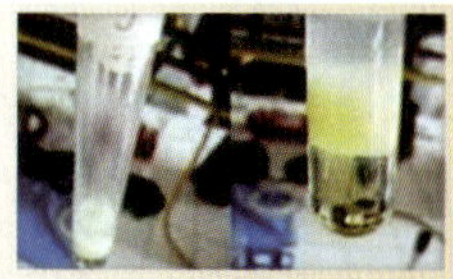

c. *Sulphosalicylic acid test*

6 drops of 20% SSA (aqueous) on 5 ml urine—if **clouds**—albumin

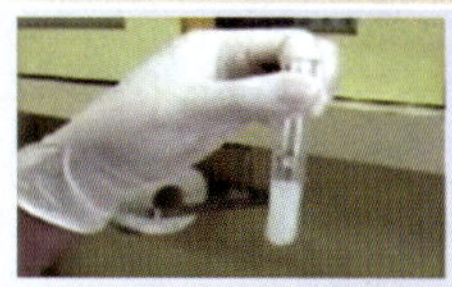

Fig. 12.5: Three methods for detection of urinary protein (albumin)

the strip in the absence of protein. Colour changes to a shade of green, depending on the type and concentration of protein present in 30–60 seconds.

Quantitative Estimation of Protein in Urine

Esbach's Method (by Albuminometer)

i. **Esbach's reagents**
   - Picric acid: 05 g (which precipitates albumin)
   - Citric acid: 10 g (which dissolves phosphates)
   - Distilled water: 500 ml

ii. **24 hours urinary sample:** Collect 24 hours urine sample in a clear container. Make the urine clear by filtering it and acidifying with 10% acetic acid. If the specific gravity is >1.025, then urine should be diluted (1:2, or 1:3, or 1:4 depending on SG), so that albumin precipitates do not float.

iii. **Esbach's albuminometer:** This is a thick-walled glass tube with 'R' mark above and 'U' mark below. At the lower part of the tube there is a few graduations with numerical markings. Also, there is a wooden stand to keep this glass tube.

Table 12.4: Comparison between reagent strip test and sulphosalicylic acid test for detection of proteinuria

Parameter	Reagent strip test	Sulphosalicylic test
1. Principle	Colorimetric	Acid precipitation
2. Sensitivity	5–10 mg/dl	20 mg/dl
3. Type of test	Screening	Confirmatory
4. Indicator	Colour change	Turbidity
5. Proteins detected	Albumin only	All (albumin, myoglobin, haemoglobin, Bence Jones protein)

Method: The albuminometer is filled with filtered and acidified urine sample (specific gravity <1.025) up to mark 'U'. Then Esbach's reagent is added up to the mark 'R'. It is then well mixed and kept in the stand in vertical position for 24 hours.

Result: The level of precipitate deposited at the bottom of the albuminometer is measured by graduation and is expressed in g/litre. To get g%, the result should be divided by 10.

Principle of the test: Albumin combines with picric acid in acid environment and forms the salt 'albumin picrate' which deposits at the bottom.

Turbidimetric Method

Here, colorimetric readings are taken against blanks and calculation done accordingly to get the result. As for example, sulfosalicylic acid turbidity method. It provides an accurate estimation of urinary protein.

Patterns of Different Proteinuria

1. **Glomerular pattern:** In healthy person, albumin is not lost in urine, because of the same negative charge of protein and glomerular capillary wall which causes repulsion. But in disease (glomerulonephritis), there is loss or reduction of the fixed negative charge on the glomerular capillary wall that allows albumin to permeate into Bowman's space in large amount, more than which can be reabsorbed by proximal tubular cells. Glomerular disease often causes heavy proteinuria (>3–4 g/day).

   When serum protein is lost in urine, other proteins of similar size or charge are also lost. As for example, transferrin, prealbumin, α_1-acid glycoprotein, α_1-antitrypsin and antithrombin. Protein with larger size or molecular weight (MW) does not appear in urine till the glomeruli are not totally damaged, e.g. β-lipoprotein and α_2-macroglobulin.

2. **Tubular pattern:** Here, glomerulus is normal but there is defective tubular reabsorption of protein. These urinary proteins are usually of low MW. As for example, light chain immunoglobulin, lysozyme, α_1-microglobulin and β-globulin like β_2-microglobulin. Tubular pattern of proteinuria is seen in renal tubular diseases like cystinosis, Wilson's disease, Fanconi's syndrome, renal transplant rejection and pyelonephritis. The amount of proteinuria is lower than with glomerular diseases and usually 1–2 g/day.

   Tubular proteinuria may be missed by the reagent strip test because of absent or very low amount of albumin and presence of other protein(s). However, it may be detected by other methods.

3. **Overflow proteinuria:** It is due to excessive production of certain proteins and subsequent loss in urine as it overflows. This overflow proteinuria is seen in haemoglobinuria, myoglobinuria and loss of immunoglobulins in urine. These proteins are not associated with glomerular or tubular disease initially but may cause renal disease later on. Myoglobinuria causes acute tubular necrosis and haemoglobinuria becomes toxic when the patient is dehydrated.

Causes of Proteinuria

Heavy Proteinuria (>3–4 g/day)

- Nephrotic syndrome: Different types of primary and secondary glomerulonephritis.
- Malignant hypertension
- Amyloidosis (primary, secondary and with multiple myeloma)
- Toxaemia of pregnancy
- Drugs (penicillamine)
- Heavy metals (gold, mercury)
- Renal transplant rejection
- Sickle cell disease

Moderate Proteinuria (1–3 g/day)

- Different chronic glomerulonephritis
- Nephrosclerosis
- Multiple myeloma
- Radiation nephritis
- Diabetes nephropathy (mild)

Minimal Proteinuria (<1 g/day)

- Chronic pyelonephritis
- Nephrosclerosis
- Chronic interstitial nephritis
- Acute diffuse post-streptococcal glomerulonephritis (nephritic syndrome)
- Congenital diseases: Polycystic kidney disease, medullary cystic disease.
- Renal tubular disease
- Hypertension (not malignant)
- Lower urinary tract infection
- Haemoglobinuria with severe haemolysis
- Fever, severe emotional stress
- Exercise

Bence Jones Proteinuria

Bence Jones protein is a group of similar proteins with molecular weight about 2500 (light chain globulin). The most characteristic of this protein is its behaviour on heating. Whereas ordinary plasma albumin and globulin begin to precipitate between 60°C and 70°C, Bence Jones protein begins to precipitate between 40°C and 60°C (lower temperature) and then redissolves as the temperature reaches boiling point. Subsequent cooling reprecipitates the protein and boiling redissolves it.

Causes of Bence Jones Proteinuria

- Multiple myeloma and other plasma cell dyscrasia (most common cause)
- Malignant lymphoma
- Other rare causes: Chronic myeloid leukaemia (CML), osteomalacia, osteosarcoma, cancer metastasis to bone.

Tests for Bence Jones Protein

1. **Heat test:** A white coagulum of Bence Jones (BJ) protein develops on heating at 40–60°C and redissolves on boiling. On cooling down, the precipitates reappear at 40–60°C. Further cooling to room temperature, the protein will be invisible.

   Albumin is often present along with BJ protein. It can be separated by filtering hot, through a hot filter funnel. BJ protein comes through leaving the albumin behind on the filter paper. On cooling the filtrate, the BJ protein reprecipitates (at 40–60°C) and can then be completely redissolved by heating to boiling point again.
2. **Bradshaw test:** Take 1 ml of concentrated hydrochloric acid in a test tube. Then add 2 ml of urine by the side of the test tube with the help of a pipette. BJ protein is precipitated by the acid giving a white ring at the junction of the two fluids.
3. **Osgood and Haskin's test:** In a test tube, mix 0.5 ml of 50% acetic acid, 1.5 ml of saturated sodium chloride solution and 2.5 ml of urine. A precipitate at room temperature on addition of the salt solution, strongly favours the presence of BJ protein. Heat the mixture gradually. If

Table 12.5: Grading of albuminuria

Condition	mg/24 hours urine	mg/litre urine	mg/g creatinine	µg/min	µg/mg creatinine
Normal	<30	<20	<20	<20	<30
Microalbuminuria	30–300	20–200	20–300	20–200	30–300
Overt albuminuria	>300	>200	>300	>200	>300

BJ protein is present in urine, then precipitate increases at 40–60°C and redissolves on boiling. Albumin and globulin usually appear only on heating, and boiling has no effect on the amount of the precipitate.

4. **Urine electrophoresis:** Urine is concentrated and run on electrophoresis just like blood. If BJ protein is present, it will appear as dense band in the gamma globulin region (M-band).
5. **Toluene sulphonic acid (TSA) test:** Add 1 ml of TSA reagent to 2 ml of urine (reagent should flow by the side of test tube). Mix well. A precipitate appears within 5 minutes, if BJ protein is present.

Test for Ketone Bodies in Urine (Ketonuria)

Ketone bodies are the products of incomplete fat metabolism, and their presence may be indicative of acidosis. Ketone bodies are synthesized in the liver by condensation of acetyl-CoA associated with impaired carbohydrate metabolism. Three types of ketone bodies are:

i. Acetone [$CH_3.CO.CH_3$]
ii. Acetoacetic acid [$CH_3.CO.CH_2.COOH$ (also known as diacetic acid)]
iii. β-hydroxybutyric acid [$CH_3.CHOH.CH_2.COOH$]

Their accumulation in blood known as ketoacidosis and presence in urine is known as ketonuria.

In ketonuria, three ketone bodies present in urine in the following percentage:

- Acetoacetic (diacetic) acid (20%)
- Acetone (20%)
- β-hydroxybutyrate (about 58%)

Acetone is formed non-reversibly from acetoacetic acid. β-hydroxybutyric acid (3-hydroxybutyrate) forms reversibly from acetoacetic acid.

$$\text{Acetoacetic acid} \xrightarrow{-CO_2} \text{acetone}$$

$$\text{Acetoacetic acid} \underset{-2H}{\overset{+2H}{\rightleftharpoons}} \beta\text{-hydroxybutyrate}$$

Causes of Ketonuria

- Uncontrolled diabetes mellitus
- Chronic starvation (due to increased tissue especially fat catabolism)
- Pregnancy toxaemia with vomiting
- In infants and children: Acute febrile diseases and toxic states accompanied by vomiting and diarrhoea.
- The use of low carbohydrates diet for weight reduction.
- Glycogen storage disease and other inherited metabolic diseases.
- Exposure to severe cold and heavy exercise.

A. Rothera's Test (Fig. 12.6)

Principle of the test: Acetone and acetoacetic acid produces a purple-coloured complex with sodium nitroprusside in an alkaline environment.

Test: Take 5 ml urine in a test tube. Saturate the urine with ammonium sulphate or ammonium chloride. A few drops of aqueous solution of sodium nitroprusside (or about 0.5 ml of 20% aqueous solution) or a pinch of powder or a crystal is added to it and well shaken to dissolve it. About 2–3 ml of concentrated ammonia (liquor ammonia) is poured down by the side of the test tube so that it forms a layer on the top of saturated urine.

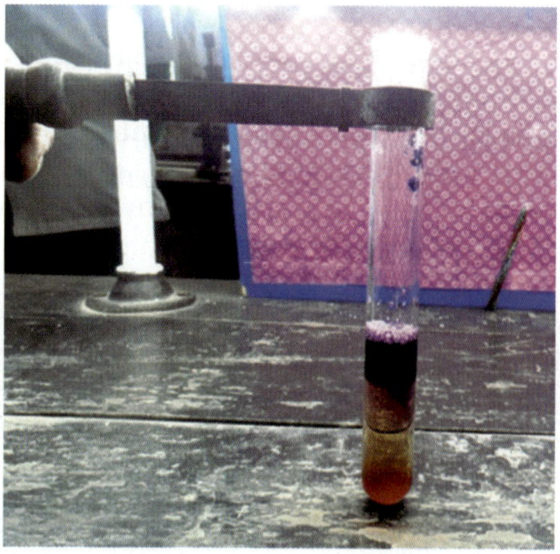

Fig. 12.6: Rothera's test

Result: Presence of acetone and acetoacetic acid is indicated by the development of a purple-coloured ring at the junction.

Sensitivity: Acetone >10–25%, acetoacetic acid >1–5 mg%

Note

β-hydroxybutyric acid cannot be detected by routine Rothera's test. For detection of it, β-hydroxybutyrate has to be oxidised by addition of H_2O_2 to acetoacetic acid.

Take 5–6 ml of diluted urine (1:10) in a test tube. Add 2–3 drops of acetic acid to it. Mix well. Then boil it for 4–5 minutes to drive away acetone and acetoacetic acid which are present in urine. Now, add 1 ml of H_2O_2 (hydrogen peroxide). Warm gently, cool it and perform the routine Rothera's test (if β-hydroxybutyric acid is present, it has been converted to acetoacetic acid).

Take 5–6 ml of diluted urine (1:10) in a test tube. Add 2–3 drops of acetic acid to it. Mix well. Then boil it for 4–5 minutes to drive away acetone and acetoacetic acid which are present in urine. Now, add 1 ml of H_2O_2 (hydrogen peroxide). Warm gently, cool it and perform the routine Rothera's test (if β-hydroxybutyric acid is present, it has been converted to acetoacetic acid).

B. Gerhardt's Ferric Chloride Test

This is not a very sensitive test. Precipitate the phosphates in 5 ml of freshly voided urine with 10% ferric chloride solution, drop by drop. Filter it and add more ferric chloride solution to the filtrate (phosphates free). If a purple-red colour appears, it indicates presence of ≥0.05% of acetoacetic acid. Sensitivity for acetoacetate <80 mg/dl.

A similar colour may be given by salicylic acid and salicylates. If the heating is done after adding the ferric chloride, the colour already formed disappears if it is due to acetoacetate (diacetic) acid but salicylates are unaffected by boiling the urine and the colour persists.

C. Salicylaldehyde Method

Behre and Benedict (1926) developed a method in which the ketone bodies of all types are converted into acetone. This acetone then reacts with salicylaldehyde in the presence of alkali. The amount of red coloured di-acetone (hydroxybenzal) thus formed is measured colorimetrically.

D. Legal's Test

Like Rothera's test, here also sodium nitroprusside is used. Take 10 ml of urine in a test tube and add a few crystals of sodium nitroprusside. Acidify the urine with glacial acetic acid, invert to mix. Pour strong liquour ammonia and wait for 5–10 minutes. A violet-coloured ring indicates a positive test.

Reagent Strip Method

The test is based on nitroprusside (sodium nitroferricyanide) reaction for ketones. **Chemstrip** contains sodium nitroferricyanide and glycine which react with acetoacetic acid and acetone in an alkaline medium to form a violet dye. The test is read at 1 minute and it detects about 10 mg/dl of acetoacetic acid and 70 mg/dl of acetone. **Multistix** (Fig. 12.7) contains buffers and sodium nitroferricyanide, which react with acetoacetic acid, producing pink-marron colour within 15 seconds. The reagent can detect 5–10 mg acetoacetic acid/dl of urine. It does not react with acetone.

Blood in Urine

Haematuria: Presence of increased number of RBCs (intact) in urine is known as haematuria.

Haemoglobinuria: Presence of haemoglobin or blood pigments (Hb) in urine in absence of RBCs is called haemoglobinuria.

Causes of Haematuria

a. **Pre-renal cause:** Blood dyscrasias (haemophilia, leukaemia, purpura), subacute bacterial endocarditis, acute febrile conditions, malignant hypertension, anticoagulant therapy, drug reactions.

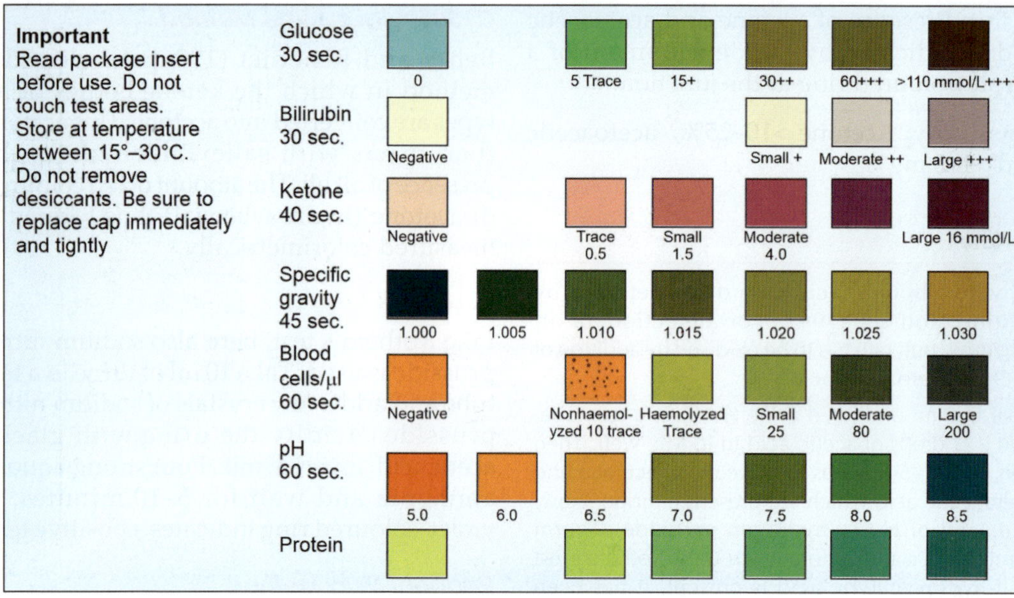

Fig. 12.7: Multistix for urine examination

b. **Renal causes:** Glomerulonephritis, acute pyelonephritis, hydronephrosis, tuberculosis of kidney, stone in kidney, renal vein thrombosis, Wilms' tumour.

c. **Post-renal causes:** Haemorrhagic cystitis, carcinoma prostate, enlarged prostate, carcinoma bladder, salpingitis.

Causes of Haemoglobinuria

- Paroxysmal nocturnal haemoglobinuria (PNH)
- Autoimmune haemolytic anaemia
- Cold haemoglobinuria
- Mismatched blood transfusion
- Black water fever
- Marching haemoglobinuria
- Gas gangrene
- Snake venom poisoning

Test for Blood (Haematuria and Haemoglobinuria)

- Orthotoluidine test
- Benzidine test
- Guaiacum test

Both orthotoluidine and benzidine tests are highly sensitive tests compared to guaiacum test.

Orthotoluidine test: Pinch of orthotoluidine is dissolved in 2 ml glacial acetic acid in a test tube. Add 10–15 drops of urine and shake well. Then 4 ml of 30% H_2O_2 is added. Development of greenish-blue colour indicates presence of blood in urine.

Principle of the test: Haemoglobin and myoglobin (iron porphyrin products) release oxygen from hydrogen peroxide. This oxygen causes oxidation of orthotoluidine and develops a blue colour.

Benzidine test: Take equal volume of saturated solution of benzidine in glacial acetic acid and hydrogen peroxide (say 4 ml each) in a test tube. Take 4 ml of urine in another test tube. Add 4 ml of the mixed reagent (from the first tube) to urine. Developement of blue colour indicates presence of haemoglobin or occult blood in urine. This is very sensitive test.

Microscopic Examination of Urine

Use a clean fresh morning sample (midstream) whenever possible. Random midstream urine is satisfactory as a screening test. Urine should be examined within one hour (preferably fresh) because cells and casts begin to lyse within 1–3 hours. If delay is presumed, then urine should be refrigerated at 2–8°C. Preservatives through not preferred but can be used during transportation and more delay is suspected.

Centrifugation of urine specimen: Take freshly void urine (10–15 ml) in a conical centrifuge tube. Centrifuge it at a moderate speed, say 2000 r.p.m. for 5 minutes. Remove the supernatant by decanting into another test tube. The centrifuged deposit along with remaining fluid is resuspended in the first tube. This is taken out by a pipette and a drop is placed on a slide and covered with a coverslip (18 mm square). Remove bubbles if any.

Microscopy: Examine urinary sediment first under low power then under high power, vary the light intensity for seeing different casts.

1. Renal epithelial cells, RBCs, WBCs are identified under HP (high power) objective and counted in 10 representative HP fields.
2. Crystals are identified under LP (low power) objective.
3. Casts are identified under LP but finer details are confirmed under HP objective.
4. Others: Yeast, bacteria, parasites are identified under HP objective and number given per HP field.

In most instances, an unstained sediment is sufficient for reporting, However, if there is difficulty, then **Sternheimer and Malbin stain** may be used.

For identifying cellular structure and bacteria a drop of **methylene blue** solution can be used. Alternatively, **crystal violet safranin** stain can be used to identify cellular elements. Sometimes a peroxidase stain (myeloperoxidase or MPO) is used to differentiate renal tubular cells and neutrophils (pus cells). Neutrophil is MPO positive while tubular cells are negative.

Urinary sediments are divided into two broad classes:

1. Organised element
2. Unorganised element

Organised element: Red blood cells (erythrocytes), white blood cells (leukocytes), epithelial cells, tubular cast, broad cast and other casts, bacteria and others (yeast, parasites, spermatozoa, etc.)

Unorganised element: Crystals in normal acid urine (amorphous urates, crystalline urates, crystalline uric acid and calcium oxalate), crystals found in normal alkaline urine (amorphous phosphate, crystalline phosphate, calcium carbonate, ammonium biurate), crystals found in abnormal urine (cysteine, leucine, tyrosine and drug crystals).

Organised Elements in Urine

Red Blood Cell (Erythrocytes)

Red cells are identified by their smaller size, round shape, often with crenated margins (due to exosmosis). It should be distinguished from yeast cells. The finding of >2 RBC/HPF is abnormal. Causes of increased RBCs in urine or haematuria are:

- Renal disease: Glomerulonephritis, interstitial nephritis, hydronephrosis, trauma, polycystic kidney, malignant nephrosclerosis, tuberculosis, calculi.
- Lower urinary tract disease: Urinary tract infection or UTI (acute and chronic), stricture ureter and urethra, urinary bladder tumour and calculus.
- Extrarenal disease: Tumour of the colon, rectum and pelvis, salpingitis, acute appendicitis, chyluria, diverticulitis.

Dysmorphic erythrocytes: Fairley in 1982, observed that aberrant or dysmorphic erythrocyte morphology is specific in detecting glomerular bleeding. These distorted cells are better visualised under phase-contrast microscopy. When ≥80% of RBCs are undistorted and uniform, then bleeding is due to non-glomerular causes (i.e. from tubular cause or associated with calculi or may be due to urinary tract disease). Fassett in 1982, pointed out that normal persons usually have a mixture of distorted and undistorted RBCs in urine.

Leukocytes (Pus Cells)

They are identified by their nucleated structure with uneven margin. Leukocytes are bigger than RBC and do not lyse with addition of 2% acetic acid like RBC. But the acid however, accentuates the nucleus that appears as dark dots inside the cell. Normal urine shows 0–5 WBC/HPF, but in female their number is a little bit higher.

An increased number of WBCs (pus cells) in urine indicates renal infection which can be in the urinary bladder (cystitis) or in the kidney (pyelonephritis).

Pyuria: When more number of WBCs is found in urine (≥10 WBC/10 HPF). Pyuria can also be detected by reagent strip (leukocyte esterase dipstick test) which has a sensitivity of 90% and specificity of 80%. The reagent strip test is specially used when neutrophils swell and exhibit Brownian movement in hypotonic urine with pyuria. Because of this Brownian movement, moving granules appear as refractile and these cells are called **glitter cells**.

Renal Epithelial Cells

In normal urine, their number is 2–3/HPF in male and 8–10/HPF in females. The renal epithelial cells are 3 types:

i. **Transitional (urothelial) cells:** These cells are originate from renal pelvis, ureter, urinary bladder and prostate (in men). These cells are 2–3 times the size of a leukocyte (from 40 to 200 mm) and they are round or pear-shaped with a tail like process.

   When stained with **Papanicolaou (Pap) stain**, transitional cells have dark blue nuclei with variable amount of pale blue cytoplasm. Another helpful clue is the presence of 'endo-ecto cytoplasmic' rim.

ii. **Squamous cells:** These cells originate from distal one-third of the urethra and vagina, vulva of women. These cells are large and flat with abundant cytoplasm and small round central nuclei. Margins are often folded. If stained with **crystal violet safranin**, nuclei are purple and cytoplasm pink to violet.

iii. **Small round or polygonal (parabasal) cells:** They originate from kidney tubules. Normally, these cells are not present in urine and their presence indicates some renal diseases.

Casts

Casts are normally formed as colourless translucent gels from protein in the tubules of nephron (e.g. hyaline cast). Cast formation is increased when larger than normal amounts of plasma proteins enter the renal tubules. Most of these excess proteins are usually albumin although Bence Jones immunoglobulin, haemoglobin and myoglobin also take part in cast formation. The plasma protein probably react or combine with Tamm-Horsfall protein to form less translucent casts and glomerular casts unlike hyaline cast which is translucent.

In a normal person, very few are seen in the urinary sediment (mostly hyaline casts). Increased number of casts is seen in widespread kidney disease when many nephrons are involved.

Classification of urinary casts

- Matrix casts: Hyaline cast, waxy cast.
- Inclusion casts: Granular casts (proteins, cell debris), fat globules, haemosiderin granules, crystal (uncommon), melanin granules (rare).
- Pigment casts: Haemoglobin, myoglobin, bilirubin, drugs.
- Cellular casts: Erythrocytes and RBC remnants, leukocytes (neutrophil, lymphocytes, monocytes, histiocyte), renal tubular epithelial cells, mixed cells (more than one above mentioned cells).

Hyaline casts: These are clear (like glass) homogenous, transparent, cylindrical with parallel walls. Hyaline casts have a low refractive index and better seen under reduced light. They dissolve rapidly in alkaline urine or standing urine. They are translucent with brightfield microscopy but are easily visualised with phase-contrast microscopy. Increased number is seen in:

- Normal person after strenuous exercise
- Chronic renal failure
- Diabetic nephropathy
- Glomerulonephritis and pyelonephritis
- Congestive heart failure

Waxy casts: These casts are more opaque than hyaline casts because of high refractive index and have yellowish tinge. With brightfield microscopy, waxy casts are homogenously smooth in appearance. Their margins are sharp even in subdued light.

- Tubular inflammation and degeneration
- Chronic renal failure
- Acute and chronic renal allograft rejection

When waxy casts are unusually broad, these are known as **renal failure casts**.

Fatty casts: These are light yellowish bodies with a transverse split, associated with chronic renal disease or amyloid disease. They contain refractile fat droplets mixed with certain amount of granular material. Commonly found in nephrotic syndrome. Visible fat droplets are triglycerides or cholesterol esters.

Granular casts: These are hyaline casts containing large granules embedded in coagulated proteins. These granules are disintegration of epithelial cells or leukocytes which are trapped into the protein matrix.

- Glomerular and tubular disease
- Tubulointerstitial disease
- Renal allograft rejection
- Pyelonephritis, viral infections, chronic lead poisoning
- Coarse granular casts with haematuria in renal papillary necrosis
- Fine granules (calcium phosphate precipitant) in hyperparathyroidism.

RBC (red blood cell or erythrocyte) casts: Glomerular injury (mostly due to immune cause) allows erythrocytes to escape into the tubules. With concomitant proteinuria, RBC casts are formed in the distal nephron. In urine, these casts appear yellow under low power objective. A prerequisite for the identification of RBC cast is that red blood cell outlines be sharply defined in at least part of the cast. If there are many RBCs, the matrix may not be visible. RBC casts are best seen with phase-contrast microscopy. With supravital staining (crystal violet or brilliant cresyl blue or new methylene blue). Erythrocytes are colourless or lavender in a pink matrix.

- Acute glomerulonephritis (nephritic syndrome)
- Subacute endocarditis
- Renal infarction
- IgA nephropathy
- Lupus nephritis

WBC (leukocyte) casts: WBCs usually enter tubular lumen from renal interstitium. They enter through and between tubular epithelial cells. So, by and large WBC casts reflect tubulointerstitial disease. WBC casts may also be present in glomerular disease owing to the chemotactic effect of complement, interstitial nephritis, lupus nephritis and even in nephritic syndrome, but most common cause is pyelonephritis.

Renal tubular epithelial cell casts: Causes of these casts are:

- Acute tubular necrosis
- Viral disease (e.g. cytomegalovirus disease)
- Exposure to various drugs
- Heavy metal poisoning
- Ethylene glycol and salicylate intoxication
- Acute allograft rejection

Unorganised Elements in Urine

Crystals are found in urine in normal as well as in abnormal condition. Phosphates, urate and oxalates are common and found in normal urine. So, presence of these crystals has a little clinical significance. Oxaluria and phosphaturia are mostly related with dietary factors and digestive disorders respectively.

Crystals Found in Acid Urine

- *Calcium oxalate:* Refractile, octahedral, folded, envelop shaped. Occasionally dumbbell shaped or spherical appearing.
- *Amorphous urates:* Reddish yellow granules. They dissolve by heat (60°C) and sodium hydroxide. But when treated with acetic acid they do not dissolve but converted to uric acid crystals.
- *Uric acid:* Reddish brown or yellow, rhombic plates or prisms.

Crystals Found in Alkaline Urine

- *Triple phosphate (crystalline phosphate):* Composed of ammonium, magnesium, phosphate. These are colourless, refractile, six-sided prisms with oblique ends referred to as coffin lids. Occasionally leaf-like or feathery forms.
- *Amorphous phosphate:* Colourless fine granular precipitate.
- *Calcium carbonate:* Small granular or colourless spherical.
- *Ammonium biurate*: Yellowish brown, apple thorn-like crystal.

Crystals Found in Abnormal Urine

- *Leucine:* Oily appearing spheres with radial and concentric striations.
- *Tyrosine:* Fine yellowish silky needles in clumps.
- *Cysteine:* Hexagonal, colourless, refractile plates.
- *Drug crystals:* Radiographic media, ampicillin (high dose), sulphonamide may be found in urine.

Chyluria

It refers to milky-white urine resulting from ruptured lymphatics in the wall of urinary bladder or kidneys. The lymph containing fat droplets enters into urine which also contains RBCs. Sometimes, there may be clot formation due to presence of excessive fibrinogen.

Composition of chyle

- *Fat:* Average 2–3 g/dl, finely dispersed. Special stain Sudan III and Oil red O. By adding equal volume of chloroform and ether, fat will be dissolved and milky colour disappears.
- *Protein:* Present in variable amount
- *Deposit:* WBCs, RBCs and microfilariae when caused by filarial infection.

Causes

i. Late stage filariasis
ii. Pregnancy or childbirth
iii. Abdominal tumours or lymph node enlargement
iv. Partial nephrectomy
v. Thermal ablation of a kidney lesion.

Urine and Pregnancy Test

There are two types of pregnancy tests; one uses a urine sample, the other uses a sample of blood.

A pregnant woman's placenta produces hCG, also called pregnancy hormone. It (hCG) is a glycoprotein produced by trophoblastic cells beginning about 10 days after conception when the fertilised egg attached to the uterine wall. hCG is a dimer, the alpha subunit is nonspecific (shared with FSH, LH and TSH) but the β-subunit is unique to hCG.

During the first 8–10 weeks of pregnancy, hCG level normally increase very rapidly. This level reaches its peak at about 10th week of pregnancy and the gradually decline until delivery.

hCG urine tests are commonly sold in kits and they detect β (beta)-subunits of hCG.

Test method: Take first morning urine sample as it contains more amount of β-hCG after 2 weeks of conception. For strip test, dip it into container containing urine sample up to maximum line. For cassette test, put 2 drops of urine in the specified sample well.

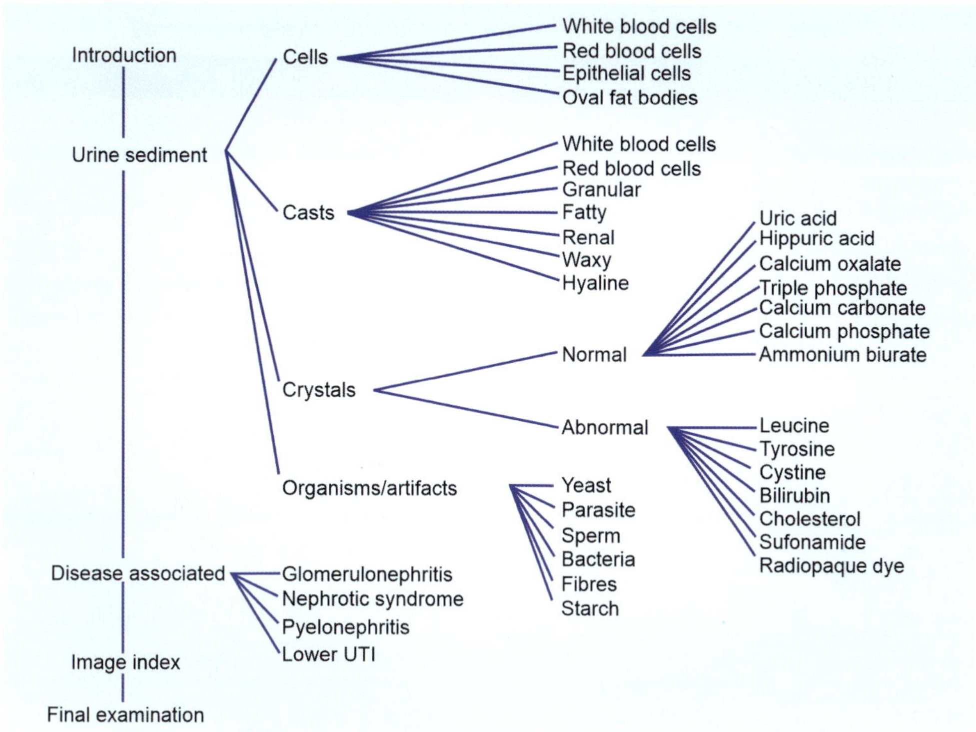

Fig. 12.8: Microscopic findings of urinary sediment

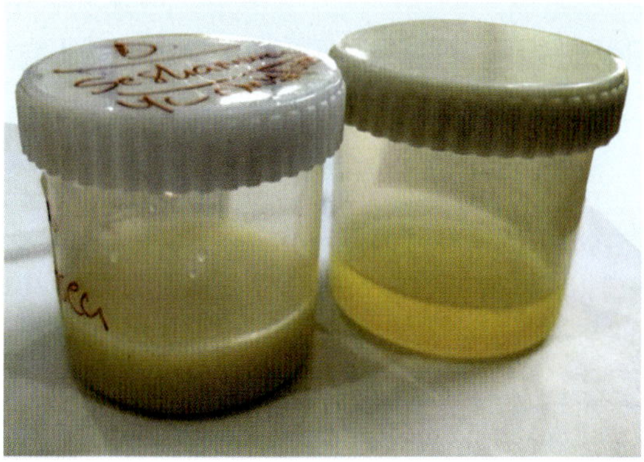

Fig. 12.9: Left container has chyluria and right container has normal urine. Note the milky-white colour of chyluria compared to pale yellow colour of normal urine

Wait for 5 minutes and notice for colour bands (red in colour) in the **control (C)** and **test (T)** area.

Interpretation

- **Positive**: When both control and test give colour band **(red in colour)**
- **Negative**: When band in control area but no band in test area
- **Invalid**: Control negative but band in test area.

Principle of test: Antiserum anti-β-hCG and enzyme conjugate used in the control and test area. If the urine contains β-hCG, it combines with anti-β-hCG and enzyme conjugate fixed on C and T areas and gives red colour band.

Table 12.6: Urinalysis in various renal/urinary system diseases

Diseases	Macroscopic urinalysis	Microscopic urinalysis
1. Acute glomerulonephritis	• Gross haematuria • Proteinuria • Smoky urine	Erythrocytes, erythrocytes and blood casts, epithelial casts, hyaline and granular casts
2. Chronic glomerulonephritis	• Haematuria • Proteinuria	Epithelial casts, granular casts, leukocytes, erythrocytes, waxy casts
3. Acute pyelonephritis	• Turbid • Occasional proteinuria • Bad smell or odour	WBC cast, numerous neutrophils (many in clumps) epithelial casts, granular and waxy casts, bacteria
4. Chronic pyelonephritis	• Occasional proteinuria	Leukocytes, broad waxy casts, granular and epithelial casts, bacteria
5. Nephrotic syndrome	• Proteinuria (heavy) • Fat droplets	Fatty and waxy casts, cellular and granular casts, oval fat bodies
6. Cystitis	• Haematuria (gross or microscopic)	Plenty of WBCs, RBCs, transitional epithelial cells, histiocytes, bacteria
7. Acute tubular neoplasm	• Haematuria • Occasional proteinuria	Necrotic and degenerated renal epithelial cells, WBC, RBC, granular cast, epithelial casts, waxy cast, broad casts
8. Urinary tract necrosis	• Haematuria	Atypical large epithelial cells with enlarged hyperchromatic nuclei, WBC, RBC

Table 12.7: Differences between haematuria and haemoglobinuria

Haematuria	Haemoglobinuria
1. Haematuria is the presence of red blood cells in urine	1. Haeglobinuria means haemoglobin (free in plasma not in red blood cells) in abnormally high in concentration in urine
2. Urine is smoky	2 Urine is coca cola/red coloured as haemoglobin is converted to acid haematin in presence of oxygen
3. After centrifugation RBC deposits are found and seen under microscope	3. After centrifugation no RBC deposit
4. Common causes are urinary tract infections, nephrolithiasis (stones in kidney, bladder or ureter), polycystic kidney disease, benign prostatic hyperplasia, glomerular causes (glomerulonephritis)	4. Common causes are any haemolytic anaemia with primarily intravascular haemolysis in which RBCs are destroyed and released haemoglobin (free haemoglobin) found in plasma
5. Tests: Orthotoluidine test, benzidine test and dipstick test	5. Same as haematuria tests

Table 12.8: Comparison of haematuria, haemoglobinuria, and myoglobinuria

Parameter	Haematuria	Haemoglobinuria	Myoglobinuria
Colour of urine	Normal/smoky/ red/brown	Pink/brown/red	Red/brown
Colour of plasma	Normal	Pink	Normal
Urine microscopy	Many RBCs	Occasional RBCs	Occasional RBCs
Urine test based on peroxidase activity	+	+	+
Serum creatine kinase	Normal	Normal	Marked increase
Serum haptoglobin	Normal	Low	Normal

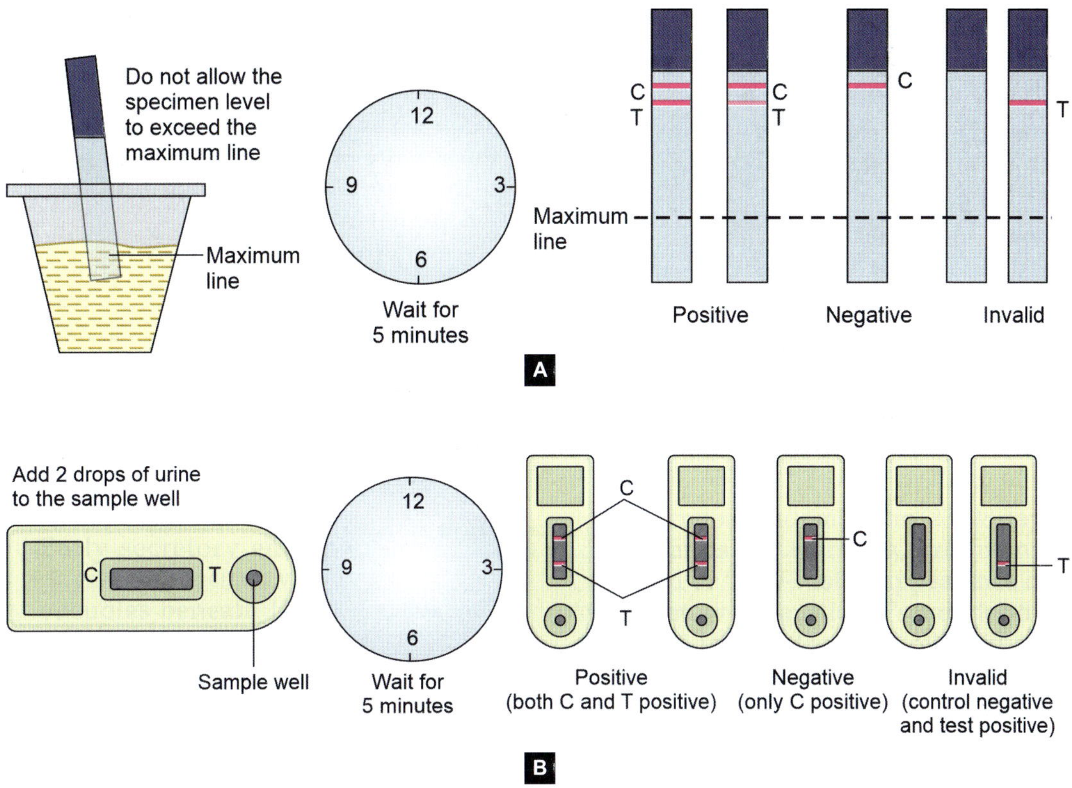

Fig. 12.10A and B: (A) Strip test; (B) Cassette test. C: Control, T: Test

TAKE HOME MESSAGE

Hematuria: Excretion of intact RBCs >3/hpf in urine.

Pyuria: Presence of >5 pus cells (WBC)/hpf in urine, typically from bacterial infection.

Sterile pyuria: Presence of elevated number of pus cells (WBCs) in urine which is sterile using standard culture techniques. Seen in renal tuberculosis.

Anuria: Complete absence of urine formation (<100 ml). It can be caused by total urinary tract obstruction, total renal artery or vein occlusion, shock, cortical necrosis, ATN and RPGN.

Oliguria: Urine output <400 ml/day, usually due to renal failure.

Polyuria: Urine output >3 L/day.

Azotemia: Increased blood (serum) value of nitrogenous waste products like urea and creatinine.

Uremia: Azotemia along with clinical manifestations (due to deranged renal function).

Microalbuminuria: Albumin (protein) excretion 30–300 mg/day in urine or 30–300 mg/g of creatinine in urine.

Macroalbuminuria (overt albuminuria): Albumin (protein) excretion 300–3500 mg/day in urine.

Nephrotic range proteinuria: Albumin (protein) excretion >3.5 g/day in urine.

Selective proteinuria: Selective excretion of low molecular weight proteins like albumin (MW 70 kD) and transferrin (MW 76 kD) in urine (seen in minimal change glomerulonephritis).

Eosinnophiluria

Definition: When >1% eosinophils among the leukocytes (WBC) in urine.

Cause: Allergic intestinal nephritis, renal transplant rejections, acute glomerulonephritis, atheroembolic disease, hypersensitivity to penicillin.

Stain used: Concentrated urine stained with Hansel stain.

Sterile Pyuria

It is defined as presence of WBCs in the urine in the absence of significant bacterial growth in urine culture. Its important causes are:

- TB, fungal infection
- Recently treated UTI (urinary tract infection)
- Perinephric abscess
- Chronic prostatitis
- Acute interstitial nephritis
- Chronic interstitial nephritis (including analgesic nephropathy)
- Chronic pyelonephritis.

Common renal stones

Calcium oxalate
- Square envelope shape, refractile colorless
- Most common renal stone
- Radio-opaque stone
- Seen in acidic urine
- Also associated with ethylene glycol poisoning and hypocitraturia
- Incidence: 0% of all renal stones

Magnesium ammonium phosphate
- Colourless prism-shaped crystals of "coffin-lid",'fern-leaf' or 'star' appearance
- Also known as triple phosphates, or struvite stones
- Occupy large part of renal pelvis. So, called as" staghorn calculi"
- Formed in alkaline urine particularly in proteus infection
- Incidence: 15% renal stones

Uric acid
- Variable in shape (diamond/barrel/rhomboid/plates)
- Seen with hyperuricaemia (gout, leukaemias)
- Seen in acidic urine (ptt <5.5)
- Radiolucent stone
- Incidence: 5–10%

Cystine
- Colourless refractile hexagonal plates with unequal plates with unequal size
- Change colour from initial yellow to green on air exposure.
- Found in cystinuria (genetic defect)
- Formed in acidic urine
- Incidence: 1–2%

VIVA VOCE

Q1. For routine examination of urine, which sample is preferred?

Ans: The morning sample is preferred as urine is concentrated and large volume of urine can be obtained. However, any fresh sample collected any time of the day is suitable but test should be done within 2 hours. If delay is anticipated, urine specimen should be refrigerated.

Q2. Which sample is preferred for culture of urine?

Ans: Midstream (clean-catch) fresh sample of urine after proper cleansing of glans penis in the male or vulva in the female.

Q3. How is 24-hour urine sample collected?

Ans: The first morning sample (say 8 AM) is discarded. All subsequent urine samples are collected in a clean and dry container (1.5 to 2 litre bottle with a cap). The last urine sample is the next day's first morning sample (say 8 AM).

Q4. What is renal glycosuria?

Ans: Normal renal threshold for glucose in humans is 180 mg/dl. This renal threshold is lowered in renal glycosuria (<180 mg/dl). So, glycosuria occurs even the blood sugar is below 180 mg/ml (normal threshold). This happens because of the defect in the tubular cells of the kidneys that decreases the reabsorption of glucose. Causes may be hereditary, cystinosis, Wilson's disease or as part of Fanconi syndrome. It may be acquired also (certain drugs, acute pyelonephritis) and sometimes in pregnancy.

Q5. What is alimentary glycosuria?

Ans: Sometimes, blood glucose level rises above renal threshold (180 mg/dl) physiologically after a meal. If may cause glycosuria. But it disappears after 2 hours of consumption of meal.

Q6. What is low and fixed specific gravity of urine?

Ans: Normal range of urine specific gravity is 1.003–1.035 (but average normal with normal water/fluid intake is 1.016–1.022). Low and fixed specific gravity is called when it becomes 1.008–1.010 and is fixed. Causes are:

i. Chronic glomerulonephritis (end stage renal disease), as the concentrating power of renal tubules are either low or lost due to damage to renal tubules.
ii. In ADH (anti-diuretic hormone) deficiency, the concentrating power of the tubules is lost. Hence, SG is low and fixed though the tubules are healthy.
iii. It is also seen in arteriosclerotic kidney, and cause is same, i.e. damaged tubules.

Q. 7. In heat test of urinary protein detection, why is upper part of the tube is heated and not the lower part of the tube?

Ans: When upper part of the tube is heated, the protein flocculate in upper part and haziness is seen. This haziness is compared to the unheated lower part which serves as control. In addition, by doing so, the convection current is not produced which may disturb the haziness. On the contrary, if lower part of the tube is heated, convection current will be produced, which will go upwards and make the whole urine specimen in the tube hazy. If there is trace or a little urinary protein is present, it will be missed as there is no control.

Q8. In Benedict's (semiquantitative) test, why is fixed volume of 5 ml Benedict's reagent and 8 drops (0.5 ml) of urine is used?

Ans: As this is a semiquantitative test and is graded from traces to 4+ based on colour changes, the ratio of reagent volume and urine volume should be fixed for accurate result and quantity of the urinary protein. If ratio is changed, the test will lose its semiquantitative nature and will be qualitative purely.

Q9. How are RBCs distinguished from air bubbles under microscope?

Ans: In unstained wet specimen of urine, RBCs are of same size, yellowish and double-contoured. But air bubbles have variable size with a dark halo and absent double-contour.

Q10. What is functional proteinuria?

Ans: When there is no organic lesion present but proteinuria occurs due to renal vasoconstriction. The causes are excessive exercise, exposure to heat and cold and emotional stress.

Q11. What is postural proteinuria?

Ans: Some people excrete more protein than normal range when they are in standing position. This proteinuria disappears, if the person lies down. The probable cause is venous vasoconstriction during standing posture.

Q12. What is microalbuminuria?

Ans: Microalbuminuria is defined as urinary albumin excretion of 30–300 mg/day, or 20–200 µg/min. It is a marker of general vascular dysfunction and nowadays is considered a predictor of both kidney and heart patients (hypertension). It is used to identify early kidney damage like diabetes mellitus. More than 300 mg albumin (macroproteinuria) indicates advanced kidney disease. In India, patients with type II diabetes of less than 1 year, the prevalence of microalbuminuria was 24.7% and macroproteinuria was 6.2%. In the US, approximately 6% of men and 9.7% of women have microalbuminuria.

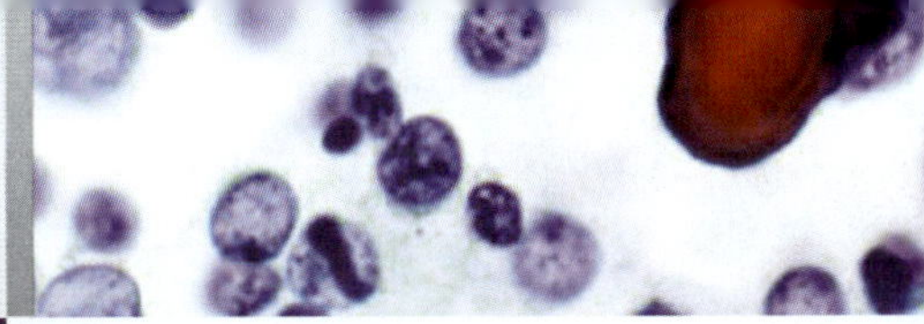

Section

III

Histopathology and Cytopathology

Chapter

13

Histological Techniques

Histological techniques are a series of processes by which the tissues are prepared for microscopic examination. It starts with fixation and continues with dehydration, clearing, embedding, cutting and staining.

When the tissues are removed from the body (e.g. surgical excision) or blood supply is cut off; tissues begin to decompose. This is due to lack of oxygen and other essential metabolites and also from the accumulation of carbon dioxide and other toxic metabolites in the cell and due to activation of different autolytic enzymes. Some tissues are decomposed rapidly, whereas others are slow to decompose. The rapidity is proportional to the natural metabolic activity of the tissue. This is the basic of rapid decomposition in liver, pancreas, convoluted tubules in kidney.

To minimize the decomposition and to preserve as nearly as possible the natural activity of the cells; the tissues are put in a suitable fixative (usually 10–20 times of volume of surgical specimens). Fixation is defined as a complex series of chemical and physical events which prevents or at least minimizes tissue decomposition and it differs for the different groups of chemical substances found in the tissues. There are other reasons of fixation. In most of the cells, there is an outer complex membrane containing the fluid protoplasm. The protoplasm is a mixed, true and colloidal solution of carbohydrates, proteins, lipids, salt, organic acid and enzymes. Many of these substances would have been lost if tissues had not been fixed.

The aims of fixation are

- Prevention of tissue autolysis and bacterial attack.
- To coagulate various tissue proteins/elements and make them insoluble.
- To maintain the shape and volume of the tissues during subsequent procedures (e.g. clearing, embedding, etc.).
- To prevent loss of tissue substances or rearrangement of tissues ingredients.
- To facilitate the staining reaction by acting as a mordant.
- To keep tissues as close to their natural state and to minimize change of natural colour and appearance.

Types of Fixatives

Fixatives may be of two types—primary and secondary.

Primary fixatives: Only one fixative or mixture of fixatives is used for specified period. Examples: 10% formalin, glutaraldehyde, Bouin's fluid, Carnoy's fixative, Zenker's fluid, etc.

Secondary fixatives: The use of two fixatives in succession. In other word, use of secondary fixative after the tissue is already fixed with previous fixative (primary fixative). As for example, after primary fixation in buffered formalin, tissues are kept in secondary fixative of mercuric chloride formaldehyde solution. Advantages of this sublimate post-fixation are that tissues are more easily cut and flatten better, also they give better staining quality. Likewise tissues fixed with glutaraldehyde may be post-fixed with osmium tetroxide which makes the membranes relatively permeable and better stained. This secondary fixation is also known as **post-fixation or post-chromatin**.

Classification of Fixatives

- **Aldehyde (protein cross-linking agents)**: Formaldehyde, glutaraldehyde
- **Protein denaturing agent**: Acetic acid, methyl alcohol, ethyl alcohol
- **Oxidizing agents**: Osmium tetroxide, potassium dichromate, potassium permanganate
- **Physical agents**: Microwave, heat
- **Other cross-linking agents**: Carbodimides
- **Miscellaneous**: Picric acid, mercuric chloride.

Routine Formalin Fixatives

This is a fixative which is most commonly used in histological laboratories. The reaction between fixative and tissue proteins is usually mild with a short reaction time. Cross-links between proteins are formed and the reaction starts with basic amino acid lysine. Lysine amino acid which is on the exterior aspect of the protein molecule can only react.

Aldehyde fixation may denature proteins to some extent apart from their primary role in forming crosslinks. As most of the proteins are not denatured, tissues fixed with aldehyde may be used for IHC (immunohistochemistry).

The commercially available solution contains 30–40% formaldehyde gas by weight and is called **formalin**. So, a 10% formalin fixative gives 4% formaldehyde gas for tissue fixation. Most laboratories prefer 10% buffered or 10% formal saline as fixative.

Formal saline (10%)
- Water (preferably distilled): 900 ml
- Sodium chloride: 9 g
- Formalin (40% formaldehyde): 100 ml

10% formalin (4% formaldehyde)
- Formalin (40% formaldehyde): 100 ml
- Distilled water or tap water: 900 ml

Neutral buffered formalin (10%)
- Water (preferably distilled): 900 ml
- Farmalin: 100 ml
- Sodium dihydrogen phosphate monohydrate ($Na_2 H_2 PO_4 . H_2O$): 4 g
- Disodium hydrogen phosphate anhydrous ($Na_2 HPO_4$.): 6.5 g.

Protein Denaturing Agents as Fixative

Alcohol: This is used as 80–100% solution. It frequently shrinks and hardens the tissue. Does not preserve chromatin well but good for demonstration of glycogen, plasma cells, amyloid, iron and uric acid. Carnoy's fluid is generally used for specific purposes. Alcohol denatures and precipitates proteins probably by disrupting hydrogen bonds. Ethyl alcohol is used as a fixative for enzymes.

Acetic acid: It is used as 1–5% aqueous solution. It is good for nuclear fixation and has rapid penetration (so, fixation time is less). Disadvantage of this fixative is that it forms pigments if used with formalin. Also, it causes haemolysis of RBCs.

Carnoy's fixative
- Absolute alcohol: 60 ml
- Chloroform: 30 ml
- Glacial acetic acid: 10 ml

Table 13.1: Advantages and disadvantages of formalin fixative

Advantages	Disadvantages
• It is cheap, relatively stable (when buffered) and easy to prepare • Tissue penetration is good • Does not make tissues very hard or brittle • Allows most routine stainings • Frozen section is possible with formalin fixed tissues • Natural colour may be restored • Most commonly used fixative and is the best fixative for the nervous system (brain)	• It may cause dermatitis and asthma in allergic individuals • It is slow to act (less tissue penetration) • There may be formation of dark brown artefact granules especially in tissues containing much blood (e.g. spleen, liver) • Reagent grade formalin (contains 10% methanol in addition to formaldehyde) is unsuitable for electron microscopy as methanol denatures protein. However, pure formalin is suitable • Gradual loss of basophilic staining of nucleus and cytoplasm. So, prolonged fixation is not advisable • Loss of myelin reactivity when Weigert iron haematoxylin stain is used

Zenker's fluid
- Distilled water: 950 ml
- Potassium dichromate: 25 g
- Mercuric chloride: 50 g
- Glacial acetic acid: 50 g
- Fixation time: 4–24 hours followed by prolonged wash.

Bouin's fluid
- Saturated aqueous picric acid solution: 75 ml
- Formalin (40% formaldehyde): 25 ml
- Glacial acetic acid: 5 ml

TISSUE PROCESSING, MICROTOMY AND PARAFFIN SECTIONS

Tissue Processing

Tissue contains intracellular as well as extracellular water which should be removed as paraffin wax (commonly used as embedding medium) is not miscible with water. Also, most fixatives are water based (like formalin). So, there must be some processes which remove this water and allow paraffin wax impregnation. The whole process is called tissue processing.

Table 13.2: Advantages and disadvantages of alcohol fixative

Advantages	Disadvantages
• Methyl alcohol (80–100%) is excellent fixative for smears • Ethyl alcohol is used as a fixative for enzymes • Carnoy's fixative is used for urgent biopsy (paraffin processing within 5 hours) • Good fixative to demonstrate glycogen, alkaline phosphatase, etc.	• Should be used at 0°C or cooler, otherwise cause marked shrinkage • Distorts morphology and hardens the tissue • Contraindicated for lipid study • Although glycogen can be demonstrated it cause polarization (steaming of protoplasm to one pole of the cell) of glycogen granules

Table 13.3: Choice of fixative for different cellular components or surgical specimens

Surgical specimens/tissue components	Choice of fixative
• Routine specimen/general surgical specimen	• 10% buffered formalin
• Glycogen	• Bouin's fluid (picric acid fixative) or alcohol fixatives (absolute alcohol)
• Fat/lipid	• Osmic acid
• Golgi bodies	• Osmic acid
• Enzymes	• Ethyl alcohol
• Smears (blood or cytologic smears)	• Methyl alcohol
• Urgent biopsies	• Carnoy's (alcohol) fixative
• Electron microscopy	• 3% glutaraldehyde, osmium tetroxide
• Nuclei	• Mercury fixative (Zenker), acetic acid
• Cytoplasm	• Potassium dichromate
• Gastrointestinal hormones	• Carbodimide
• Metachromasia	• Mercury fixative (Zenker's fluid)
• Testis	• Bouin's fluid, buffered formalin
• Nucleic acid (DNA and RNA)	• Carnoy's fluid
• Mucoprotein	• Glutaraldehyde
• Neuroendocrine granules	• Ethanol, methanol, acetone
• Cholesterol and its esters	• Bouin's fluid, Zenker's fluid
• Glycoprotein	• Chromates
• Gouty crystals (monosodium urate)	• Absolute alcohol
• Intermediate filaments	• Carnoy's fluid, Methacar n
• Trephine/bone marrow biopsy	• Zenker's formalin (previously called B_5)

The steps in tissue processing are:

- **Dehydration:** Common agents are ethyl alcohol/ethanol/acetone, methyl alcohol, isopropyl alcohol and dioxane.
- **Clearing:** Common agents are xylene (xylol), toluene (toluol), chloroform, citrus fruits oil, paraffin and Histoclear.
- **Impregnation:** Common agents are paraffin wax, other waxes (like ester wax, polyester wax), resins (acrylic, epoxy), agar, gelatin, and celloidin.
- **Embedding:** Final stage with paraffin blocks.

Dehydration

This step removes water and fixative from the tissue and replaces then with dehydrating fluid. Naturally dehydrating fluid should mix with and has water affinity so that it can easily penetrate the tissue cells. The best reagent is ethanol or ethyl alcohol.

1. **Ethyl alcohol (ethanol):** It is a clear colourless flammable liquid. It is used as graded alcohol beginning with 70%, then to higher grades, e.g. 85% or 95%. But for delicate tissues like embryo, animal tissues or brain it should be more gradual (begins with 50%). As it is hydrophilic, it is miscible with water and many other organic solvents.
2. **Acetone:** This is also a clear and volatile, colourless, flammable fluid which is miscible with water, ethanol and many organic solvents. Through it has rapid action, it has poor tissue penetration and prolonged use may cause tissue brittleness. It is cheaper than ethanol but more amount (at least 10 times the volume of tissue) is needed.

3. **Methanol:** It is highly toxic but can substitute ethanol, rarely used nowadays.
4. **Isopropyl alcohol:** Becoming very popular as it is cheaper and no excise duty is required as in alcohol. It is miscible with water, ethanol and most organic solvents It is recommended for microwave over processing method.
5. **Dioxane (diethyl dioxide):** It has the advantage of being miscible with water, alcohol, xylene, balsam and paraffin wax. The dioxane can be reused after removing the water from dehydrating fluid with calcium chloride or quick lime ($CaOH_2$). But it is toxic and in not recommended for routine use.

Clearing

This step replaces the dehydrating fluid and embedding medium (paraffin wax). So, this stage acts as a bridge between dehydration and subsequent embedding. When the dehydrating fluid is totally replaced by these agents, the tissue looks translucent, hence the name clearing agent came.

1. **Xylene (xylol)**: This is an excellent clearing agent but immersion must not be prolonged (>3 hours) as it makes tissue hard and brittle. It is cheap and can be used with celloidion section. This is not suitable for lymph nodes and brain, as it makes them very brittle.
2. **Toluene (toluol):** It has almost similar properties to xylene but has the advantage of not making the tissues hard and brittle.
3. **Chloroform:** It is slower in action than xylene. It causes a little brittleness and is recommended for nervous tissue, eye, granulation tissue, lymph nodes and larger tissue block (up to 1 cm) can be processed. It is non-inflammable but highly toxic. Unlike other clearing agents it does not make tissues translucent.
4. **Citrus fruit oils:** It is extracted from orange and lemon rinds. It is nontoxic and miscible with water. But it has the disadvantage of dissolving out small mineral deposits in tissues (copper, calcium).
5. **Paraffin wax:** Recently introduced as a clearing agent because of its cheapness. Time of immersion is similar to chloroform.
6. **Histoclear:** It has been recently introduced. This nontoxic agent is derivative of food-grade material and has much promise.

Impregnation

This step involves replacement and clearing agent with the embedding medium. This impregnating medium fills all natural cavities, interstices and spaces of the tissue. It makes the tissues sufficiently firm to allow thin section cutting but without alteration of the spatial relationship of the tissues and cellular components and also not to distort the tissues. Subsequently, making of blocks is done with embedding medium. Usual duration is 1–3 hours. Paraffin is the most commonly used impregnating medium used in the routine histological laboratory.

Embedding

Tissues which have been impregnated in paraffin wax is put in freshly melted paraffin wax is put in freshly melted paraffin wax and allowed to solidify. This can be done by using metal containers like tissue Tek, Leukhart's L or paper boats, etc. The tissues should be carefully oriented so that the surface to be cut is placed downwards. Commonly two methods are used in histology namely paraffin wax, resins and celloidion method.

- **Paraffin wax:** It is probably the most popular embedding medium as it is cheap, easily handled and section cutting is easier. Melting point ranging between 40–70° C. Wax with higher melting point has higher hardness. Wax with a melting point of 54–58° C is preferred for routing use. Sometimes, substance like bee wax, rubber ceresin, dental wax, diethylene glycol are added as additive to increase the hardness of paraffin wax hence, more thin sections can be cut.

- **Resins:** This is particularly used for thin sections for high resolution for electron microscopy and for undecalcified bone.
- **Celloidion:** Celloidion or its variant **low viscosity nitrocellulose (LVN)** was popular large tissue and for nervous tissue (like eye). Sections are cut by base sledge or a sliding microtome.
- **Agar:** It does not have sufficient support for sectioning friable tissue pieces after fixation. After solidification in molten agar, tissues are embedded in paraffin wax.
- **Gelatin:** Its main use is in frozen sectioning.
- **Paraplast:** It is a mixture of purified paraffin wax and synthetic plastic polymers whose melting point is 56–57°C. Sections can be cut without cooling the block face by ice. Ribbon like sections are more easy to cut and does not tend to crack. Large blocks and bone blocks may be cut easily as it is more resilient than paraffin wax.
- **Carbowax:** Alcohols with more carbon atoms (≥12) are solid at room temperature and may be used in tissue embedding. Alcohol with 12–18 carbon atoms are suitable for this purpose. Carbowax (polyethylene glycol) is good for this purpose. Carbowax is soluble in and miscible with water, hence embedding may be done directly from the formalin fixation bypassing the first dehydration and second clearing steps of normal tissue processing. Normally, four changes of carbowax (70%, 90% and two changes of 100%) are used at 56° C for 30 minutes, 45 minutes and 1 hour respectively with agitation.

The specimens are then put in fresh carbowax at 50° C for blocking and the blocks are immediately cooled in the refrigerator.

Table 13.4: Manual processing (2 days)

Container No.	Fluid	Time (hours)
1.	70% alcohol	1 hr (9.00 AM–10.00 AM)
2.	95% alcohol	1 hr (10.00 AM–11.00 AM)
3.	95% alcohol	2 hr (11.00 AM–1.00 PM)
4.	100% alcohol	1.5 hr (1.00 PM–2.30 PM)
5.	100% alcohol	1.5 hr (2.30 PM–4.00 PM)
6.	100% alcohol	1.5 hr (4.00 PM–5.30 PM)
7.	100% alcohol	**Over night**
8.	Xylene	1 hr (9.00 PM–10.00 PM)
9.	Xylene	1.5 hr (10.00 PM–11.30 PM)
10.	Paraffin wax	1.5 hr (11.30 PM–1.00 AM)
11.	Paraffin wax	1.5 hr (1.00 AM–2.30 AM)
12.	Paraffin wax	2.5 hr (2.30 AM–5.00 AM)
		Total = 16.5 hours

As carbowax is very hygroscopic, blocks and sustained sections must not come in contact with water or ice and are stored in dry, airtight containers.

Automated Tissue Processing

Many histopathological laboratories nowadays use automatic tissue processors to process tissues. These machines have reduced the processing time compared to manual time (at least 24 hours). Other advantage is superior quality of tissue processing due to constant agitation.

There are two types of automated tissue processor:

- Open (hydraulic)
- Closed (vacuum)

Open (hydraulic) type: Usually there are 11 to 12 stations.

- 1 jar: Formalin (optional)
- 6 jars: Graded alcohol
- 3 jars: Xylene
- 2 jars: Molted paraffin wax

Closed (vacuum) type: Different processing fluids are moved in and out of a single station sequentially. Enclosed tissue processor is advantageous over open type, as in case of any electric fault, this machine sounds an alarm and automatically stop.

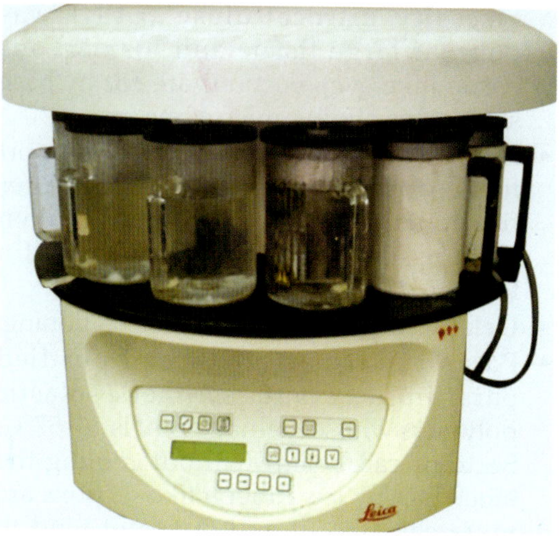

Fig. 13.1: Automatic tissue processor (closed or vacuum type) with different jars (stations) containing processing fluid

Table 13.5: Overnight schedule (automation technique)

Container No.	Fluid	Time
1.	10% formalin	0
2.	70% alcohol	½ hours
3.	95% alcohol	½ hours
4.	100% alcohol	½ hours
5.	100% alcohol	1 hours
6.	100% alcohol	1 hours
7.	100% alcohol	1 hours
8.	100% alcohol/xylene	½ hours
9.	Xylene	1 hours
10.	Xylene	2 hours
11.	Paraffin wax (molted)	2 ½ hours
12.	Paraffin wax (molted)	4 hours
		Total time = 14½ hours

Most laboratories use an overnight schedule of approximately 14–18 hours. In case of weekend and holidays, when delay is required, then the tissues are kept in first container with 10% formalin.

Microtomy

Microtomy is the process by which tissues are sectioned by microtomes and these sections are attach to a surface for visualization by microscopes. A microtome (from Greek *micros*, meaning ''small'' and *temmein*, meaning 'to cut') is a tool used to cut extremely thin slices of material, known in histology as **sections**.

Microtomes are basic instruments for microtomy and are designed for accurate cutting of sections (thin slices). Generally there are several types of microtome:

- Rotary microtome
- Rocking microtome
- Sliding microtome
- Freezing microtome
- Ultrathin microtome
- Rotary rocking microtome
- Base sledge microtome
- Vibrotome

Rotary microtome: This microtome was invented by Minot in 1885-1886. Probably this is the most popular microtome for routine paraffin wax embedded tissues. Serial sections can be cut conveniently. A large number of paraffin blocks can be cut. Electrically driven rotary microtomes are costlier compared to manual microtomes and are used when the control is necessary to produce ribbons for serial sections. Electrically driven or manual rotary microtomes are used in cryostats for frozen sections.

Disadvantages

i. Only a small length of knife is available for cutting, so large blocks cannot be cut (cutting facet base sledge microtome).
ii. Celloidion embedded blocks cannot be cut (cutting facet sliding microtome).

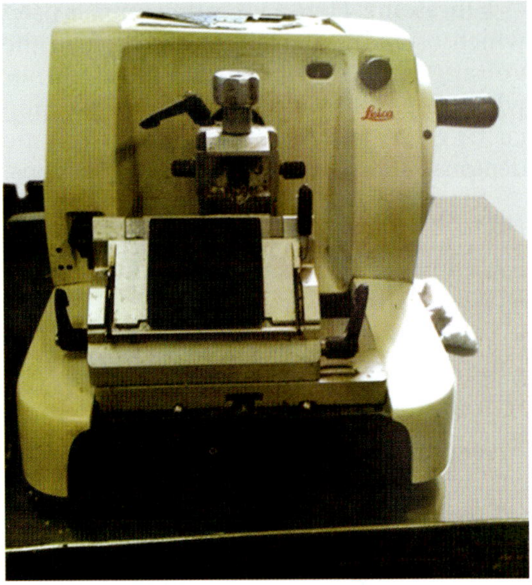

Fig. 13.2: Rotary microtome (manual type)

iii. Relatively costlier than other microtomes.

Rocking microtome: It was used in the past and Cambridge rocking microtome was most commonly used. It is cheap and was also used in cryostats first. But hard tissue cannot be cut and size of block should be small.

Base sledge microtome: This microtome is favoured when large blocks and very hard tissues should be sectioned. In neuropathology, this microtome is preferred as large blocks of brain are made. It is also good for resin embedded undecalcified bone. But consistent thin sections are difficult to cut unlike in rotary microtome.

Sliding microtome: This machine is dangerous as knife is taken along with runners to the block and knife guards cannot be attached. It was used in the past for celloidion embedded blocks cutting.

Rotary rocking microtome: This microtome has the advantage of making flat surface to the tissue block. It is usually used in cryostat though paraffin embedded blocks can also be cut.

Vibratome: Here a vibrating knife is used which oscillates variably according to the voltage supplied through a transformer when passed through a tissue during section cutting, its main use in some enzyme demonstration in unfixed, unfrozen sections.

Microtome Knives

Four types of microtome knives in use are:
- Wedge shaped
- Plano concave
- Biconcave
- Tool edge

Wedge-shaped knife: This is the most common microtome knife used nowadays for section cutting. The sides of the wedge knives are inclined at an angle of approximately 15° **(wedge angle)**. Surfaces of these knives are highly polished so that sections will move on surface and will not adhere to surface. This minimizes chances of folding, distortion and facilitates ribbon formation.

Plano concave: This knife is used in sliding microtome for sectioning celloidion embedded material.

Biconcave: This is not recommended for normal routine work as rigidity is sacrificed because of its shape. But a very keen edge can be produced.

Tool edge: This kind of knife is rigid and is recommended for use in hardest of tissues and embedding media. So, it is preferred for resin embedded undecalcified bone. This type is used in Jung K microtome.

Knife Materials

Knives used for microtomy are made from good quality tool steel or high carbon, tempered from the tip inwards for one-third of the width of knife. Hardness preferred for these knives is about 700 on **Vickers hardness**. Knives with higher hardness are difficult to sharpen and knife edges become brittle.

Disposable blade (made of steel) is the most common type used for routine paraffin embedded sectioning. Other types are glass knives, Tungsten carbide tipped knives, diamond knives, stellite tipped knives.

Paraffin Section Cutting

The numbered paraffin block is secured in place in the microtome object clamp. The object holders are adjusted so that top of the paraffin block just touches the knife edge. After placing the knife in position, both the **clearance angle** and **angle of slope** should be adjusted. A clearance angle of 3–4° and angle of slope of 40° are found to be satisfactory.

After trimming the paraffin block (10–15 µm thickness), melting ice is placed on suitable area of the block for few minutes. This is to give the tissue and paraffin wax a similar consistency so that sections can be cut with ease. For routine purpose, sections are cut at 4–5 µm thickness. Some tissues are cut at 3 µm (e.g. kidney, bone marrow, trephine and lymph node biopsies) and other thicker at 5–6 µm (e.g. bone and brain).

The sections are taken out and placed in floating out bath. Usually water bath is used and temperature of water should be 10° C below the melting point of paraffin wax.

After that, the whole length of section (ribbon which contains 6–8 sections) is placed on a slide coated with adhesive. As adhesive Mayer's egg albumin—glycerol, poly-L-lysine or **3-aminopropyltriethoxy-silane (APES)** is used.

Note

Stromal granulocytes once thought to derive from the endometrial stroma, now believed to originate from endometrial granular lymphocytes (NK cells).

Blocking out Moulds

For making paraffin blocks, tissues after processing (impregnation) are placed within liquid paraffin and to solidify to prepare paraffin blocks. These paraffin blocks are prepared in several containers.

- **Leuckhart's embedding irons:** These consist of two L-shaped pieces of heavy brass or similar metal. Advantages are adjustability to give wide variety of block sizes, even blocks with parallel sides.
- **Tissue-Tek system:** This system has stainless steel base moulds in which the tissue block is embedded. A plastic mould is then placed on top and filled with wax.
- **Peel-A-Way:** These are disposable thin plastic embedding molds. When paraffin wax has solidified, the plastic walls are simply peeled off, hence the name.
- **Plastic moulds:** Convenient for use.

Mounting Media and the Sections

After cut paraffin sections are placed on slides with adhesives, the sections are stained. These stained sections are covered with mounting media and covered with coverslips. ***Mounting*** *is the placing of mounting media on the stained tissue section and covering it with coverslips.*

The main function of mounting media is to make stained sections visible under microscope. Therefore, it should have refractory index (RI). close to the glass (RI 1.5) as light passes through glass slides and coverslips. Other functions are: To fill the tissue and tissue cavities, to prevent damage to the section, easy handling, storage and to release entrapped air bubbles. Common

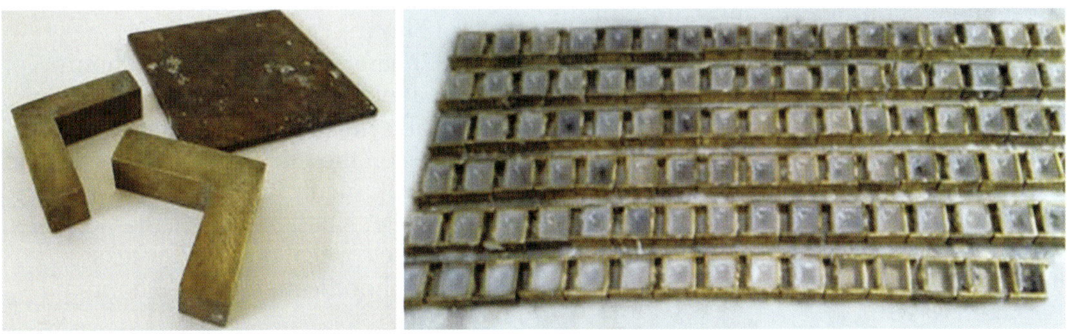

A B

Fig. 13.3A and B: (A) Leuckhart's embedding iron without paraffin (embedding medium); (B) Leuckhart's embedding iron after proper arrangements with paraffin (embedding medium)

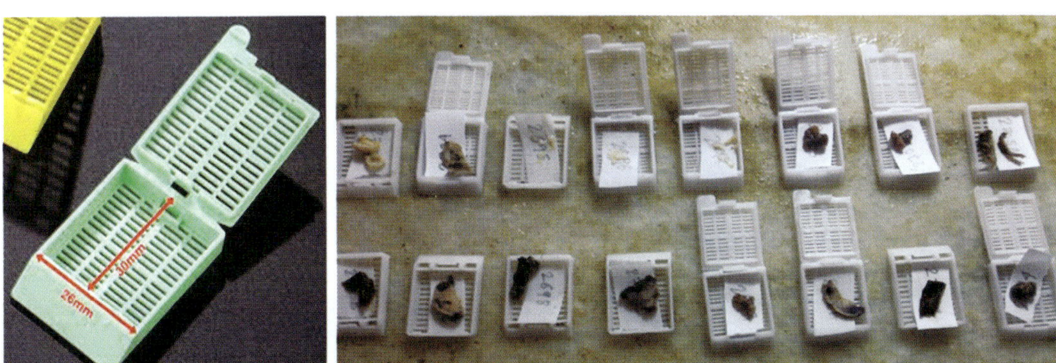

A B

Fig. 13.4A and B: (A) Plastic mould with open lid; (B) Plastic moulds containing surgical specimens after grossing mounting media are Canada balsam (RI 1.5) and **DPX or distrene dibutylpthalate xylol** (RI 1.52). Others are glycerine jelly, Apathy's medium, Farrant's medium, etc.

Decalcification

The presence of calcium salts and other minerals in bone and other calcified tissues prevents the preparation of good histologic sections by routine methods. Incomplete removal of these minerals results in ragged and torn sections and in damage to the cutting edge of the microtome knife.

Decalcification is a routine procedure which makes bone and calcified tissue compatible with the embedding media for cutting a microslide (section) and the subsequent staining. The most ubiquitous media is paraffin wax. Decalcification adjusts the hard substance of bones to the softness of paraffin. Some media, like resins do not require decalcification at all. Bones are the main object of decalcification but other surgical specimens like calcified tumors, atheromatous plaques, calcified heart valves also require decalcification.

Classification of Decalcifying Agents

1. **Acid solutions**
   A. Strong or inorganic acids: Nitric acid (HNO_3), hydrochloric acid (HCl), formalin—nitric acid, Perenyi's fluid.
   B. Weak or organic acid: Aqueous formic acid, formic acid—formalin, buffered formic acid, others like acetic acid and picric acid as components in Bouin's, Carnoy's fixative or Zenker's fixative.
2. **Chelating agents**: Ethylenediaminetetra-acetic acid (EDTA), formalin EDTA.
3. **Ion exchange resins**
4. **Electrophoretic method or electrolytic ionization**
5. **Microwave technique.**

Time Requirement for Decalcification

- Aqueous nitric acid (5–10% solutions): 24–48 hours
- von Ebner's fluid (HCl): 36–37 hours
- Formalin (formol) nitric acid: 24–48 hours
- Formic acid (5–10%): 1–10 days depending upon the thickness of the tissue and degree of calcification.
- EDTA: For small bone/spicules <1 week, for dense cortical bone 6–8 weeks
- Electrophoretic method: 6–8 hours.

VIVA VOCE

Q1. Why the tissues are fixed in fixative(s)?

Ans:

i. Prevention of tissue autolysis and bacterial attack (putrefaction).
ii. To preserve the cell elements, most importantly nuclei and cytoplasm. Fixative coagulates, various tissue proteins/elements and make them insoluble.
iii. To maintain the shape and volume of the tissues during subsequent procedures (e.g. clearing, embedding, etc.)
iv. To facilitate the staining reaction by acting as mordant.
v. To keep tissues as close to their natural state and to minimize change of natural colour and appearance.

Q2. Why 10% formalin or neutral buffered formalin is most commonly used as fixative?

Ans:

i. It is relatively cheaper and easy to prepare.
ii. The reaction between fixative and tissue proteins are usually mild with a short reaction time.
iii. It penetrates well and cause a little cell shrinkage. It maintains normal colour of large specimen.
iv. It permits many staining methods in histologic sections.

Q3. What is secondary fixation (post-fixation/post-chromatin)?

Ans: It is use of two fixatives in succession. The first one is the primary fixatives and the second one is the secondary fixative. The primary fixative is usually 10% formalin and secondary fixatives are often those contain mercuric chloride, such as formal sublimate or Helly's solution.

The second fixative reflexes the tissue so that some of its characteristics can be obtained. It must be remembered that secondary fixation does not give same results as would have been obtained if the secondary fixative had been applied to fresh, unfixed tissue.

Advantage of this sublimate post-fixation (secondary fixation) is that tissues are more easily cut and flatten better. Also, they give better staining quality.

Q4. What is the role of clearing agent in tissue processing?

Ans: Clearing agent (xylene or toluene) is a solvent of wax, helps to replace alcohol in dehydrated tissue and thus it facilitate paraffin wax penetration into tissue. Clearing agent must be miscible with alcohol. It usually makes the tissue transparent, hence the name. But some clearing agents do not make tissue transparent, so the better terminology would be 'de-alcoholisation agent'.

Q5. What is decalcification?

Ans: The presence of calcium salts and other minerals in bone and other tissue prevents the preparation of good histologic sections by routine methods. Incomplete removal of these minerals results in ragged and torn sections and in damage to the cutting edge of the microtome knife.

Decalcifying agents remove those minerals and adjust the hard substance of bone to the softness of paraffin wax. Apart from bones, other surgical specimens like calcified tumours, atheromatous plaques, calcified heart valves also require decalcification.

Common decalcifying agents are strong acids (nitric acid, hydrochloric acid), weak acids (aqueous formic acid, acetic acid, picric acid) and EDTA (ethylenediaminetetra-acetic acid).

Q6. What is microtome?

Ans: A microtome (from the Greek *mikos*, meaning "small" and *temmein*, meaning "to cut") is a tool used to cut extremely thin sections (4–5 microns thickness routinely). Uses are:

- Traditional histology techniques, sections are stained and viewed under microscopes.
- Frozen sections procedures: Uses freezing microtome or microtome cryostat.
- Electron microscope: Usually transmission electron microscope (TEM).
- Botanical microtomy: Sledge microtomy is used.
- Spectroscopy (especially infrared spectroscopy or FTIR)
- Fluorescent microscopy
- Recently laser microtome: It uses femtosecond laser instead of mechanical knife.

Q7. Why rotary microtome is most commonly used?

Ans: Although most rotary microtomes are manual, some are automatic or semi-automatic, where the advancement of the block and speed of cutting are controlled by a foot pedal or a digitally keypad at one's fingertips. Main advantages are:

i. Ideal for cutting serial section and making ribbons
ii. Heavier knife is use, so less vibration
iii. Cutting angle to knife is adjustable
iv. Ability to cope with harder tissue
v. Can be used in cryostat for frozen sections
vi. Heavier, so more stable.

Q8. What are the disadvantages of rotary microtome?

Ans: i. Only a small length of knife is available for cutting, so large blocks cannot be cut.

ii. Celloidion embedded blocks cannot be cut.

iii. It is relatively costlier.

Q9. What is frozen section?

Ans: The basic principle in frozen section is to freeze the tissue (–5° to –25°C commonly –23°C), so that the water within the tissue transforms into ice. The tissue becomes firm. The ice acts as embedding medium (like paraffin wax in routine tissue processing) and sections are cut by a special microtome known as cryostat.

The frozen section was pioneered by the Dr Louis B. Wilson in 1905.

Q10. What are advantages of frozen sections?

Ans: i. They are indispensable for rapid diagnosis during operations (to know the tumour type, margin involvement, etc.), i.e. 'on-table' diagnosis of malignancy.

ii. For certain staining procedures these are essential, e.g. fat staining by Oil red O, some methods in CNS and silver impregnation methods.

iii. Ideal to demonstrate enzymes in tissues.

iv. Also used in immunofluorescent method and in immunocytochemical method.

Q11. What are the disadvantages of frozen section?

Ans: i. Only individual section is obtained. No serial section or ribbon possible.

ii. Staining of unfixed tissues is not as satisfactory as paraffin embedded permanent sections.

iii. Structural details are somewhat distorted during section cutting as no embedding medium (like paraffin) is used.

iv. Sometimes freezing artefacts are produced due to improper techniques. These include presence of ice crystals in tissues, separation of mucosal and other epithelial surfaces, nuclear vacuolization and ballooning.

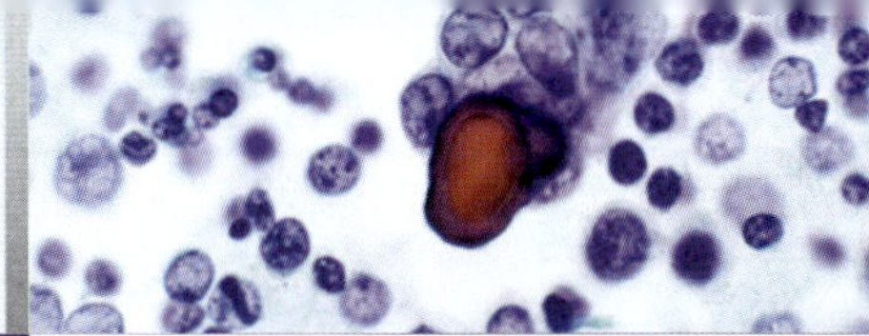

Chapter 14

H and E (Haematoxylin and Eosin) and Other Special Stains

A good routine histologic stain must be able to stain nuclei and cytoplasm but also connective tissue. A properly stained histologic section by haematoxylin and eosin differentiates and distinguishes the nuclei, the cytoplasm and connective tissue. The nuclei appear blue, whereas the cytoplasm and connective tissue fibres will have shades of pink. As it can stain and differentiate well all these structures, so it is the most popular routine stain.

Haematoxylin is used in conjunction with eosin as routine stain. Usually 0.5–1% aqueous solution of eosin is used as a counterstain, though some prefer phloxine (0.5–1%) as a counter stain. Phloxine gives a brighter and vivid red stain but eosin is more informative as it differentiates better. Some other counterstains are orange G, Bordeaux red and Biebrich scarlet.

Haematin (oxidation product of hematoxylin) is inadequate as a nuclear stain without the presence of a mordant. So, Haematoxylin solutions are classified according to which mordant is used.

- **Alum haematoxylin:** Ehrlich's hematoxylin, Harris's hematoxylin, Mayer's hematoxylin, Cole's hematoxylin, Gill's haematoxylin and Carazzi's haematoxylin.
- **Iron haematoxylin:** Weigert's haematoxylin, Verhoeff's hematoxylin, Loyez's hematoxylin, heidenhain hematoxylin.
- **Tungsten hematoxylin:** Phosphotungstic acid Haematoxylin (PTAH)
- **Lead hematoxylin**
- **Molybdenum Haematoxylin**
- **Haematoxylin without mordant.**

PRINCIPLE OF ALUM HAEMATOXYLIN STAINING

The mordant used in alum Haematoxylin is aluminum either potash alum (aluminium potash sulfate) or ammonium alum (aluminium ammonium sulfate).

Initially, the nuclei become red after staining, which turn blue or blue black when stained sections are washed in weak alkali. Practically, tap water can be used for washing as it is alkaline enough to produce desired colour change. Sometimes, alkaline solutions like Scott's tap water, saturated lithium carbonate or 0.5% ammonia in distilled water is used for this colour change. *This process of changing colour from red to blue is called 'blueing'*.

Progressive staining: Here, the sections are stained for a predetermined time, so that the nuclei become well stained but the background is relatively under stained.

Regressive staining: In this procedure, the sections are first over stained, and then excess stain is selectively removed in acid alcohol. Advantage of this staining procedure is that the degree of staining is controlled (some tissue elements retain more stain/dye compared with others. Hence, the nuclei take good staining, whereas the cytoplasm and background are perfectly clear.

Harris Alum Haematoxylin

Composition of alum haematoxylin

- Hematoxylin: 2.5 g
- Absolute alcohol: 50 ml
- Ammonia or potassium alum: 50 g
- Distilled water: 500 ml
- Mercuric oxide: 1.5 g or sodium iodate: 0.5 g
- Glacial acetic acid: 20 ml.

Preparation: The Haematoxylin is dissolved in the absolute alcohol and it is then added to previously prepared alum solution (alum in distilled water). The two solutions are mixed well. The mixture is now heated to boiling point and mercuric oxide or sodium iodide is added. Then the mixture is rapidly cooled by plunging the flask in cold water or into a sink containing ice pieces. The solution is ready for staining.

Addition of glacial acetic acid is optional but is preferred, because this gives more precise and selective nuclear staining. Filter before use when previously made solutions are used.

Advantages: It is a good nuclear stain and is used for general purpose. As the nuclear staining is very clear, it is also used in exfoliative cytology. In routine histologic sections, Harris's Haematoxylin is used regressively but in exfoliative cytology it is used progressively.

Disadvantages: Nuclear stain fades after a few months which is also seen in other chemically ripened alum Haematoxylin (of natural ripening of Ehrlich's alum hematoxylin). In stored solution, there is formation of a precipitate after few months and the solution is not good for staining. At this stage, the stain can be used by filtering the precipitate and increasing the staining time. But best thing is to use freshly prepared stain.

Standing time

- Progressive in exfoliative cytology: 4–30 seconds
- Regressive method: 5–15 minutes.

Staining Method Using Alum Haematoxylin and Eosin

- Dewax histologic sections.
- Hydrate through graded alcohol first, then to water.
- Stain the nuclei with preferred alum Haematoxylin (Harris hematoxylin) for required time.
- Wash the stained sections for 5 minutes in tap water till the blueing of the nuclei.
- Differentiate the sections, in 1% acid alcohol (1% HCl in 70% ethyl alcohol) for 5–10 seconds.
- Wash again in tap water until the sections are 'blue' for 5 minutes or less.
- Stain in 1% eosin (eosin Y is preferred) for 10 minutes.
- Wash in tap water for 1–5 minutes.
- Dehydrate through graded alcohol (70%, 95% and then 100%).
- Clearing in xylene, then mount it DPX or Canada balsam.

Result of Alum Haematoxylin and Eosin Stain

- Nuclei → Blue/black
- Cytoplasm → Varying shades of pink
- Fibrin → Deep pink
- Red blood cells → Orange/red
- Muscle fiber → Deep pink/red
- Fungal hyphae → Faintly blue
- Calcium deposits → Deep blue-black.

Iron Haematoxylin

Here iron salts are used both as oxidizing agent and as mordant in the haematoxylin solutions. Ferric chloride and ferric ammonium sulphate are commonly used as iron salts.

In comparison to alum haematoxylin, iron haematoxylin can demonstrate wide range of tissue structures but staining technique is time-consuming and also it needs microscope evaluation during differentiation stage.

Weigert's Iron Haematoxylin

Composition of staining solution

i. Haematoxylin solutions
   - Haematoxylin: 1 g
   - Absolute alcohol: 100 ml

ii. Iron solution
   - 30% aqueous ferric chloride solution (anhydrous): 4 ml
   - Hydrochloric acid (concentrated): 1 ml
   - Distilled water: 95 ml

Preparation: First the solution (i) or haematoxylin solution must be allowed to ripen. For natural ripening, it takes 4–5 weeks time. It may also be prepared from a stock solution of 5% Haematoxylin in absolute alcohol (previously ripened solution). Now, mix equal part of solution (i) and solution (ii) immediately before use. When mixing is done in a test tube, it is advisable to pour solution (i) in the tube first, and then add solution (ii) as it contains concentration of HCl. The staining solution/mixture ideally should be violet-black in colour. If the colour becomes brown, then the mixture should be discarded.

Advantage: Main use is as a nuclear stain in techniques, where acid is used subsequently (e.g. picric acid in van Gieson stain). It resists removal of counterstain containing differentiating agent like picric acid. It stains nuclei black unlike blue/blue-black in alum hematoxylin. The stained nuclei will not be decolourized by light. So, it is a more permanent stain than alum haematoxylin.

Disadvantage: More time consuming and needs microscopic control for accuracy. It has been replaced by more convenient Celestine blue-alum hematoxylin. Still it is in use for CNS tissues.

Staining time: 20–30 minutes.

Heidenhain Haematoxylin

Composition of staining solution

- Iron alum solutions
  - Ferric ammonium sulfate (violet crystals): 5 g
  - Distilled water: 100 ml
- Haematoxylin solutions
  - Hematoxylin: 0.5 g
  - Absolute alcohol: 10 ml
  - Distilled water: 90 ml
- This solution must be kept ready for 4–5 weeks for natural ripening, or 5% stock solution (ripened) alcoholic hematoxylin: 10 ml
- Distilled water: 90 ml
- This solution is ready for immediate use.

Staining methods

1. Dewax histologic sections (either putting into xylol for 1–2 minutes or by heating).
2. Hydrate through graded alcohol to water.
3. Mordant in 5% iron alum/iron alum solution for 1 hour.
4. Rinse in distilled water (10–20 seconds).
5. Stain in Heidenhain haematoxylin solution for 1 hour.
6. Wash in running tap water until the sections are blue (usually takes 10 minutes in tap water of pH 8). Lithium carbonate may be added to water if it is not sufficiently alkaline.
7. Differentiate in 5% iron alum until the desired structure is clearly demonstrated under microscope.
8. Wash in running tap water for 8–10 minutes.
9. Dehydrate in graded alcohol (70%, 95% and then 100%).
10. Clear and mount in DPX or Canada balsam.

Advantage: It can be used to demonstrate many structures as per degree of differentiation. mitochondria, muscle striations, myelin, nuclear membrane, chromatin, chromosomes, nucleoli, centrioles, yolk and ground cytoplasm can be demonstrated which become jet black or grey black. Good for photography. The stain is permanent, if the alum is properly removed. It is applicable after use of any fixative.

Disadvantage: It is used only regressively and experience is required for good staining quality. For beginners use half-strength iron alum is advisable until they again experience.

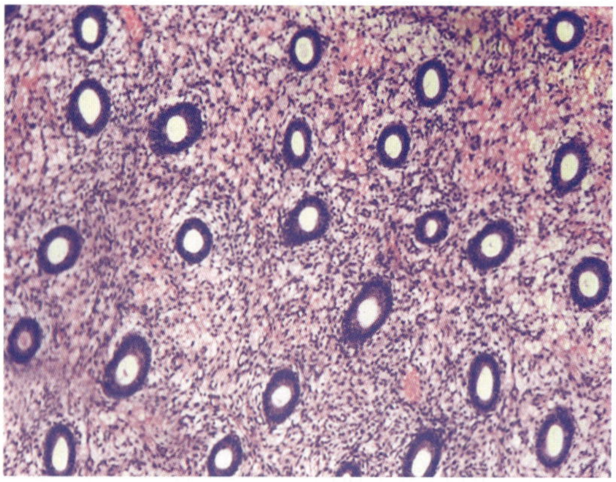

Fig. 14.1: Haematoxylin and eosin stain showing proliferative endometrium (H and E, 100X)

PERIODIC ACID-SCHIFF (PAS) STAIN

Periodic acid is a very strong oxidizing agent and under the controlled condition of the staining reaction, it reacts with the aldehyde group of the carbohydrates. This periodic acid cleaves the carbon-carbon bond in amino or alkyl amino derivatives or 1.2 glycols to form aldehydes. These aldehydes will react with fuchsin-sulfurous acid and this product combines the basic pararosaniline to give a positive result (magenta-coloured compound). This compound is chemically alkyl sulfate.

Any substance that fulfils the following criteria will give a positive result during PAS reaction (Hotchkiss, 1948).

- The substance must not diffuse away during fixation.
- It must produce an oxidation product which is not diffusible.
- The substance must have the 1.2 glycol grouping or the equivalent amino or alkyl amino derivative or the oxidation product CHOH-CO.
- Sufficient concentration of the substance must be present in the tissue to give a positive reaction (magenta color).

PAS (Periodic Acid-Schiff) Reagents

- Periodic acid solution (0.5%)
  Periodic acid: 1 g
  Distilled water: 200 ml
- Schiff's reagent: Dissolve 1 g basic fuchsin in 200 ml of boiling distilled water. When dissolved; cool it to 50–60°C. Add 2 g of potassium metabisulfite and mix it. Bring the mixture to room temperature and then add 2 ml of hydrochloric acid and mix it. Also add 2 g of activated charcoal and this chemical solution is kept at room temperature in a dark place overnight. Next morning, filter it (Whatman paper No. 1). The ideal solution after filtration should be pale yellow or clear. Store this solution at 4°C in dark container.

Staining Method

1. Deparaffinize histologic sections and bring the section to water. If Zenker's fluid is used as a fixative, remove mercury precipitate in iodine. Wash in water and decolourize in hypo solution.
2. Rinse in distilled water.
3. Oxidize in 0.5% periodic acid for 5–10 minutes.
4. Wash in running tap water for 5 minutes and rinse in distilled water.
5. Treat with Schiff reagent for 10–30 minutes.

6. Wash in running tap water for 5–10 minutes.
7. Counterstain (optional) with Harris's haematoxylin for 1–3 minutes to stain the nuclei. Differentiate in 1% acid alcohol (3–5 dips). Blueing the sections in running tap water.
8. Wash in water.
9. Rinse in absolute alcohol.
10. Clear in xylene and mount in DPX or Canada balsam.

Results

- Glycogen and other PAS positive substances: Magenta/bright red.
- Nuclei: Blue
- Other tissue constituents: Yellow.

PAS Positive Substances

- Glycogen, most basement membrane, amyloid, fibrin of thrombi, colloid of thyroid.
- Mucins: Intestinal glands, gastric glands, endocervical glands, salivary glands, bronchial glands, conjunctiva, prostatic gland secretion, corpora amylacea.
- Adrenal lipofuscin, many fungi, actinomycosis (clubs only), hyaline casts of kidney, cartilage matrix, ocular lens capsule, starch, zymogen granules of pancreas, beta cells of pituitary.
- Russel bodies of plasma cells, megakaryocyte granules.

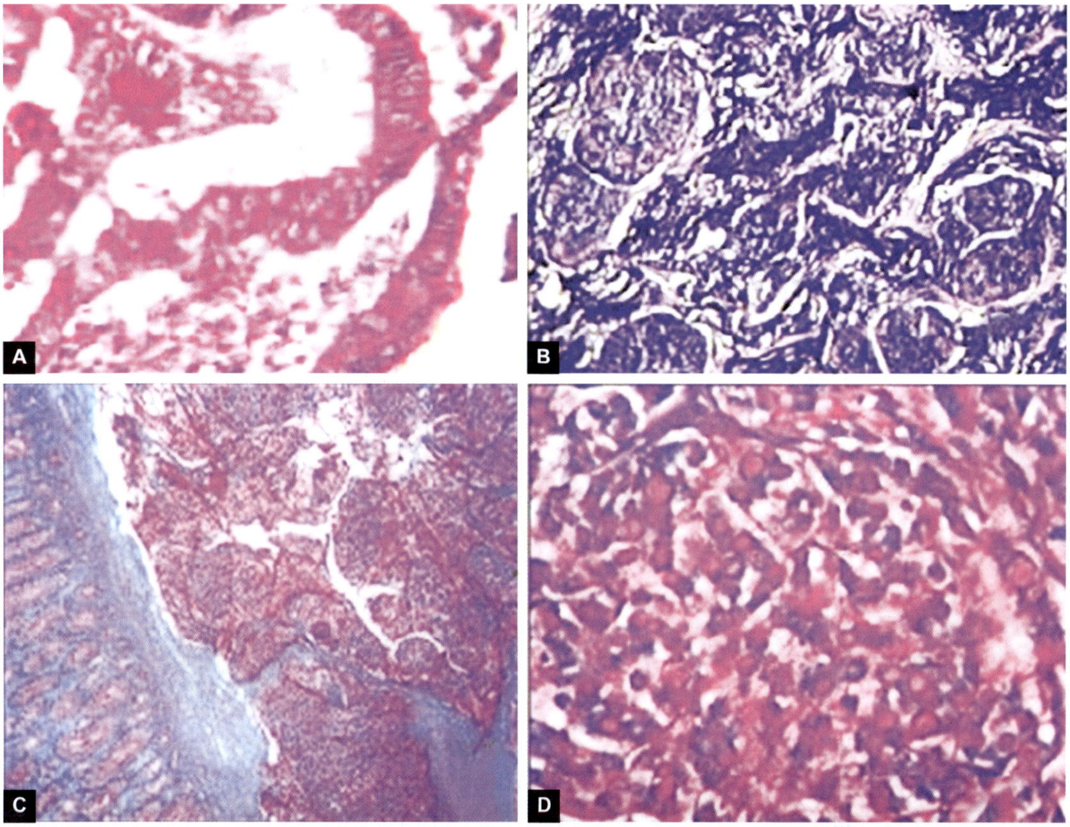

Fig. 14.2A to D: (A) Adenocarcinoma of colon showing malignant cells with neutral mucins (PAS, 400X); (B) Mucinous carcinoma showing pools of acidic mucin (alcian blue, 400X); (C) Mucinous carcinoma showing acidic and neutral mucins (combined alcian blue and PAS, 100X); (D) Signet ring cell carcinoma showing neutral mucin (combined alcian blue and PAS, 400X)

SUDAN BLACK B STAIN

Sudan black B is known as the most sensitive lipid stain. It was introduced by Lison and Dagnelie in 1935. Unlike the other Sudan dyes it can stain both phospholipid and neutral fat (compound lipids). It also can stain myelin and mitochondria.

The ability of formalin and calcium to make these lipids insoluble in acetone and other reagents used in paraffin processing, make them unsuitable for Sudan III or osmium tetroxide staining. But Sudan black B stain can be used. Ideal sections for Sudan IV staining are unfixed cryostat sections, short fixed frozen sections and cryostat sections, post-fixed in formol-calcium. Use of solvents like ethanol or acetone is not recommended for this dye, as these solvents remove a significant portion of the lipid. So, small fat droplets are dissolved out and are not detected by stain. Propylene, propylene glycol, isopropyl alcohol or ethylene glycol are better as a solvent. But 70% ethanol is still used for general purpose.

Standing Methods

1. Rinse cryostat sections in 70% ethanol.
2. Stain the slides in saturated Sudan black B in 70% ethanol for 30–120 minutes. Sections of routine formol saline-fixed tissue should be stained for 30–180 minutes at 60°C.
3. Rinse in 70% ethanol to remove excess surface dye.
4. Wash in tap water and differentiate in 70% alcohol (or in 85% propylene glycol solution for 2–3 minutes).
5. Wash in distilled water.
6. Counterstain in Mayer's carmalum for 2–3 minutes. (Mayer's carmalum: Dissolve 2 g of carmine in 100 ml of 0.5% ammonium alum by boiling for 1 hour. Add a few crystals of thymol to prevent fungal growth, filter before use.)
7. Wash well in water.
8. Mount in glycerine jelly.

Results

- Compound lipids (phospholipids, cerebrosides): Blue black
- Nuclei: Red.

OIL RED O STAIN

For this staining technique, cryostat sections, short-fixed frozen sections, unfixed in formol calcium is chosen.

Staining Solution

A saturated solution of Oil red O (0.25–0.5%) in isopropyl alcohol is kept in stock. Working solution is made by adding 6 ml of stock solution with 4 ml of distilled water. Allow the mixture to stand for 5–10 minutes and then filter it.

Staining methods

1. Cut frozen sections (relatively thick section of 8–10 μm).
2. Wash well in distilled water.
3. Rinse in 70% ethanol.
4. Stain in Oil red O staining solution for 10–35 minutes.
5. Differentiate in 70% alcohol to remove excess stain.
6. Counterstain nuclei lightly in Harris Haematoxylin for 1–2 minutes.
7. Blueing in tap water (alternatively, ammonia water may be used).
8. Mount in glycerine jelly.

Results

- Lipids: Orange to red
- Nuclei: Blue

VERHOEFF'S VAN GIESON STAIN FOR ELASTIC FIBRES

Composition of Staining Solution

- Verhoeff's staining solution
  - Stock 5% alcoholic haematoxylin: 20 ml
  - 10% ferric chloride: 8 ml
  - Verhoeff's iodine (10 dine 2 g, potassium iodide 4 g, water 100 ml): 8 ml

- Reagents are added as given above, then mix well; solution should be freshly prepared before use.
- van Gieson's staining solution
  - Saturated aqueous solution of picric acid: 100 ml
  - 1% acid fuchsin: 10 ml
  - Freshly prepared solution is better

Staining Methods

1. Bring histologic sections to water.
2. Stain in Verhoeff's staining solution for 15–30 minutes until sections are jet-black.
3. Differentiate in 2% ferric chloride until elastic fibres are clearly visible (rinse in water and examine under low power microscope).
4. Wash in water.
5. Place in 95% alcohol to remove iodine staining.
6. Wash in water for 5–10 minutes.
7. Counterstain in van Gieson's staining solution for 3 minutes. Blot it.
8. Dehydrate in graded alcohol.
9. Clear in xylene and mount in DPX.

Results

- Elastic fibres and nuclei: Black to blue black
- RBC, cytoplasm, background and muscle: Yellow
- Collagen: Red

Note

Do not wash the sections after van Gieson's staining (step 7). Put them directly in graded alcohol for dehydration. Otherwise, it will impair staining quality (if washed in water).

GOMORI'S SILVER IMPREGNATION STAIN FOR RETICULIN

Gomori's Silver Solution Preparation

In a test tube or flask, add 4 parts of 10% aqueous silver nitrate and 1 part of 10% potassium hydroxide. The potassium hydroxide will cause silver to deposit. Mark the volume of the fluid with a pencil/marker. Remove the supernatant fluid and wash the deposit several times with distilled water to make up to its original volume (previously marked by pencil/marker). Now, add strong ammonia drop by drop until the deposit is just dissolved. Again add 10% silver nitrate solution, to produce a light precipitate. Make the volume of this solution twice with addition of distilled water. Store in dark bottle. Filter before use. Preferably, solution should be freshly prepared but it can used for 24–35 hours.

Staining Methods

1. Bring the deparaffinized sections to water.
2. Oxidize with 1% potassium permanganate for 1–2 minutes.
3. Rinse in tap water.
4. Decolourize with 3% potassium metabisulfite for 1 minute.
5. Rinse in tap water.
6. Sensitize in 2% iron alum for 1 minute.
7. Wash in tap water for 2–3 minutes, then rise in distilled water 2–3 changes.
8. Impregnate in silver solution for 3 minutes.
9. Rinse quickly in distilled water.
10. Reduce in 10% formalin in tap water for 3 minutes.
11. Wash in running tap water for 3–4 minutes, then rinse in distilled water.
12. Tone in 1:500 gold chloride (yellow) for 5–15 minutes.
13. Rinse in distilled water
14. Place in 3% potassium metabisulfite for 1 minute to reduce toning.
15. Fix in 3% sodium thiosulfate for 1 minute.
16. Rinse in distilled water
17. Wash in water.
18. Dehydrate through graded alcohol.
19. Clear in xylene and mount in DPX.

Results

- Reticulin fibres: Black
- Collagen fibres: Purple
- Nuclei and cytoplasm: Grayish/shades of gray.

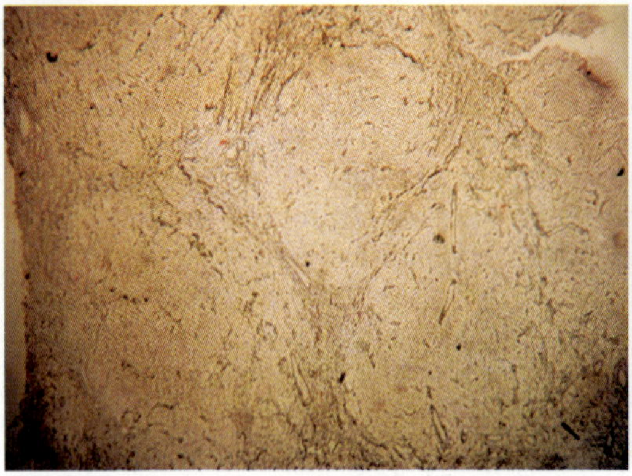

A

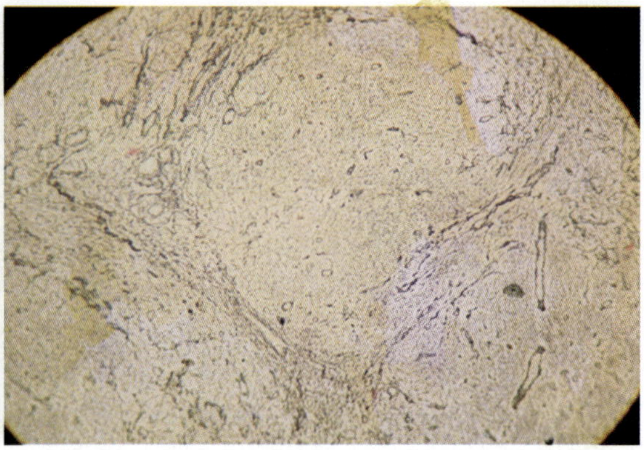

B

Fig. 14.3A and B: (A) Microphotograph showing reticulin fibres in cirrhotic nodules of liver (reticulin stain, low power view, 100X); (B) Microphotograph showing reticulin fibres in a cirrhotic nodule (reticulin stain, high power view, 400X).

Table 14.1: Common stains used for different connective tissues and its colour

Tissue Type	Masson trichrome	Reticulin silver	Methenamine silver	van Gieson	PTAH	H and E	PAS
Collagen	Blue green	Pale gray	Unstained	Red	Orange red	Deep pink	Pale pink
Reticulin fibres	Blue green	Black	Unstained	Yellow	Orange brown	Unstained	Pink
Elastic fibres	Pale red	Unstained	Unstained	Yellow	Orange brown	Pink	Unstained
Fibrin	Red	Unstained/ grey	Unstained	Variable yellow	Variable blue	Pink	Pink or unstained
Muscle	Red	Pale grey	Pale grey	Yellow	Blue	Deep pink	Pale pink
Cartilage	Variable	Variable	Variable	Variable	Variable	Purple	Pink
Basement membrane	Blue green	Pale grey	Black	Yellow	Orange	Pink	Magenta

VIVA VOCE

Q1. What is the basic principle of H and E stain?

Ans: This stain has two components; haematoxylin and eosin. Staining of nuclei is done by oxidized haematoxylin (haematin) through mordant bonds and make nuclei blue in colour. Nuclear staining is followed by counterstaining with the xanthene dye, the eosin, which colours the cytoplasm in varying shades of pink.

Q2. What are the results (colour) after H and E staining?

Ans: Nuclei: Blue/black

Cytoplasm: Varying shades of pink

Fibrin: Deep pink

Red blood cells: Orange/red

Muscle fibre: Deep pink/red.

Q3. What is the principle of PAS staining?

Ans: Substances which contain vicinal glycol group or their amino or alkyl amino derivatives are oxidized by periodic acid to form dialdehydes. It combines with Schiff's reagent to form an insoluble magenta-coloured compound.

Q4. Which tissue components are stained by PAS staining?

Ans: It stains glycogen, neutral mucin and carbohydrate portions of glycoproteins and glycolipids.

Positive stains (magenta colour) are seen in glycogen, basement membrane, starch, neutral mucin, colloid, fungi, amoeba, cellulose, collagen (weak positive) and amyloid (weak positive).

Q5. What is the principle of reticulin staining?

Ans: Reticulin fibres mainly consist of type III collagen in a glycoprotein complex. It can be stained by several techniques but Gordon-Sweet's silver impregnantion method is most sensitive and most widely used stain. In this technique, hydroxyl group of adjacent hexose sugars are oxidized to aldehydes by potassium permanganate. These newly formed aldehydes then reduce silver diamine to metallic silver. This reaction can be further modified by use of silver chloride as a toner.

Q6. What are the results (colour) after reticulin staining?

Ans: Reticulin fibres: Black

Collagen fibres: Purple

Nuclei and cytoplasm: Grayish/shades of gray.

Q7. How reticulin fibres are differentiated from collagen fibres?

Ans: Reticulin fibres are fine and delicate fibres which are found along with a stronger and coarser collagen fibre, i.e. type III collagen fibre. Reticulin fibres form a delicate supporting framework for highly cellular organs like lymph nodes, liver and endocrine glands.

Reticulin fibres are gram-negative, coloured black by silver stain and isotropic (not birefringent), whereas collagen fibres are slight gram-positive, stained purple, or brown to mauve by silver stain and is anisotropic (birefringent).

Q8. What are elastic fibres? How are they stained?

Ans: Elastic fibres consist of elastin and glycoprotein. They are found throughout the body but most common locations are skin, respiratory system (lung, pleura), urinary bladder, ligaments, circulatory system (blood vessels).

In the Verhoeff staining technique, elastic fibres are stained black due to formation of metallic (iron)—dye (haematin) is called lake. Weigert's resorcin fuchsin also stains elastic fibres blue to black. In aldehyde fuchsin, elastin fibres are stained purple and it becomes dark brown in orcein stain.

Q9. When is Masson's trichrome staining used?

Ans: This is a three-step staining technique (hence the name trichrome). It stains three different categories of cell components: Nucleus, muscle and collagen.

In the first step, nucleus is stained by Weigert's iron-Haematoxylin stain followed by the second step of staining of cytoplasm and muscles with a red cytoplasmic staining of cytoplasm and muscles with a red cytoplasmic stain differentiated in phosphomolybdic acid. Lastly, staining of fibres with aniline blue or light green.

- Nuclei: Bluish black or black
- Muscle, cytoplasm, keratin: Red
- Collagen, cartilage, mucus: Blue (if aniline dye is used) or green (if light green is used).

Q10. What is a mordant?

Ans: The mordants form a link between the tissue and the stain. The combination of the dye and the mordant forms a compound which is capable of attracting itself to the tissue firmly. This compound is sometimes called 'lake'. The mordants are salts, usually sulpfates of aluminium, iron or chromium. Generally, double sulphates or alums are used.

Chapter

15

HP (Histopathology) Slides, Light Microscopy

Tuberculosis of Lung

- Section shows structure of lung parenchyma.

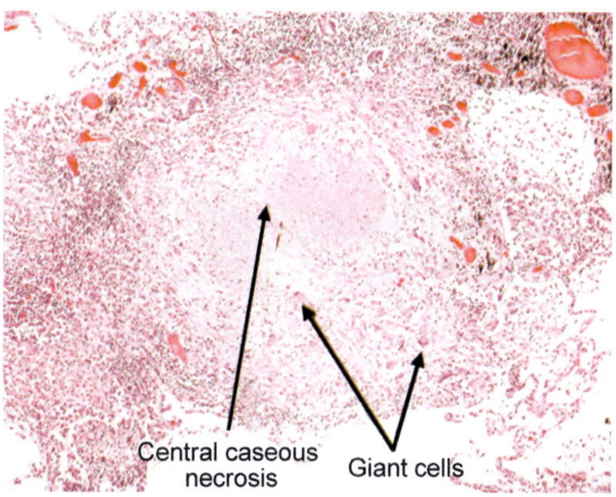

- Central granular caseation (caseation necrosis) is surrounded by epithelioid histiocytes (modified macrophages) and Langhans giant cells. Foreign body giant cells are also found.
- The tubercles are surrounded by lymphocytes and fibroblasts.

Emphysema of Lung

- There is marked enlargement of airspaces.
- Alveolar walls show thinning and destruction. Adjacent alveoli become confluent, creating large airspaces.

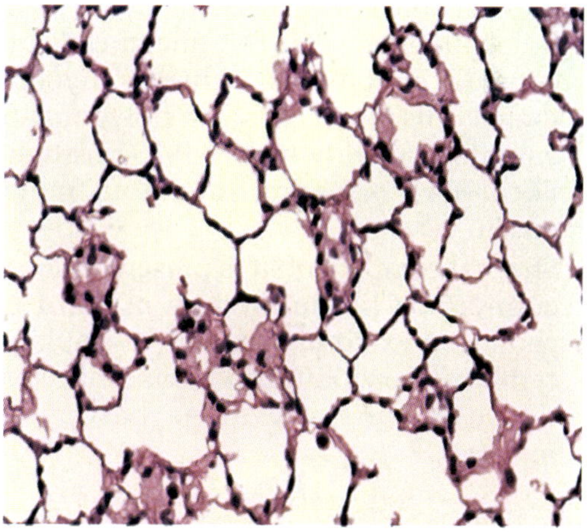

Normal lung (control)

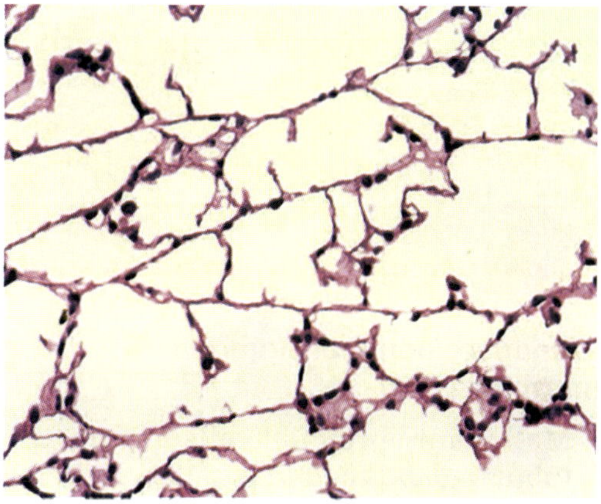

Emphysematous lung (due to cigarette smoking)

- There is loss of elastic tissue in the surrounding alveolar septae.
- Alveolar capillaries are reduced in number.

Pleomorphic Salivary Adenoma

- There is considerable variation or great heterogeneity in the histologic features within the tumour.
- It is characterized by pleomorphic or 'mixed' appearance in which both epithelial and stromal components are seen in varying proportions.
- Epithelial component: It forms various patterns like ducts, acini, tubules, sheets and strands of cells of ductal or myoepithelial cells. The ductal cells are cuboidal or columnar, whereas myoepithelial cells (basal cells) are polygonal or spindle shaped (which is PAS-positive). Focal areas showing squamous metaplasia.
- Stromal component: It is present as loose connective tissue, and as myxoid or chondromyxoid matrix which simulates cartilage (pseudocartilage). This connective tissue mucins appear as basophilic material.

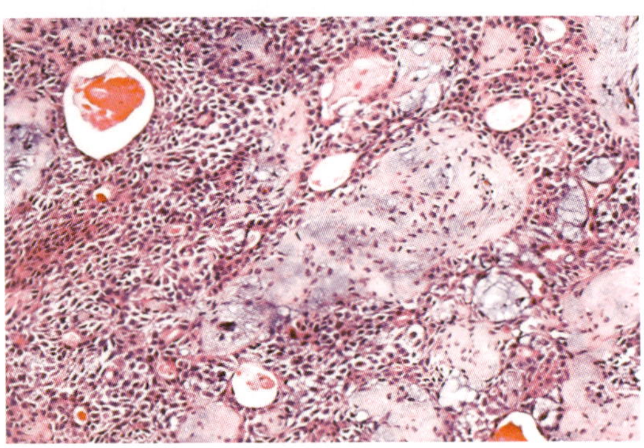

Adenocarcinoma of Stomach (Intestinal Type)

- Malignant epithelial cells arranged in tubular glands and in papillary pattern.
- Malignant epithelial cells are also arranged in sheets.

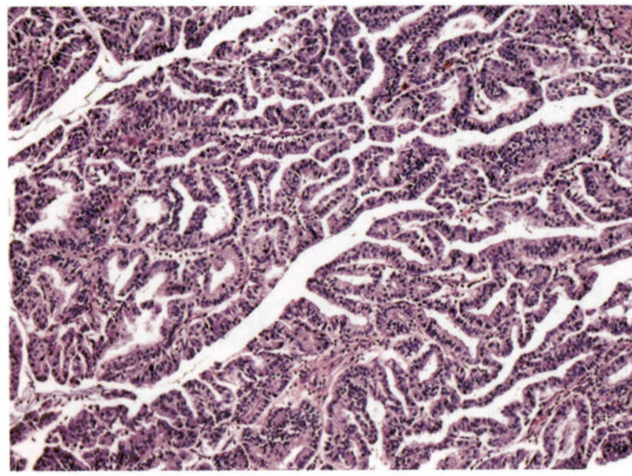

- The malignant cells have large vesicular nuclei with prominent nucleoli.
- The malignant glands are lined by tall columnar cells containing mucin resembling colonic adenocarcinoma.
- There is chronic inflammatory cell infiltration into stroma.

TB Intestine (Ileocaecal)

- There is mucosal and submucosal ulcerations.
- There is moderate to severe infiltration of chronic inflammatory cells.
- Against this background, many epithelioid granulomas are seen in all the layers of intestine, i.e mucosa, submucosa, muscularis layer and serosa.
- Both caseating and non-caseating granulomas are seen.

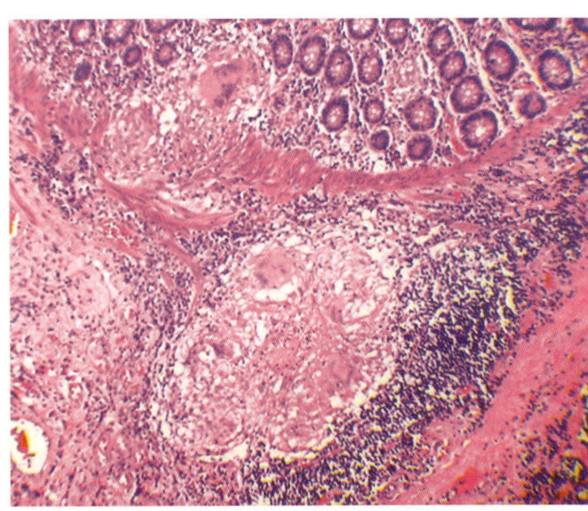

- Multinucleated giant cells of both Langhans and foreign body type are found.
- Most of the mucosal glands are unremarkable while some glands show pyloric metaplasia.

Acute Appendicitis

- There is an acute inflammatory infiltrate (neutrophilic infiltration) which extends from mucosa through the full thickness of the appendiceal wall.
- Neutrophilic infiltration is present in the muscularis layer.
- Acute inflammatory exudate is seen in the lumen.
- Focal superficial (mucosal) ulceration is noted.
- Subserosal vessels are dilated.
- Serosal layer is granular and erythematous (organized).

Clear Cell Carcinoma of Kidney

- Tumour cells with clear cytoplasm arranged in solid sheets, in trabecular (cord-like) pattern and in tubular pattern.
- Slightly irregular nuclei and nucleoli are seen in high power (40X) only. Nuclear diameter 15 μm and chromatin is open (Fuhrman nuclear grade 2).
- Mitoses are not seen.
- The tumour has delicate branching vasculature.
- The cytoplasm is abundant and clear or granular due to presence of glycogen and lipids.

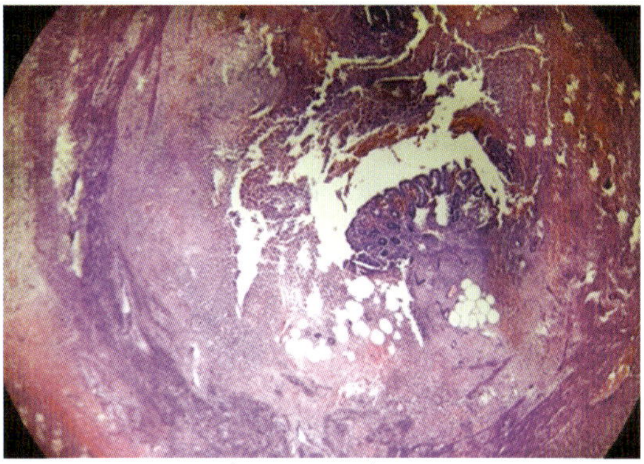

Low power view

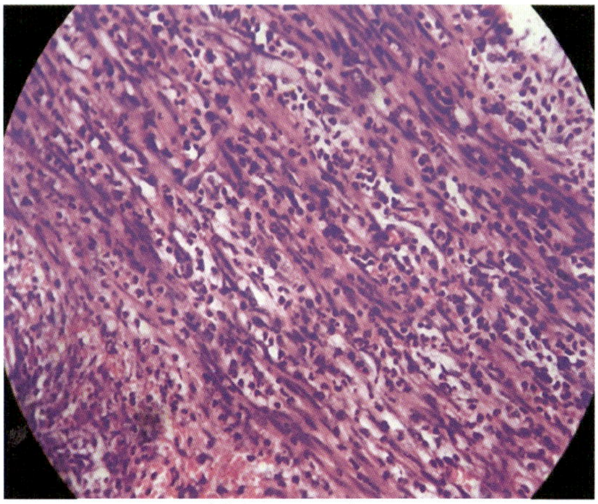

High power view

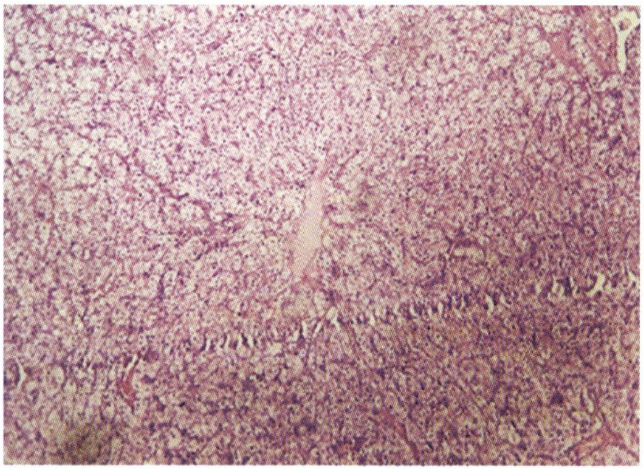

Low power view

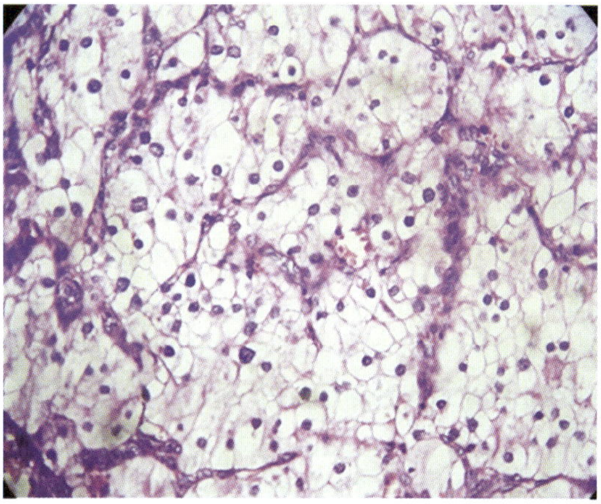

High power view

Osteogenic Sarcoma

- Tumour is composed of pleomorphic polyhedral or spindle-shaped neoplastic cells.
- The tumour cells have hyperchromatic nuclei and frequent mitoses.
- These neoplastic cells form islands of reactive new women bone (pinkish lace-like osteoid and calcified bone spicules).
- Other matrices, including cartilage or fibrous tissue, are present in varying amount.
- Bizarre tumour giant cells are present.

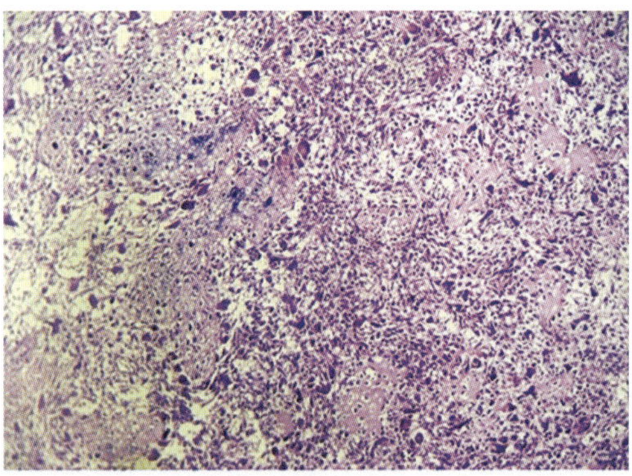

Low power view

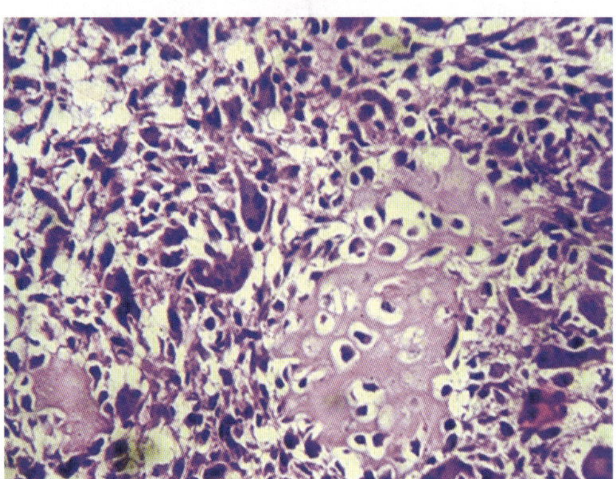

High power view

Giant Cell Tumour (of Bone)

It is a biphasic tumour composed of mononuclear uniform tumour cells (stromal cells) and giant cells.

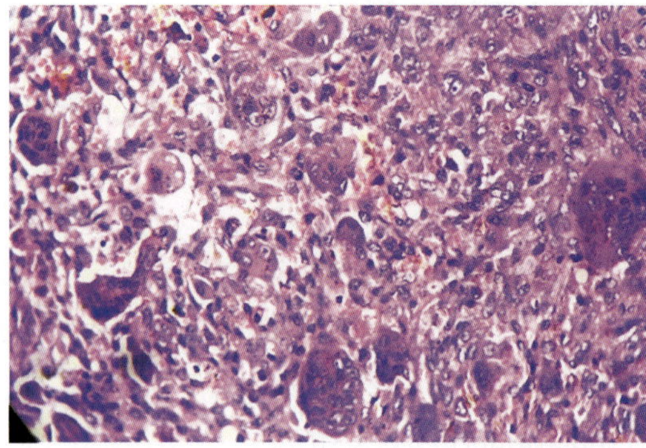

- **Tumour cells:** They are uniform cells with indistinct cell membrane growing in a syncytium as stromal cells. The tumour cells are usually oval or round in shape.
- **Giant cells:** Numerous multinucleated osteoclast-like giant cells containing >100 nuclei are uniformly scattered among mononuclear tumour (stromal) cells. The nuclei of stromal cells resemble those of the mononuclear stromal cells. Mitoses are infrequent.

Proliferative Endometrium

- Early proliferative endometrium (days 4–7): Thin surface epithelium. Glands are small, round and straight (tubular glands) having columnar living with basal nuclei. Stroma is compact and composed of spindle-shaped cells that have scant

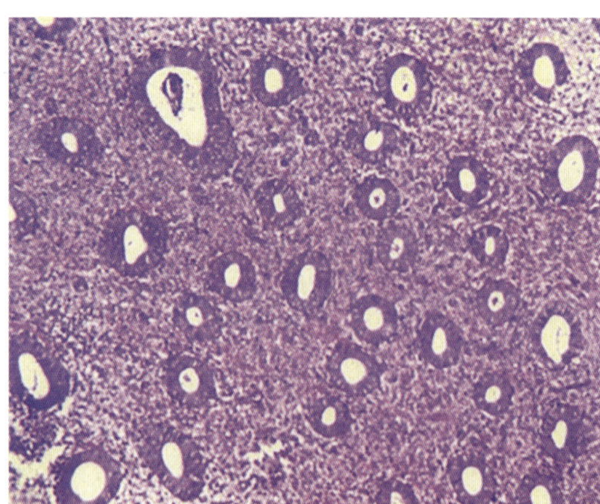

Early proliferative endometrium

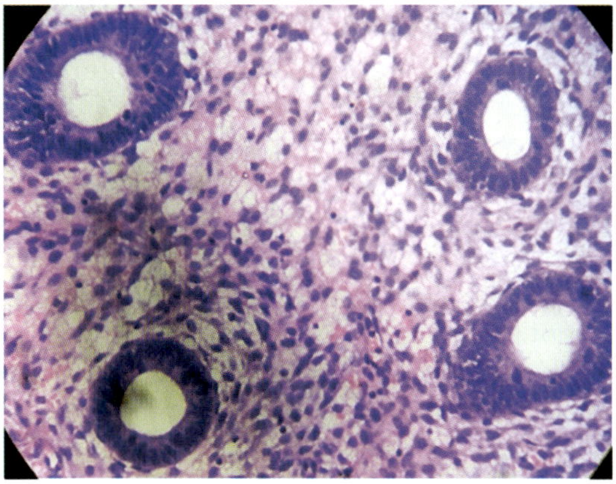

Mid-proliferative endometrium

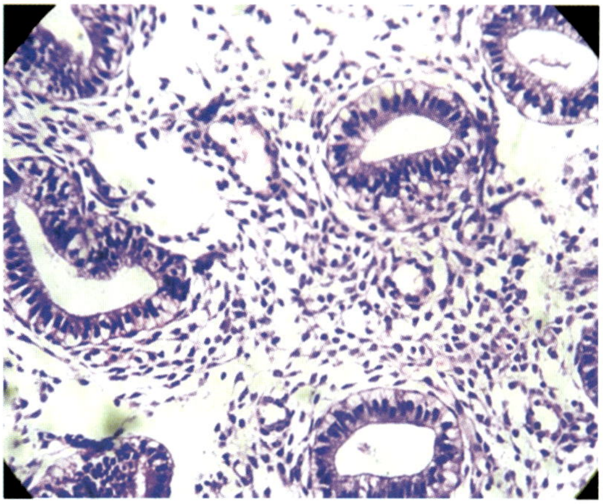

Early secretory endometrium

cytoplasm. Mitoses are seen both within glands and stroma. No oedema is seen within stroma. Stroma contains small, regularly distributed blood vessels.

- Mid-proliferative endometrium (8–10 days): Columnar surface epithelium. The endometrial glands are longer and curving. Variable stroma, oedema and numerous mitotic figures are seen within stroma.
- Late proliferative endometrium (11–14 days): Undulant surface epithelium. The glands are tortuous and crowded with prominent mitotic activity and pseudostratification. Subnuclear vacuoles are seen in less than 50% of glands. Stromal oedema is variable but present.

Secretory Endometrium

- Early secretory endometrium (16–19 days): Subnuclear vacuoles (secretory vacuoles beneath the nuclei) are seen >50% of glands. The glands are usually longer and tortuous. Stroma is edematous.
- Mid-secretory endometrium (20–22 days): The glands are fully coiled **(corkscrew appearance)** and lined by cells with round often vesicular nuclei. Basal vacuoles (subnuclear vacuoles) progressively push past the nuclei and become **supranuclear vacuoles**. Glandular secretion is prominent. Stromal oedema is prominent. Pseudodecidual changes seen only around spiral arterioles.

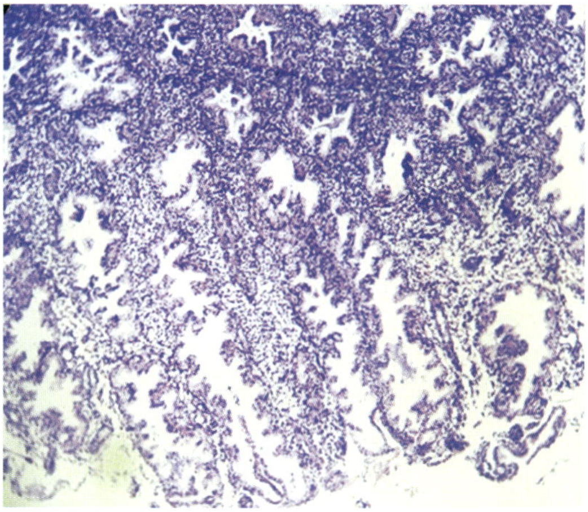

Mid-secretory endometrium

- Late secretory endometrium (23–28 days): The glands are tortuous, producing a serrated or **"saw-tooth" appearance** due to secretory exhaustion. Pseudodecidual changes in the stroma is marked as is stromal edema. Spiral arterioles become prominent as is stromal edema. Spiral arterioles become prominent as a result of thickness of their walls and cuff of predecidual stromal cells around them. There is increase in the number of **stromal granulocytes** (bean-shaped, dense nuclei, inconspicuous cytoplasm). Scattered neutrophils and occasional lymphocytes are seen in the stroma which do not imply inflammation.

> **Note**
>
> Stromal granulocytes once thought to derive from the endometrial stroma, now believed to originate from endometrial granular lymphocytes (NK cells).

Leiomyoma

- It is composed of smooth muscle cells which are arranged in whorls and fascicles.
- The individual smooth muscle cells are uniform in size and shape and have the characteristic oval nucleus and long, slender bipolar cytoplasmic processes.
- Mitotic figures are sparse (rare).
- Hyaline degeneration is present.

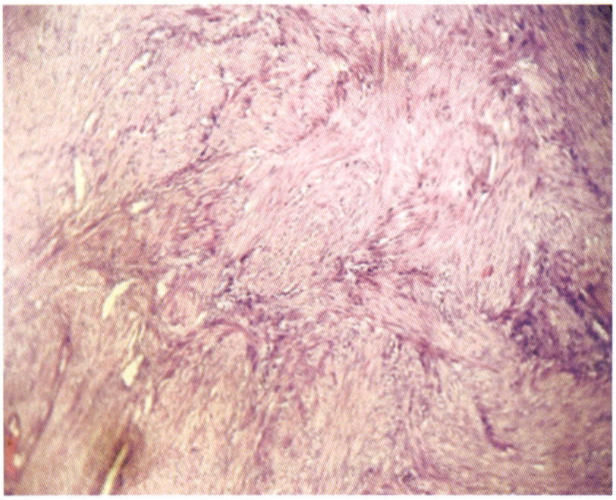

Low power

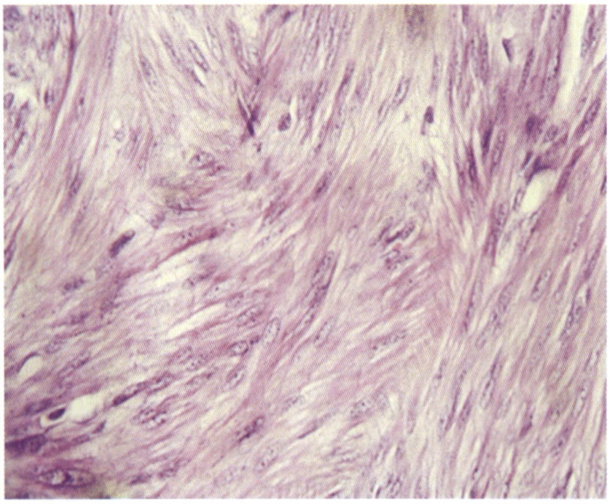

High power

Mucinous Cystadenoma

- It is lined by a single layer of tall columnar nonciliated epithelium similar to intestinal type or endocervical (müllerian) type.
- These lining columnar cells have basally placed nuclei and large apical mucinous vacuoles.
- Nuclear stratification or nuclear atypia not present.
- Stromal invasion by tumour cells is absent and basement membrane is intact.

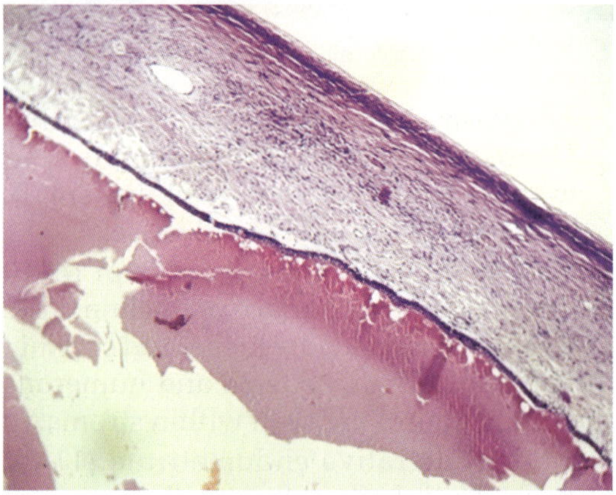

Low power view

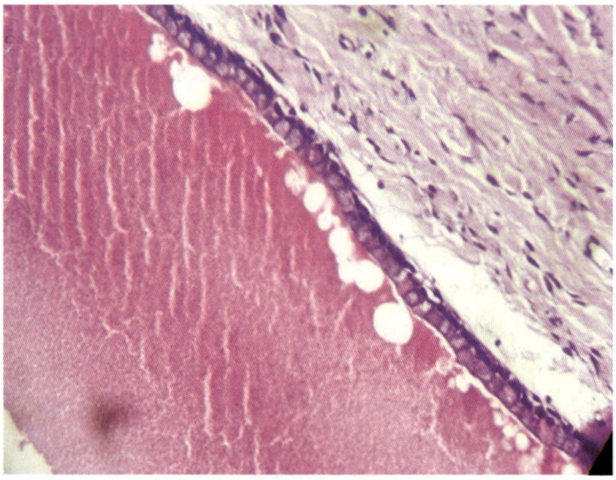

High power view

Portal Cirrhosis (Laennec's Cirrhosis or Hobnail Cirrhosis Related to Alcohol)

- Diffuse disruption in architecture of entire liver (loss of normal central vein–portal tract relationship).

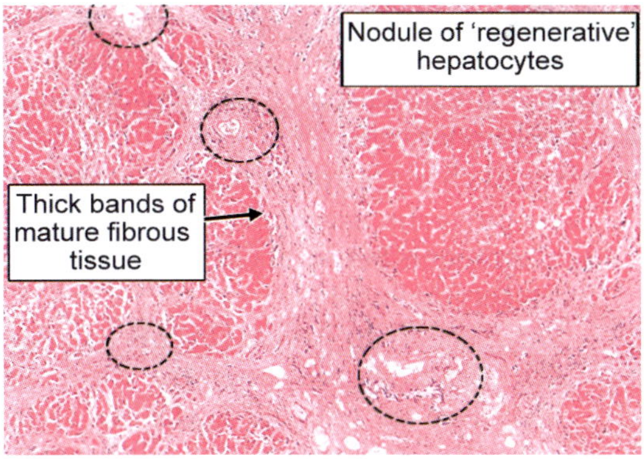

- Round-shaped parenchymal nodules of regenerating hepatocytes, i.e. regenerating nodules are seen. These nodules are small (micronodule).
- These regenerating nodules are separated by fibrous septa that bridge between portal tracts (dotted circles).
- This fibrosis occurs due to synthesis of collagen by perisinusoidal hepatic stellate cells (Ito cells).
- Within this fibrous tissue (collagenous tissue) scattered lymphocytes and proliferating bile ducts seen.

Fatty Liver

- Presence of numerous fat (lipid) vacuoles in the cytoplasm of hepatocytes around the nucleus.
- Some of these vacuoles are small and present around the nucleus (microvesicular).

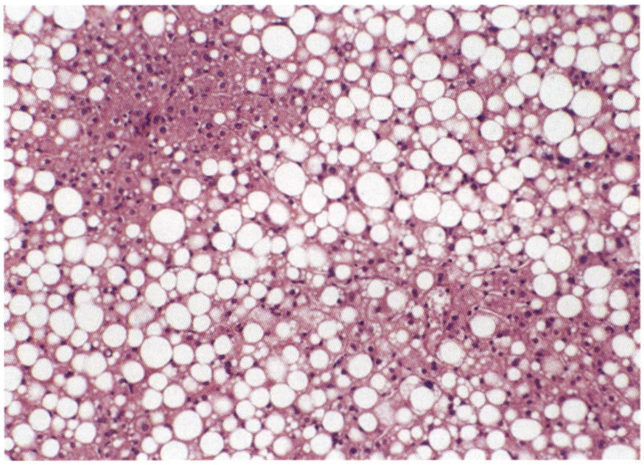

- Most of these vacuoles are large, creating cleared spaces that displace the nucleus to the periphery of the cell (macrovesicular).

Note

i. Fat can be stained and demonstrated in fresh unfixed tissue by frozen section by fat stains like Sudan III, IV, Sudan black and Oil red O. [Remember in routine paraffin embedding technique fats are dissolved by organic solvents/alcohols used.]

ii. Alternatively, osmic acid can be used which acts both as fixed and fat stain.

iii. In fatty liver, **triglycerides** are deposited.

Chronic Cholecystitis

- There is chronic inflammatory cell infiltration into mucosa and other layers of gallbladder wall.
- The predominant chronic inflammatory cell is lymphocyte though plasma cells and macrophages (histiocytes) are also present.
- Focal erosion and ulceration are seen in the mucosal layer.
- Variable degree of fibrosis is noted in the subserosal and subepithelial layers.

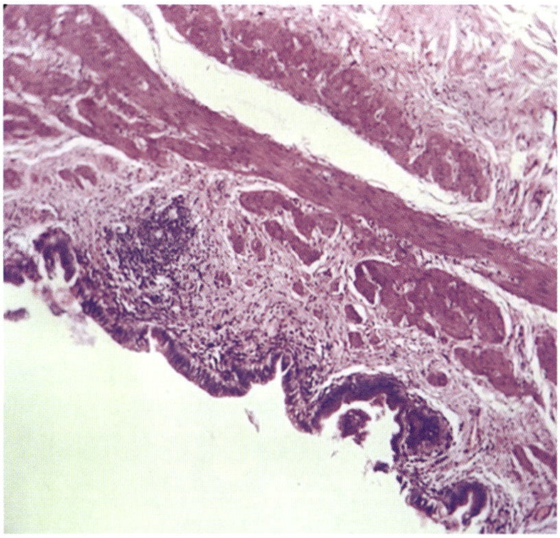

Low power view

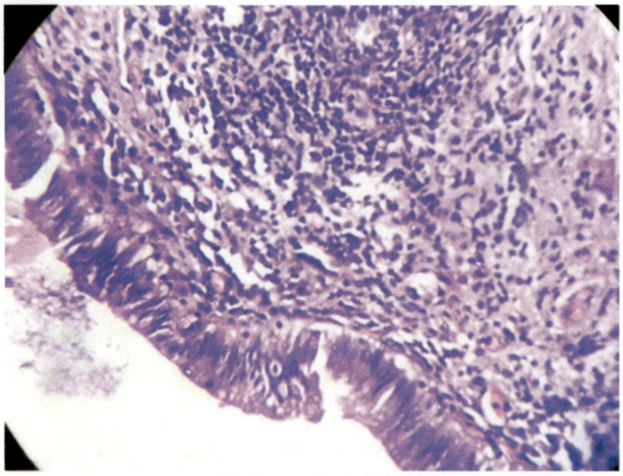

High power view

Fibroadenoma of Breast

- The tumour has a fibrous capsule (see low power view, right side).
- The tumour is biphasic which is composed of fibrous tissue element as stroma and epithelial component (ducts).
- Fibrous tissue comprises most of the tumour.

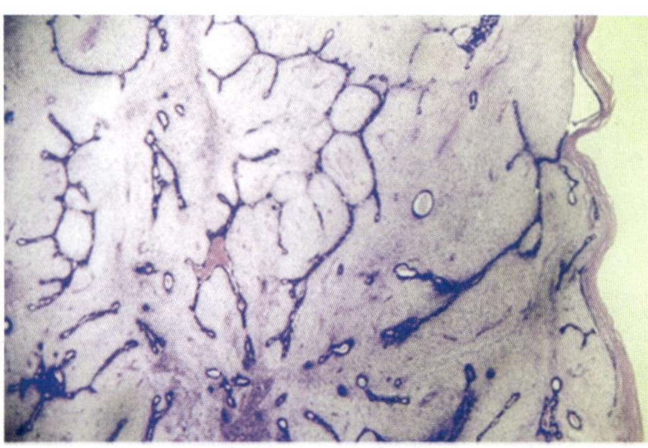

Low power view

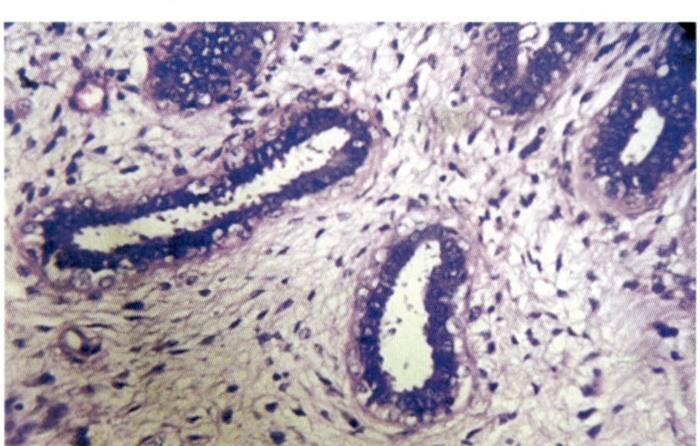

High power view

- Delicate loose fibrous stroma encloses the epithelial component consisting of gland-like or duct-like spaces lined by cuboidal or columnar cells.
- Myxoid changes are seen in the stroma.
- Two patterns are observed based on arrangements between fibrous tissue and ducts (epithelial element).
  - *Intracanalicular pattern*: In this pattern, the stroma compresses the ducts so that they are reduced to slit-like clefts lined by ductal epithelium or may appear as cards of epithelium or may appear as cards of epithelial elements surrounding masses of fibrous stroma.
  - *Pericanalicular pattern*: In this pattern, fibrous stroma encircles around patent or dilated ducts and the ducts are not compressed.
- Nuclear atypia or mitosis is not seen.

Duct Carcinoma of Breast (Moderately Differentiated)

- Malignant epithelial cells arranged in tubular glands, in cards, in sheets and in trabecular pattern.
- Malignant epithelial cells infiltrate the surrounding stroma.
- Tubule (malignant gland) formation is seen in 70% of the tumour area.
- Nuclear pleomorphism is moderate.
- Mitotic figures are increased.
- Focal necrosis and microcalcification are noted.

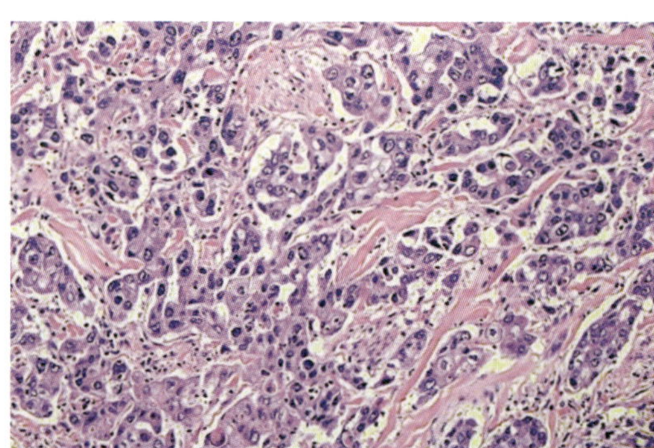

Seminoma of Testis (Classic Type)

- Sheets of uniform tumour cells divided into poorly demarcated lobules by delicate septa of fibrous tissue containing a moderate amount of lymphocytes.
- The tumour cell is large and round to polyhedral in shape.
- Tumour cell has distinct cell membrane or well defined cytoplasmic border.
- Tumour cell has abundant clear cytoplasm.
- Tumour cell has large, central nucleus with one or two prominent nucleoli.

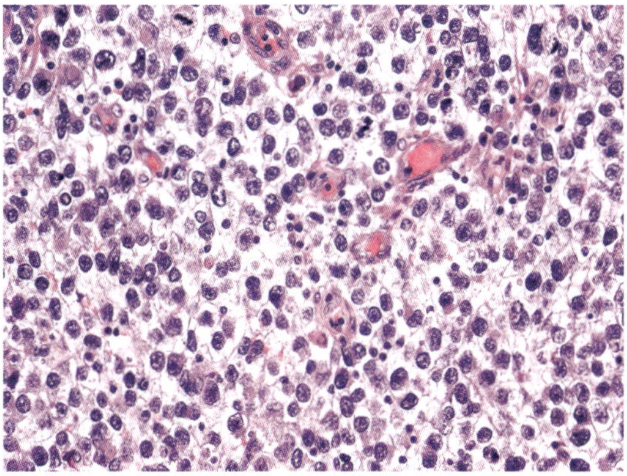

High power

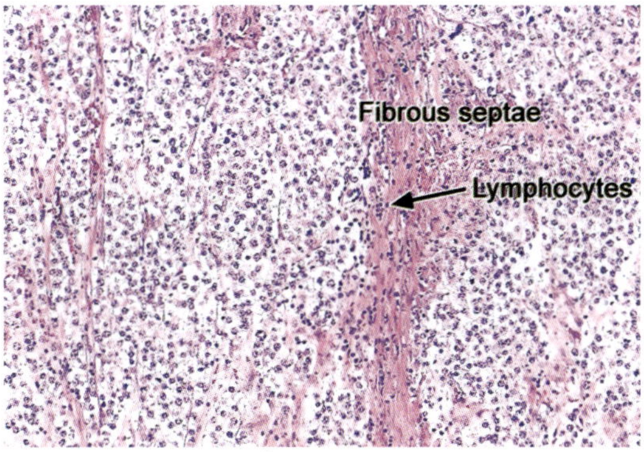

Low power

Benign Hyperplasia of Prostate (BHP) or Nodular Hyperplasia of Prostate

- There is hyperplasia of all three tissue elements in varying degree—glandular, fibrous and muscular tissue (smooth muscles).

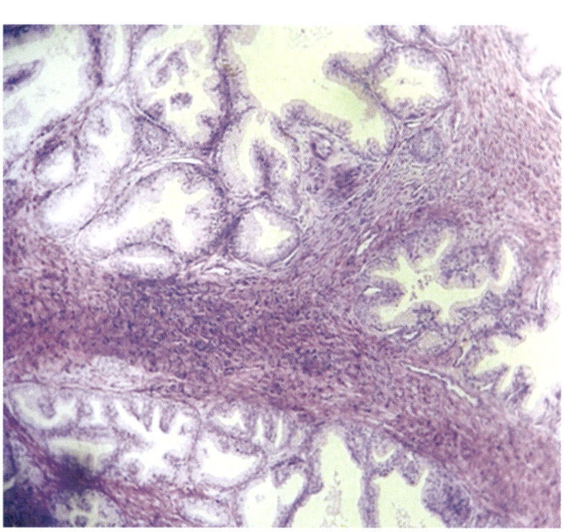

Low power view

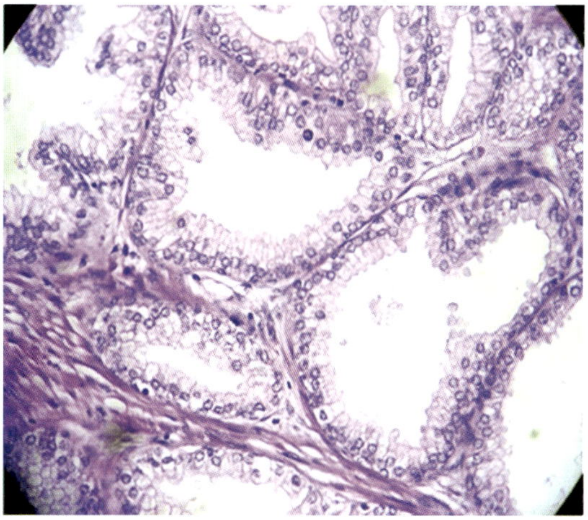

High power view

- Glandular hyperplasia predominates and is recognized by exaggerated intra-acinar papillary infoldings with delicate fibrovascular cores.
- The glands are of benign type and the lining epithelium is two-layered: The inner tall columnar mucus-secreting with poorly-defined borders and the outer cuboidal or flattened epithelium with basal nuclei.
- Some of the glands contain eosinophilic material within lumen (corpora amylacea).
- Lymphocytotic infiltration and foci of lymphoid aggregates present.

Metastatic Deposit in Lymph Node (Metastatic Adenocarcinoma)

- There is effacement of normal lymph node architecture.
- Lymphoid tissue of normal lymph node is replaced by turmour cells.
- The tumour cells are arranged in diffuse sheets, in cords, in trabecular pattern and in glandular pattern.
- Tumour cells are also observed in subcapsular sinuses.
- The tumour cells have high nucleocytoplasmic ratio (N:C ratio) anisonucleosis, and prominent nucleoli.

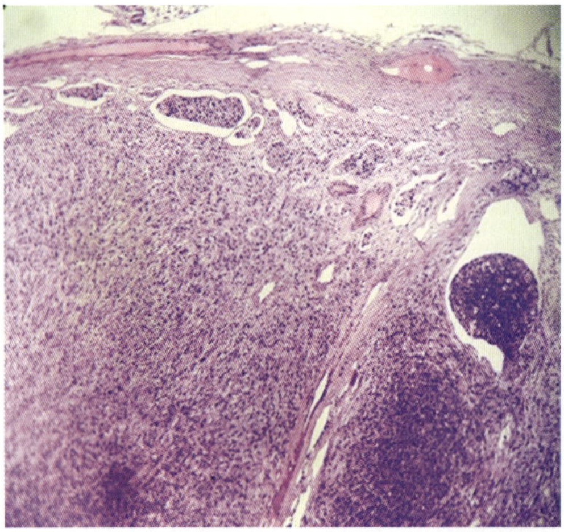
Low power view

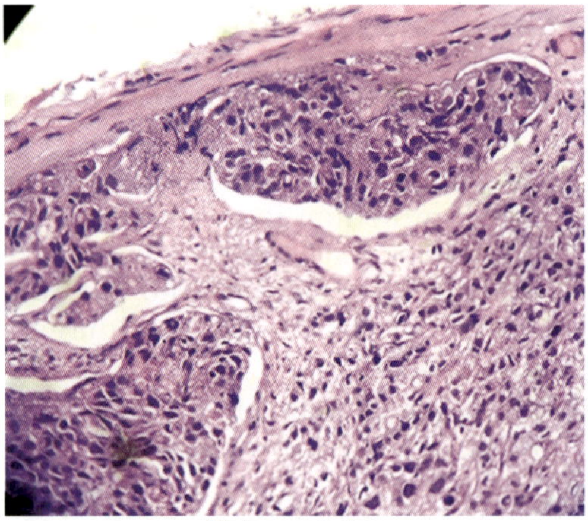
High power view

Tuberculosis of Lymph Node

- There is effacement of normal lymph node architecture.
- Many epithelioid granulomas are noted surrounded by lymphocytes and fibroblasts.
- Multinucleated giant cells of both Langhans and foreign body type are seen.
- Some of the granulomas contain eosinophilic, granular material (caseation necrosis) in the central area.

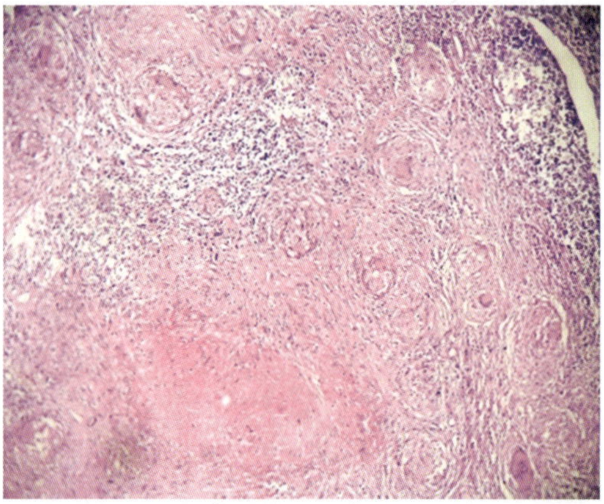
Low power view

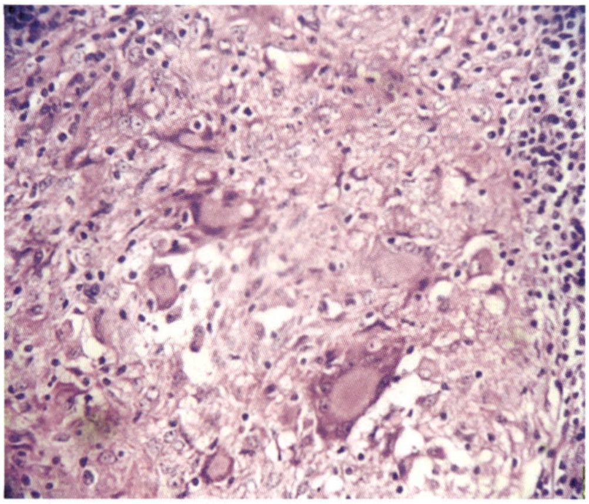
High power view

Colloid Goitre (Nodular Goitre)

- Numerous colloid filled follicles forming ill-defined nodules.

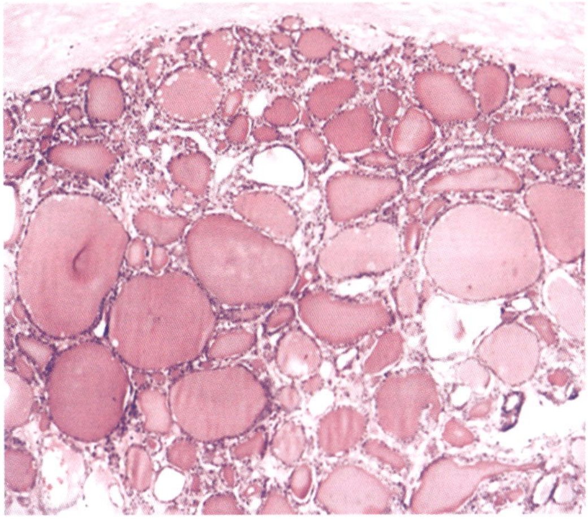

Low power view

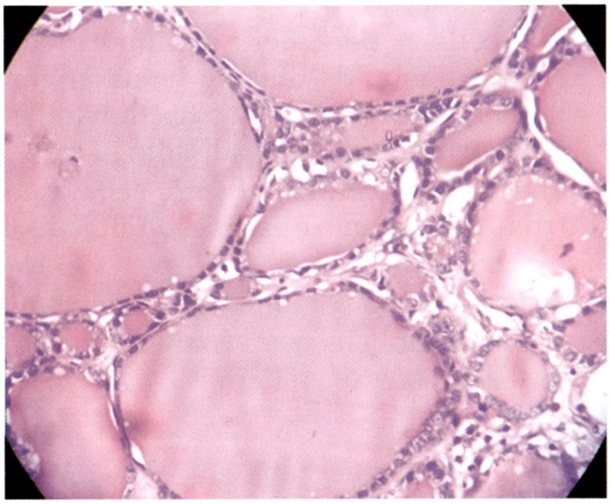

High power view

- The follicles are variably-sized (large distended to small) and are lined by flat to high epithelium.
- Few follicles show micropapillary formation.
- Colloid inside the follicles is abundant thin, pale and eosinophilic.
- Fibrous tissue deposition and scarring are noted surrounding the follicles and forming nodular appearance.
- Thin capsule is noted which separates it from surrounding compressed thyroid parenchyma.
- Foci of microcalcification are seen.

Papilloma/Squamous Papilloma of Skin (Skin Tag, Acrochondron, Fibroepithelial Polyp)

- Papillomatosis, hyperkeratosis and acanthosis of epidermis.
- It has a central fibrovascular core covered by benign squamous epithelium.
- Stroma is edematous and hypocellular.

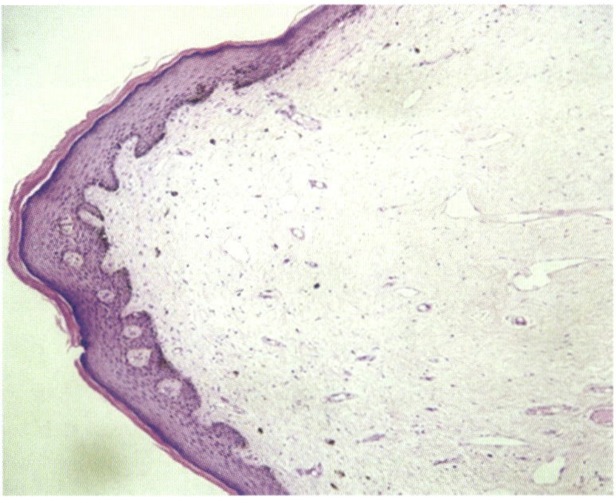

Low power view

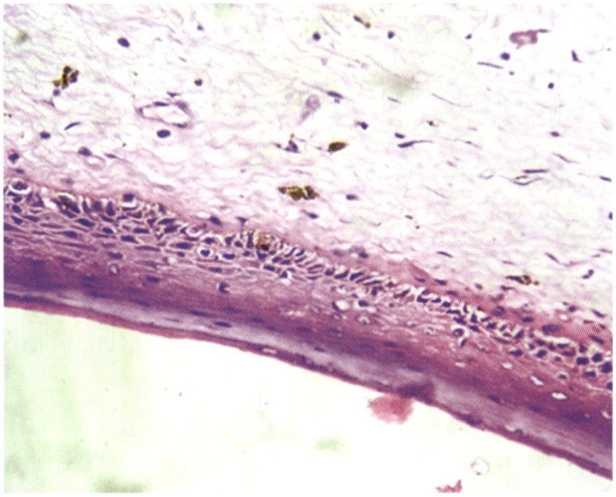

High power view

Melanoma/Malignant Melanoma of Skin

- The tumour has marked junctional activity at the dermoepidermal junction with pagetoid spread.
- From junctional layer tumour cells grow downwards into the dermis.
- Individual melanoma cells are considerably larger than normal melanocytes.

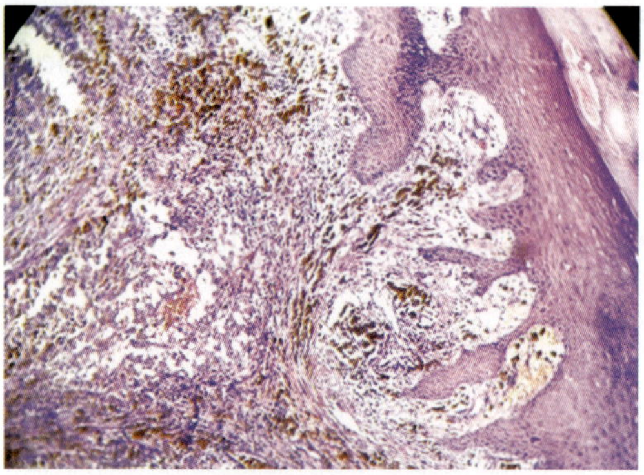

Low power view

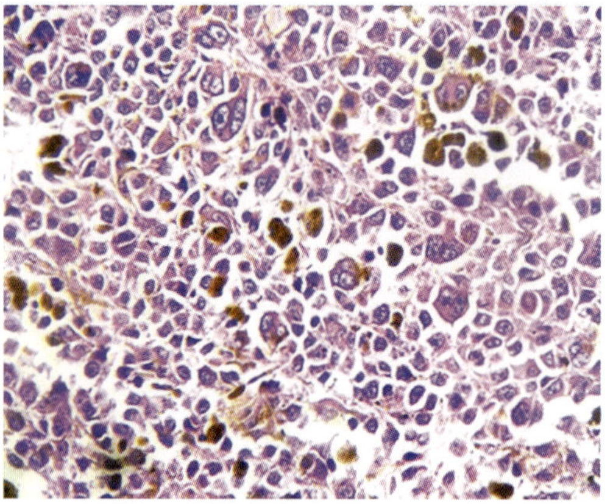

High power view

- Melanoma cells contain large nuclei with irregular nuclear contours.
- Chromatin is characteristically clumped at the periphery of the nuclear membrane.
- Nucleoli are red (eosinophilic) and prominent.
- Melanin pigments are seen both within tumour cells and in-between tumour cells.
- These brown-coloured melanin pigments in melanoma cells are fine granules unlike the benign nevi in which coarse irregular clumps of melanin are seen.
- Chronic inflammatory cell infiltrates (lymphocytes) are seen.

Basal Cell Carcinoma (Rodent Ulcer)

- There is proliferation of basaloid cells (resembling basal layer of epidermis).

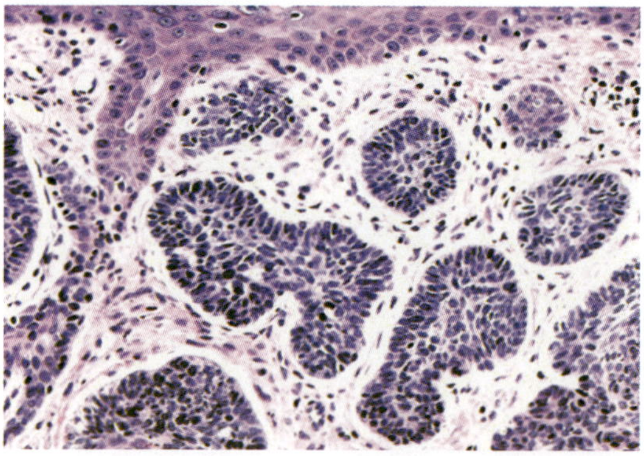

- The tumour cells (basaloid cells) are arranged in lobules and clusters which are separated by stroma.
- The tumour cells have hyperchromatic nuclei and conspicuous small nucleoli.
- The cells at periphery of tumour cell clusters/islands tend to be arranged radially with their long axes in parallel alignment (peripheral palisading).
- The tumour cell islands are separated from dermal fibrous tissue (cleft-like retraction artefact).
- A few mitoses are found (sparse mitoses).
- The tumour cells have connection with the basal layer of epidermis.

Lipoma

- Lobules of mature adipose tissue (fatty tissue) cells separated by delicate fibrous septa.

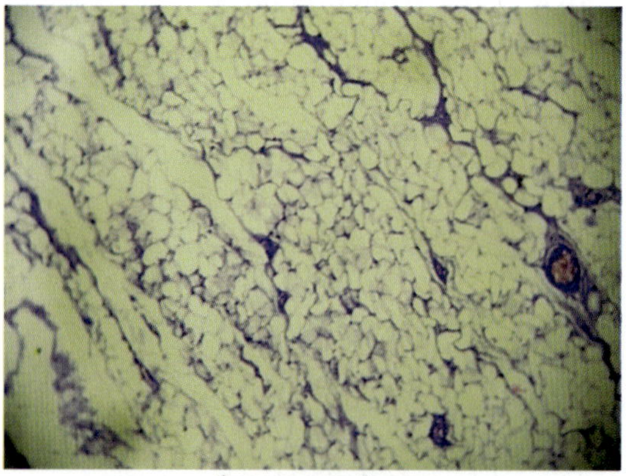

Low power view

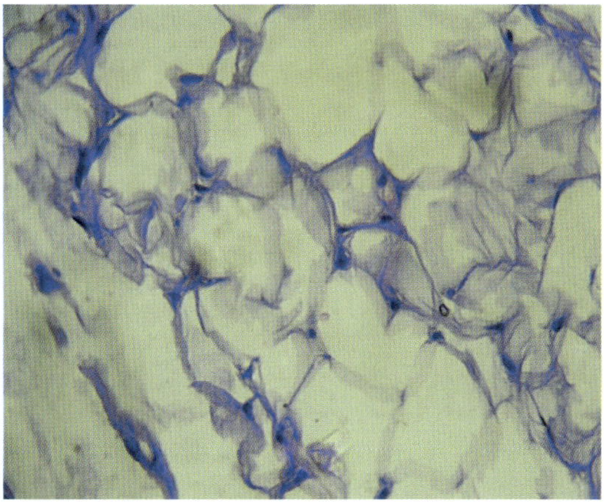

High power view

- The fat cells (adipocytes) have abundant clear lipid (fat) vacuoles and small nuclei pushed to periphery.
- Pleomorphism and nuclear atypia are absent.

Capillary Haemangioma

- Well defined lesion but lacking capsule.
- It is made up of aggregates of closely packed, thin-walled capillaries.
- These capillaries are lined by scant connective tissue stroma.

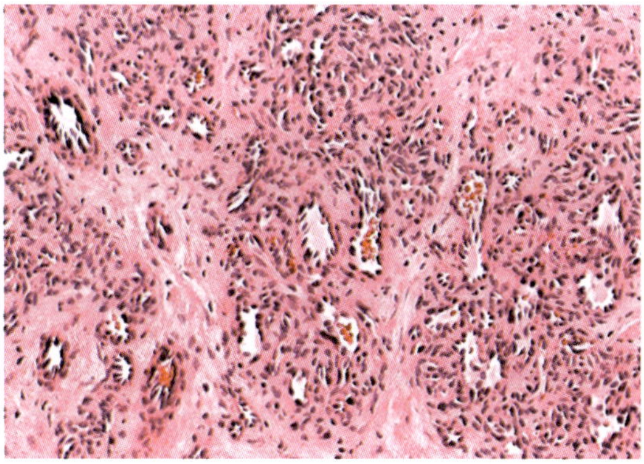

- Some of the capillaries are partially or completely thrombosed and organized.

Cavernous Haemangioma

- It is sharply defined but not encapsulated.
- It is composed of large, cavernous blood-filled vascular spaces, filled partially or completely with blood.
- The vascular spaces (dilated blood vessels) are lined by flattened endothelial cells.
- They are separated by scanty connective tissue stroma.

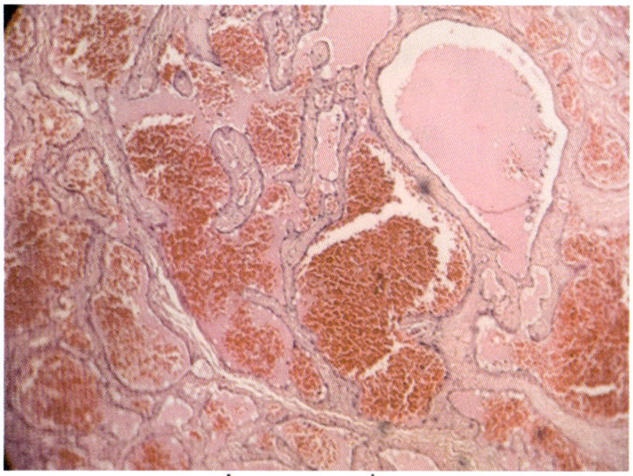

Low power view

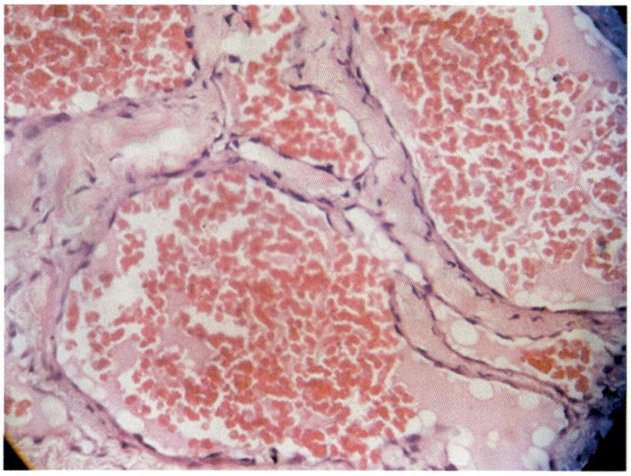

High power view

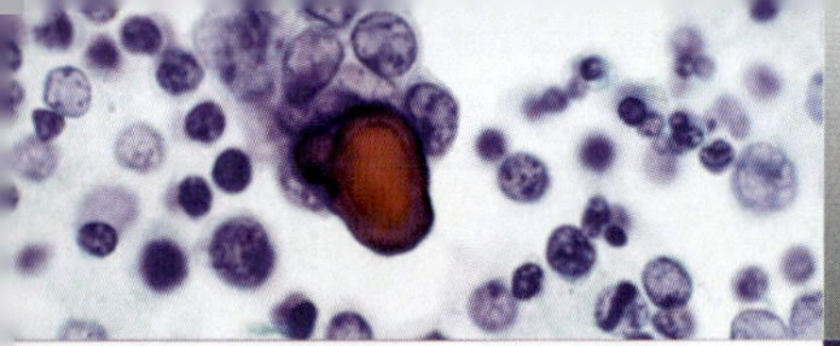

Chapter

16

Cytology: Exfoliative and FNAC

Cytology is the branch of laboratory (diagnostic) medicine which deals with the study of individual cell and/or tissue fragments (microfragments) spreaded on glass slides and stained with stain(s).

Cytology came from Greek words; kytos means a hollow and *logia* means study of the cells. Robert Hooke (1635–1703) is considered sometimes father of cytology. But George Papanicolaou (1883–1962) was a Greek pioneer in cytopathology and inventor of Papanicolaou stain for 'Pap smear' in 1940.

Cytopathology: It is the study of cellular disease and the use of cellular changes for the diagnosis of disease.

EXFOLIATIVE CYTOLOGY

Definition

Exfoliative cytology is the microscopic examination of shed, desquamated cells from body surfaces or cells collected by rubbing, scrapping or brushing a lesional tissue surface or by tapping fluid.

The importance of exfoliative cytology in cancer diagnosis started as early as in 1950s. Exfoliative cytology means, cytological examination of stained smears of the cells, which have exfoliated, fallen or appeared in the body fluid from superficial surfaces of mother tissue.

Collection of Exfoliated Cells

1. **By collection of body fluids**
   - Mouth washings or gurgle: For oral cavity lesions
   - Gastric juice collection by Ryle's tube and syringe: For stomach lesions
   - Peritoneal fluid collection by tapping ascitic fluid or by paracentesis: For lesions of liver, ovaries and peritoneum itself.
   - Pleural fluid collection from pleural effusion: For lesions in the lung and pleura.
   - Urine collection in a clean tube: For urinary tract lesions.
   - Collection of sputum or bronchial washing: For lesions in the lungs or the bronchus
   - Joint effusions: For lesions in the joint cavity
   - Cerebrospinal fluid obtained by lumbar puncture: For lesions in the brain or the spinal cord.
2. **Scrape method:** Scraping is done by means of a wooden or spatula from the superficial surface of the tissue. Used for buccal, vaginal and cervical mucosa.
3. **Brushing:** Endoscopic brushing from lung, stomach, etc.

Exfoliated cells degenerate and distort rapidly. Hence, smears should be prepared and fixed in fixative immediately. For thick cellular discharges/fluids no centrifugation is required. But if it is watery, thin and hypocellular fluid, then it needs centrifugation. Centrifugation is done at 2000 r.p.m. for 5–15 minutes (depending on the size and concentration of suspending cells). Half of the smears are air-dried and other half of the smears are fixed.

Imprint Cytology

Procedure: On a clean glass slide, freshly cut surface of unfixed surgical specimen is gently pressed. Then these slides are fixed in 95% alcohol for a brief period and stained with Pap or H and E stain. Air-dried smears can be stained with MGG or LG stain.

Uses

1. In diagnosis of benign and malignant tumours
2. In determining parathyroid tissue, sentinel lymph nodes and adenomatous goitre
3. In certain CNS tumours like meningiomas and gliomas
4. Useful in determining the surgical resection margins.

Advantages

1. Useful as an intraoperative diagnosis and resection margin and lymph node status.
2. Immediate result.
3. Costly infrastructure or trained technician not required.
4. Tissue and cell architecture preserved.

Disadvantages

1. The depth of infiltration cannot be analysed.
2. Tumours with dense fibrous stroma cannot be interpreted.

Scrape or Brush Cytology

Another cytology technique is to gently scrape or brush some cells from the organ or tissue being tested. It may be from lesions or tumours from living persons or it may be from surgically resected unfixed specimens.

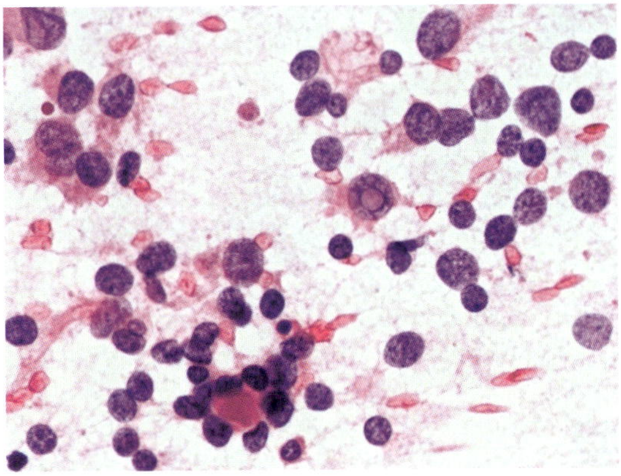

Fig. 16.1: Imprint cytology of papillary carcinoma of thyroid showing microfollicles, single cells, powdery chromatin of nuclei and intranuclear inclusions (Pap, 400X)

The best known cytology test which samples this way is the Pap test. A small spatula and/or brush is used to remove cells from the cervix for Pap test. Other areas which can be brushed or scraped include oesophagus, bronchi, mouth, bladder in living persons and ovarian tumours/other tumours as surgical specimens.

Procedure: Scrape can be done by gentle scraping over the tumour surface by scalpel blade/glass slide. For living persons, brush cytology is done by special endoscopic/bronchoscopic/cytoscopic instruments.

Barr Body (Sex Chromosome) Determination

The sex chromosome or Barr body (found in 1949 by Murray Barr and his co-workers) is the small basophilic body presents in the nuclei of epithelial cells (somatic cells) of females. The Barr body is located in the inner surface of nuclear membrane.

As per Lyon hypothesis, one of the two X chromosomes becomes inactivated in early embryonic life (blastocyst stage) and remains as **Barr body**.

There are two methods for Barr body determination:

1. Buccal smear method
2. Neutrophil method.

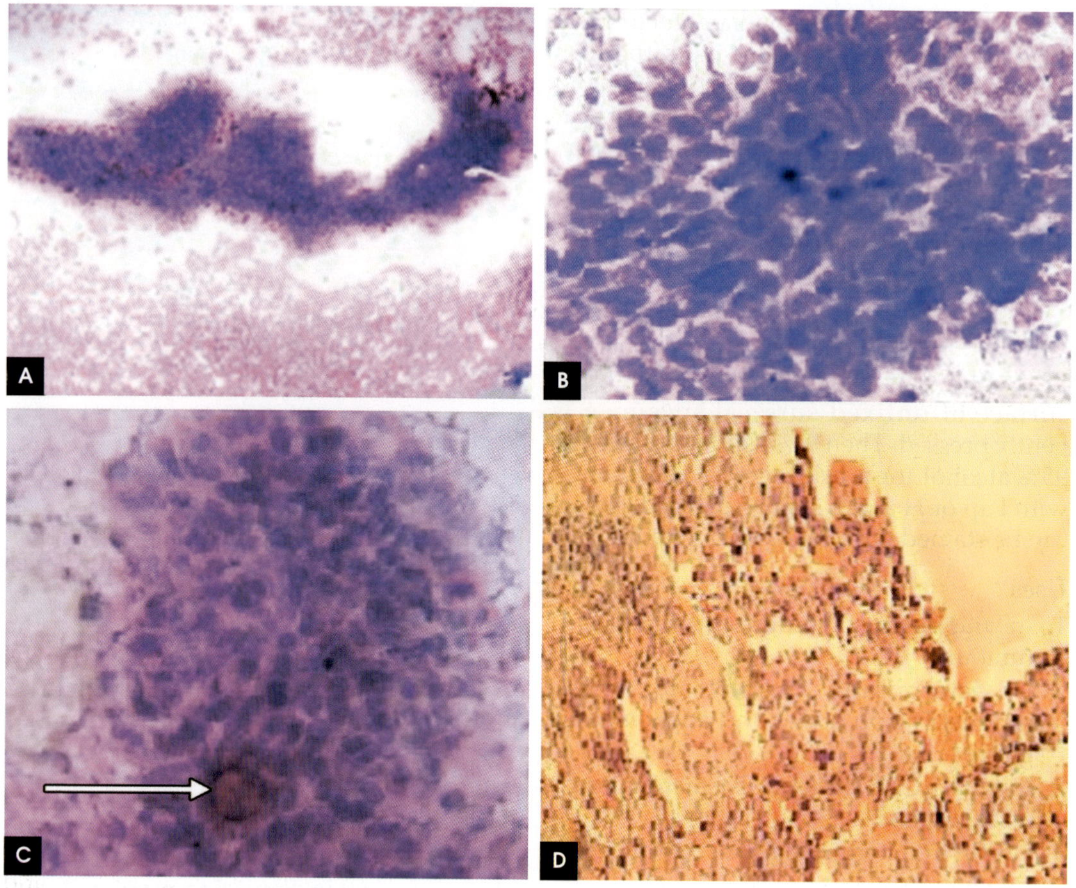

Fig. 16.2A to D: Scraping of conjunctival sqamous cell carcinoma. (A) Low power view (MGG stain); (b) High power view; (C) High power view showing a keratin pearl, marked by arrow (Pap stain); (d) Subsequent histopathological confirmation

Buccal Smear Method

Procedure: After brushing teeth, patient is asked to rinse mouth several times. The inner surface of cheek is scraped gently by edge of a tongue depressor or by Ayre's spatula. Smears are prepared on a clean glass slide and immediately fixed with alcohol. A control smear should be prepared from normal female and fixed with alcohol (95%).

Staining reagent: Orcein 0.1 gm

Glacial acetic acid solution (50% and warm): – 10 ml

Solution is cooled and mixture is prepared by shaking the bottle under running tap water. Then mixture is filtered several times to remove precipitate and debris.

Fixation of smears: Smears are fixed in at last 2 hours in acetic acid and alcohol mixture (1 ml acetic acid + 9 ml of ethyl alcohol/ methanol).

Staining: Fixed smears are covered with Orcein stain for 10–20 minutes. Mount the smears with coverslips for oil immersion examination.

Microscopic examination: Only the chromatin components of nuclei are stained. Other parts of squamous epithelial cells are not stained. At least 200–300 epithelial cells of both patient and control are examined (well stained cells with chromosomes are selected for examination).

Result: Barr body (sex chromosome or X chromatin) is seen as a darkly staining small mass in contact with the nuclear membrane in the interphase nuclei of buccal cells. In normal females (XX), one Barr body is seen in 20–80% of the cells. The number of sex chromatin equals the number of X chromosome minus 1.

Interpretation: In XXX females, two Barr bodies are found. In Klinefelter syndrome (47, XXY), one Barr body is seen. In Turner syndrome (45, XO) no Barr body is seen.

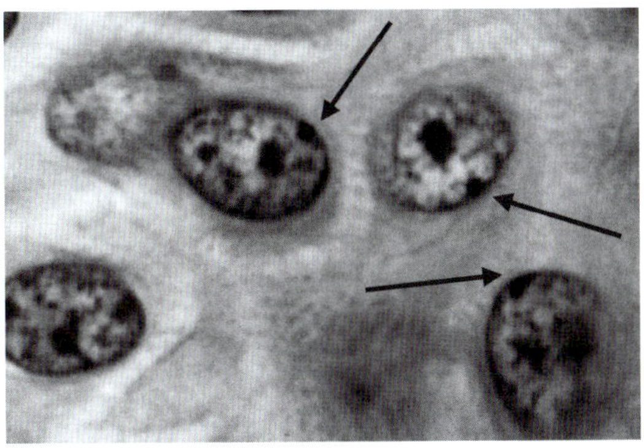

Fig. 16.3: Barr bodies (marked by arrows) in squamous epithelial cells of buccal smear (oil immersion, 1000X)

Neutrophil (Leukocyte) Method

In neutrophils, one X chromosome is visualized as a drumstick in normal females (46, XX) but not in males (46, XY). In Turner syndrome (45, XO) no drumstick is present while in Klinefelter syndrome (47, XXY), one drumstick is seen.

Procedure

1. Make few good peripheral blood smears.
2. Fix the blood smears in methanol and stain them in Giemsa stain well.
3. "Drumstick" is visualised as 1.5 micron round to oval nuclear material attached to nuclear lobes of the neutrophils by a stick like nuclear thread (stalk).
4. Examine 100–200 neutrophils (at least 100 neutrophils).

Result: In normal females, 5–7 drumsticks/100 neutrophils are visualised.

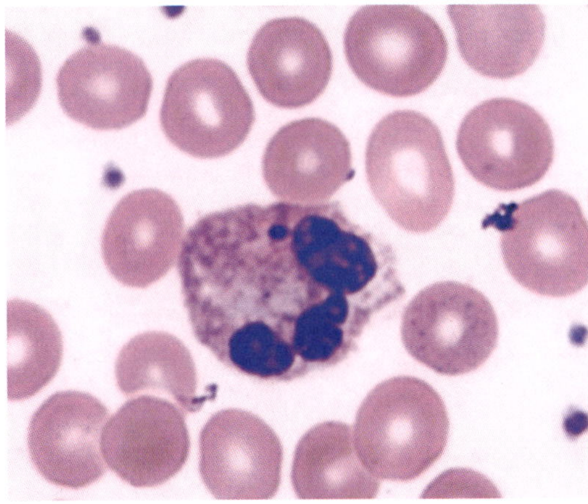

Fig. 16.4: Neutrophil of normal female (XX) showing Barr body (drumstick) in peripheral smear

Fixatives used in Cytology (Cytological Smears or Cytosmear)

In order to prevent distortion of cells as the smears dries up, the specimen must be immediately fixed in Koplin jar while the smears are moist. Common fixatives are:

1. Alcohol–ether fixative: Most commonly used. Absolute or 95% ethyl alcohol and ether in 1:1 volume (say 50 ml of alcohol and 50 ml of ether).
2. 95% ethyl alcohol
3. Carnoy's fluid: It permits good nuclear staining and has the advantage of lysing red blood cells. But it is more expensive and cannot be reused.
4. Spray fixatives: Fix it at least 30 minutes. But preferably >2 hours. But can be done up to 1 week.

Air-dried smears: MGG (May-Grünwald Giemsa) and LG (Leishman Giemsa) stains are used.

Wet-fixed smears: Papanicolaou (Pap) and/or H and E (haematoxylin and eosin) stains are used.

Fixation time: 30 minutes to 2 hours (minimum 15 minutes). Can also be fixed overnight.

Table 16.1: Papanicolaou stain (regressive method)

Staining steps	Papanicolaou laboratory	Memorial Solan Kettering
1. Fixation	95% ethyl alcohol	95% ethyl alcohol
2. Hydration	80%, 70%, 50% ethyl alcohol—six to eight dips each Distilled water—six to ten dips each	70%, 50% ethyl alcohol—five dips each Distilled water—five dips
3. Nuclear stain (DNA specific)	Harris haematoxylin (without acetic acid)—6 minutes	Harris haematoxylin (without acetic acid)—6 minutes
4. Rinse	Distilled water (× 2, i.e. two times)	Distilled water—five dips
5. Removal of haematoxylin	0.25% HCl—six dips	0.5% HCl aqueous solution—three to five dips slowly
6. Rinse	Running tap water (lukewarm)—6 minutes	Running tap water—6 minutes
7. Dehydration	50%, 70%, 80%, 95% ethyl alcohol—six to eight dips each	50%, 70%, 80%, 95% ethyl alcohol—five dips each
8. Cytoplasmic stain	OG 6—1.5 minutes	OG 6—3 minutes
9. Rinse	95% ethyl alcohol (× 2)—rinse gently, do not keep in alcohol, otherwise cells will be discoloured	95% ethyl alcohol (× 2)—five dips each (slowly)
10. Cytoplasmic and nuclear stain (RNA specific)	EA 36 (EA 50 or EA 36)—1.5 minutes	EA 50—3 minutes (drain or paper towel)
11. Rinse	95% ethyl alcohol (× 3), rinse gently but thoroughly	95% ethyl alcohol (× 3)—five dips each (slowly)
12. Dehydration	Absolute ethyl alcohol (× 2)—six to eight dips each	Absolute ethyl alcohol (× 2)—five dips each (slowly)
13. Clearing	Absolute ethyl alcohol and xylene—six to eight dips each Xylene (× 4)—six to eight dips each	Absolute ethyl alcohol and xylene (1:1)—five dips
14. Mounting	Permount (DPX or Canada balsam)	Histoclear (× 7)—five dips each (slowly)

Results in cervical smear

- Nucleus: Blue
- Superficial squamous cells (cytoplasm): Red to orange
- Intermediate and parabasal cells (cytoplasm): Green to greenish blue
- Red blood cells: Orange to orange—green.

Cervical Smear

Currently three types of squamous cells are given importance during cervical smear reporting—superficial cells, intermediate cells and basal–parabasal cells.

1. **Superficial squamous cells:** These cells are mature, usually polygonal, squamous epithelial cells. The cytoplasm stains

either cyanophilic or eosinophilic and nucleus is pyknotic. All nuclei with diameter smaller than 6 µm (less than that of a RBC diameter for comparison) should be called pyknotic. Many superficial cells exhibit an eosinophilic, orange-yellow or orangeophilic cytoplasmic staining due to presence of intracellular cytoplasmic keratin.

2. **Intermediate squamous cells:** Intermediate cells are also mature but they contain nonpyknotic vesicular nuclei, i.e. nuclei which exhibit structural details.

   The most important feature which distinguishes a superficial cell from an intermediate cell is the nuclear appearance. The former has pyknotic nuclei (compressed, smaller nuclei with condensed chromatin), whereas the intermediate cell has vesicular (large, oval or rounded non-pyknotic nuclei).

   Intermediate cells usually have folding, and these cells are present in small or large clusters. However, most mature intermediate cells are flat and lie discretely. In presence of *Bacillus vaginalis* Döderlein, these cells tend to show cytolysis of the cytoplasm due to peptolytic but normal process (not seen in superficial cells).

3. **Basal–parabasal cells:** These cells are small, round or oval, immature (no keratin) squamous epithelial cells. These

Table 16.2: Different types of squamous epithelial cells seen in cervical/vaginal Pap (Papanicolaou) smear

Cell type	Size	Nuclei	Cytoplasm	Morphology
1. Superficial	30–60 µm	<6 µm, clear and pyknotic	Polyhedral, either cyanophilic or eosinophilic. Keratinising cells have keratohyaline granules in cytoplasm and are orange-yellow or orangeophilic. No cytoplasmic fold	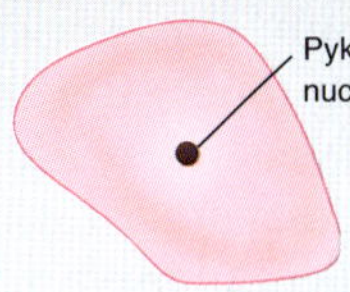
2. Intermediate	20–40 µm	6–9 µm vesicular	Polyhedral or elongated, cyanophilic. Cytoplasmic folds	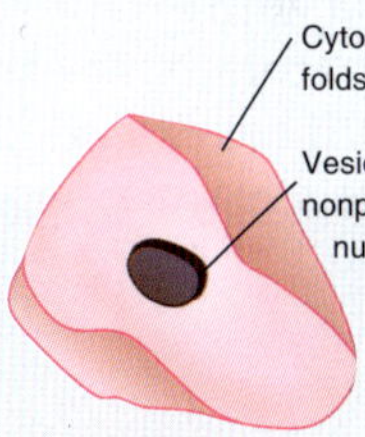
3. Parabasal	15–25 µm	6–12 µm vesicular	Oval to round cells, well defined cytoplasmic border. Basophilic with occasional small vacuoles	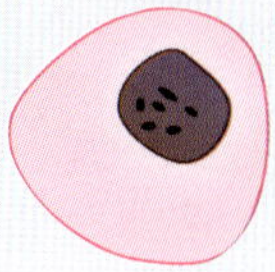
4. Basal	14–20 µm	8–12 µm hyperchromatic, may have small nucleoli	Oval to round, deeply basophilic	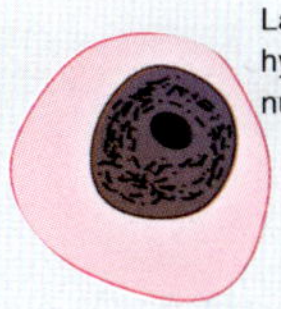

cells usually contain relatively large nuclei. The staining pattern is cyanophilic or indistinct.

Ayre's Spatula

Ayre spatula is a device used to collect Pap smear. It is a wooden spatula with U-shaped openings on one side and a flat surface on another. The broad end is for vaginal sample collection, whereas narrow end is used for cervical sample collection. It is rotated 360° (clockwise or anticlockwise) to obtain exfoliated cells from all quadrants.

Recent studies have shown that long-tipped spatulas **(Aylesbury device)** cervical brush or a **cytobrush** along with an extended tip spatula are better than Ayre's spatula in collecting endocervical cells.

However, Ayre's spatula is still popular in developing (less-income) countries. Ayre's spatula is introduced into the cervix after visualizing the external os using a vaginal speculum. The cervical cells are collected by rotating (360°) the spatula firmly over the ectocervix and quickly transferring the cells onto slides or jar for wet fixation (alcohol or ether-alcohol mixture).

Another device which is popular for cervical sample collection is **Szalay cyto-spatula** with extended tip. The advantage of this spatula is, it can collect endocervical cells as it has extended tip (longer) compared to Ayre's spatula. Ready to use Pap smear kit (CMB-2020) is also available in market which contains microscope slides, wooden spatula, cervical cytobrush and plastic Maller tray. The UK screening programmes changed their cervical screening method from the Pap (Papanicolaou) test to liquid-based cytology (LBC) in 2008.

New Technologies in Cervical Smear

Over the years, several methods have been proposed to improve the cytological specimens. Neubauer et al in 1981 described a **sedimentation velocity separation method**; and Naslund proposed a **pulse wash method**. Then Steven et al suggested **chemical depolymerization of cervical mucin** to help produce monolayers.

But in practice, new technology which is most useful is **liquid-based cytology (LBC)**. But automated scanning devices and computer assisted microscopy are also helpful.

Liquid-based cytology: Liquid-based cytology (LBC) technique involves rinsing all the materials collected on the sampling device into a preservative fluid, creating a cell suspension. This specimen in fluid is sent to laboratory rather than a glass slide pre-smeared with cellular material. In the laboratory, the cell suspension can be processed to remove excess blood and inflammatory cells and to get only representative epithelial (cervical) cells. The technique allows more accurate result.

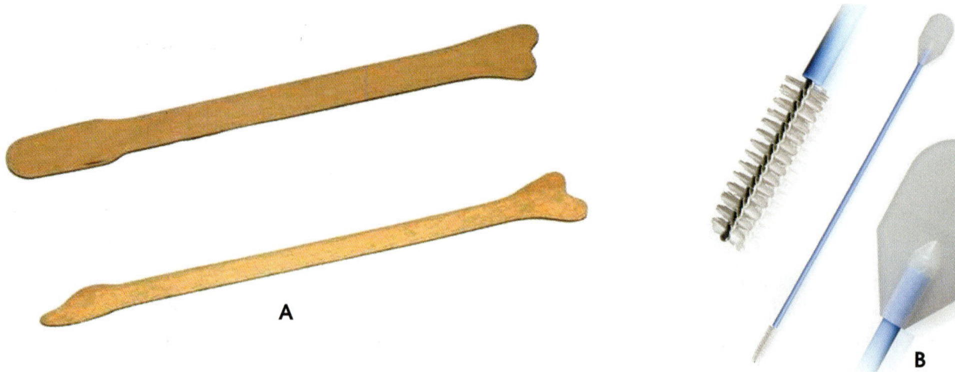

Fig. 16.5A and B: (A) Ayre's spatula (normal and the other with extended tip); (B) Cytobrush with handle

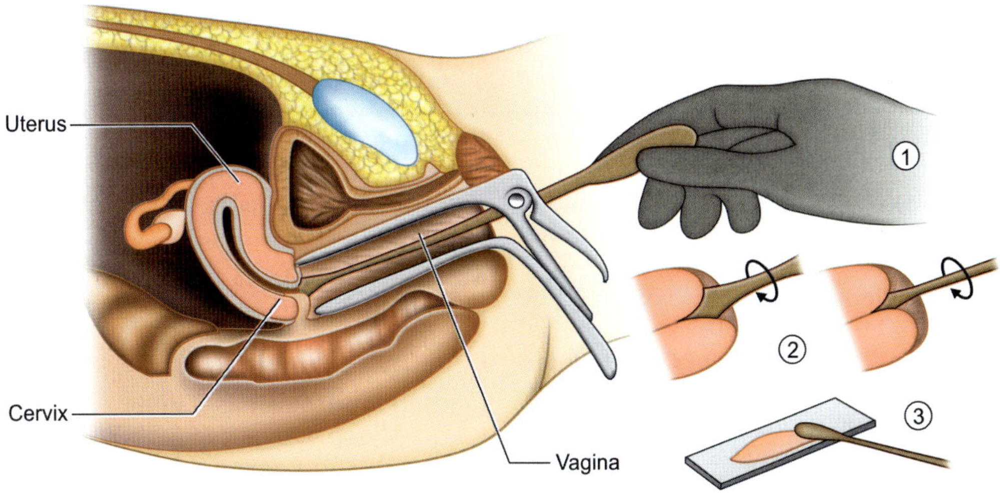

Fig. 16.6: Collection of cervical Pap smear by using Ayre's spatula (different steps, 1, 2 and 3)

Automated scanning devices: Screening of cervical smears manually is a very laborious and monotonous method. Due to tiredness and monotony of job, rare abnormal cells may be overlooked. Automated primary screening devices have been tried over the years. Two systems were eventually approved by the FDA in USA in 1990s. One is AutoPap 300 (Neopath, Seatle, USA) and another is PAPNET (Neuromedical Systems Inc., New York, USA).

Computer assisted microscopy: In the 1990s, there was a practice to attach microscope with the computer which would support cytotechnologists with conventional microscopy. One of the most successful was Pathfinder, manufactured by Compucyte. The system connected sensors to the microscope stage to a computer and monitor display. Zeiss microscopes produced a similar system called the Highly Optimized Microscope Environment (HOME). Another company Acumed had a system called ACcell.

Unfortunately those systems were very costly and commercially unsuccessful. Most are no longer being developed nowadays.

SurePath and **ThinPrep 2000 system** are two such systems currently approved by the US Food and Drug Administration (FDA) for cervicovaginal testing.

1. **SurePath method:** In the SurePath method, the sample is vortexed, stained, layered onto a density gradient and is centrifuged. Instruments required are a computer-controlled robotic pipette and a centrifuge. The cells form a circle of 12.5 mm in diameter.
2. **ThinPrep method:** This method requires an instrument and special polycarbonate filters. After the instrument immerses the filter into the vial, the filter is rotated to homogenize the sample. Cells are collected on the surface of the filter when a vacuum is applied. The filter is then pressed against a glass slide to transfer the processed cells into a **20 mm diameter circle**.

Both methods (SurePath and ThinPrep) result in a well-preserved approximate monolayer of cells, with a background devoid of blood, mucus or parasites. But current high cost of these patented, commercial systems required of trained cytotechnologists and pathologists to interpret the ThinPrep slides, leads to search for alternative, less costly newer methods.

One such method is **SpinThin method**, developed by Khalbuss et al in 2000. It uses a modified electric toothbrush to release the cells into suspension from the collecting device. The cell are then spun directly onto a (20 × 10 mm) area of glass slide using a Cytospin II centrifuge with mega-funnel. Results correlate well with conventional smears and follow-up histology.

Another method has been developed by Johnson et al in 2000. It places the cervical collection device into 15 ml of **CytoRich red** (Tripath Imaging Inc.), a proprietary formula of buffering agents, emulsifiers, formaldehyde and alcohol. After it comes to laboratory, cell suspensions are vortexed, poured through tulle (oridal veil fabric) and centrifuged. After that, the supernatant is discarded and the sediment is vortexed. A drop of sediment is placed into an 8 ml of Hettich cytocentrifuge chamber which is filled with 2 ml of **CytoRich yellow** (Tripath Imaging Inc.), a fixative that prevents dehydration and collapse of three-dimensional structures when slides are air-dried and then spun onto adhesive-coated slides.

Abnormal Cells in Cervical Smear

Nuclear characteristics are the main determinants for the grading of an epithelial abnormality although cytoplasmic features may provide additional inflammation.

Nuclear atypia should be classified as mild, moderate and severe. Cytoplasmic changes should be classified according to quantity, staining pattern/quality, density and shape.

Papanicolaou introduced the term dyskaryosis in cervical smear. He described dyskaryotic cells as follow, "The nuclei show distinct abnormal features such as enlargement, hyperchromasia, anisokaryosis, bi- or multinucleation, etc."

Mild dysplasia/cervical intraepithelial neoplasia (CIN) grade 1 or low grade SIL (squamous intraepithelial lesion): These cells have plentiful clear, translucent cytoplasm with well-defined angular borders. Cells resemble superficial and intermediate type squamous cells and a slightly enlarged nucleus, occupying less than one-third of the total area of the cell. Nuclear chromatin is evenly distributed, finely granular and slightly hyperchromatic. Cells are distributed singly.

Moderate dysplasia (CIN grade II, high grade SIL): The size of abnormal cells varies. Abnormal cells of the superficial squamous cell type as well as smaller cells of intermediate and parabasal cells are usually found. Cytoplasm is cyanophilic but a few cells may show eosinophilia. Nuclei are enlarged and round to oval, sometimes irregular in shape. The nucleus usually occupies less than half of total area of the cell. Nuclear chromatin is evenly distributed and slightly to moderately hyperchromatic. Nucleoli are either absent or inconspicuous. Cells are distributed singly and in small loose aggregates.

Severe dysplasia (CIN grade III, high grade SIL): These abnormal cells look like parabasal cells. Cytoplasm is usually sparse and represents a small rim around the nucleus. Cells are distributed singly as well as in aggregates. The nucleus usually occupies more than two-thirds of the total area of the cell. Nuclei have hyperchromatic, irregularly distributed, coarsely granular chromatin. Nucleoli are usually seen in actively proliferating lesion which is eosinophilic. But may be obscured by dense hyperchromatic chromatin.

Carcinoma *in situ*

Cells occur singly but predominantly in syncytial (tight) aggregates. In a syncytial group, cells are arranged irregularly and have indistinct cell borders and overlapping nuclei. The latter two features are absent in dysplastic cells. The neoplastic cells are relatively small. Nuclei vary in size and shape. Nuclear chromatin is hyperchromatic, irregularly distributed and coarsely

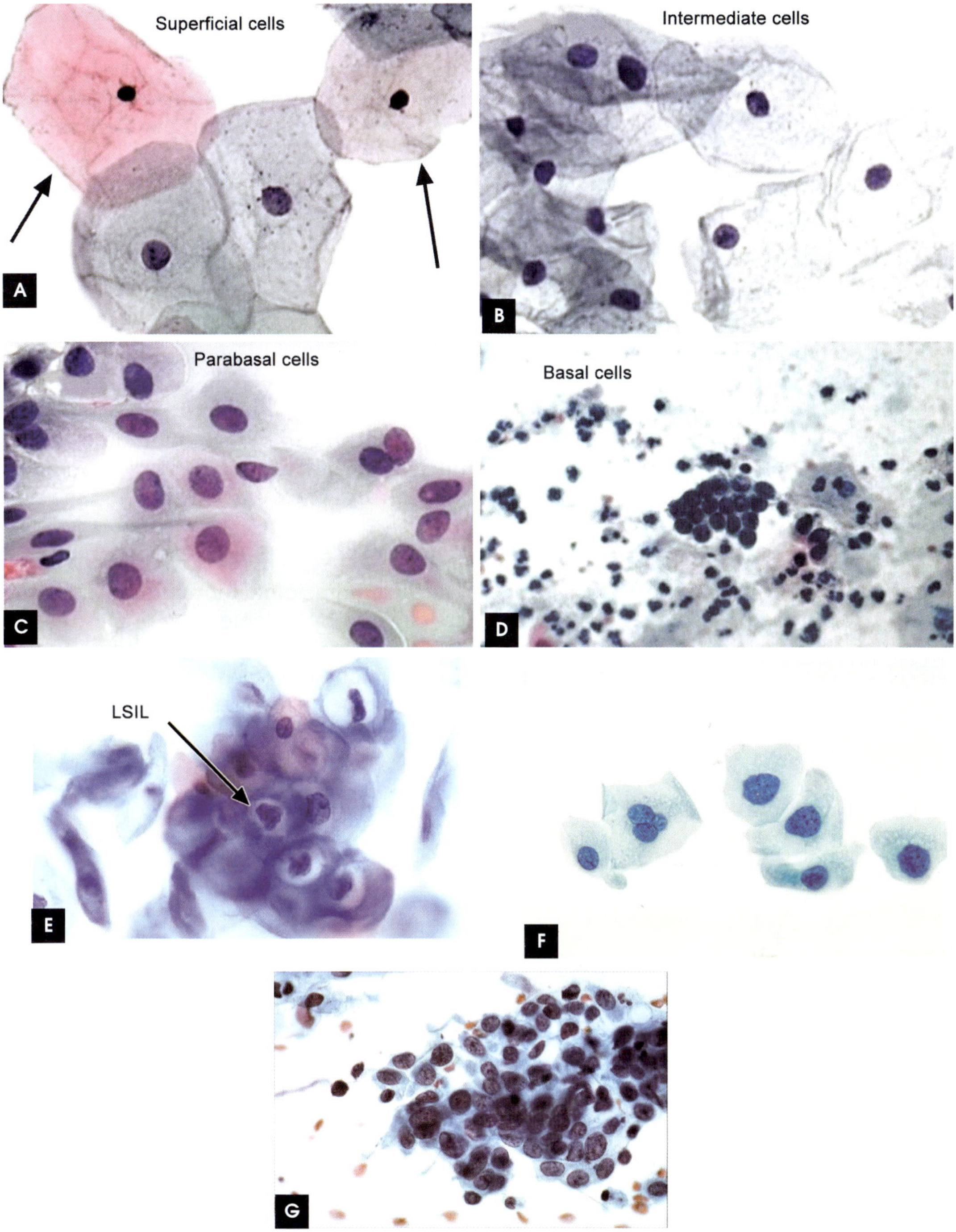

Fig. 16.7: Cervical Pap smear. A to D: Normal smear showing superficial, intermediate, parabasal and basal cells; (E) Mild dysplasia/cervical intraepithelial neoplasia (CIN) grade I or low grade SIL (squamous intraepithelial lesion); (F) Moderate dysplasia (CIN grade II, high grade SIL); (G) Serve dysplasia (CIN grade III, high grade SIL)

granular. Nuclear grooves may be seen occasionally. It is rare to find eosinophilic nucleoli. Macronucleoli which are found in invasive carcinomas, are very rarely seen in in situ carcinomas.

Invasive squamous cell carcinoma: This may be of two types—nonkeratinizing and keratinizing.

Nonkeratinizing squamous cell carcinoma: High power view (Pap smear) tadpole cell

Syncytial aggregates of tumour cells with indistinct cell border and moderate amount of cytoplasm. Nuclei are round to oval or irregularly shaped. Nuclear chromatin is moderately hyperchromatic, coarsely granular, and irregularly distributed. Nucleoli are conspicuous. "Tadpole" like malignant squamous epithelial cell in the background.

Keratinizing squamous cell carcinoma: Tumour cells frequently appear singly. Elongated caudate, bizarre cells or binucleated cells are seen. Cells have relatively large amount of cytoplasm. Cytoplasmic orangeophilia is characteristic of keratinizing cancer. Nuclei may be round to oval but most of the times elongated or irregular. Nuclear chromatin is hyperchromatic and coarsely granular. Occasionally "keratin pearl" may be observed.

Adenocarcinoma (Endocervical or Endometrial)

Sometimes adenocarcinoma arising from endocervix or from endometrium may also be diagnosed by cervical smear.

These malignant cells are arranged in sheets, in papillary pattern and in glandular pattern. Discretely arranged cells are also found. The cells have high nucleocytoplasmic ratio and oval to round nuclei. The nuclear chromatin is vesicular. Prominent nucleoli and macronucleoli are also seen.

Cytology of Body Fluids (Effusions)

The intrathoracic and intraperitoneal organs are covered by a single layer of mesothelial cells (flattened cuboidal epithelium), which is continuous with the lining of the thoracic and peritoneal cavities. The potential space

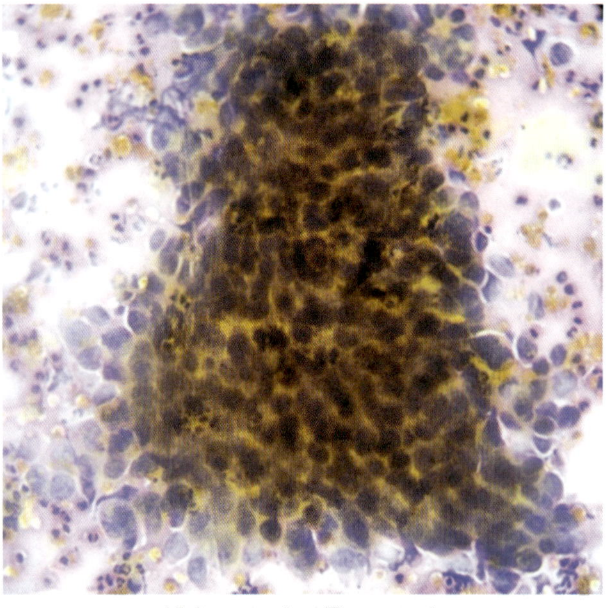

High power view (Pap smear)

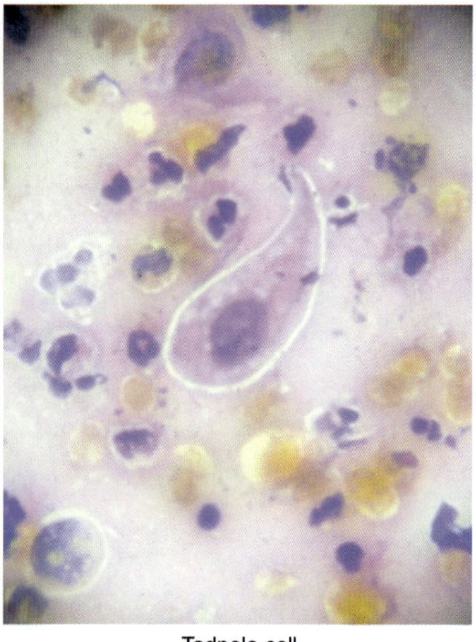

Tadpole cell

Fig. 16.8: Non-keratinising squamous cell carcinoma

between the two layers of epithelium (visceral and parietal) contains a small amount (few ml) of lubricating fluid, known as serous fluid.

An accumulation of fluid, called an effusion, results from an imbalance of fluid production and reabsorption. This fluid accumulation in the pleural, pericardial, and peritoneal cavities is known as serous effusion. These effusions may be infectious effusions, noninfectious inflammatory effusions and malignant effusions.

Infectious effusions: It is due to direct effects of infective organism or as by-product of inflammation. Varying types of inflammatory cells may be present. Cultures and/or Gram and AFB stains may be useful to identify an organism.

Noninfectious inflammatory effusions: This is due to conditions or reaction to a stimulus like autoimmune conditions (rheumatoid arthritis or SLE) or reactive conditions (tissue necrosis, radiation therapy).

Malignant effusions: It is due to a primary tumour of mesothelium (mesothelioma) or a metastatic tumour (most commonly metastatic adenocarcinoma). The fluid may be cloudy, bloody or partially clotted.

The fluid is aspirated from body cavities and is centrifuged. The deposit is smeared on glass slides and stained with Papanicolaou's stain and examined microscopically. Sometimes, MGG and H and E stains are also used.

Normal Cells in Fluid Cytology

- Lymphocytes
- Mesothelial cells
- Histiocytes/monocytes
- Occasional neutrophils or eosinophils
- Reactive mesothelial cells.

Mesothelial cells: Bland cells forming a monolayer covering serous surfaces of body cavities. It is 20–40 µm in diameter.

Nuclei

- Single or binucleated
- Centrally located but can be eccentric
- Round to oval with well defined, smooth nuclear borders
- Fine chromatin
- Inconspicuous nucleoli

Cytoplasm

- Dense centre with pale periphery
- Lacy "skirt" cell borders
- Blunt cytoplasmic process due to degeneration.

The mesothelial cells appear in smears as broad and flat sheets. There is gap between cells called 'window'.

Histiocytes: They have smaller nuclei than mesothelial cells and nuclei are vesicular often with nuclear indentation. The cytoplasm is abundant and may be vacuolated or granular.

Abnormal findings

- Lymphocytes (>50%)
- Neutrophils (>50%)
- Eosinophils (>10%)
- Presence of microorganisms, LE cells, sickle cells, Charcot-Leyden crystals, psammoma bodies, collagen balls.

Reactive mesothelial cells: Varying cell size and increased number of mesothelial cells. Central or paracentral nuclei are enlarged. Coarse chromatins which are evenly distributed. Binucleation or multinucleation may be seen. Nuclear membrane is regular.

***Mesothelioma*:** One cell population of malignant mesothelial cells. Larger clusters with irregular, knobby flower-like borders. Dense endoplasm with delicate, lacy ectoplasm. Central enlarged nucleus with macronucleoli and irregular borders. Abnormal mitotic figures may be seen.

Metastatic adenocarcinoma: Most adenocarcinoma cells in serous fluids originate in neoplasms of the breast, lung or ovary. The cells may show the classic feature of adeno-

Table 16.3: Suggested immunocytochemistry (ICC) markers

	Reactive mesothelial cells	Mesothelioma
• Calretinin	+	+
• CK 5/6	+	+
• p53	–	+
• Desmin	+	–
• EMA	–	+

Table 16.4: Tumours causing malignant effusions

Primary	Secondary/metastatic
• Malignant mesothelioma • Effusion lymphoma	• Metastatic adenocarcinoma • Metastatic squamous cell carcinoma • Neuroendocrine tumours • Lymphoma/leukaemia • Melanoma • Sarcoma • Other cancers/neoplasm

carcinoma: A tendency to form smoothly contoured cohesive group composed of large cells with eccentric, malignant-appearing nuclei, prominent nucleoli and vacuolated cytoplasm. However, there may be great variation in adenocarcinoma cells in effusions.

Differences between adenocarcinoma and mesothelioma: Adenocarcinoma cells may be single or may form clusters composed of only few cells or large papillary fragments or cell balls/spheroids. Such cell balls may also be seen in mesothelioma. But the mesothelial cells have irregular knobby border and they have windows (intercellular gaps). The N–C ratio is more in adenocarcinoma cells and nuclei are more vesicular. The nuclear outline of adenocarcinoma cells are more angulated than mesothelioma which are smoothly round or oval. Prominent nucleoli though seen in both the cases, but macronucleoli are seen in adenocarcinoma.

Immunocytochemistry: Adenocarcinoma cells express GLUT 1, CA 19–9, CEA (carcinoembryonic antigen) which is negative in mesothelioma cells. On the other hand, calretinin, WT-1, D2-40 are positive in mesothelial cells but negative for adenocarcinoma cells. Acid mucopolysaccharide is also positive in mesothelial cells.

Electron microscopy: Adenocarcinoma cells are characterized by short, plump microvilli

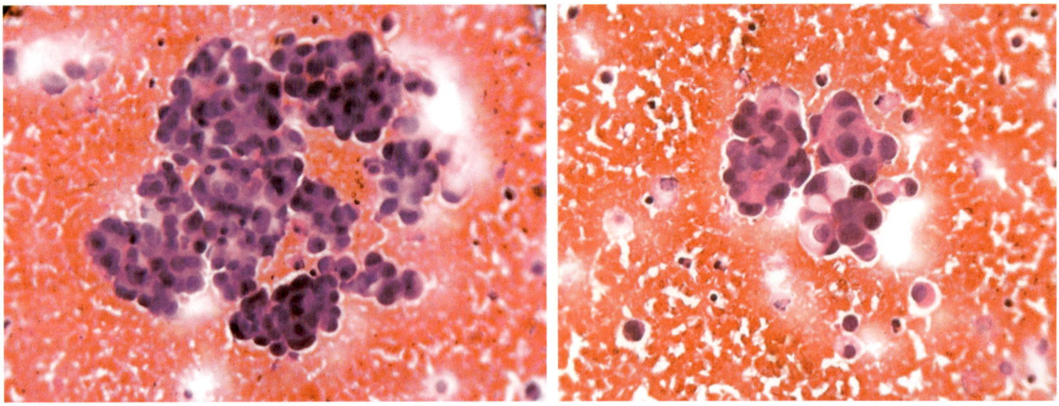

A B

Fig. 16.9A and B: Adenocarcinoma in peritoneal fluid cytology. (A) Malignant cells arranged in papillary configuration (MGG, 400X); (B) Malignant cells arranged in acinar/pseudoglandular pattern. Also some tumour cells showing cytoplasmic mucin vacuoles (Pap, 400X)

in contrast to mesothelial cells which have numerous, long and slender microvilli.

Fine Needle Aspiration Cytology (FNAC)

Equipment

i. *Needles fitted in syringes*: Standard disposable 20–23 gauge needles are commonly used. For highly vascular (thyroid) and/or highly cellular tissue (lymph node) 24–25 gauge needle are preferred. For very hard tissue (bone) 20 gauge needle is recommended.

ii. *Syringes*: Good quality disposable plastic syringes, 5–20 ml of strong rigid material with a good negative pressure is used. Routinely 10 ml syringe is used. For fibrotic and hypocellular lesion 20 ml syringe may be used. For highly vascular and/or cellular lesion 5 ml syringe may be used.

iii. *Syringe holder*: Made of stainless steel, commercially available (Cameco syringe pistol).

iv. *Glass slides*: Thoroughly cleaned, dry and grease free.

v. *Fixative*: For wet fixation of smears, 70–90% ethanol in Coplin jars. Alternatively, Carnoy's fixative is used.

vi. *Stains*: For wet fixed smears Papanicolaou (Pap) stain and/or H and E stain are used. For air-dried smear MGG (May Grunwald-Giemsa) or LG (Leishman-Giemsa) stain is used.

FNAC Technique

The syringe (with needle) is fitted with a syringe holder which permits a single hand operation during aspiration. Then follow these steps:

1. Skin overlying the lesion is properly cleaned with antiseptic solution.
2. Immobilize the site to aspirated (breast, thyroid, lymph node, soft tissue, etc.) with thumb and index finger of left hand. Then insert the needle to the target area/lesion while holding the syringe holder by right hand.
3. Once the needle is in the mass, retract the piston of syringe holder to create a negative pressure in the syringe.
4. Move the needle back and forth several times (usually 3–4, up to 6 passes) in various directions for a few seconds.
5. Withdraw the needle slowly while maintaining a negative pressure until the subcutaneous tissue is reached. Then the piston of the syringe is released to equalize the pressure.
6. Withdraw the needle completely and disconnect from the syringe.
7. Fill the syringe with air and reconnect to the needle.
8. The content of the needle is expressed on glass slides and smears are prepared (air dried and wet fixed).

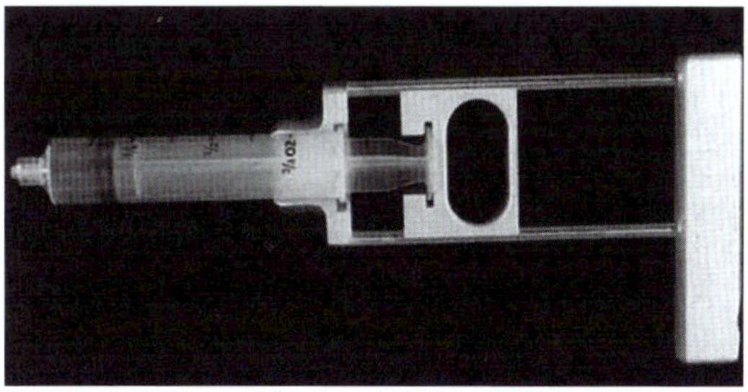

Fig. 16.10: Syringe fitted in a syringe holder before doing FNAC

Indications of FNAC

- In the rapid diagnosis of neoplastic conditions especially cancers and metastasis.
- In the diagnosis of inflammatory, infectious and degenerative conditions.
- Also, useful in the diagnosis and monitoring of graft rejections in transplantation surgery.

MGG Stain

Reagents: (i) May-Grunwalds's stain, (ii) Giemsa stain, (iii) methanol, (iv) phosphate buffer (pH 6.8), (v) conical flask (200–250 ml).

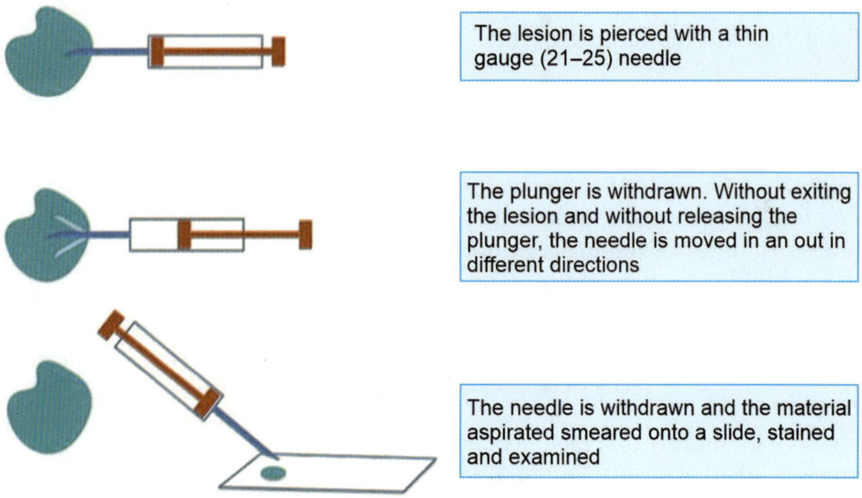

Fig. 16.11: Steps in FNAC

Table 16.5: Advantages and disadvantages of FNAC

Advantages	Disadvantages
• The diagnosis is rapid (few minutes) compared to conventional histological (biopsy) diagnosis • This procedure is easy and cost effective • Modern imaging techniques like USG and CT scan allowed guided FNAC for deep-seated lesions, lung, mediastinum, abdominal, retroperitoneal and pelvic organs. Surgical biopsy may not be easily accessible • No need of hospital stays and paying hefty bills • Less traumatic than usual knife biopsy. • The samples can be used for microbiological and biochemical analysis in addition to cytological preparations	• Rare chances of needle tract seedling and possibility of cancer cells being disseminated along the needle tract • Preoperative FNA (fine needle aspirate) may cause changes in the tissue which may cause subsequent histological diagnosis difficult • Changes like haematoma, infarction, capsular pseudoinvasion, and pseudomalignant reparative reactions may occur • Complications like pneumothorax, air emboli and internal bleeding may occur rarely

Preparation of May-Grunwald stain: 0.3 gm of powdered dye and 100 ml of methanol is mixed in a conical flask. The mixture is warmed to 50° C. The flask is allowed to cool at room temperature and mixture is shaken several times during the day. After standing for 24 hours, the solution is filtered.

Staining procedure

- Air-dried smears are fixed in methanol in a Coplin jar for 5 minutes.
- Stain with diluted May-Grunwald stain (1:1 dilution with phosphate buffer) for 5 minutes.
- Stain with diluted Giemsa stain (1:9 dilutions with buffer) for 15–20 minutes.

Table 16.6: Comparison between wet-fixed (Pap) and air-dried (MGG) smears

	Wet-fixed (Pap stain) smear	Air-dried smear (MGG stain)
• Cell and nuclear size	Comparable to tissue fragments	Size more than tissue
• Cytoplasmic detail	Poorly demonstrated	Well demonstrated
• Nuclear detail	Excellently demonstrated	Different and not well demonstrated
• Nucleoli	Well demonstrated	Not demonstrated always
• Stromal components	Poorly demonstrated	Well demonstrated and differently stained often
• The 'wet' smear	Good fixation	Artefacts common
• The 'dry' smear	Drying artefacts seen	Good fixation

- Wash with phosphate buffer (pH 6.8).
- Dried in air
- Mount in DPX or Canada balsam.

Some Common FNAC Findings (Microscopic)

Reactive Hyperplasia of Lymph Node

- Smears show high cellular yield (hypercellular)
- A mixed population of lymphoid cells with a predominance of small mature lymphocytes.
- Centrocytes, centroblasts and immunoblast are present but in "logical" proportions.
- The ratio of small lymphocytes and other large cells are approximately 80:20.
- Plasma cells are increased.
- Tingible body macrophages (scattered histiocytes with intracytoplasmic nuclear debris) are seen.
- Background reveals lymphoid globules or lymphoglandular bodies (pale-blue rounded cytoplasmic fragments up to 8 μm (in Giemsa/MGG stain).

Granulomatous Lymphadenitis

- Clusters of cohesive epithelioid histiocytes surrounded by lymphocytes.
- These epithelioid histiocytes (cells) have elongated nuclei like the sole of a shoe.

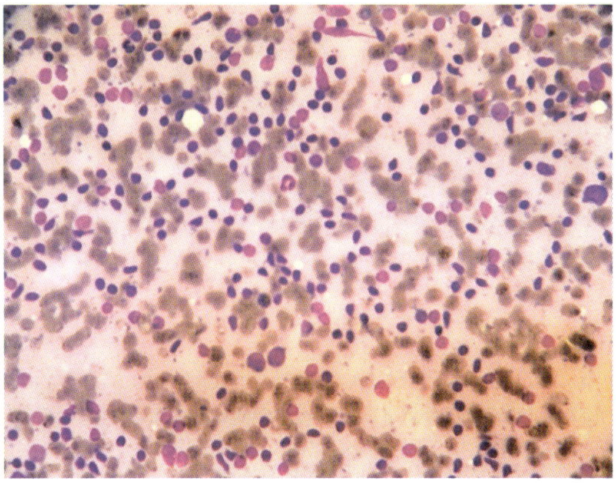

Fig. 16.12: Reactive hyperplasia of lymph node (MGG, 100X)

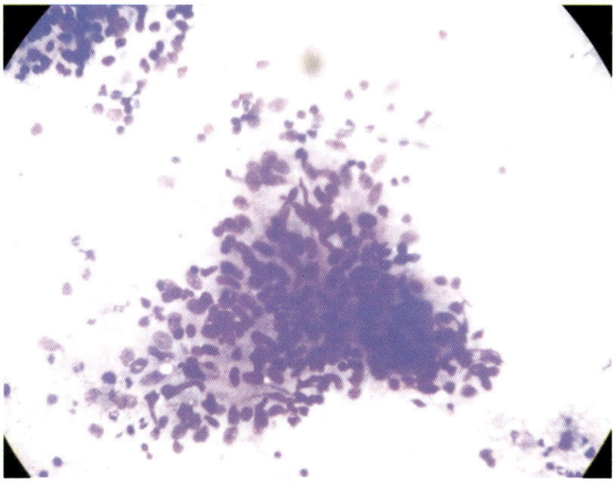

Fig. 16.13: Low power view of granulomatous lymphadenitis (MGG stain)

The nuclear chromatin is finely granular and pale with a small nucleolus. The cytoplasm is pale and lacks distinct cell border.

- Multinucleated giant cells of both Langhans and foreign body types are found with typical arrangement of nuclei.
- Caseation (necrosis) may or may not be present.
- Background reveals mixed population of lymphoid cells of lymph node.

Nodular Colloid Goitre

- Abundant colloid material (usually thin colloid).
- Follicular epithelial cells (benign type) present in monolayered sheets and in cohesive groups.
- Many bare nuclei of benign follicular epithelial cells (lymphocyte like) in a background of thin colloid.
- Cyst macrophages in the background when there is colloid goitre with cystic degeneration.

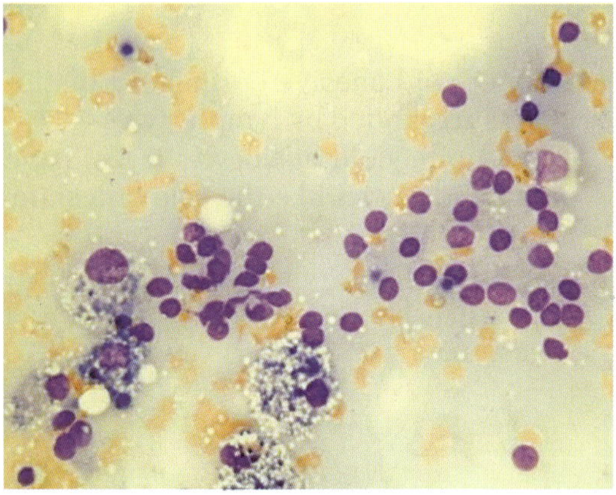

Fig. 16.14: High power view of nodular colloid goitre with cystic degeneration (MGG stain)

Papillary Carcinoma of Thyroid

- Highly cellular smear.
- The epithelial cells are arranged in papillary, in monolayered sheets or dispersely.
- Finger-like papillae have anatomical borders, nuclear crowding and overlapping. Vascular core may or may not be present in the papillae.
- Nuclei are enlarged, ovoid with finely granular, powdery chromatin (Pap stain).
- Nucleoli are small and inconspicuous.
- Nuclear cytoplasmic inclusions and longitudinal grooves/folds are frequently present. The cytoplasmic inclusions are present in more than 5% of cells and in 90% of cases.
- Dispersed cells (single cells) have dense cytoplasm and distinct cell borders.

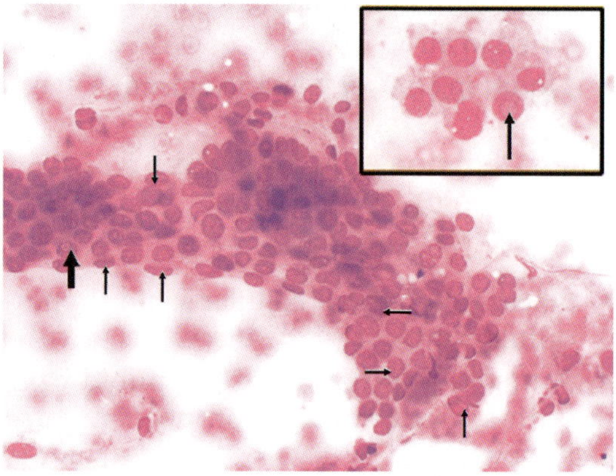

A

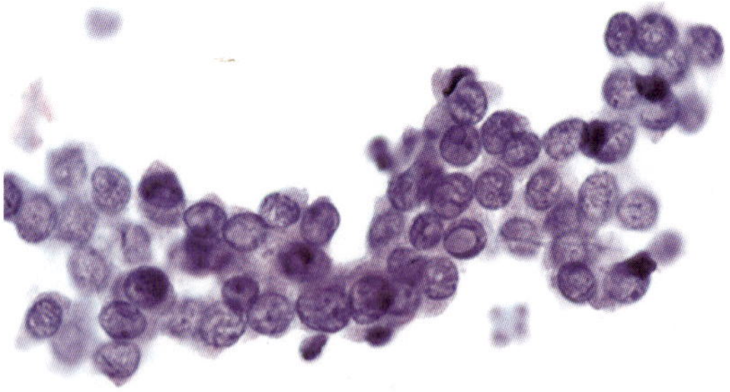

B

Fig. 16.15A and B: (A) FNA smear showing many nuclear grooves (thin arrow), whereas thick arrow and inset showing intranuclear cytoplasmic inclusions (MGG, 400X); (B) Papillary structure, intranuclear grooves, intranuclear cytoplasmic inclusions and granular, powdery chromatin (Pap, 400X).

- Scanty, viscous, stringy colloid (chewing gum colloid).
- Macrophages, giant cells and psammoma bodies may be present.

Fibroadenoma of Breast

- Moderate to high cellular yield (depending upon the fibrosis).
- Large, branching, monolayered sheets of benign ductal epithelial cells. Smaller, darker nuclei of myoepithelial cells are present in between the ductal epithelial cells.
- Numerous, single bare bipolar nuclei of benign type in the background.
- Scanty fragments of fibromyxoid stroma. They stain pink to magenta with MGG stain, have fibrillary appearance and contain spindle fibroblasts.

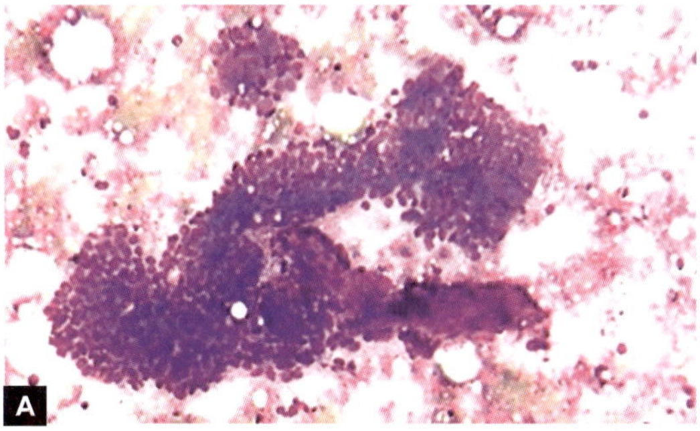

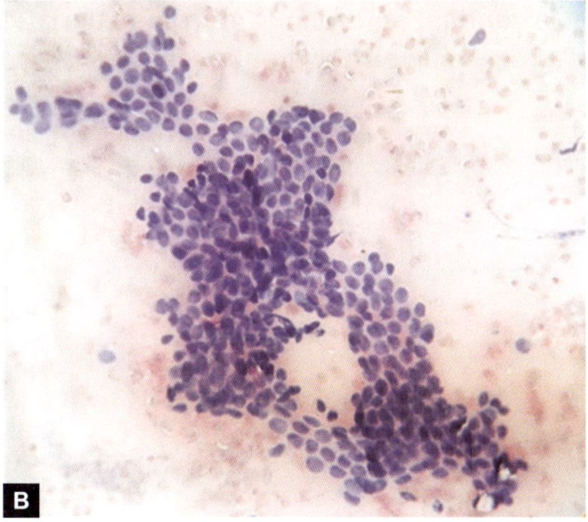

Fig. 16.16A and B: (A) Fibroadenoma of breast (MGG × 100); (B) Fibroadenoma of breast (Pap × 100)

Note

In fibrocystic disease (FCD) or fibroadenosis, apocrine changes in the epithelial cells and macrophages in the background are seen in addition to above finding.

Duct Carcinoma of Breast

- Highly cellular smears (high cellular yield).
- Loosely cohesive and individual scattered malignant cells.
- Malignant epithelial cells arranged in three dimensional clusters, syncytial groupings and occasional acinar/glandular patterns.

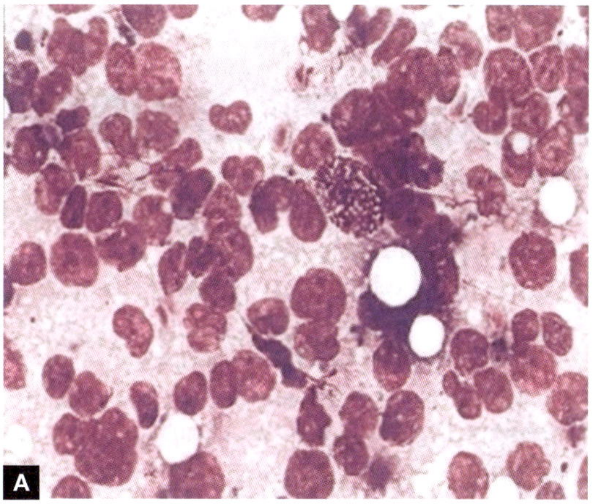

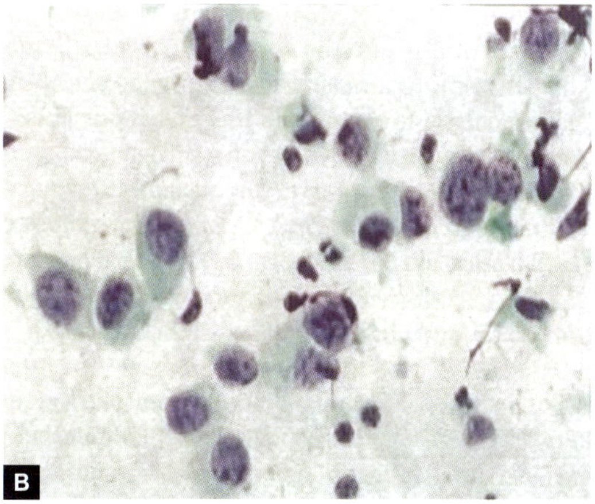

Fig. 16.17A and B: Invasive duct carcinoma of breast. (A) MGG stain, high power view; (B) Pap stain, high power view

- Absence of single bare nuclei of benign type.
- Nuclear atypia like irregular shape, irregular contours (buds, indentations, sharp angles, folds, etc.) and chromatin irregularities are present.
- Necrosis if present is important clue.
- Tumour diathesis may be seen.

Lipoma

- Fragments of mature adipose tissue, a few single fat cells (adipocytes) and fat droplets.
- These fat cells (adipocytes) are large and have abundant empty cytoplasm with eccentrically placed small, dark nucleus.
- Few strands of anastomosing or branching capillary vessels are seen.

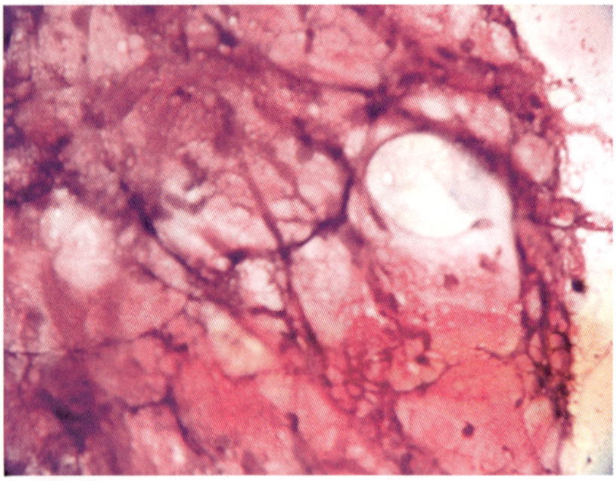

A

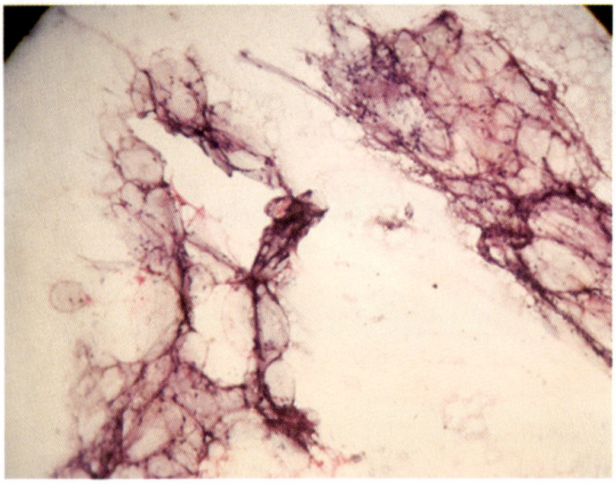

B

Fig. 16.18A and B: (A) Lipoma (MGG × 400); (B) Lipoma (Pap × 100)

Neurofibroma/Benign Peripheral Nerve Sheath Tumour

- Slender spindle cells within fibrillary mesenchymal tissue fragments.
- These spindle cells have long hair like cytoplasmic processes and pale nuclei with pointed ends. The nuclei are pyknotic.
- The cytoplasmic processes of several cells may form bundles and can be tangled.
- The nuclei often form a parallel row or palisade (in case of neurilemmoma or schawannoma).

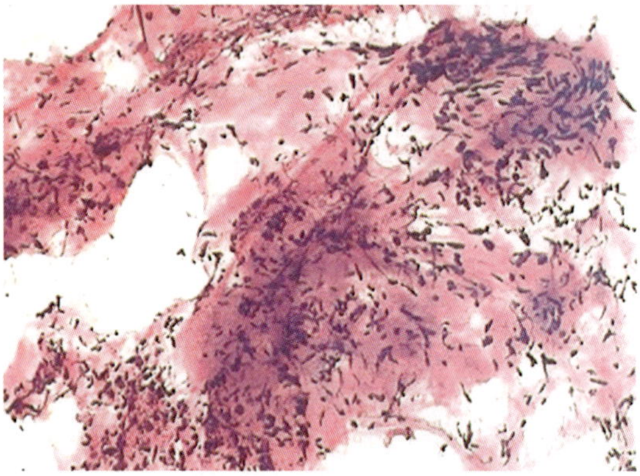

Fig. 16.19: Neurofibroma (MGG, 100X)

Ganglion (Ganglion Cyst)

- Abundant amorphous mucoid material.
- A few pale histiocyte-like cells.

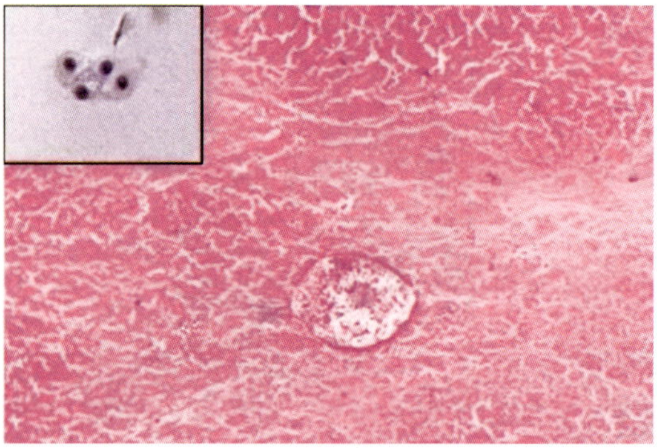

Fig. 16.20: Ganglion cyst, MGG × 400 (inset shows Pap stain)

Pleomorphic Salivary Adenoma of Salivary Gland

- Fibrillary chodromyxoid or myxoid stromal substance.
- In MGG stained smears, this stromal substance appears as an intensely red to dark purple, fibrillar material.
- Rounded, monomorphic epithelial cells with a well defined sometimes eccentric cytoplasm are seen together with spindled myoepithelial cells.
- These epithelial and myoepithelial cells are seen single and in poorly cohesive clusters and sheets.
- Nuclei of these cells are oval with bland nuclear chromatin.

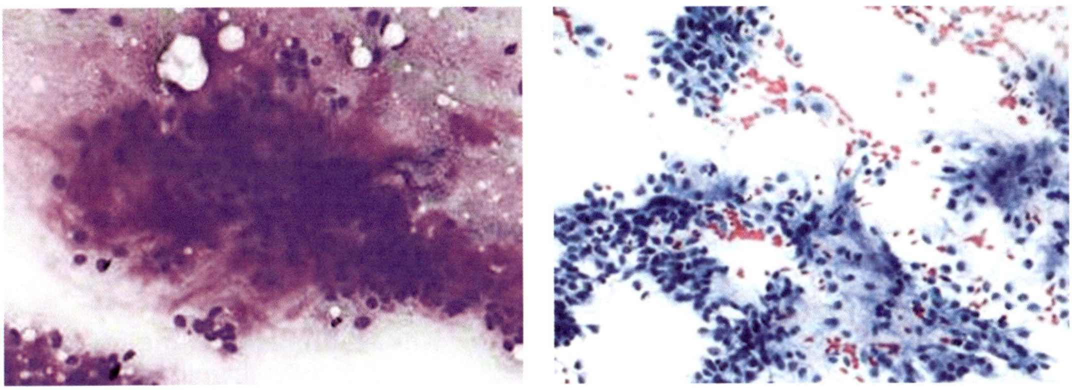

A B

Fig. 16.21A and B: (A) MGG stain, low power view; (B) Pap stain, low power view

VIVA VOCE

Q1. What are the other names of FNAC?

Ans: i. The terminology FNAC or fine needle aspiration cytology was popular among some British and American workers. They also called **needle biopsy cytology (NBC)**.

ii. Other terminologies are **aspiration biopsy cytology (ABC)** and **fine needle aspiration biopsy (FNAB)** which were used by Scandinavian and American workers.

Q2. What is usual fixative for Pap smears?

Ans: Usually 95% ethyl alcohol, 100% methanol or 85% isopropyl alcohol are used as fixative. A mixture of ether and ethyl alcohol (1:1 v/v) is also used.

Q3. What are the indications for Barr body detection in buccal smear?

Ans: i. To determine the genotypic sex in children who have ambiguous external genitalia (phenotypic sex) like male or female pseudohermaphrodites.

ii. In Turner's syndrome (45, XO), Klinefelter syndrome (47, XXY) or super females (47, XXX).

Q4. What are the different stains used for buccal smear staining?

Ans: Orcein stain, basic fuchsin stain and Shorr's stain.

Among these first two stains are commonly used.

Q5. What is F body or Y chromatin?

Ans: The fluorescent dye, quinacrine, binds strongly to the Y chromosome and only to a lesser extent to the other chromosome in cells of humans. A bright fluorescent spot (F body), which is presumed to be the Y chromosome, is clearly visible in quinacrine stained interphase cells from various tissues and spermatozoa of human males.

Spermatozoa bearing one F body (~ 45% of total) are taken to be Y spermatozoa. Spermatozoa having two F bodies (about 1.3% of the total) are YY spermatozoa. If number of YY spermatozoa is high, then there is high non-disjunction rates during spermatogenesis.

The intensely fluorescent F body is seen under fluorescent microscope in about 60% of interphase nuclei in human males and <8% in nuclei of females. This F body is also observed in the nuclei of lymphocytes in blood smears if stained with quinacrine mustard.

Q6. What are interventional cytology and exfoliative cytology? What are their differences?

Ans: In **interventional cytology**, materials are obtained by aspiration technique or surgical biopsy. These include FNAC, imprint cytology, crush smear cytology and biopsy sediment cytology.

In **exfoliative cytology**, cells which are shed off from epithelial surfaces into body fluids or body cavities are used. Beside the representative cells are also obtainable from scraping, brushing or washing mucosal surfaces (abrasive cytology) (*see* table on page 285).

Q7. What is biopsy sediment cytology?

Ans: First the sample deposit of the fixative (neutral buffered formalin or 10% formalin) in which the biopsy specimen has been sent is centrifuged. Then smear is prepared.

It is used in some causes of bone tumours and diagnostic criteria are same as in exfoliative cytology.

Parameters	Interventional cytology	Exfoliative cytology
1. Smears	Abundant cellular material in clumps, aggregates and discrete.	Cells are discrete. Particular cell has to be find out by screening
2. Method of sample collection	Obtained by aspiration/intervention	Cells are exfoliated from epithelial cells.
3. Basis of diagnosis	Cellular pattern and morphologic evaluation of groups of cells	By evaluating particular cell of interest
4. Morphologic evaluation for diagnosis	Though nuclear features are very important, cytoplasmic features are also important	Nuclear features more important than cytoplasmic features

Q8. What are the contraindications of doing FNAC?

Ans:
- Bleeding diathesis: Coagulopathies like haemophilia, von Willebrand's disease.
- Testis: Acute epididymo-orchitis as FNAC is extremely painful.
- Pancreas: Acute pancreatitis
- Prostate: Acute prostatitis
- Lung: Elderly patients with emphysema or pulmonary hypertension
- Adrenal: Suspected pheochromocytoma because of fluctuations in blood pressure.
- Liver: Prothrombin time should be checked
- Malignant melanoma: Extreme precautions should be taken, because some fear that there is chance of needle seedling and spread of tumour through needle tract.

Q9. What is the ideal needle size for doing FNAC?

Ans: Usually for most of the sites (soft tissue, breast, etc.), needle size of 21 gauge or 22 gauge needle is used. For highly vascular tumours like thyroid, lymph node and in children; 24 gauge or 25 gauge needles are suitable. For very hard tissue like bone 18 gauge or 20 gauge needles are used.

Needle gauge	Outer diameter in inch	Outer diameter in mm
• 18 Gauge	0.050	1.270
• 19 Gauge	0.042	1.067
• 20 Gauge	0.03575	0.9081
• 21 Gauge	0.03225	0.8192
• 22 Gauge	0.02825	0.7176
• 23 Gauge	0.02525	0.6414
• 24 Gauge	0.02225	0.5652
• 25 Gauge	0.02025	0.5144

The standard 21 gauge needle has a length of 38 mm while 24 to 25 gauge needle has a length of 25 mm.

For guided FNAC longer needles (80–160 mm long) are needed.

For guided FNAC of abdominal organs and lung, Chiba spinal needle of 20–22 gauge needles are used. For transrectal FNAC of prostate and transvaginal FNAC of ovary needles of up to 200 mm length are employed.

Q10. What are the infective organisms that can be detected in Pap smears?

Ans:
- Bacteria: *Neisseria gonorrhoeae, Gardnerella vaginalis, Mycobacterium tuberculosis.*
- Virus: Cytomegalovirus, herpes simplex, human papillomavirus (HPV)
- Fungus: Candida, Aspergillosis
- Parasites: *Trichomonas vaginalis, Entamoeba histolytica.*

Section IV

Museum Techniques and Mounted Surgical Specimens

Chapter

17

Museum Specimens

CARDIOVASCULAR SYSTEM SPECIMENS

Mitral Stenosis

Description: Mounted specimen of heart in a jar which is cut transversely showing following features:

- Ventricles, atrium and valves of the heart.
- Left ventricle is recognized by its thick wall compared to right ventricle.
- Mitral valve is seen in-between left ventricle and left atrium which has become thickened, puckered, fibrosed and deformed.
- Focal dystrophic calcification is noted in mitral valve.
- Commissures are fused resulting in stenosis and having **'fish-mouth' appearance**.
- Left atrium is dilated.
- Left ventricle is slightly smaller in size compared to normal left ventricle.

Diagnosis: Mitral stenosis.

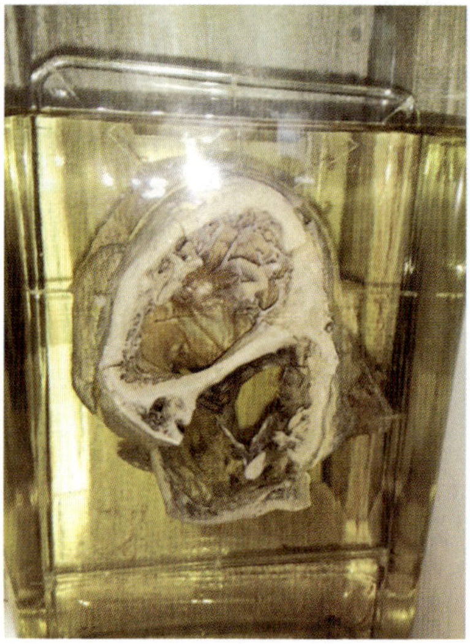

A

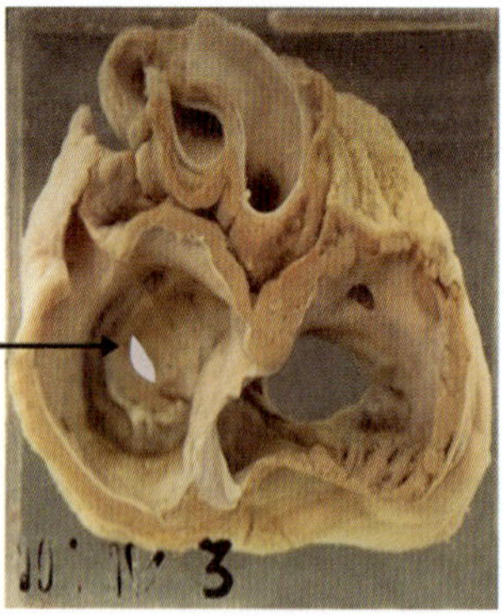

B

Fig. 17.1A and B: Button hole; (B) Fish mouth

Q. What are the clinical features of mitral stenosis and what is the most common cause?

Ans: Rheumatic fever is the most common cause. Clinical features are pulmonary hypertension, left atrial and left ventricular hypertrophy, opening snap and diastolic murmur.

Q. What are the complications of mitral valve stenosis?

Ans: Congestive cardiac failure, atrial fibrillation, recurrent haemoptysis, subacute bacterial endocarditis and embolism.

Q. What are the consequences of mitral valve stenosis?

Ans: Mitral valve stenosis hampers normal blood flow from left atrium to left ventricle during diastolic period. This leads to hypertrophy of left atrium, pulmonary congestion, brown induration of lungs and right ventricle hypertrophy (cor pulmonale).

Atheroma of Aorta

Description: Mounted specimen of a large artery (abdominal aorta) in a jar showing following features:

- Intimal surface which is identified by many small holes which are actually ostia of branch vessels.
- Elevated white to yellowish fibrous or fibrofatty patchy or plaques (0.3–1.5 cm to long in size) are seen close/surrounding to the opening of ostia of branch vessels.

Diagnosis: Atheroma of artery (aorta).

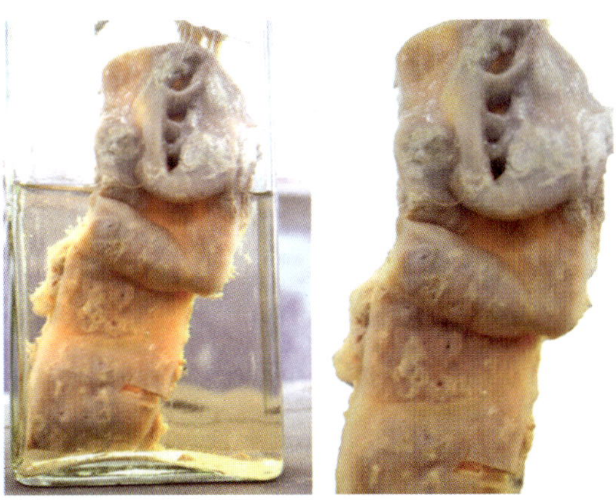

A B

Fig. 17.2A and B: (A) Mounted specimen of atheroma; (B) The lesions

Q. What are the arteries commonly affected by atheroma?

Ans:

i. Large elastic arteries (abdominal aorta, carotid, iliac).

ii. Large to medium-sized muscular arteries (coronary, popliteal, anterior and posterior tibial, mesenteric, renal and circle of Willis).

Q. Which vessels are spared by atherosclerosis?

Ans: Internal mammary arteries and arteries of upper extremities are spared. As internal mammary arteries are not affected, these are used as graft in coronary bypass surgery.

Q. What are the different stages in the evolution?

Ans: **Fatty streaks** are the earliest lesions in atherosclerosis. Then formation of **atheromatous plaques** occurs in which there are intimal thickening and lipid accumulation. Plaques vary from 0.3 to 1.5 cm in diameter but may from larger masses when they coalesce.

Complications like erosion, ulceration and rupture may occur which may lead to thrombosis. Other complications are aneurysm formation.

Q. What are the components of atheromatous plaques?

Ans: They have three layers or zones. Inner layer contains **necrotic core** (lipid, cholesterol clefts, fibrin, foam cells or foamy macrophages, cell debris). Outer layer is **fibrous cap** composed of smooth muscle and collagen. In-between is the **cellular layer** (smooth muscle, lymphocytes, macrophages with less connective tissue).

Left Ventricular Hypertrophy (LVH)

Description: Mounted specimen of heart in a jar and has following features:

- Thickness of left ventricular wall is increased (>1.5 cm) and decreased in size of left ventricular chamber. Normal

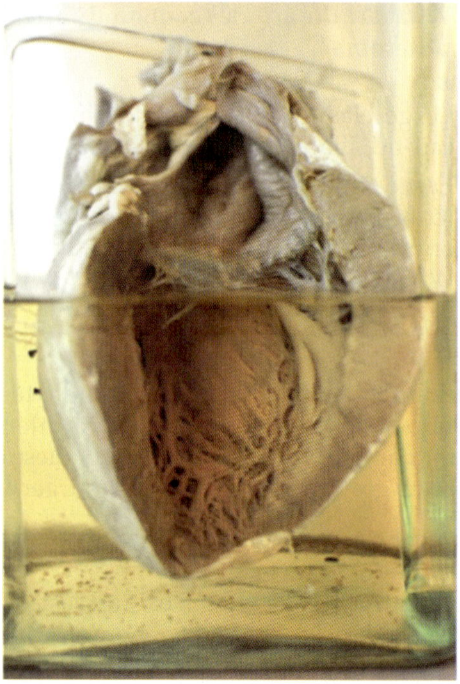

Fig. 17.3: Left ventricular hypertrophy

thickness of left ventricular wall is 1.2–1.5 cm.

- Papillary muscles and trabeculae carneae are prominent.
- Heart may be massively enlarged sometimes (corbovium).

Diagnosis: Left ventricular hypertrophy.

Q. What are the common causes of LVH?

Ans: It occurs due to systemic hypertension and aortic valvular disease. The overall weight of heart increases >375 g in males and >350 g in females. Congestive heart failure is the most common cause of death in untreated patients.

Q. What are the light microscopic features?

Ans: Microscopically, hypertrophic myocardial cells (cardiac myocytes) exhibit an increased in diameter with enlarged, hyperchromatic, **rectangular (boxcar) nuclei**.

Also, there are focal interstitial fibrosis and myofibre degeneration.

Fibrinous Pericarditis

Description: Mounted specimen of heart in a jar showing following features:

- There is deposition of fibrin over pericardium and it ranges from barely visible fibrin ridges to massive, velvety deposit.
- Fibrin deposited in-between two layers of pericardium (viscreral and parietal layers) exhibits **bread and butter** appearance.
- At places, mesothelium below fibrin is destroyed. In these areas, fibrinous coating is adherent so firmly that it becomes progressively difficult to pull off fibrinous coating.
- The surface is dry, with a fine granular roughening.

Diagnosis: Fibrinous pericarditis.

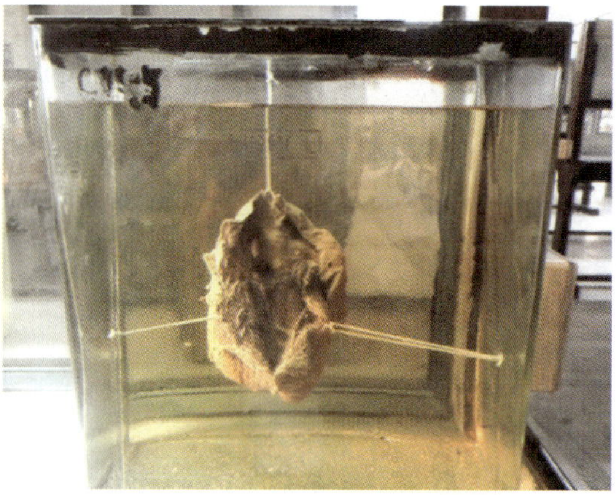

Fig. 17.4: Fibrinous pericarditis

Q. What are the causes of fibrinous pericarditis?

Ans: Fibrinous or serofibrinous pericarditis is characterized by a fibrin-rich exudate due to increased vascular permeabilility. Causes are chronic renal failure (uraemia), myocardial infarction, acute rheumatic fever, SLE, postinfarction (Dressler) syndrome, chest radiation and trauma.

Q. What are the clinical features?

Ans: Development of a loud pericardial friction rub is very characteristic of fibrinous pericarditis. Also, there are pain, systemic febrile reactions and signs of cardiac failure.

Q. What are the components of fluid in serofibrinous pericarditis?

Ans: There is accumulation of larger amounts of yellow to brown turbid fluid, which is made brown and cloudy by the presence of leukocytes and red cells (may be bloody in appearance) and fibrin. Over time, fibrin may be lysed with resolution or it may be organized.

Verrucous Lesions Mitral Valve in Rheumatic Heart Disease (RHD)

Description: Mounted specimen of heart in a jar showing following features:

- There are many small, warty, vegetations along the lines of closure of mitral valve leaflets (arrow on right side picture). Also seen on the rest of the valvular surface.
- These verrucae (actually small thrombi and composed of fibrin and platelets) are greyish or reddish-brown.

Diagnosis: Verrucous lesions of mitral valve.

Q. What are the differences of vegetations, seen in RHD, infective endocarditis, nonbacterial thrombotic endocarditis, Libman-Sacks endocarditis of SLE?

Ans: In RHD, vegetations are small (1–2 mm) warty and seen mainly along the lines of closure of the valve leaflets. In infective endocarditis, vegetations are large, irregular masses which are seen on the valve cusps that can extend onto the chordae. In nonbacterial thrombotic endocarditis, vegetations are small, bland and attached at the line of closure of valve leaflets. In SLE, vegetations are small or medium-sized which are seen on both sides of valve leaflets.

Q. Which valve is most commonly involved in RHD?

Ans: The mitral valve is affected most commonly (65–70%) followed by aortic valve involvement (25% of cases). Tricuspid valve involvement is uncommon and involvement of pulmonary valve is very rare.

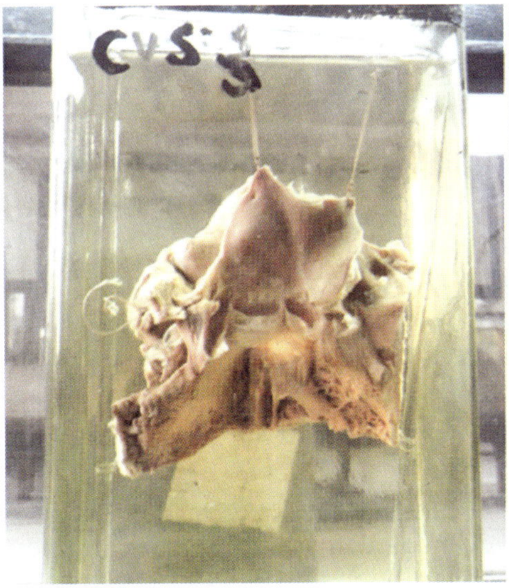

A

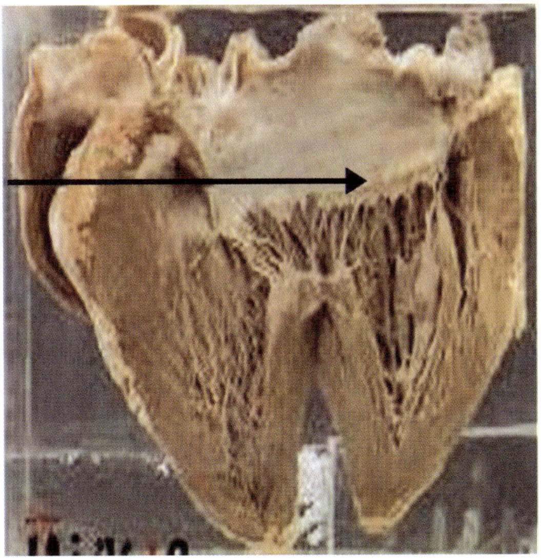

B

Fig. 17.5A and B: Rheumatic heart disease (verrucous lesions)

RESPIRATORY SYSTEM SPECIMENS

Lobar Pneumonia

Description: Mounted specimen of cut section of lung in a jar showing following features:

- Solidification of a lobe of lung (diffuse homogenous consolidation).
- This area of consolidation, looks gray-brown or yellowish-gray in colour.
- The pleura is thickened and covered by fibrinosuppurative exudate.
- Other portion of the lung is unaffected and appears normal.

Diagnosis: Lobar pneumonia (gray hepatization).

Q. What are the different stages of lobar pneumonia?

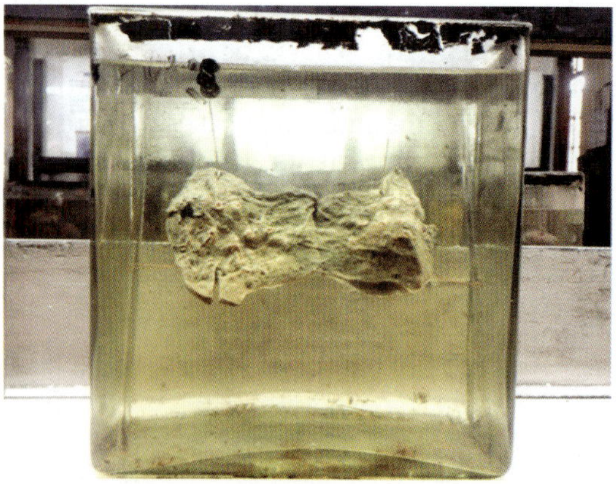

Fig. 17.6: Lobar pneumonia

Ans:

i. Stage of **congestion** (12–24 hours)
ii. Stage of **red hepatization** (2–4 hours)
iii. Stage of **gray hepatization** (4–8 days)
iv. Stage of **resolution** (8–10 days)

Q. Why has it been named as hepatization, though it is a lung tissue?

Ans: During autopsy, the affected lobe/ portion of lung feels like hepatic tissue (liver) in consistency. Also, the affected lobe sinks in water unlike unaffected lung tissue which floats in water due to entrapped air within it.

Q. Why the lower lobes of lung are commonly affected?

Ans: This is because of the tendency of secretions to gravitate into the lower lobes.

Q. Why the affected portion looks gray during gray hepatization?

Ans: In this stage, there is progressive disintegration of red cells and the persistence of a fibrinosuppurative exudate (neutrophil rich), giving the gross appearance of grayish brown, dry surface.

Q. What do you mean by the term "consolidation"?

Ans: Consolidation literally means the process of becoming or the condition of being solid. In lobar pneumonia this means replacement of alveolar air by neutrophil-rich fibrinosuppurative exudate and to became solidified or consolidated.

Q. Why is it not a case of bronchopneumonia (lobular pneumonia)?

Ans: The lesion is patchy in bronchopneumonia and does not involve an entire lobe unlike lobar pneumonia. Also, bronchopneumonia is associated with area of emphysaema and collapse.

Q. What are the complications of lobar pneumonia?

Ans: Lung abscess, empyema, septicaemia (bacterial dissemination), pleuritis and delayed resolution.

Bronchiectasis

Description: Mounted specimen of cut section of lung in a jar showing following features:

- Marked dilatation of bronchi and bronchioles with fibrosis in the adjoining areas.
- Dilated airways take various shapes, i.e. cylindrical, fusiform, varicose (numerous constriction and dilation) and saccular (bead-like bulge on one side). But it is predominantly cylindrical.

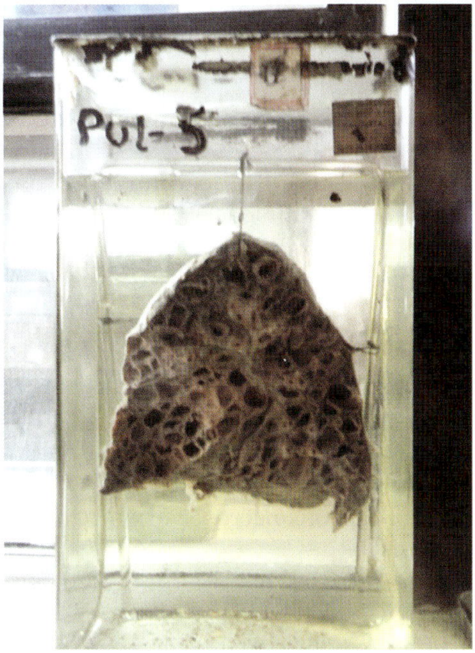

Fig. 17.7: Bronchiectasis

- These dilated airways are easily visible up to <3 mm from the pleural surface (normally, bronchioles are traceable up to 2–3 cm from pleural surface).
- Dilated bronchi and bronchioles are filled with pus.
- Unaffected lung parenchyma is compressed.

Diagnosis: Bronchiectasis.

Q. What is bronchiectasis?

Ans: Bronchiectasis is a disease characterized by permanent dilation of bronchi and bronchioles caused by destruction of the elastic tissue, resulting from or associated with chronic necrotizing infections.

Q. What are different types of bronchiectasis?

Ans: Obstructive (tumour, foreign body, etc.) and non-obstructive (postinfectious, congenital or hereditary, others).

Obstruction and infection are the major conditions associated with bronchiectasis.

Q. What are the complications of bronchiectasis?

Ans: Lung abscess, pneumonia, bronchopleural fistula, cor pulmonale, necrotizing brain abscess, meningitis, squamous cell carcinoma, and amyloidosis.

Emphysema

Description: Mounted specimen of cut section of lung in a jar showing following features:

- Central or proximal area shows marked dilatation of respiratory bronchioles surrounded by relatively spared alveolar spaces.
- The lesion is more severe in the upper lobes, particularly in the apical segments.
- The walls of emphysematous spaces contain large amount of black pigment (due to heavy smoking nicotine and other).

Diagnosis: Centriacinar (centrilobular) emphysema.

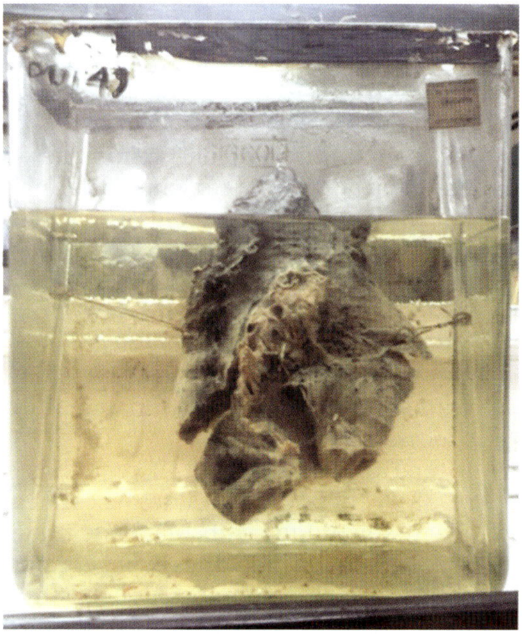

Fig. 17.8A

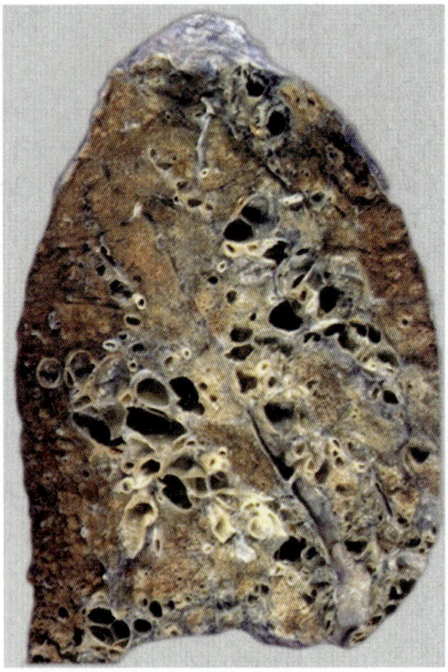

Fig. 17.8B

Fig. 17.8A and B: Emphysema

Q. What are the different types of emphysema?

Ans:

i. **Centriacinar (centrilobular) emphysema:** Respiratory bronchioles are dilated. Cause is heavy smoking, often associated with chronic bronchitis.

ii. **Panacinar (panlobular) emphysema:** Alveoli and alveolar ducts are dilated. Cause α_1-antitrypsin (antiprotease) deficiency.

iii. **Paraseptal (distal acinar) emphysema:** Proximal portion of the acinus is normal, but distal portion of acinus is dilated. Seen adjacent to areas of fibrosis, scarring or atelectasis.

iv. **Irregular emphysema:** Acini are irregularly involved and are almost invariably associated with scarring. Seen along with scars from a healed inflammatory process.

v. **Interstitial emphysema**: It occurs as a result of entrance of air into the connective tissue of lung, subcutaneous tissue or mediastinum in settings of penetrating chest injury, chronic bronchitis or obstruction. Also seen in children with whooping cough.

Q. What are the light microscopic findings of emphysema?

Ans:

- Abnormally large alveoli separated by thin septa.
- Adjacent alveoli become confluent, creating large airspaces.
- As alveolar walls are destroyed, there is decrease in the capillary bed.

Fibrocaseous Tuberculosis of Lung

Description: Mounted specimen of lung in a jar showing following features:

- Yellowish caseous necrosis area of variable size.
- Foci of caseous necrosis accompanied by fibrosis
- Acute cavities have irregular, ragged yellowish-gray walls.
- Chronic cavities have regular, smooth and thick wall lining.
- Fibrosis of lung accompanied by thickened pleura, thickened wall of bronchi and thickening of blood vessels.

Diagnosis: Fibrocaseous (cavitating) tuberculosis of lung.

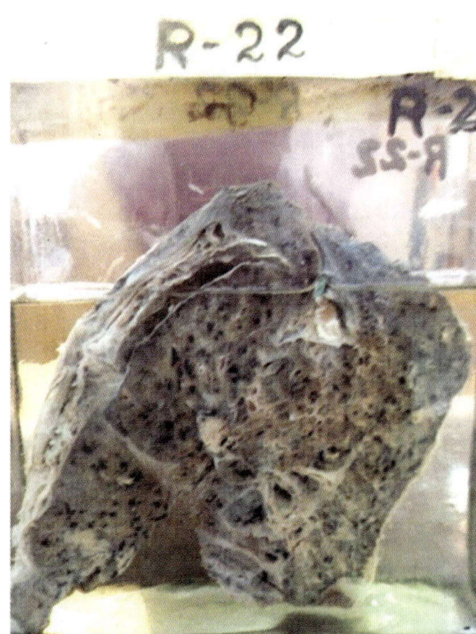

Fig. 17.9: Fibrocaseous tuberculosis of lung

Q. What is primary tuberculosis?

Ans: Primary infection may occur in any organ such as lung, intestine or skin. But in children, the usual site is lung and is called primary tuberculosis. Exposure to AFB occurs first time and consolidation is usually solitary. There is formation of **Ghon's focus** in subpleural location and midzone of lung is involved. Lymphadenopathy is common. Cavitation is rare.

Q. What is secondary tuberculosis?

Ans: It is usually caused by reinfection or reactivation of an old infection. Any age group may suffer. Multifocal lesions (consolidations) are seen. Upper lobes or apical regions are usually affected. Cavitation is common but lymphadenopathy is rare. **Simon's focus** (2 cm gray white to yellowish well circumscribed consolidation in apical regions) may be seen.

Q. What are Ghon's focus and Ghon's complex?

Ans: Ghon's focus: 1–1.5 cm area of gray-white inflammation with consolidation. Seen in lower part of upper lobe and upper part of lower lobe. The centre of this focus undergoes caseous necrosis.

Ghon's complex: Combination of parenchymal lung lesion of tuberculosis and regional hilar lymph nodes involvement is referred to as Ghon's complex.

Q. What are the different types (morphological) of pulmonary tuberculosis?

Ans:

i. Fibrocaseous
ii. Cavitary (ulcerative)
iii. Tuberculous bronchopneumonia
iv. Miliary tuberculosis with haematogenous infection.

Miliary Tuberculosis of Lung

Description: Mounted specimen of longitudinal section of lung in a jar showing following features:

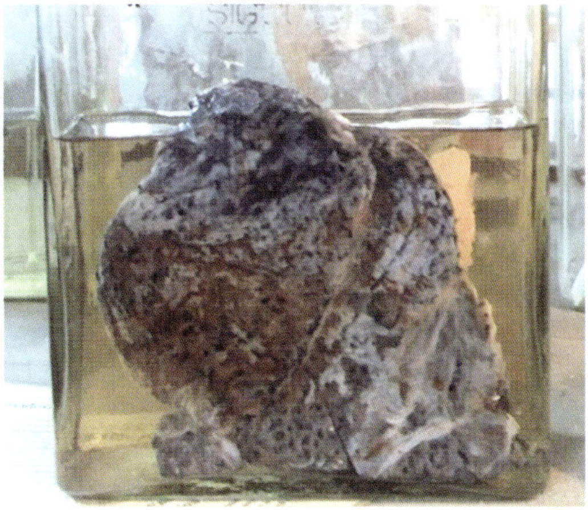

A

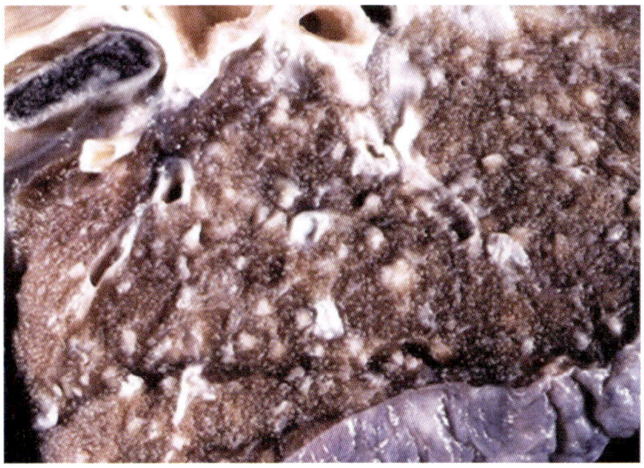

B

Fig. 17.10A and B: Miliary tuberculosis of lung

- The lung is studded with numerous uniform small **millet-size white spots (tubercles)** surrounded by intense congestion.
- These small spots (1–3 mm in diameter) are seen both in subpleural location and in section.

Diagnosis: Miliary tuberculosis of lung

Q. Why does miliary tuberculosis occur?

Ans: This is due to rupture of caseous parenchymatous or glandular lesion and when organisms draining through lymphatics enter the venous blood organisms enter systemic circulation and dissemination occurs.

Q. What are light microscopic features of miliary tuberculosis of lung?

Ans:

- Tubercles are usually located in inter-alveolar septa and usually no change is seen in the alveoli.
- In the granulomas, giant cells are a few in number.
- Peripheral fibrotic zone is absent.
- Vessels present in septa undergo dilatation.

Bronchogenic Carcinoma

Description: Mounted specimen of a section of lung in a jar showing following features:

- Gray-white growth arising from major bronchus, spreading both within and outside the bronchus and in the walls. Also, the tumour is infiltrating the lung substance.
- Focal areas of haemorrhage and necrosis which produce red or yellow-white mottling and softening.
- The tumour is arising from the hilum.
- Uninvolved lung tissue is compressed.

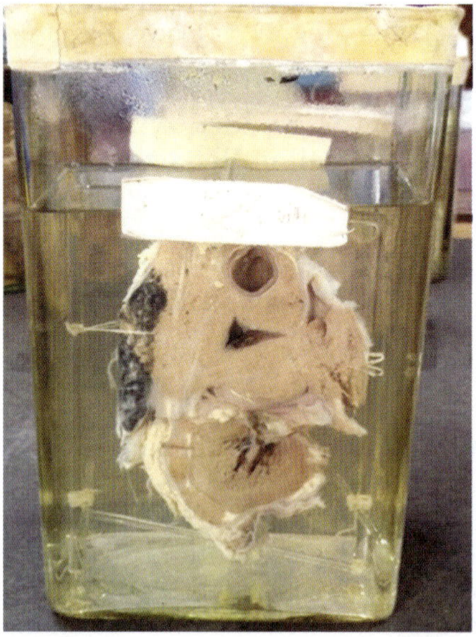

Fig. 17.11: Bronchogenic carcinoma

Diagnosis: Bronchogenic carcinoma (squamous cell carcinoma).

Note

Most lung carcinomas arise in and about the hilus of the lung. About three-fourths of the tumours originate from first-order, second-order, and third-order bronchi.

As most of the carcinomas of lung arise from bronchi, the term 'Cancer lung' and bronchogenic carcinoma are used synonymously.

Q. What are the different types of lung carcinomas?

Ans:

- Adenocarcinoma (males 37%, females 47%)
- Squamous cell carcinoma (males 32%, females 25%)
- Small cell carcinoma (males 14%, females 18%)
- Large cell carcinoma (males 18%, females 10%)

Q. What are the risk factors of bronchogenic carcinoma?

Ans: Tobacco smoking accounts from 80 to 90% of lung cancers. High-dose ionizing radiation, uranium, asbestos and air-pollutants are other risk factors. Genetic predisposition and p53 mutation also play an important role.

Q. What are precursor lesions of lung cancers?

Ans: Four types of epithelial precursor lesion:

- Squamous dysplasia and carcinoma *in situ*
- Atypical adenomatous hyperplasia
- Adenocarcinoma *in situ*
- Diffuse idiopathic pulmonary neuroendocrine hyperplasia

Q. Lepidic pattern of growth is seen in which lung carcinoma?

Ans: It is seen in bronchoalveolar carcinoma during light microscopic examination. The tumour grows along preexisting structures without destruction of alveolar architecture. This pattern of growth is known as **lepidic**, and the neoplastic cells resembling butter flies sitting on a fence. Bronchoalveolar carcinomas have two subtypes: Mucinous and nonmucinous.

GASTROINTESTINAL SYSTEM SPECIMEN

Peptic Ulcer

Description: Mounted specimen of stomach in a jar showing following features:

- Stomach is cut open along greater curvature.
- An ulcer is seen in lesser curvature with the antrum.
- The ulcer is <2 cm in diameter, oval to round and sharply delineated.
- Edge is thickened and overhanging.
- Margin of ulcer sharply punched out.
- Base of ulcer is smooth and clean.

Diagnosis: Chronic peptic ulcer.

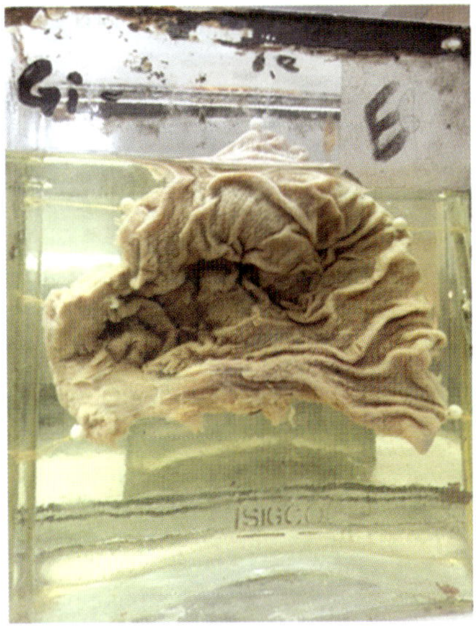

A

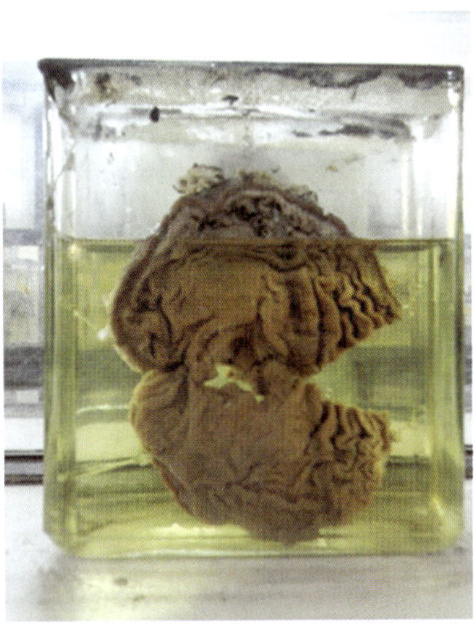

B

Fig. 17.12A and B: (A) Peptic ulcer; (B) Peptic ulcer with perforation

Q. What are the common sites of peptic ulcer?

Ans: It occurs in duodenum, stomach, lower end of oesophagus, Meckel's diverticulum and jejunum after gastrojejunostomy. Gastric peptic ulcers are usually located along the lesser curvature near the interface of the body and antrum. Duodenal ulcers usually occur within few centimeters of the pyloric valve and involve the anterior duodenal wall. Peptic ulcers are four times commoner in proximal (1st part) of duodenum than in the stomach.

Q. What are the risk factors of peptic ulcers?

Ans: *Helicobacter pylori* infection, bile reflux and delayed gastric emptying, alcohol and spicy food, use of NSAIDs, tobacco smoking, hyperparathyroidism, multiple endocrine neoplasia 1, genetic factors (blood group O for duodenal ulcer and blood group A for gastric ulcer).

Q. What are the complications of peptic ulcers?

Ans: Perforation, hourglass deformity and pyloric stenosis, pancreatitis and rarely malignant transformation.

Q. What are differences between gastric and duodenal ulcer?
Ans:

Features	Gastric Ulcer	Duodenal Ulcer
Incidence	Less common	More common
Male: Female ratio	1.5–2.1	3:1
Age	Older patients (>60 years)	Younger patients (20–40 years)
Common locations	First part of duodenum (anterior wall)	Lesser curvature and pyloric antrum
Acid level	Usually, high	Usually normal; but increased when gastrin level is increased.
H. Pylori	Less strong association (present in 70% cases)	Strong association (present almost in all cases)
Pain	Aggravates after taking food	Relieved after taking food
Night pain	No night pain	Common
Vomiting and hematemesis	More common	Less common
Melena	Less common	More common
Microscopy	Almost similar. From the lumen outward four layers , also known as **Askanazy zones:** (i) Necrotic zones, (ii) Superficial exudative zones (fibrinopurulent exudates with neutrophils), (iii) Granulation tissue zone, and (iv) Zone of cicatrization (fibrous tissue or collagenous scar).	From the lumen outward four layers , also known as **Askanazy zones**: (i) Necrotic zones, (ii) Superficial exudative zones (fibrinopurulent exudates with neutrophils), (iii) Granulation tissue zone, and (iv) Zone of cicatrization (fibrous tissue or collagenous scar)

Q. What are the differences between benign and malignant peptic ulcer?
Ans:

Features	Benign Ulcer	Malignant Ulcer
Site	Usually along lesser curvature of pylorus and antrum	Along greater curvature of stomach
Ulcer base	Clear	Necrotic and haemorrhagic
Size	Generally, ?3 cm	Usually more than 3 cm
Mucosal folds	Radiating from ulcer crater	Interrupted; flattening of the rugae around the ulcer due to infiltration of malignant cells.
Margins	No heaping	Heaping prominent
Age	Younger age	Older age
Sex	Obvious male preponderance	slight male preponderance

Gastric Carcinoma

Description: Mounted specimen of stomach in a jar showing following features:

- A large ulceroproliferative growth projecting in the lumen from the mucosa. The growth is situated body of stomach.
- There is also a large ulcer (>3 cm in diameter)
- Margin of ulcer is heaped up and irregular.
- Base of ulcer is haemorrhagic and necrotic. Also, it is hard and indurated.

Diagnosis: Gastric carcinoma.

Q. What are the common sites of gastric carcinoma?

Ans:

- Pylo-antrum region (lesser curvature): 50–60%
- Cardiac region of stomach: 25%
- Body and fundus: 25%
- Greater curvature of stomach: 12%.

Q. What are the different types of gastric carcinomas?

Ans: It may be classified on the basis of depth of invasion (e.g. early and advanced carcinoma); macroscopic growth pattern (e.g. flat mucosal lesions, exophytic, ulcerative and diffuse infiltrative type) and histologic types (intestinal type and diffuse type). Signet-ring carcinoma and linitis plastica are variants of diffuse type of gastric adenocarcinoma.

Q. What are the primary tumours of stomach?

Ans: They may be benign and malignant. These include adenocarcinoma (95%), lymphoma (3%), carcinoid and neuroendocrine carcinoma (1%), stromal tumour and leiomyoma (1%).

Leiomyoma is the most common benign tumour and adenocarcinoma is the most common malignant tumour.

Typhoid Ulcer of Small Intestine

Description: Mounted specimen of stomach in a jar showing following features:

- Multiple small ulcers on the mucosa of small intestine.
- Long axis of ulcers oriented parallel to the long axis of the intestine.
- Margins are regular and well circumscribed. Edges are of undermined.
- Ulcers are round to oval with foci of haemorrhage.
- The Peyer's patches are prominent.

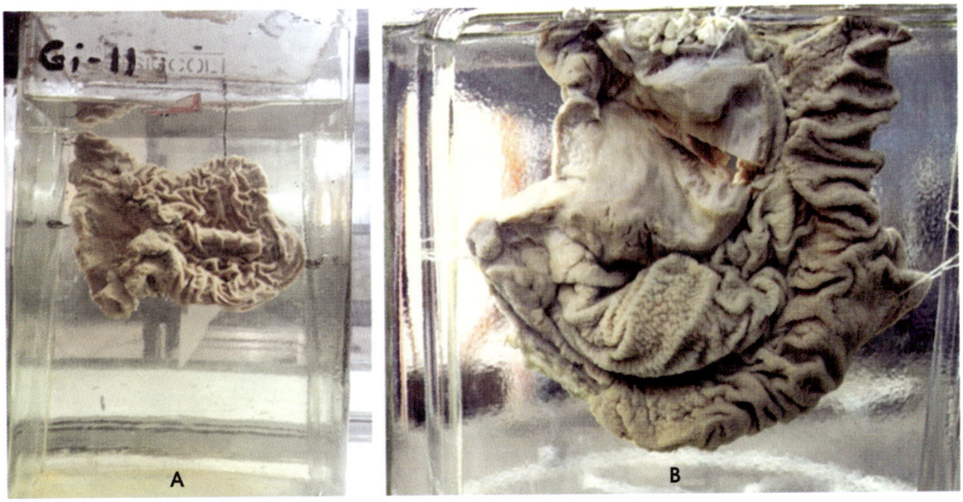

Fig. 17.13A and B: Gastric carcinoma

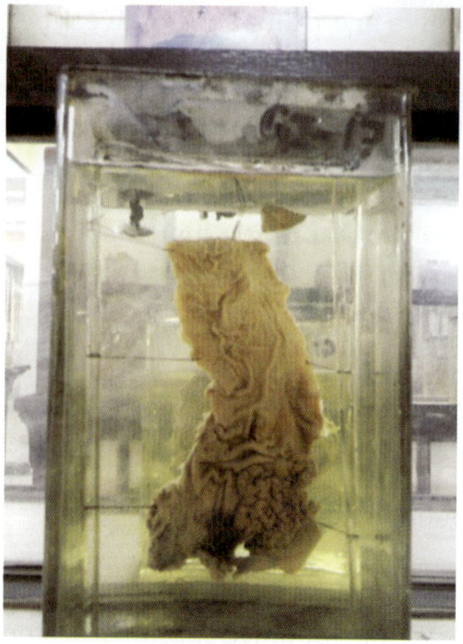

Fig. 17.14: Typhoid ulcer

Diagnosis: Typhoid ulcer of small intestine.

Q. What are the stages of intestinal pathology in typhoid infection?

Ans: There are **four stages** and usually terminal ileum and caecum are involved. Four stages last for 4 weeks:

i. Hyperplasia of Peyer's patches (first week)
ii. Necrosis of Peyer's patches (second week)
iii. Ulceration of intestinal mucosa (third week)
iv. Healing of ulcers (fourth week)

Q. What are the extraintestinal lesion?

Ans: Proliferation of reticuloendothelial cells (monocytes/histiocytes) seen in spleen (sinus histiocytes), liver (Kupffer's cells), lymph nodes and bone marrow. So, patients develop splenomegaly, hepatomegaly and lymphadenopathy.

Q. What are the complications of typhoid ulcer?

Ans: Haemorrhage and perforation may occur at the end of 2nd week. Septicaemic complications like pneumonia, myocarditis, meningitis, arthritis and cholecystitis may be noticed.

Q. Describe briefly intestinal pathogenesis of typhoid infection?

Ans: Intestinal pathogens (*Salmonella typhi* bacilli invade the intestinal mucosa, engulfed by macrophages and transported to reginal lymph nodes. In the lymphoid tissue multiplication of pathogen occurs resulting in bacteremia. These pathogens reinfect lymphoid tissue and liberate endotoxin leading to delayed hypersensitivity reaction. After a few days of bacteremia, the bacteria localize in lymphoid tissue of small intestine, mesenteric nodes, gallbladder, spleen and liver. Typically, lesions are seen in Peyer's patches and follicles.

Tubercular Ulcer of Small Intestine

Description: Mounted specimen of small intestine in a jar showing following features:

- Multiple large ulcers on the mucosa of small intestine.

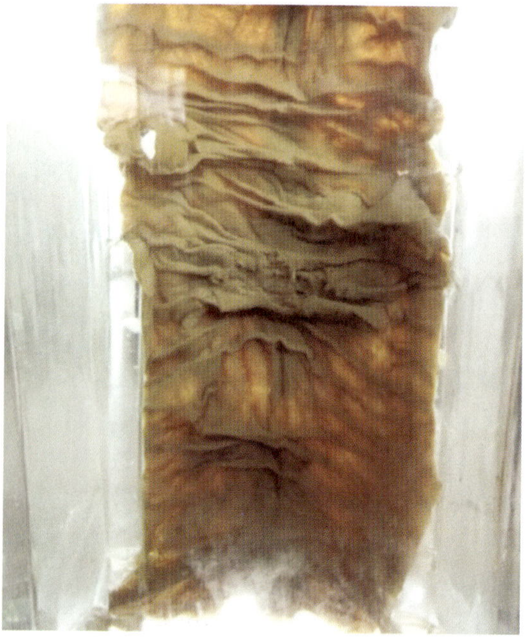

Fig. 17.15: Tubercular ulcer of small intestine

- Long axis of ulcers oriented transversely to the intestinal axis.
- Margins are irregular and may encircle the intestine (circumferential).
- Size of ulcers are large.
- Stricture formation and narrowing of intestinal lumen seen.
- Peyer's patches are not prominent.

Diagnosis: Tubercular ulcer of small intestine.

Q. What are the different ulcerative lesions of small intestine?

Ans: Peptic ulcer in duodenum, typhoid ulcer, tubercular ulcer, Crohn's disease and bacillary dysentery ulcers.

Q. What are the differences between typhoid ulcer and tubercular ulcer of small intestine?

Ans:

Q. What are the different types of intestinal tuberculosis?

Ans:

i. **Primary intestinal tuberculosis**: Mycobacterium tubercle bacilli (bovis strain) reach the intestine due to ingestion of unpasteurized milk. Draining lymph nodes of small intestine are enlarged which may be matted with caseous necrosis, known as **tabes mesenterica**. Most of them heals by fibrosis and dystrophic calcification.

ii. **Secondary tuberculosis**: The pathogens (*M. tuberculosis*) enter the intestine by swallowing of infected sputum in a case of pulmonary tuberculosis. Intestinal lesions are prominent compared to draining lymph nodes.

Parameters	Typhoid ulcer	Tubercular ulcer
• Causative organism	*Salmonella typhi*	*Mycobacterium tuberculosis* bacilli
• Site of involvement	Terminal ileum (most common), also jejunum or colon	Ileo-caecal region
• Axis of ulcer	Longitudinal axis of intestine	Transverse axis of intestine
• Size of ulcer	Small	Large
• Base of ulcer	Black due to sloughing of mucosa	Creamy white due to presence of caseous material
• Margin	Regular well circumscribed	Irregular and may encircle gut (circumferential)
• Bleeding from ulcer	Common	Absent
• Stricture formation	Absent	Present due to fibrosis
• Perforation of ulcer	Common	Absent
• Light microscopy	Erythrophagocytosis and presence of pathogens in macrophages. Absence of neutrophils	Epithelioid granulomas, Langhans and foreign body type giant cells, caseous necrosis. Zn stain shows AFB
• Lymphoid involvement	Peyer's patches—follicles and regional lymph nodes	Lymph nodes in primary and Peyer's patches in secondary tuberculosis

Q. What are the complications of tubercular ulcer?

Ans: Stricture, peforation and fistula are known complications.

Q. What is hyperplastic ileocaecal tuberculosis?

Ans: It is variant of intestinal TB characterized by thickening of terminal ileum, caecum and ascending colon along with mucosal ulceration. Clinically, a mass is papable and may be misdiagnosed as ileocaecal carcinoma.

Colorectal Cancer (Rectosigmoid)

Description: Mounted specimen of cut open sigmoid colon and rectum in a jar showing following features:

- A circumferential annular/napkin ring configuration mass is seen in the rectosigmoid region.
- Tumour is firm with gray-white appearance.

Diagnosis: Carcinoma of rectosigmoid.

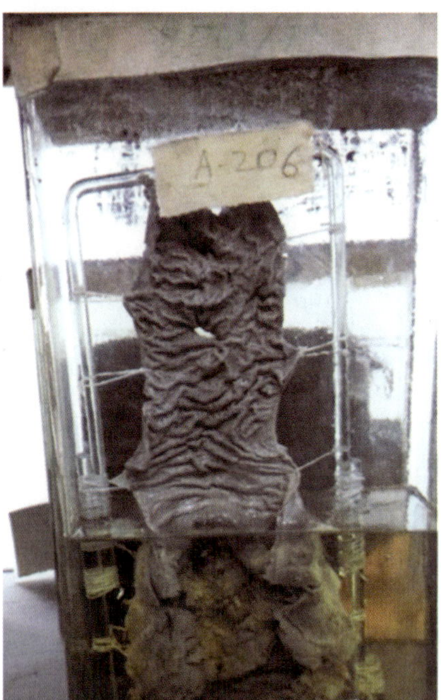

Fig. 17.16: Rectosigmoid cancer

Colorectal Cancer (Colon)

Description: Mounted specimen of cut open ascending colon and part of transverse colon in a jar showing following features:

- An ulceroproliferative, exophytic polypoid mass is seen in the ascending colon.
- Crater-like ulcerations with raised margins are noted.
- The mass is cauliflower-like, soft and friable projecting into the lumen.

Diagnosis: Carcinoma of colon.

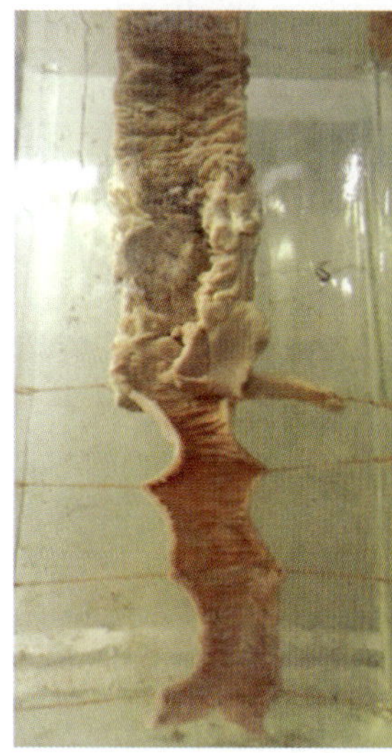

Fig. 17.17: Colon cancer

Q. What are the risk factors for colorectal cancer?

Ans: Elderly persons, familial adenomatosis polyposis, inflammatory bowel disease; dietary factors (consumption of excessive red meat, animal fat, refined carbohydrate), NSAIDs, obesity, tobacco smoking and chronic alcoholism.

Q. What are the common sites of colorectal cancer?

Ans: Rectosigmoid is the commonest site (38%) followed by sigmoid colon (20%), descending colon (10%), caecum (8%), hepatic flexure (8%), transverse colon (5%), ascending colon (3%) and anus (3%).

Q. What are the differences between right- sided and left-sided colorectal carcinoma?
Ans:

Parameters	Right-sided colorectal carcinoma	Left-sided colorectal carcinoma
• Site	Caecum and ascending colon	Rectosigmoid area and descending colon
• Growth pattern	Ulceroproliferative, exophytic, polypoid soft to firm mass	Circumferential, napkin-ring firm mass
• Invasiveness	More invasive	Less invasive
• Involvement of other structures	Common like mesentery, lymph nodes, distant metastasis	Lesson common
• Clinical presentation	Silent and diagnosed late	Obstructive features, so diagnosed early
• Prognosis	Poor	Good

KIDNEY (RENAL) SPECIMENS

Granular Contracted Kidney

Outer surface showing granularity and inner surface (cut section)

Description: Mounted specimens of cut section of kidneys in a jar showing following features:

- Kidneys are symmetrically contracted.
- Surface is finely granular.
- Capsule is adherent to cortex.
- Cortex is thin with an increase in peri-pelvic fat.
- Consistency seems to be firm.

Diagnosis: Granular contracted kidney.

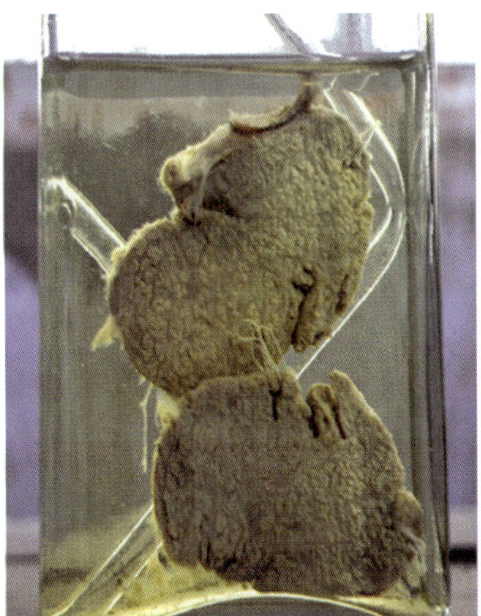

A Outer surface showing granularity

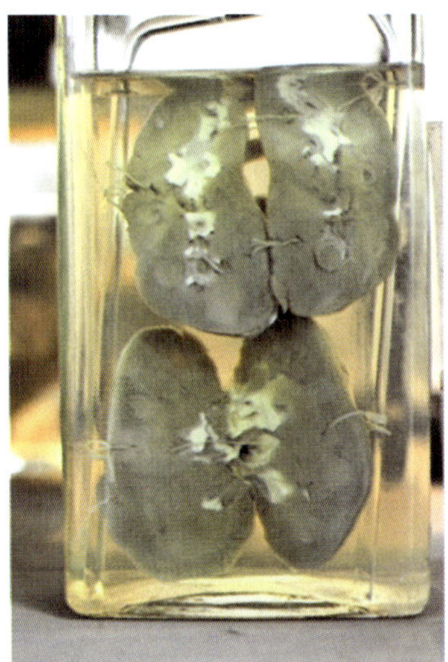

B Inner surface (cut section)

Fig. 17.18A and B: Granular contracted kidney

Q. What are the causes of granular contracted kidney?

Ans:

i. Chronic glomerulonephritis
ii. Chronic pyelonephritis (U-shaped scar)
iii. Benign nephrosclerosis (benign hypertension, V-shaped scar)
iv. Less common causes are diabetic nephropathy, myeloma kidney and amyloid kidney.

Q. What are the differences between chronic glomerulonephritis and chronic pyelonephritis?

Ans:

Large White Kidney (RPGN)

Description: Mounted specimen of kidney in a jar showing following features:

- Kidney is enlarged, pale and soft
- Surface is smooth
- Capsule is thin
- Petechial (pin-point) haemorrhages seen or cortical surface

Diagnosis: Large white kidney (rapidly progressive glomerulonephritis)

Q. What are the causes of large white kidney (RPGN)?

Ans: RPGN may be classified into 3 groups as per causes

Parameters	Chronic glomerulonephritis	Chronic pyelonephritis
• Causes	Different types of glomerulonephritis	Reflux nephropathy or chronic obstructive pyelonephritis
• Pathogenesis	End stage glomerular disease due to specific glomerulonephritis	Chronic tubulointerstitial inflammation and fibrosis associated with renal disease
• Gross appearance of kidney surface	Diffusely, granular, cortical surfaces	Depressed area on dilated and blunted calyx
• Nature of scar	Fine and symmetrical	Coarse and asymmetrical
• Glomeruli	Reduced in number and atrophic	Normal; may show periglomerular fibrosis
• Tubules	Atrophied	Atrophy in some and hypertrophy in others. Filled with colloid casts (thyroidisation)
• Interstitial and periglomerular fibrosis	Mild	More severe
• Renal calyx and pelvis	Normal	Dilated
• Clinical features	Onset is insidious. Proteinuria, oedema, azotemia, hypertension	May be asymptomatic. Some present with back pain, fever, pyuria, polyuria, nocturia, bacteria, with gradual onset of hypertension and renal insufficiency

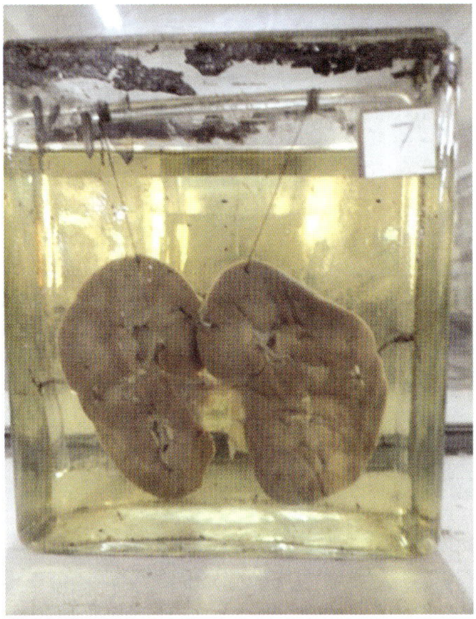

Fig. 17.19: Large white kidney

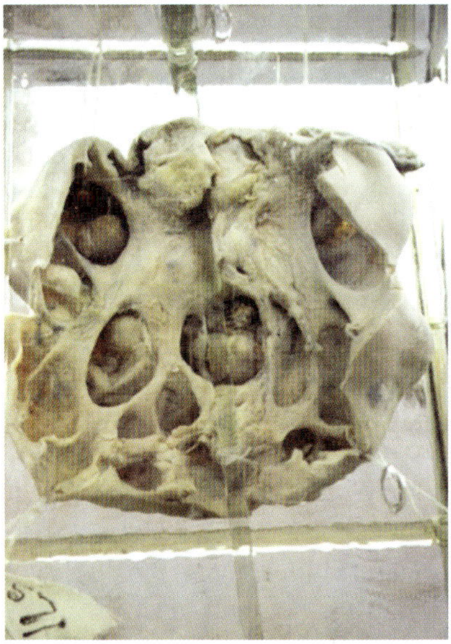

Fig. 17.20: Hydronephrosis

i. Idiopathic RPGN: Nearly half of all cases
ii. Glomerulonephritis (GN) associated with systemic disease such as SLE, diabetes, polyarteritis nodosa and Goodpasture's syndrome.
iii. Postinfectious (post-streptococcal GN)

Other causes of large white kidney (uncommon): Membranous GN, membranoproliferative GN, amyloidosis.

Q. What are light microscopic features of RPGN?

Ans: Depending on underlying cause, the glomeruli may show diffuse or focal endothelial proliferation, mesangial proliferation and focal necrosis.

But the important finding is distinctive **crescents**. Crescents are formed by proliferation of parietal cells and migration of macrophages and monocytes into Bowman's (urinary) space. Fibrin strands are frequently seen between cellular layers of crescents.

Hydronephrosis

Description: Mounted specimen of cut section of kidney in a jar showing following features:

- Kidney is enlarged and outer surface is irregular.
- Multiple cystic cavities are seen in the cut surface which is present in the renal pelvis and calyces.
- Wall of these cystic spaces communicate with renal pelvis.
- Cyst wall is thin and devoid of congestion.
- Many of these cystic spaces contain whitish stones.
- Cortex and renal tissue are compressed and atrophic.

Diagnosis: Hydronephrosis with renal stones.

Q. What is hydronephrosis?

Ans: It is the permanent dilation of the renal pelvis and calyces associated with progressive atrophy of the kidney due to obstruction to the outflow of urine.

Q. Why these multiple cysts are not part of polycystic kidney?

Ans: Here, these cysts communicate with renal pelvis. But in polycystic kidney, the cysts do not communicate with renal pelvis.

Also, here stones within cystic spaces are found, which are the cause of obstruction and leading to hydronephrosis.

Q. What are the causes of hydronephrosis?
Ans:

i. Renal pelvis: Calculi, tumours, uretero-pelvic stricture
ii. Intrinsic ureter: Calculi, tumours, blood clot, inflammation
iii. Extrinsic ureter: Tumour compression (e.g cervix), pregnancy, retroperitoneal fibrosis
iv. Urinary bladder: Vesicoureteral reflux, calculi, tumours, neurogenic
v. Prostate: Hyperplasia (BHP), carcinoma, prostatitis
vi. Urethra: Posterior valve stricture, rarely tumours

Q. What is flea-beaten kidney? What are the causes?

Ans: Kidney is enlarged. The cortex shows tiny petechial haemorrhage visible through capsule giving the characteristic appearance of flea-bitten kidney. Cut surface also shows this haemorrhage.

Causes are: Acute post-streptococcal glomerulonephritis, malignant nephrosclerosis, rapidly progressive GN (RPGN), haemolytic-uraemic syndrome, thrombotic thrombocytopenic purpura and Henoch-Schönlein purpura.

Polycystic Kidney

Description: Mounted specimen of cut section of kidney in a jar showing following features:

- Kidney shows marked multicystic nodulations with transparent walls, visible on surface.
- Both small and large cysts are seen resembling bunches of grapes.
- In cut section, almost entire renal parenchyma (both cortex and medulla) is replaced by multiple smooth-walled dilated cysts.

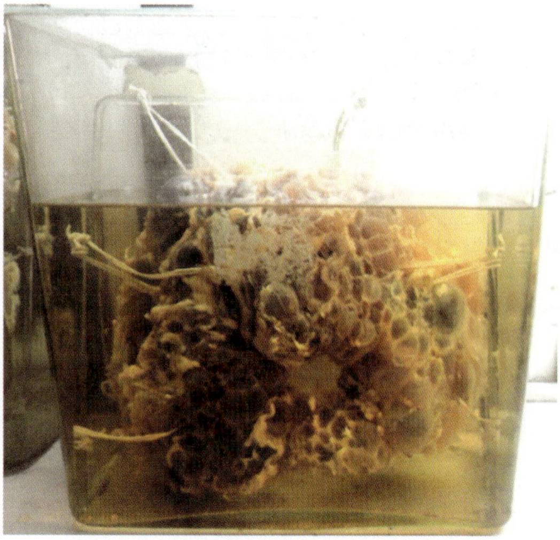

Fig. 17.21: Polycystic kidney

- All these cysts fail to communicate with renal pelvis and renal pelvis is not dilated.
- Occasional cysts communicate with each other producing a larger cyst.
- Renal tissue presents in-between the cysts is compressed and atrophic.

Diagnosis: Polycystic kidney: Adult type

Q. What are the different types of cysts in kidney?

Ans: Polycystic kidney disease, renal dysplasia, medullary cystic disease, acquired (dialysis-associated) cystic disease, simple renal cyst, renal cysts in hereditary malformation syndrome (e.g. tuberous sclerosis), glomerulocystic disease.

Q. What are differences between adult and childhood polycystic kidney disease?

Ans: Adult polycystic kidney disease (ADPKD) is autosomal dominant and mutations in gene located on chromosome 16p13.3 (PKD1) and 4q21 (PKD).

Childhood polycystic kidney disease (CHPKD) is autosomal recessive and mutations seen on chromosome region 6p21–p23 (PKHD1 gene).

Also, in CHPKD, the cysts are smaller which give the kidney a sponge-like appearance. Dilated elongated channels seen in CHPKD which are present at right angles to the cortical surface replacing the cortex and medulla.

Renal Cell Carcinoma (Hypernephroma)

Description: Mounted specimen of cut section of kidney in a jar showing following features:

- A solitary large well circumscribed rounded tumour is seen in the upper pole.
- The tumour has a variegated appearance due to areas of haemorrhage necrosis and cystic spaces (solid-cystic).
- Cut surface of the tumour is yellowish-gray or golden yellow in colour.
- Peripherally kidney tissue is compressed to form an incomplete capsule.

Diagnosis: Renal cell carcinoma (hypernephroma, Grawtiz's tumour)

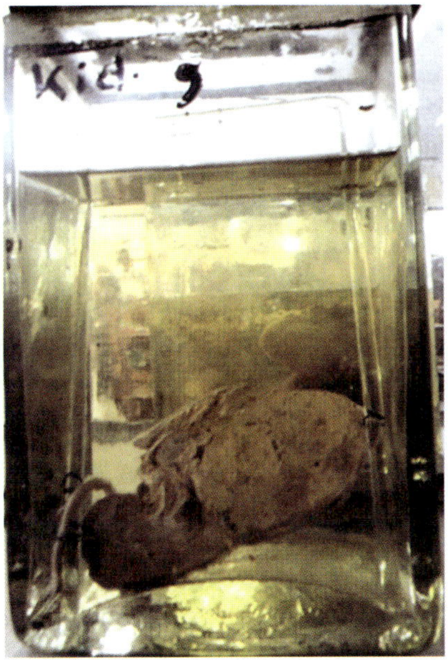

Fig. 17.22: Renal cell carcinoma

Q. What are the light microscopic features of renal cell carcinoma?

Ans: The most common variant is clear cell variant RCC (70–80%). Other variants are RCC papillary (chromophil) type (10–15%), RCC chromophobe type (5%), Bellini duct carcinoma (rare) and Xp11 translocation RCC (rare).

In clear cell carcinoma the tumour cells are arranged in sheets to trabecular (cord like) or tubular (resembling tubules) pattern. The tumour cells are round or polygonal in shape. They have abundant clear cytoplasm, which contains glycogen and lipid. The tumour has delicate branching vasculature. Centrally placed round nuclei with nucleoli seen with vasculature. Centrally placed round nuclei with nucleoli seen within tumour cells.

Q. What special stains may be used to demonstrate constituents in clear cytoplasm of carcinoma cells?

Ans: Tumour cells are rich in glycogen which may be demonstrated by PAS (Periodic acid–Schiff) stain on formalin-fixed paraffin-embedded (FFPE) tissue sections.

Lipids (fats) are dissolved during processing of tissue in paraffin-embedded tissue sections. Hence, cannot be demonstrated in FFPE. Lipids can be identified by frozen section technique by applying fat stains (Sudan III, Sudan IV, Sudan black or Oil red O). There is no mucin in the cytoplasm of the tumour cells.

Q. What are the classic diagnostic features of RCC?

Ans: There are three classic diagnostic features: Haematuria, palpable renal mass and costovertebral pain. But these features combinedly seen only in 10% of cases. Haematuria which is intermittent in nature is the most reliable feature of these triads.

Renal Tuberculosis

Description: Mounted specimen of cut section of kidney in a jar showing following features:

- Kidney is slightly enlarged
- Cut section shows foci of caseous with formation of cavities in some. The caseous

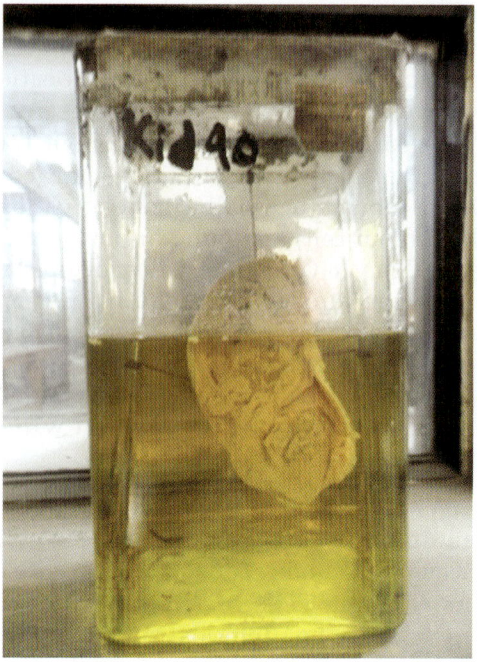

Fig. 17.23: Renal tuberculosis

areas are seen specially near base of pyramid. Wall of the cavities is irregular and caseous.
- Caseous material present within the cavities.
- Renal capsule and perinephric fat are adherent.

Diagnosis: Renal tuberculosis (caseous type)

Q. What are the different morphological types of renal tuberculosis?

Ans:
- Acute miliary tuberculosis
- Chronic ulcerative and caseous type
- Tuberculous pyonephrosis

Q. What is the pathogenesis of renal tuberculosis?

Ans: It is usually blood-borne and almost always secondary to an active tuberculosis lesion elsewhere. Infection starts at renal cortex and then it spreads to glomeruli. Later on, tuberculosis bacilli may progress to the adjacent tubules and peritubular tissues.

Q. What are urinary findings in renal tuberculosis?

Ans: Urine analysis reveals acidic pH, proteinuria and pus cells. It can cause asymptomatic pyuria or it may produce **sterile pyuria** (no organism detected in ordinary culture medium). LJ media or Bactec culture media will demonstrate *M. tuberculosis*.

BONE

Osteomyelitis and Sequestrum

Description: Mounted specimen of tibia in a jar showing following features:
- Tubular tibial bone with fragile bone and a large hole **(cloaca)**.
- Dry, irregular piece of dead bone with granular surface **(sequestrum)** is seen through cloaca.
- Also seen sheath of living reactive oven or lamellar bone deposited around sequestrum. This is **involucrum**.

Diagnosis: Osteomyelits with sequestrum.

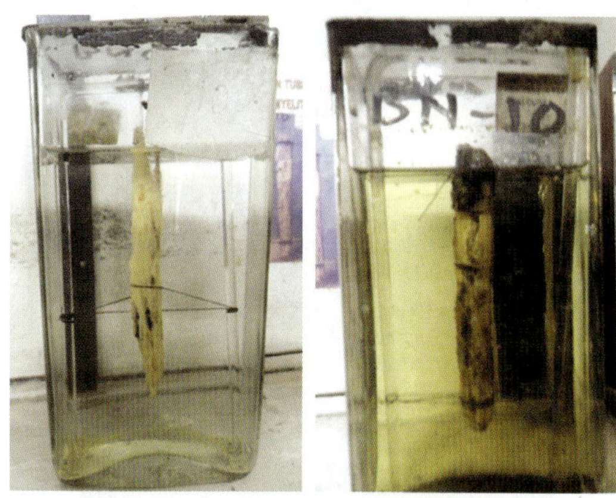

A B

Fig. 17.24A and B: Chronic osteomyelitis and sequestrum

Q. What is sequestrum?

Ans: Due to rigid structure and limited space with bone, inflammatory exudates in bone cavity compress the endosteal blood vessels and impair the blood flow to the bone.

As a result erosion, thinning and infarction necrosis of cortical bone occurs which is known as **sequestrum.** Frequently, this dead bone detaches from main bone and floats inside the abscess cavity due to action of lytic enzymes.

Q. What is involucrum?

Ans: With passage of time, there is new bone formation beneath the periosteum over the infected bone which is known as **involucrum.** This involucrum has irregular surface and has perforations through which discharging sinus tract pass.

Q. What is Brodie's abscess?

Ans: Sometimes, acute osteomyelitis may be contained (limited) to a localized area and walled off by fibrous tissue and granulation tissue. This is known as Brodie's abscess.

Q. What are the causative organisms of osteomyelitis?

Ans: Pyogenic osteomyelitis is caused by *Staphylococcus aureus* (commonly), *E. coli*, Pseudomonas, Klebsiella and anaerobes. Tuberculous osteomyelitis is caused by *Mycobacterium tuberculosis*. Osteomyelitis also may occur in systemic infectious diseases like enteric fever (typhoid), actinomycosis, mycetoma (Madura foot), syphilis and brucellosis.

Q. What are the common sites of osteomyelitis?

Ans: It primarily affects the metaphyseal area of long bones of extremities around knee, hip and ankle joints. Tuberculous osteomyelitis usually involves vertebral column and less commonly hip bone, long bones (femur, tibia) and small bones of hands and feet.

TB (Tuberculosis) Spine

Description: Mounted specimen of a portion of spine (hemisection) in a jar showing following features:

- Destruction of a part of vertebral body and intervertebral disc.

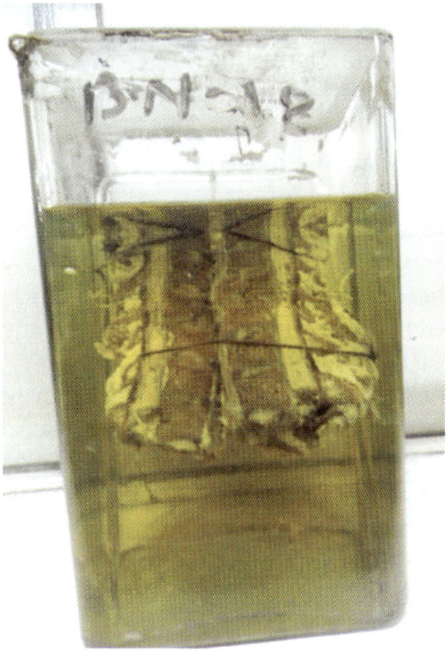

Fig. 17.25: TB spine

- The lesion starts in the bodies and spread through medullary cavity and breaks through intervertebral discs involving multiple vertebrae.
- It also extends into soft tissues forming cold abscess.
- The affected vertebrae are weak and tend to collapse, producing an acute anteflexion or angular kyphosis.
- Intervertebral space is diminished.

Diagnosis: Tuberculosis of spine (Pott's disease) with kyphosis.

Q. What is Caries spine or Pott's disease?

Ans: Tuberculosis of spine is known as Pott's disease. It often commences in the vertebral body and may be associated with compression fractures and destruction of intervertebral discs, producing permanent damage and paraplegia.

Q. What is cold abscess?

Ans: Extension of caseous material and pus from vertebrae (commonly lumbar) to the sheaths of psoas muscle produces cold abscess or psoas abscess.

Osteogenic Sarcoma

Description: Mounted specimen of lower end of femur in a jar showing following features:

- A bulk gray-white solid mass is seen at the lower end of femur.
- Cut surface is grayish-white with areas of haemorrhage and necrosis.
- The cortical bone is involved and destroyed. The tumour involves the medullary cavity.
- The tumour looks fleshy with irregular fusiform shape and located at the end of a long bone (femur) gives the lesion so-called **'leg of mutton' appearance**.
- Periosteum is elevated due to pressure of growth producing a triangle—**Codman's triangle.**

Diagnosis: Osteogenic sarcoma of femur (conventional intramedullary).

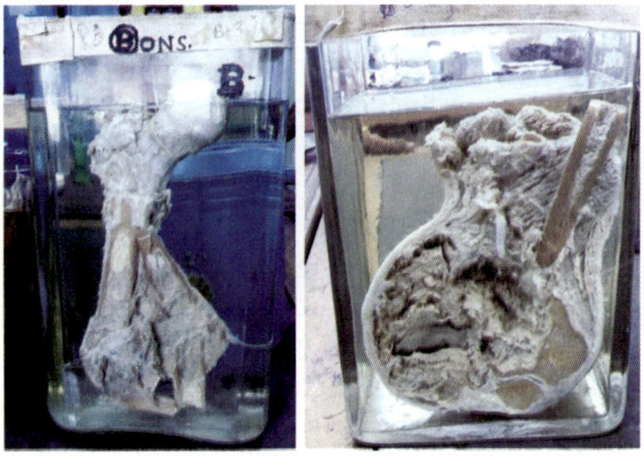

A B

Fig. 17.26A and B: Osteogenic sarcoma

Q. What are the types of osteosarcoma as per site of origin?

Ans: Osteosarcomas are classified into 3 types: Intramedullary, intracortical, surface.

Q. What are the different histologic variants?

Ans: Conventional type (osteoblastic, chondroblastic, fibroblastic); telangiectatic, small cell, giant cell, fibrohistiocytic, anaplastic and well differentiated osteosarcoma.

Q. What are the sites of osteosarcoma?

Ans: Most common sites, in descending order of frequency, lower end of femur and upper end of tibia (i.e. around the knee joint about 80%); the upper end of humerus (10%), pelvis and upper end of femur (i.e. around hip joint about 15%); and less often in jaw bones, skull and vertebrae.

Q. What is secondary osteosarcoma?

Ans: It develops following pre-existing bone disease, e.g. Paget's disease of bone, fibrous dysplasia, chronic osteomyelitis, multiple osteochondromas, bone infarcts and prior irradiation.

Giant Cell Tumour of Bone (Osteoclastoma)

Description: Mounted specimen of lower end of radius and ulna in a jar showing following features:

- A fusiform growth involving lower end of radius and ulna (epiphysis).
- The growth is red-brown, friable mass with areas of cystic degeneration due to necrosis.
- Foci of haemorrhage and necrosis seen.
- Due to presence of many small cystic spaces (degeneration), it has a honeycomb appearance.
- Cortex is thinned and eroded.

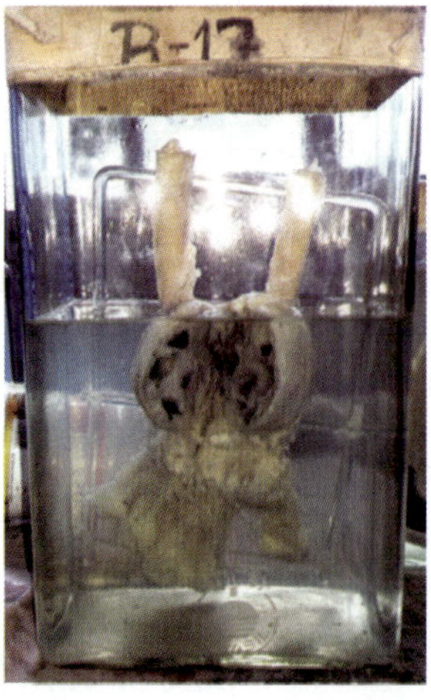

Fig. 17.27: Giant cell tumour of bone (osteoclastoma)

Diagnosis: Giant cell tumour of bone (osteoclastoma).

Q. What are the light microscopic features of GCT?

Ans: It is a biphasic tumour-composed of mononuclear stromal cells and multinucleated giant cells. The mononuclear stromal cells (tumour cells) are round to oval in shape, uniform with indistinct cell membrane. Multinucleated giant cells of osteoclastic type (>100 nuclei) are uniformly scattered among mononuclear stromal cells. The nuclei of stromal cells have identical features to that of the mononuclear cells.

Q. What are the common sites of GCT?

Ans: GCT arises in the epiphysis of long bones close to the articular cartilage. Most common sites are lower end of femur, upper end of tibia, lower end of radius and upper end of fibula.

Q. What are the other giant cells containing benign bone tumours?

Ans: Aneurysmal bone cyst, chondroblastoma, metaphyseal fibrous defect (non-ossifying fibroma), simple bone cyst, brown tumour of hyperparathyroidism, giant cell reparative granuloma and chondromyxoid fibroma.

Q. What are the radiographic findings?

Ans: On radiography, GCT gives **soap-bubble appearance**. It shows a large osteolytic eccentric lesion, which erodes into the subendosteal bone plate.

FEMALE GENITAL AND BREAST SPECIMENS

Fibroid Uterus (Leiomyoma)

Description: Mounted specimen of uterus in a jar showing following features:

- Hemisection of uterus and cervix showing one large nodular growth.
- These growths are well-circumscribed, whitish, glistening and encircled by fibrous capsule.

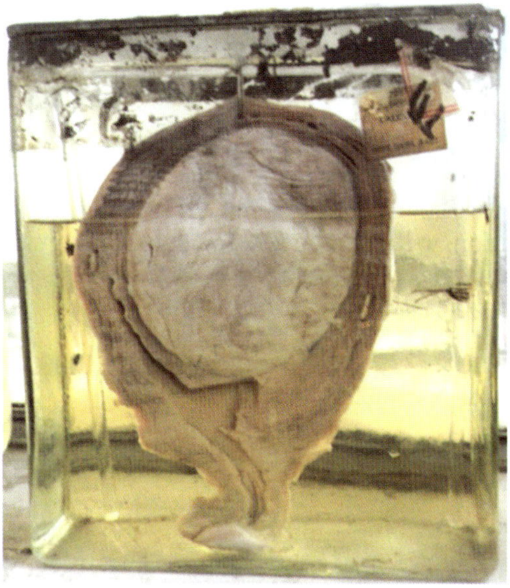

Fig. 17.28: Fibroid uterus

- These nodules have a typical whorled or so-called **'watered silk' appearances**.
- This growth is found within myometrium (intramural).
- Rest of the uterine muscle appears to be reddish-brown.

Diagnosis: Fibroid (leiomyoma) of uterus.

Q. What are the common sites of leiomyoma?

Ans: Most commonly it occurs in the uterus. It also occurs in the cervix, broad-ligament, ovary, gastrointestinal tract, retroperitoneum, skin, etc.

Q. What are the light microscopic features?

Ans: Leiomyoma (fibroid) comprised of whorled bundles of well differentiated smooth muscle cells. Individual smooth muscle cells are uniform in size and shape containing oval nucleus and long slender bipolar cytoplasmic processes. Mitotic figures are sparse (rare).

Q. What are the other histological variants apart from common form?

Ans: Cellular leiomyoma or apoleptic leiomyoma, symplastic (bizarre) leiomyoma, epithelioid leiomyoma, lipoleiomyoma, benign metastasizing leiomyoma and disseminated peritoneal leiomyomatosis.

Q. What are the secondary changes in leiomyoma (fibroid)?

Ans: These are hyaline change/degeneration, yellow-brown to red softening (cystic degeneration), atrophy, fatty change, red degeneration, dystrophic calcification and chondroid/osseous metaplasia.

Hyaline degeneration is the commonest secondary change in leiomyoma.

Carcinoma of Cervix

Description: Mounted specimen of uterus and cervix in a jar showing following features:

- A gray-white exophytic solid mass which projects above the surrounding mucosa.
- The surface is irregular
- The tumour involves the ectocervix and also lower part of endocervix.

Diagnosis: Carcinoma of cervix.

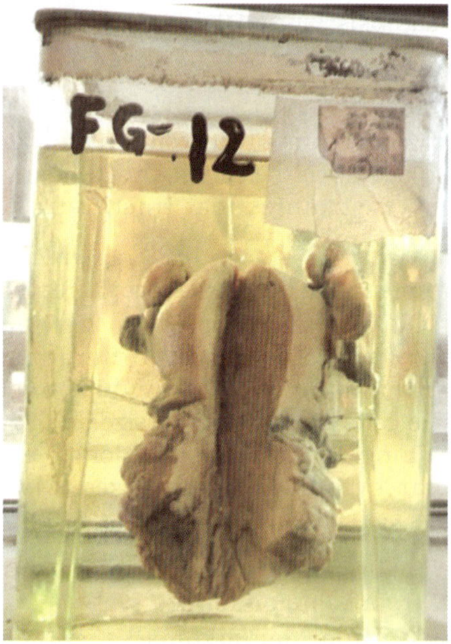

Fig. 17.29: Carcinoma of cervix

Q. What are the histologic variants of carcinoma of cervix?

Ans: Squamous cell carcinoma (80–90%), adenocarcinoma (10–20%), adenosquamous carcinoma (4%) and small cell carcinoma (rare).

Q. What are the risk factors for cervical carcinoma?

Ans:

i. Early sexual activity <16 years of age with multiple sexual partners.
ii. Human papillomavirus (HPV), type 16, 18, 31, 33; oncoproteins E6 and E7.
iii. Herpes simplex virus II and HPV: Synergetic.
iv. Molecular genetics: Mutation of p53 and RB tumour suppressor gene by HPV (16, 18, 31, 33) oncoproteins E6 and E7.
v. Cigarette smoking, immunosuppression, multiple pregnancies and oral contraceptive use.

Q. What are the modes of spread of cervical carcinoma?

Ans:

i. Lymphatic route: To pelvic lymph nodes (paracervical, obturator, external iliac, internal iliac, common iliac and aortic lymph nodes).
ii. Direct invasion: To parametrium. Compression of ureter.
iii. Haematogenous route: Distant metastases to lung, liver, bones and brain.

Dermoid (Teratoma) Tumour of Ovary

Description: Mounted specimen of already cut open ovarian cyst in a jar showing following features:

- External surface is smooth and ovary is enlarged.
- Already cut open ovary, showing a multilocular cyst containing sebaceous, greasy pultaceous/chessy material and tufts of hairs.
- Teeth are present in a well-defined nipple-like structure covered with hair, known as **Rokitansky's protuberance**.
- One firm to hard bony area is also present.

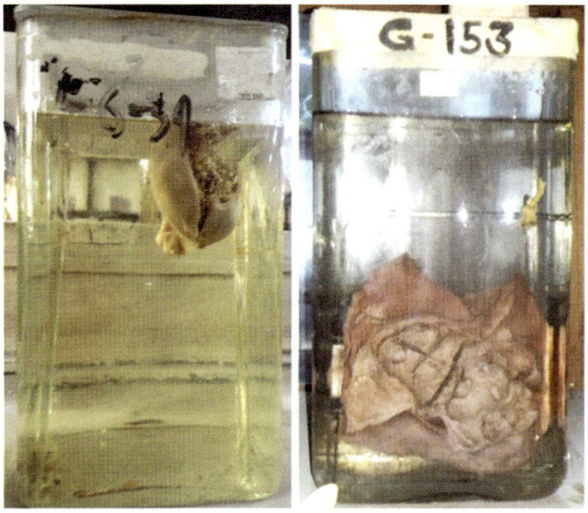

A B

Fig. 17.30A and B: Dermoid (teratoma) of ovary

Diagnosis: Mature cystic teratoma (dermoid cyst) of ovary.

Q. What are the light microscopic features of mature cystic teratoma?

Ans: The cyst is lined by stratified squamous epithelium, sebaceous glands, hair shaft and other adnexal structures. Many tumours also exhibit cartilage, bone, teeth, smooth muscles and respiratory epithelium.

Q. What is immature teratoma?

Ans: This teratoma is composed of a mixture of embryonal and adult tissues derived from all three germ layers. Embryonal component of the tumour resembles tissues from an embryo or fetus. Immature cartilage, glands, muscle, bone and neural rosettes are present.

Q. What is malignant transformation of mature cystic teratoma?

Ans: Rarely (<1%) mature cystic teratoma may undergo malignant transformation. Malignancy is usually squamous cell carcinoma followed by carcinoid tumour, adenocarcinoma, thyroid carcinoma, melanoma, osteosarcoma, carcinosarcoma or glioblastoma multiforme.

Q. What are the other sites of teratoma?

Ans: Sacrococcygeal teratoma is the commonest site for embryonal teratoma and single most common tumour found in newborns of humans. Other sites are mediastinum, retroperitoneum, floor of mouth, urinary bladder, kidney, nasopharynx and base of skull.

Carcinoma of Breast

Description: Mounted specimen of breast (mastectomy) in a jar showing following features:

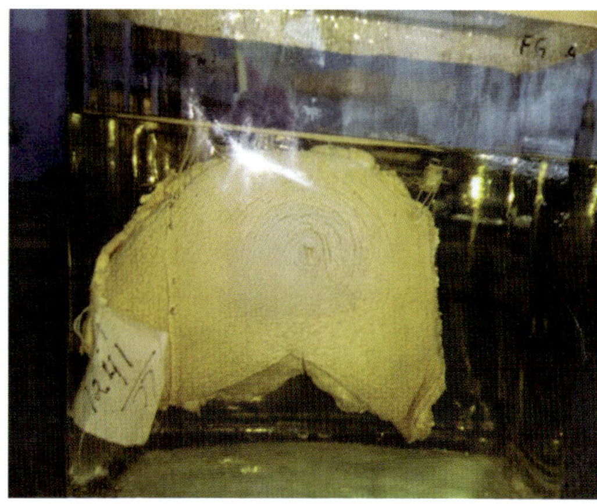

A

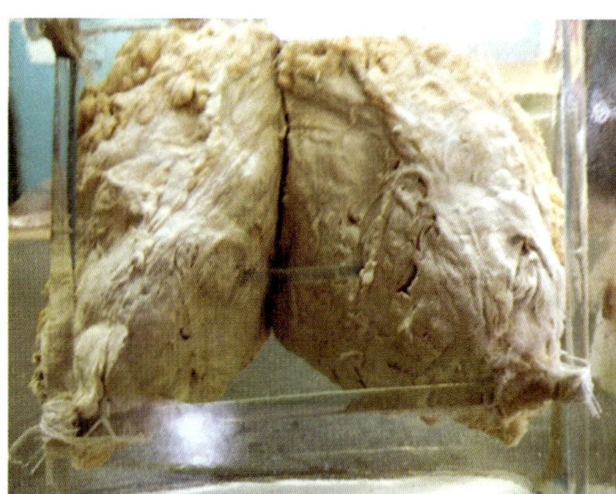

B

Fig. 17.31A and B: Carcinoma of breast

- A solid grayish-yellow growth is seen.
- The growth is irregular, poorly circumscribed and poorly defined margins.
- Foci of haemorrhage and necrosis are present.
- The growth extends or radiates through surrounding parenchyma into fat (crab-like configuration)
- Nipple is retracted.

Diagnosis: Carcinoma of breast.

Q. What are the different histologic types of breast carcinoma?

Ans: It can be classified into two broad groups:

i. **Carcinoma *in situ* (15–30%)**: Ductal carcinoma *in situ* (80%) and lobular carcinoma *in situ* (20%)
ii. **Invasive carcinoma (70–85%):** No special-type carcinoma (79%), lobular carcinoma (10%), tubular/cribriform carcinoma (6%), mucinous (colloid) carcinoma (2%), medullary carcinoma (2%), papillary carcinoma (1%), metaplastic carcinoma (<1%).

Q. What are the common locations of breast carcinoma?

Ans: In decreasing frequency it is located in upper outer quadrant (50%), central region beneath nipple (20%), lower outer quadrant (10%), upper inner quadrant (10%) and lower inner quadrant (10%) respectively.

Q. What are the risk factors of breast cancers?

Ans: Older age (>50 years), family history of breast cancer, genetic mutations (such as BRCA1 and BRCA2), early menarche (<12 years), late menopause (>55 years), late or no pregnancy, taking oral contraceptive pills, using combination therapy as hormone replacement, drinking alcohol, smoking, physical inactivity, obesity after menopause, etc.

Q. What are the major prognostic factors?

Ans:

i. Tumour size: <1 cm good prognosis, >2 cm bad prognosis
ii. Invasive carcinoma has worse prognosis than *in situ* carcinoma
iii. Involvement of axillary lymph nodes is associated with worse prognosis.
iv. Distant metastasis indicates bad prognosis.
v. Inflammatory carcinoma carries poor prognosis
vi. Local invasion into adjacent skeletal muscle carries poor prognosis.

Q. What are the good prognostic factors?

Ans: Age group 30–50 years, early diagnosis, early treatment, certain histologic types (ductal carcinoma *in situ*, lobular carcinoma *in situ*, low grade invasive ductal carcinoma (NOS)—luminal type A, cribriform carcinoma—luminal type A, tubular carcinoma—luminal type A, papillary carcinoma, colloid carcinoma), negative expression of C-erB2, p53, Srp27, cathepsin D and EGFR, tumor size <2 cm, estrogen and progesterone receptor positivity.

MALE GENITAL SPECIMENS

Carcinoma of Penis

Description: Mounted specimen of penis in a jar has following features:

- A large cauliflower-like fungating mass having rolled out and everted margin.
- The mass arises from the glans penis and inner surface of the prepuce.
- The surface of the mass is ulcerated
- Resected margin of penis (opposite side of growth) is grossly unremarkable.

Diagnosis: Carcinoma of penis (squamous cell carcinoma)

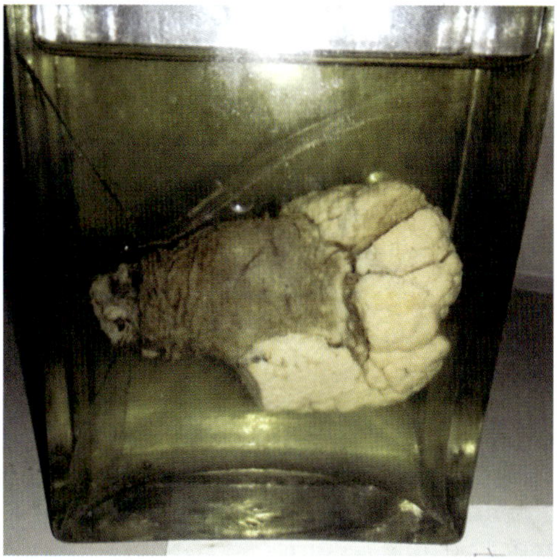

Fig. 17.32: Carcinoma of penis

Q. What are the risk factors of carcinoma of penis?

Ans: HPV type 16, type 18 and cigarette smoking are risk factors. HPV DNA can be detected in penile squamous cell carcinoma in about 50% of patients.

Males with bad genital hygiene and without circumcision have more chances to exposure to carcinogens and subsequently developing carcinoma of penis.

Q. What is verrucous carcinoma?

Ans: This is an exophytic well-differentiated variant of squamous cell carcinoma which has low malignant potential. These tumours are locally invasive but they rarely metastasize.

Q. What are the histologic subtypes of squamous cell carcinoma?

Ans: Keratinising squamous cell carcinoma (SCC), non-keratinising SCC, basaloid SCC, warty carcinoma and papillary variants of SCC.

Seminoma of Testis

Description: Mounted specimen of bisected testis in a jar has following features:

- Large homogeneous gray-white mass.
- The mass has lobulated cut surface.
- No haemorrhage or necrosis.
- Tunica albuginea is not penetrated by the tumour.

Diagnosis: Seminoma of testis.

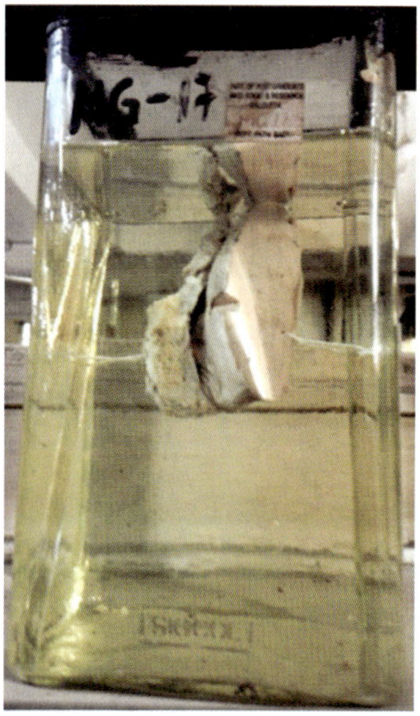

Fig. 17.33: Seminoma of testis

Q. What are the histologic variants of seminoma?

Ans: Classic seminoma is the most common variant (85–90%) of all cases. Other variants are anaplastic seminoma, spermatocytic seminoma, seminoma with syncytiotrophoblastic element and seminoma with yolk sac element.

Q. What are the light microscopic features of classic seminoma?

Ans: Monomorphic polyhedral large cells arranged in sheets and divided by fibrous septa. The tumour cells have distinct cell membrane and abundant clear cytoplasm and a large central nucleus with one or two prominent nucleoli. The fibrous septa is infiltrated by lymphocytes. Mitoses are scant.

Occasionally granulomas with giant cells may be present.

Q. What are the routes of metastasis?

Ans:

i. Lymphatic route: To retroperitoneal/ para-aortic, mediastinal and supraclavicular lymph nodes.

ii. Blood or haematogenous route: To lungs, liver and brains.

Benign Hyperplasia of Prostate

Description: Mounted specimen of prostate in a jar having following features:

- Enlarged prostate with multiple gray-white rubbery nodules of variable sizes.
- Cut surface shows solid mass with a few microcysts.
- Nodules compress the urethra (prostatic) into a slit-like lumen.

Diagnosis: Benign hyperplasia of prostate (BHP) or nodular hyperplasia.

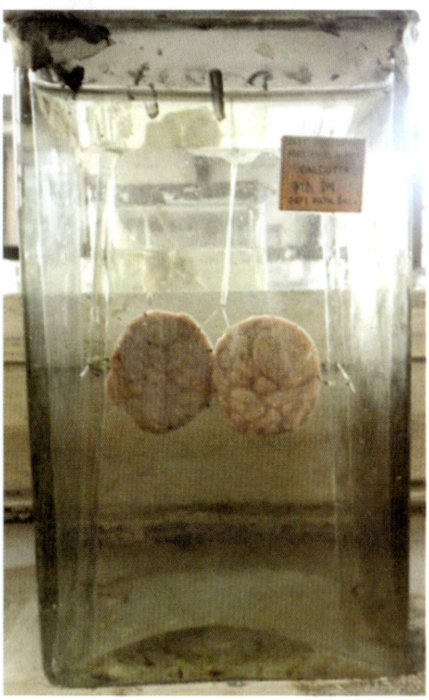

Fig. 17.34: Benign hyperplasia of prostate (BHP)

Q. What are the clinical features of BHP?

Ans: Male patients are usually elderly (>60 years). They experience increased urinary frequency, nocturia, difficulty and in starting and stopping the stream of urine, overflow dribbling, dysuria (painful micturition) and have an increased risk of developing bacterial infection of the bladder and kidney (UTI).

Q. What are the light microscopic features of BHP?

Ans: There is adenoleiomyomatous hyperplasia of prostate, i.e. hyperplasia of smooth muscles and glands. The glands are of different sizes and are lined by two layers of epithelium—inner columner and outer flattened myoepithelial cell layer (basal cell layer). Stroma is composed of fibromuscular tissue.

Q. Which zone is affected by BHP?

Ans: Prostate has 3 zones: Central zone, transition zone and peripheral zone. Transition zone is the site for BHP, whereas peripheral zone is the site for prostatic cancer.

HEPATOBILIARY SYSTEM SPECIMENS

Micronodular Cirrhosis

Description: Mounted specimen of liver in a jar has following features:

- Liver is shrunken and atrophic. Approximate weight would be 900 g (normal 1440–1660 g or 3.2–3.7 pounds).
- Surface is irregular and multiple small nodules of <3 mm in size are seen.
- Colour of liver is yellowish-orange.
- Consistency of liver is firm
- Gallbladder is seen in the gallbladder fossa of liver (inferior surface).

Diagnosis: Cirrhosis of liver (micronodular variant)

Q. What are the different types of cirrhosis based on morphology?

Ans: There are 3 types of cirrhosis:

i. Micronodular: Nodules measuring <3 mm in size.

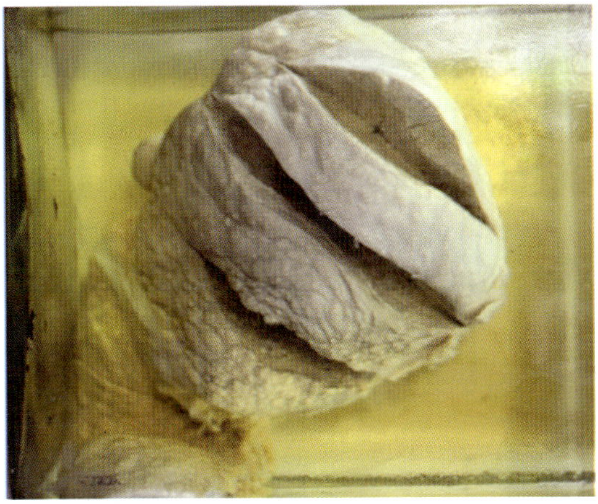

A

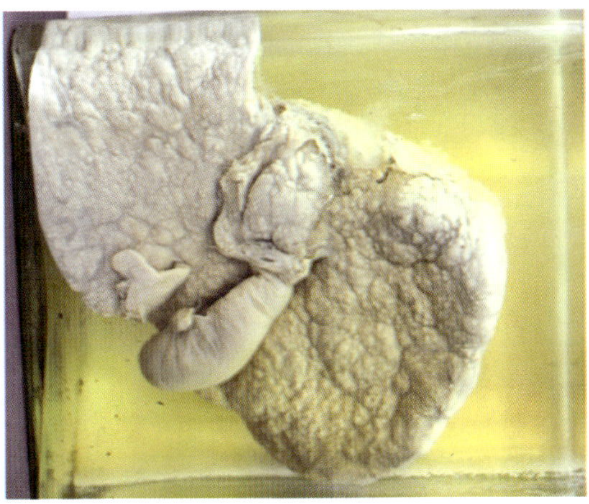

B

Fig. 17.35A and B: Micronodular cirrhosis

ii. Macronodular: Nodules measuring >3 mm in size.
iii. Mixed or micro-macronodular cirrhosis: Both micronodules (<3 mm) and macronodules (>3 mm) are present.

Q. What are the causes of micronodular cirrhosis?

Ans: Alcoholic cirrhosis, hereditary haemochromatosis, hepatic venous outflow obstruction (Budd-Chiari syndrome, veno-occlusive disease), large bile duct obstruction, Indian childhood cirrhosis, Hepatitis D.

Q. What are the causes of macronodular cirrhosis?

Ans: Alcohol, Chronic viral hepatitis (HBV or HCV), cryptogenic cirrhosis, Wilson's disease, α1-antitrypsin deficiency, drugs and toxins, primary biliary cirrhosis.

Q. What are the causes of mixed nodular cirrhosis?

Ans: Most common cause is alcoholic liver disease. Other causes are viral hepatitis (B, C, D), haemochromatosis, biliary disease and Wilsons's disease.

Q. What are the light microscopic features of cirrhosis?

Ans:

- Liver architecture is disrupted. Initially the developing fibrous septa are delicate and extend through sinusoids from central to portal tract or portal to portal tract.
- Regenerative activity of entrapped parenchymal hepatocytes generate uniform micronodules. Later on, these micronodules become larger and none prominent to produce macronodules. These scattered larger nodules create a 'hobnail' appearance on the surface of liver.
- Hepatocytes look normal in some nodules while they may be irregular with dysplastic changes in other nodules.

FATTY LIVER

Description: Mounted specimen of liver in a jar has following feature:

- The liver is enlarged and approximate weight is 5 kg.
- Liver is soft in consistency.
- It is yellow and greasy.

Diagnosis: Fatty liver

Q. What is microvesicular and macrovesicular hepatic steatosis (fatty liver)?

Ans: With moderate intake of alcohol, initially small droplets of lipid (triglyceride) accumulate within cytoplasm of hepatocytes and produce **microvesicular steatosis**.

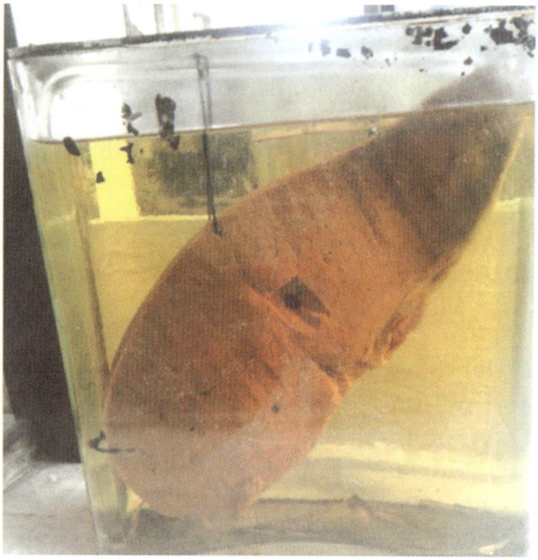

Fig. 17.36: Fatty liver

With chronic intake of alcohol, accumulated lipid droplets create large, clear globules that compress and displace the hepatocyte nucleus. These larger lipid droplets in cytoplasm produce **macrovesicular steatosis**.

Q. What are the causes of microvesicular steatosis?

Ans: Apart from alcoholism, other causes are tetracyclines, acute fatty liver of pregnancy, Reye's syndrome and hepatitis C.

Q. What are the causes of macrovesicular steatosis?

Ans: Apart from alcoholism (ethanol), other causes are obesity, diabetes, corticosteroids, methotrexate and total parenteral nutrition.

Q. What are the light microscopic features of fatty liver?

Ans: Initially there is a little or no fibrosis at the outset. But with continues alcohol intake (commonest cause) fibrous septa develop around the terminal hepatic veins and extend into the adjacent sinusoids. But this fatty change is completely reversible if the cause/injury is withdrawn (commonly alcohol intake).

Metastatic Liver

Description: Mounted specimen of cut section of liver in a jar has following features:

- Liver shows multiple nodular growths of different sizes.

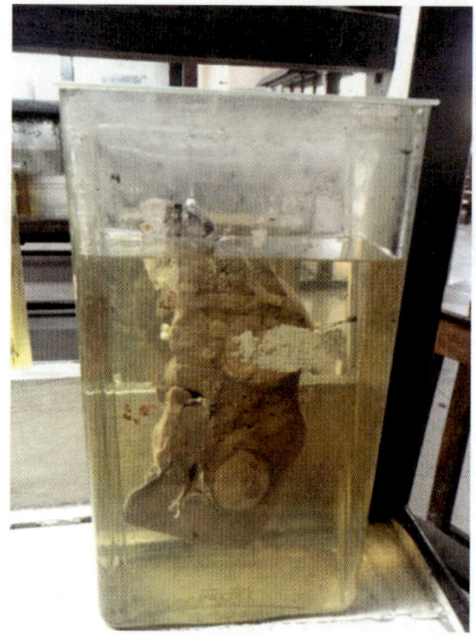

A

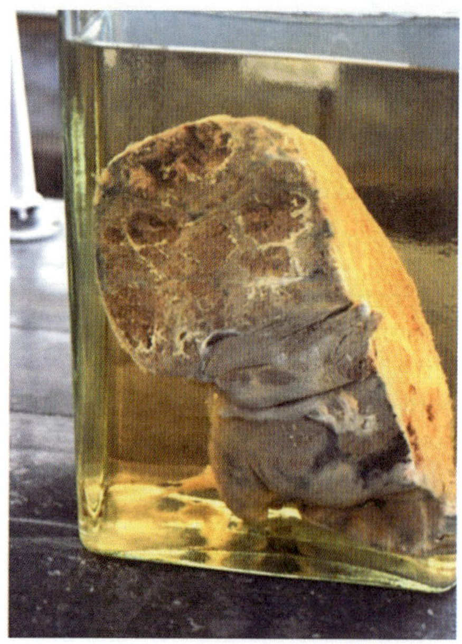

B

Fig. 17.37A and B: Metastatic liver

- These nodules are yellowish-white in colour.
- Central part of many of these nodules is depressed (umbilication).
- There are areas of haemorrhage (blackish) and necrosis.
- Cystic changes are also seen.

Diagnosis: Metastatic carcinoma of liver.

Q. What are the primary sites which cause liver metastasis?

Ans:

i. **Metastasis from epithelial cancer:** Breast, lung, stomach, colon, rectum, pancreas, kidney, prostate, endometrium, thyroid.

ii. **Metastasis from mesenchymal malignancies:** Angiosarcoma, rhabdomyosarcoma.

iii. **Metastasis from round cell tumours:** Wilms' tumour, neuroblastoma, Ewing's sarcoma, bronchial carcinoid.

iv. **Haematolymphoid malignancies:** Leukaemic infiltration (common), NHL (non-Hodgkin lymphoma)

Q. How IHC (immunohistochemistry) can help for confirmatory diagnosis?

Ans:

- Epethial cancer (carcinoma): EMA (epithelial membrane antigen) and pan-CK (cytokeratin)
- Rhabdomyosarcoma: MyoD1, desmin, vimentin, myogenin
- Wilms' tumour: WT1 and WT2
- Neuroblastoma: NSE (neuron-specific enolase), synaptophysin, chromogranin, neurofilament
- Ewing's sarcoma: CD99 (MIC2), vimentin and NSE
- Bronchial carcinoid: NSE, synaptophysin, chromogranin
- NHL B cell: CD45, CD20, CD19
- NHL T cell: CD45, CD3, CD5
- Leukaemia: B or T cell markers, immunophenotyping (flow cytometry)

Gallstones

Description: Mounted specimen of cut open gallbladder in a jar has following features:

- Multiple faceted, round to ovoid, pale yellow stones are seen.
- These stones have finely granular, hard external surface
- Gallbladder wall is thick.
- Gallbladder mucosa is reddened and irregular as a result of coexistent chronic cholecystitis.

Diagnosis: Cholesterol gallstones with chronic cholecystitis.

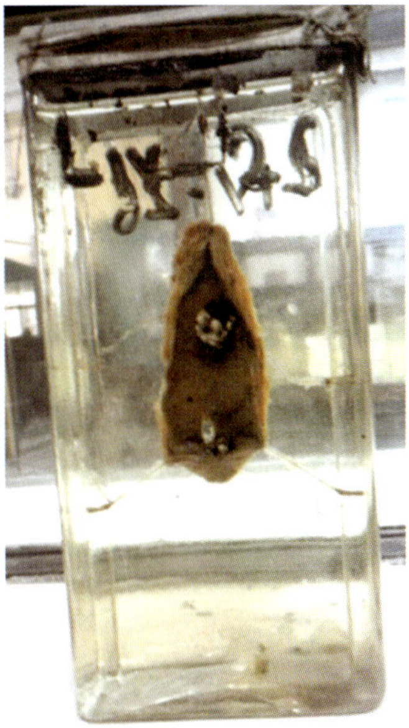

Fig. 17.38: Gallstones

Q. What are the different types of gallstones?

There are two main types—cholesterol stones and pigment stones. More than 90% are gallstones which contain >50% of crystalline cholesterol monohydrate.

The remaining are pigment stones composed predominantly of bilirubin calcium salts.

There are mixed cholesterol stones also. These mixed stones contain 50% cholesterol and rest mucoprotein, calcium and bilirubin.

Q. What are the predisposing factors for gallstone formation?

Ans: Risk factors for cholesterol stones are female sex, diabetes mellitus, pregnancy, hyperlipidaemia, estrogen therapy, bile stasis and inborn errors of bile acid metabolism.

Risk factors for pigmented stones are haemolytic syndromes, severe ileal dysfunction (or bypass) and bacterial contamination of biliary tree. Also, some parasitic infections of bilary tract like *Ascaris lumbricoides* and liver fluke O may lead to pigmented gallstone formation.

Q. Which gallstones are radio-opaque?

Ans: Black pigmented gallstones are radio-opaque due to presence of calcium carbonate and phosphates and approximately 50–75% black stones are radio-opaque.

Q. Which gallstones are radiolucent?

Ans: Pure cholesterol stones and stones composed largely of cholesterol are radiolucent. Also, brown pigmented gallstones are radiolucent.

Q. What are the complications of gallstone?

Ans: Most common complication is severe biliary colic or pain which tends to be excruciating and constant or ''colicky'' (spasmodic). Other complications include obstructive jaundice, ascending cholangitis and acute pancreatitis.

Less common complications are acute cholecystitis, empyema, perforation of gallbladder, porcelain gallbladder, mucocele of gallbladder, gallstone ileus and rarely squamous cell carcinoma.

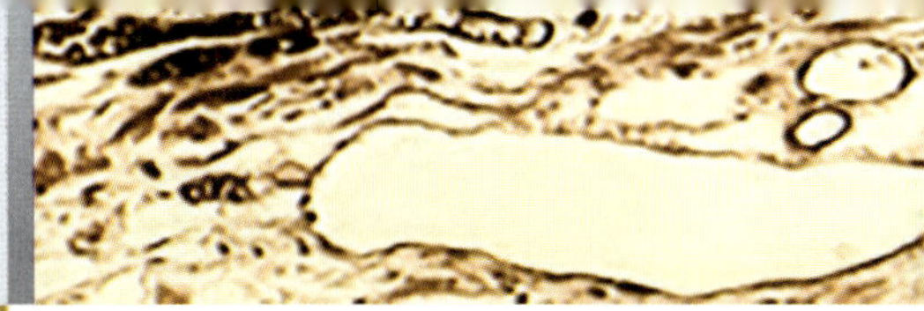

Section

V

Problem Cards and Discussion

Chapter

18

Problem Cards

PC 1

Q1. What is this black discolouration? 1

Q2. Define this pathological process. 1

Q3. What are the causes? 1

Q4. What are the different types of this pathological process? 1

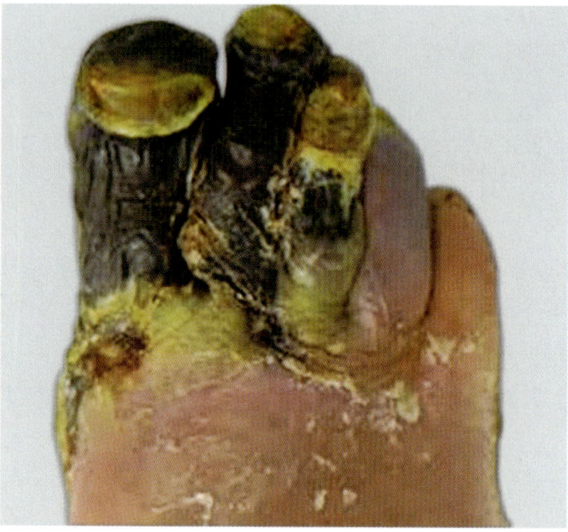

Fig. 18.1

PC 2

Q1. What is this intensely eosinophilic cell in the epidermis? 1

Q2. Give two examples of physiological conditions of this process? 1

Q3. Give two examples of pathological conditions of this process. 1

Q4. What is the most characteristic morphological feature? 1

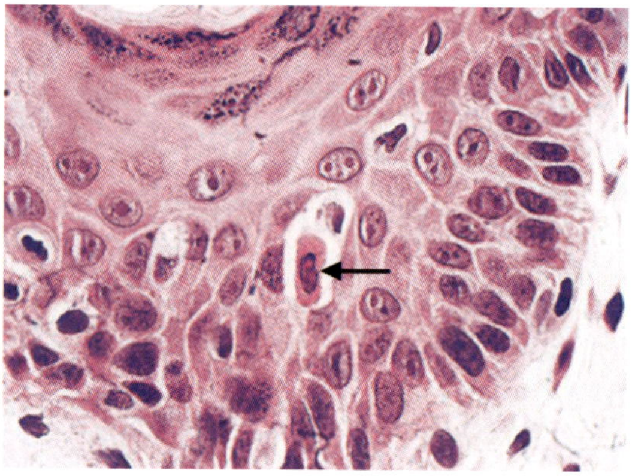

Fig. 18.2

PC 3

A 52-year-old poor man suffering from fever and cough for 2 months with cervical lymphadenopathy. Cervical lymph node shows following histological features:

Q1. What is the diagnosis of the disease? 1

Q2. What particular cells have been focused by arrows? 1

Q3. Which cytokines play an important role in pathogenesis? 2

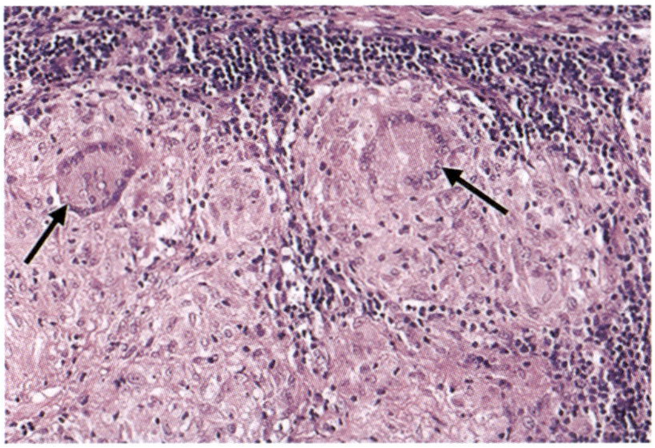

Fig. 18.3

PC 4

A 47-year-old female who had varicose veins in left leg and was on prolonged rest after hysterectomy. She suddenly developed swelling of left leg, pain and red or discoloured skin of left leg.

Q1. What is the diagnosis? 1

Q2. Name the triad and component which predisposes to the pathophysiology. 1

Q3. Name some hereditary (primary) factors which can cause it. 1

Q4. What are the microscopic features of this pathologic lesion? 1

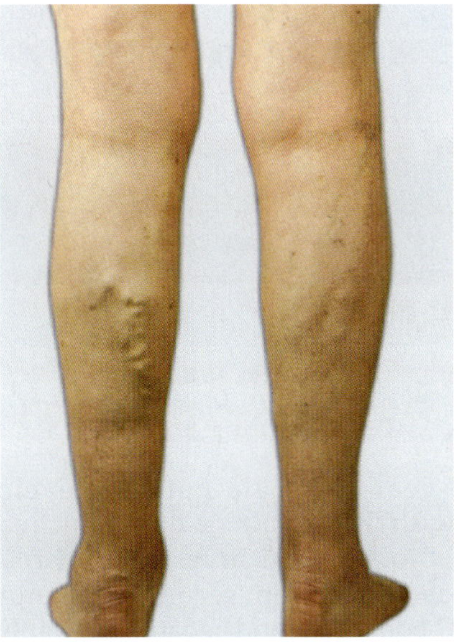

Fig. 18.4

PC 5

A patient had clinical diagnosis of splenic artery occlusion following thromboembolism. Cut section of the spleen shows following morphological features:

Q1. What is the diagnosis? 1

Q2. Why this pathologic lesions are white? 1

Q3. In which organs red-coloured lesions of same pathologic process are seen? 1

Q4. What are the properties of this pathologic lesion? 1

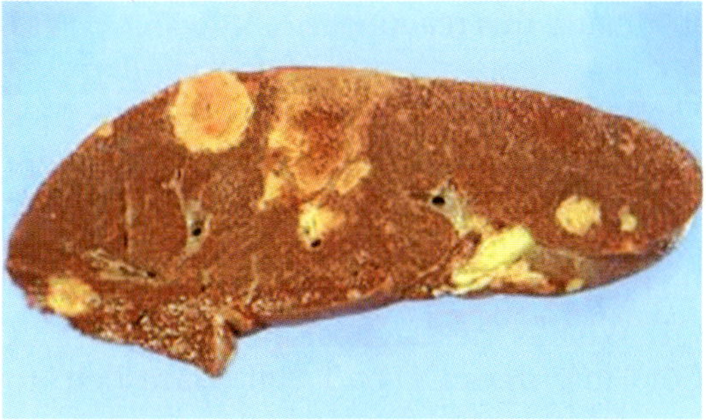

Fig. 18.5

PC 6

A baby was born with severe mental retardation (IQ 30) with flat facial profile, oblique palpebral fissures, epicanthic folds and congenital heart defects.

Q1. What is this genetic disorder? 1

Q2. What are the chromosomal changes? 1

Q3. What is the most common cause? 1

Q4. What are the future complications? 1

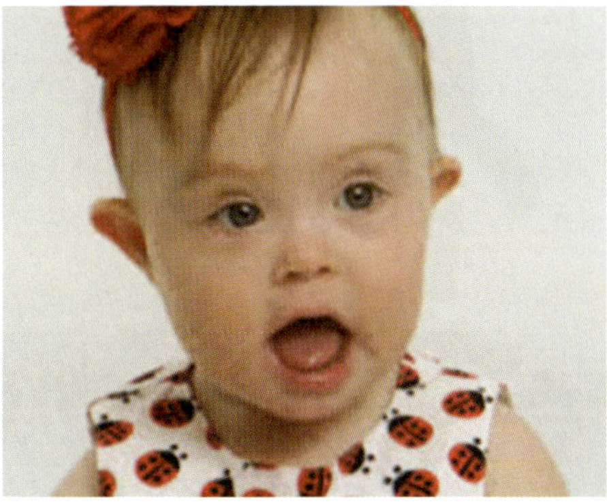

Fig. 18.6

PC 7

A person was given penicillin injection for treatment without a test dose. Within a few minutes (10 minutes) he develops mucosal secretion (nasal, conjunctival), smooth muscle contraction and oedema.

Q1. What is the diagnosis? 1
Q2. Which cell is responsible for this reaction? 1
Q3. Which chemical mediators are responsible for this? 1
Q4. Which antibody is most important to cause this reaction? 1

PC 8

An adult person presents with fever, severe weight loss, generalized lymphadenopathy and opportunistic infections. History reveals that he had unprotected sex in brothels.

Q1. What is the diagnosis? 1
Q2. How does CD4+ T cell count help to diagnose the disease? 1
Q3. What neoplasms may develop in these patients? 1
Q4. What are the most sensitive and specific tests? 1

PC 9

A patient had died of multiple myeloma and chronic inflammatory diseases. During autopsy, liver was found to be enlarged. Cut section of liver was firm and had a waxy appearance. Painting the cut surface with iodine imparts a yellow colour which transformed to blue violet after application of sulphuric acid (H_2SO_4).

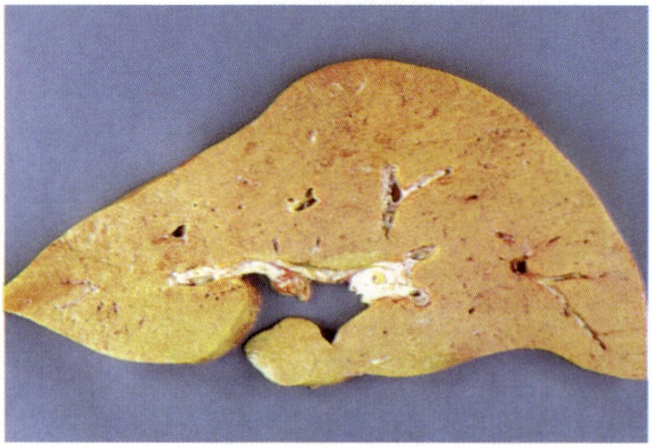

Fig. 18.7

Q1. What is the diagnosis? 1
Q2. What other organs may be involved? 1
Q3. Name two special stains to diagnose this disease and their colours. 1
Q4. What are the biopsy sites for microscopic examinations?

PC 10

A patient had a small firm tumour (1.5 × 1.3 cm) on arm for several years. It was surgically resected. Grossly, the tumour is well circumscribed and white-glistening. Microscopically it is found to be nerve sheath origin.

Q1. From history and gross, is it a benign tumour or malignant tumour? 1
Q2. What morphological features (microscopical) differentiate a benign and malignant tumour? 2
Q3. Mention two differences between carcinoma and sarcoma. 1

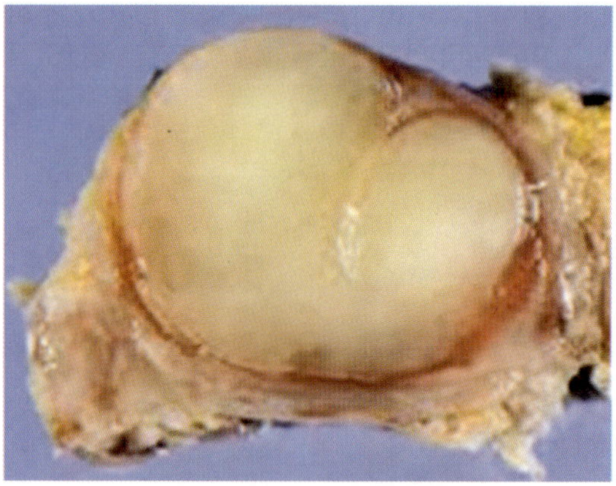

Fig. 18.8

PC 11

A 58-year-old male patient developed yellowish discolouration of conjunctiva and skin. Biochemical investigation reveals increased bilirubin, serum transaminases (SGOT and SGPT) and hepatitis viral antigens and antibodies.

Q1. What is this clinical condition?
Q2. What is the normal value of bilirubin in adults? 1
Q3. Mention some causes of unconjugated hyperbilirubinaemia. 1
Q4. Mention some causes of conjugated hyperbilirubinaemia. 1

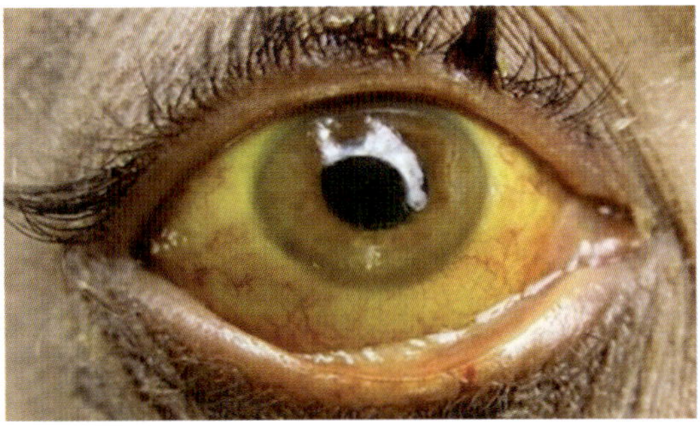

Fig. 18.9

PC 12

A 52-year-old patient had tuberculosis and chest X-ray show following features.

Q1. What is the provisional diagnosis based on chest X-ray? 1
Q2. What will be glucose and protein value in this fluid compared to plasma? 1
Q3. What will be LDH content and fluid LDH/serum LDH ratio? 1
Q4. What is anasarca? 1

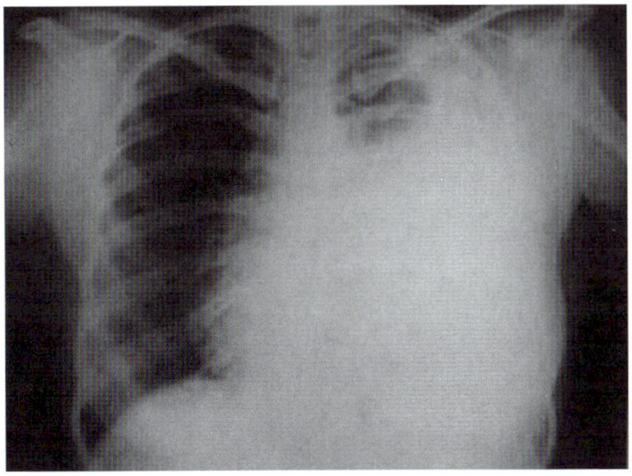

Fig. 18.10

PC 13

A 5-year-old girl is suffering from fever, anaemia, bone pain and generalised lymphadenopathy. Peripheral blood smear and flow cytometry reveal the following features.

Q1. What is the diagnosis? 1
Q2. What will be the bone marrow picture? 1
Q3. Which marker/markers are positive in the flow cytometry? 1
Q4. Which special stain can be used for these abnormal cells? 1

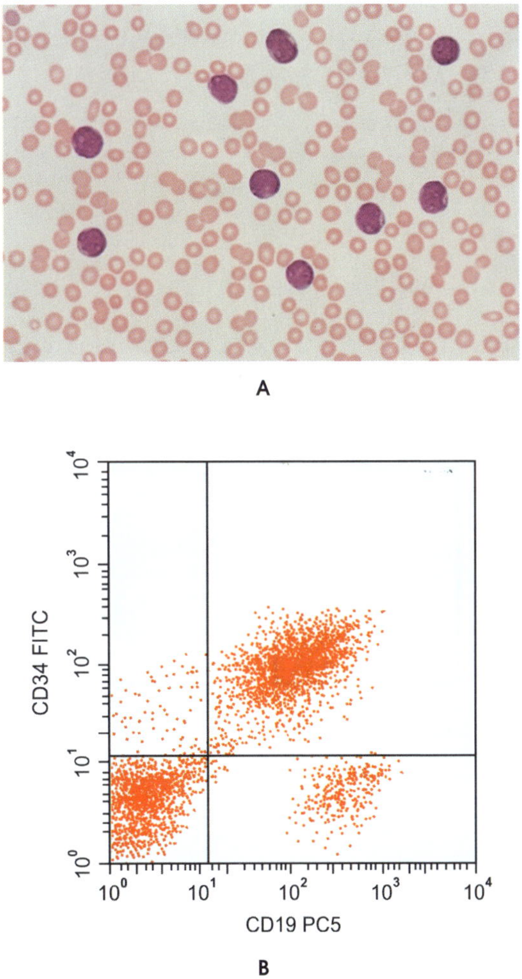

Fig. 18.11A and B

PC 14

A middle-aged man suffering from fatigue, fever and gum bleeding. His bone marrow smear shows the following features:

Q1. What is the diagnosis? 1

Q2. What is that constituent in the cytoplasm of cells indicated by arrow? 1

Q3. Why there is gum bleeding? 1

Q4. What markers are positive in flow cytometry (immunophenotyping)? 1

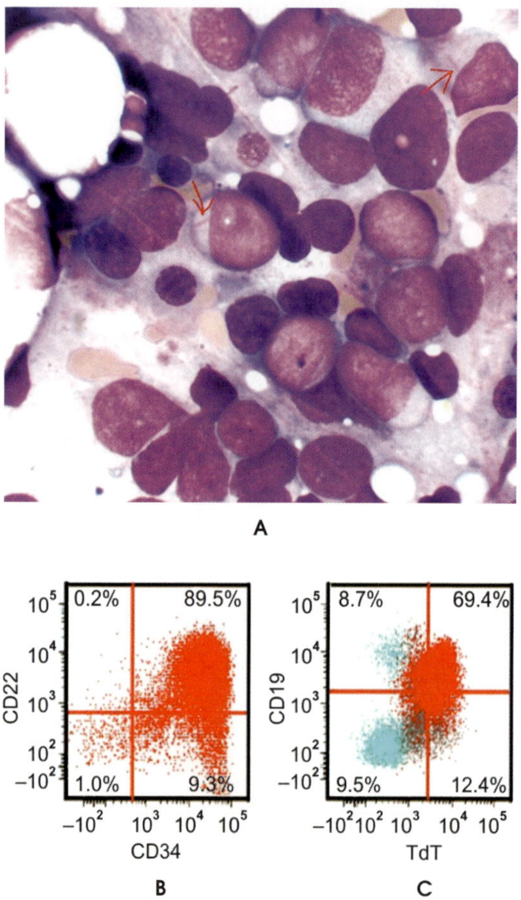

Fig. 18.12A to C

PC 15

A 56-year-old female patient is suffering from moderate anaemia, weakness, fatigability and dragging sensation in the abdomen. TLC is 108,000/mm^3.

Peripheral blood smear has following features:

Q1. What is the diagnosis? 1

Q2. Why there is dragging sensation in the abdomen? 1

Q3. Which particular chromosome can be detected in this case? 1

Q4. What will be the NAP (neutrophil alkaline phosphatase) score? 1

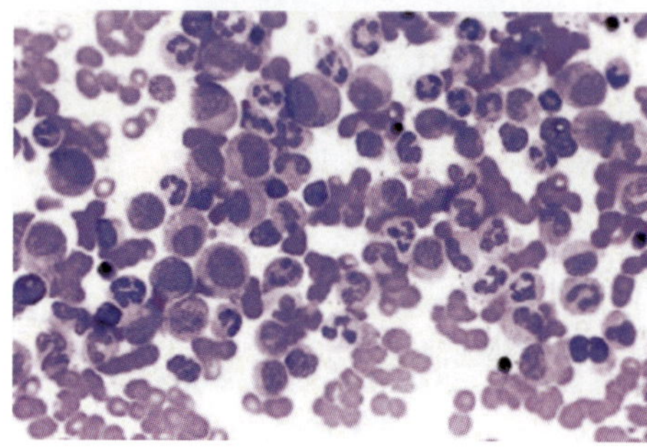

Fig. 18.13

PC 16

A 60-year-old male patient is suffering from anaemia and symmetrically enlarged, discrete and non-tender lymph nodes. Peripheral blood smear shows the following features:

Q1. What is the diagnosis? 1

Q2. Why 10–15% of these patients develop haemolytic anaemia?

Q3. What aggressive tumour may develop in these patients? 1

Q4. What immunomarkers will be positive? 1

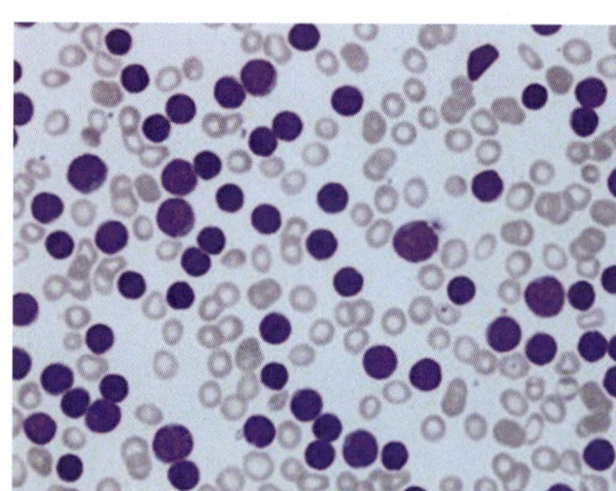

Fig. 18.14

PC 17

A young adult presented with painless lymphadenopathy (potato size cervical lymph node). He also had constitutional symptoms like fever, night sweats and weight loss. Microscopy of lymph node and IHC staining have following features:

Q1. What is the diagnosis? 1

Q2. Which variant of the disease is shown in the upper right picture? 1

Q3. Which markers are positive for the neoplastic cells (lower left)? 1

Q4. Which variant of the disease is shown in the lower right picture? 1

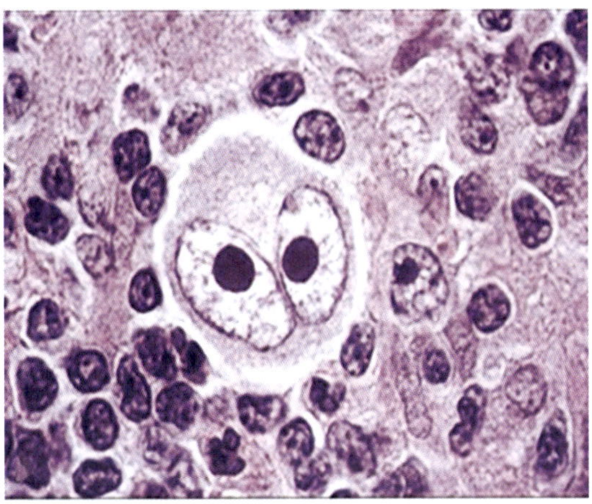

A

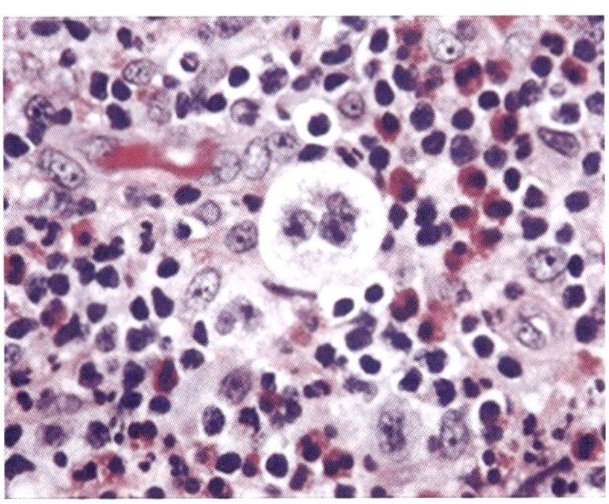

B

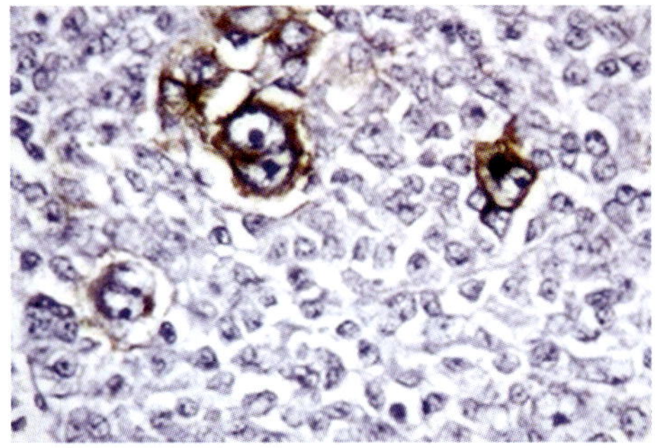

C

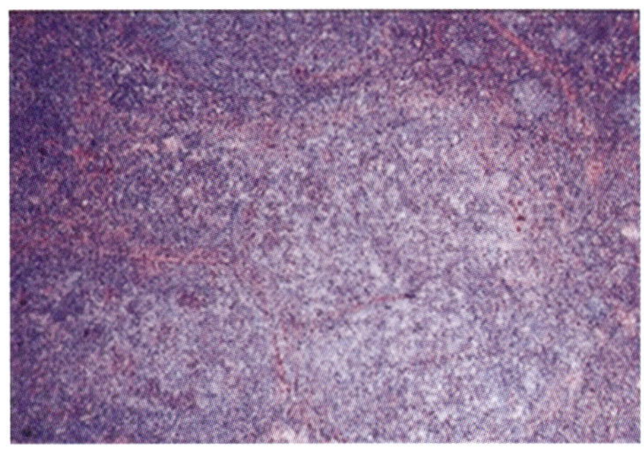

D

Fig. 18.15A to D

PC 18

An elderly woman suffering from bone pain, pathologic fractures and renal failure. Bone marrow aspirates have following microscopic features:

Q1. What is the diagnosis? 1

Q2. What will be found in serum electrophoresis? 1

Q3. What may be found in X-ray of skull? 1

Q4. What will be urinary findings? 1

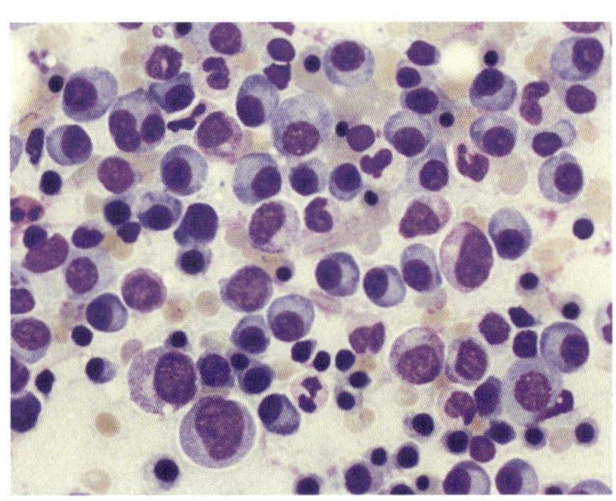

Fig. 18.16

PC 19

A 38-year-old female presented with pinpoint haemorrhages (petechiae) in the dependent areas and ecchymoses. Spleen is of normal size. But microscopy of spleen has following features:

Q1. What is the diagnosis? 1

Q2. What will be the peripheral blood picture? 1

Q3. What will be bone marrow picture? 1

Q4. Is there any antibody for the pathogenesis? 1

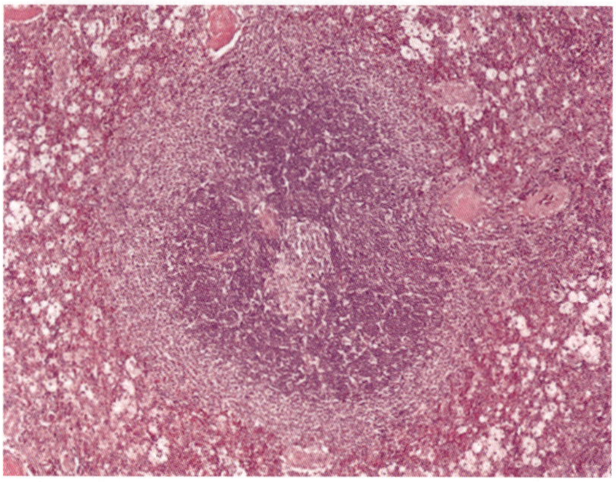

Fig. 18.17

PC 20

A pregnant lady is suffering from weakness, extreme fatigue and skin pallor. Peripheral blood smear shows the following features:

Q1. What is your diagnosis? 1

Q2. What will be bone marrow findings? 1

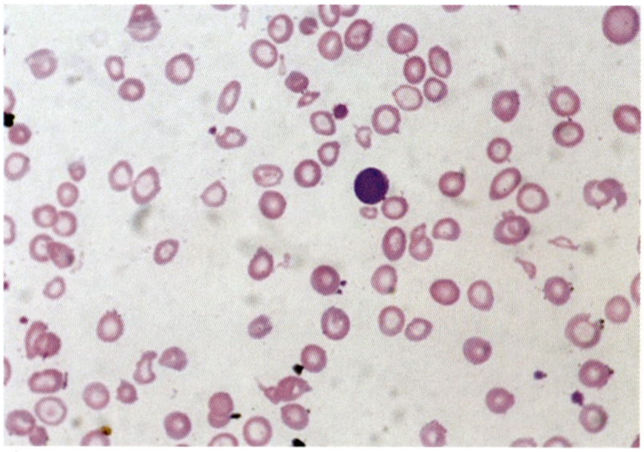

Fig. 18.18

Q3. What biochemical investigations will help to reach the diagnosis? 2

PC 21

A 62-year-old female is suffering from anaemia. Bone marrow has following features:

Q1. What is the diagnosis? 1

Q2. What are the features seen in peripheral blood? 2

Q3. Describe the particular cell in the bone marrow. 1

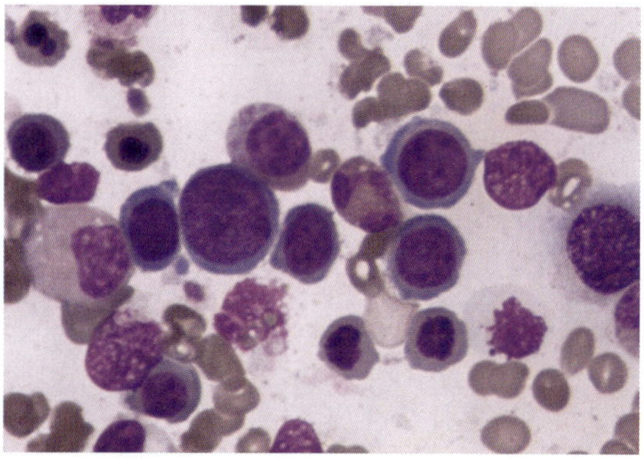

Fig. 18.19

PC 22

A 7-year-old child is suffering from anaemia, priapism and bone pain. Peripheral blood smear has the following features:

Q1. What is the diagnosis? 1

Q2. What is the molecular defect? 1

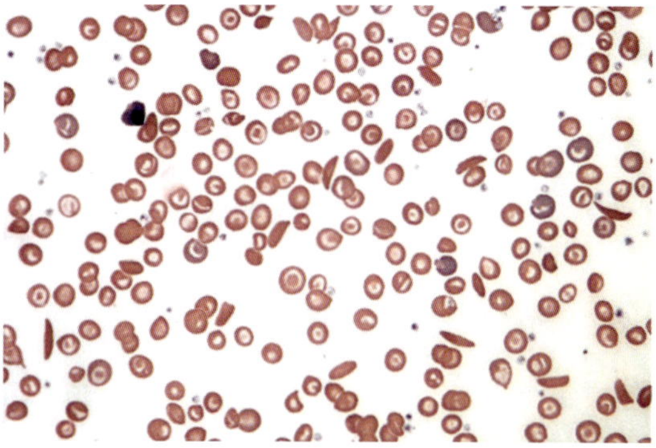

Fig. 18.20

Q3. Which organs are affected by vaso-occlusive or pain crises? 1

Q4. What particular blood test is helpful? 1

PC 23

A patient presented with anaemia, splenomegaly and jaundice. Peripheral blood smear has following features:

Q1. What is the diagnosis?

Q2. What is the molecular defect? 1

Q3. What is the cause of aplastic crises in these patients? 1

Q4. Which particular laboratory test (simple and cost-effective) will help to diagnose? 1

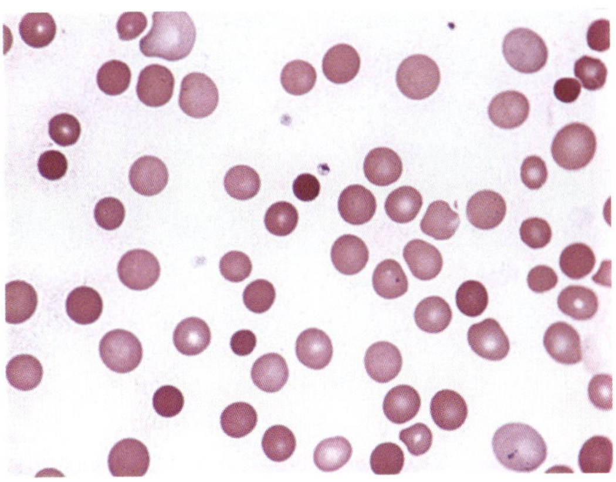

Fig. 18.21

PC 24

A child is suffering from growth retardation, severe anaemia, hepatosplenomegaly and prominent cheek bones. Mother is also known to suffer from the disease. Haemoglobin electrophoresis shows the following features:

a. Upper panel—normal control
b. Middle panel—affected mother
c. Lower panel—affected child

Q1. What is the disease in child? 1

Q2. What is the disease in affected mother? 1

Q3. What will be peripheral blood pictures? 1

Q4. Why there is crew-cut appearance on X-ray? 1

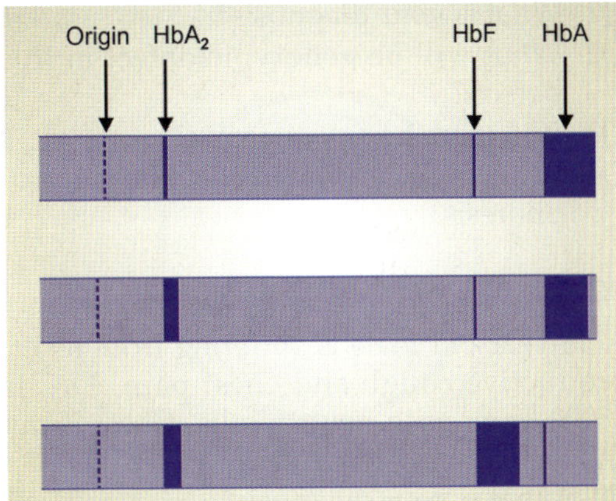

Fig. 18.22

PC 25

During marriage negotiation both the bride and groom underwent blood testing for HPLC. The groom has the following HPLC features:

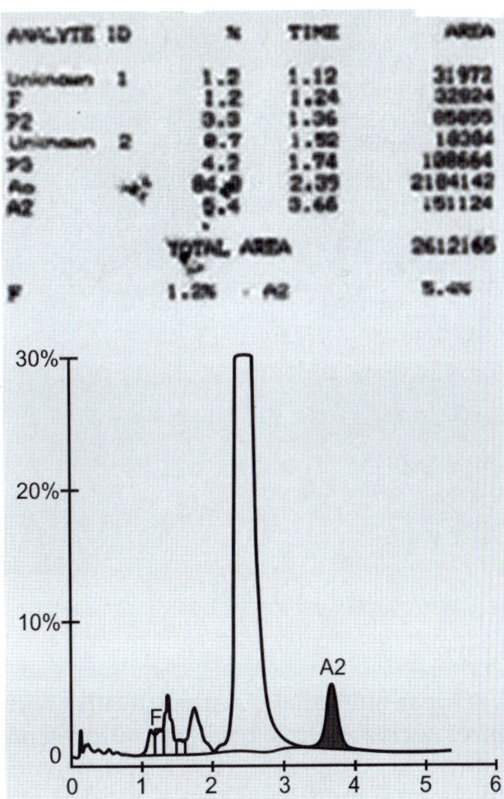

ANALYTE ID		%	TIME	AREA
Unknown	1	1.2	1.12	31972
F		1.2	1.24	32024
P2		3.3	1.36	[illegible]
Unknown	2	0.7	1.52	18304
P3		4.2	1.74	108664
Ao		[illegible]	2.39	2104142
A2		5.4	3.66	151124
		TOTAL AREA		2612165
F		1.2%	A2	5.4%

Fig. 18.23

Q1. What is your diagnosis? 1

Q2. What will be genotypic defect in this person? 1

Q3. Will there be any anaemia? 1

Q4. What will be finding in Hb electrophoresis? 1

PC 26

A 56-year-old male is suffering from fever, productive cough and chest pain. TLC is 18000/mm^3 with neutrophilia. Chest X-ray shows following features:

Q1. What is your diagnosis? 1

Q2. What is the finding in air bronchogram (chest X-ray)? 1

Q3. What is the commonest organism in nosocomial form of this disease? 1

Q4. What will be histologic findings in lung biopsy? 1

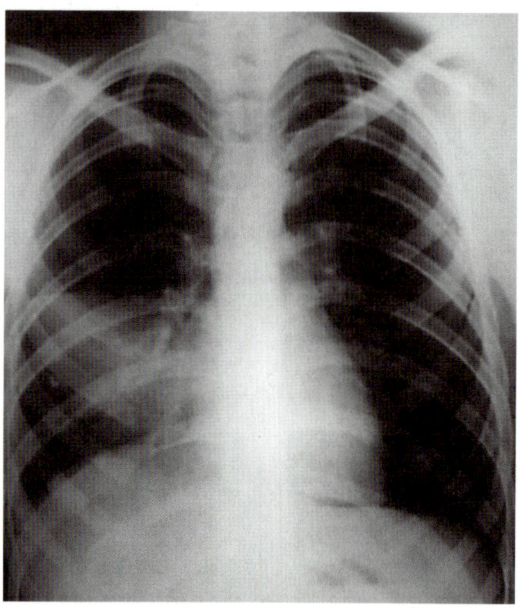

Fig. 18.24

PC 27

A 45-year-old female, a slum dweller with lower socioeconomic background presents with fever, dyspnoea, cough and haemoptysis for 3 months. Chest X-ray has the following features:

Q1. What are the radiological features and your diagnosis? 1

Q2. What is the source of haemoptysis in this patent? 1

Q3. Which special stain is commonly used to diagnose the case? Why causative organisms give positive colour with this stain? 2

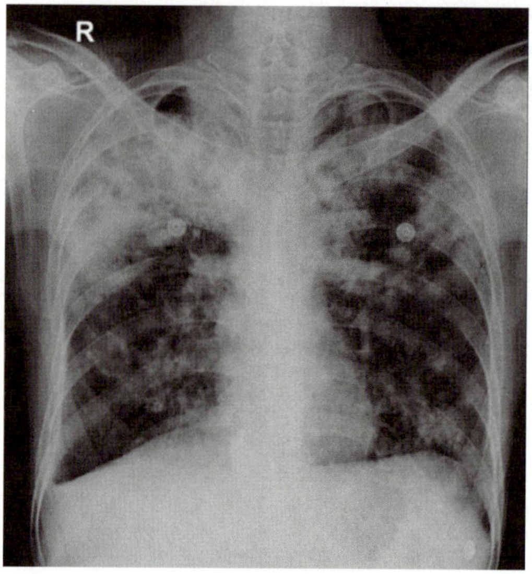

Fig. 18.25

PC 28

An elderly patient had barrel-shaped chest and presents with dyspnoea, prolonged expiration, and sits forward. Spirometry reveals the following features:

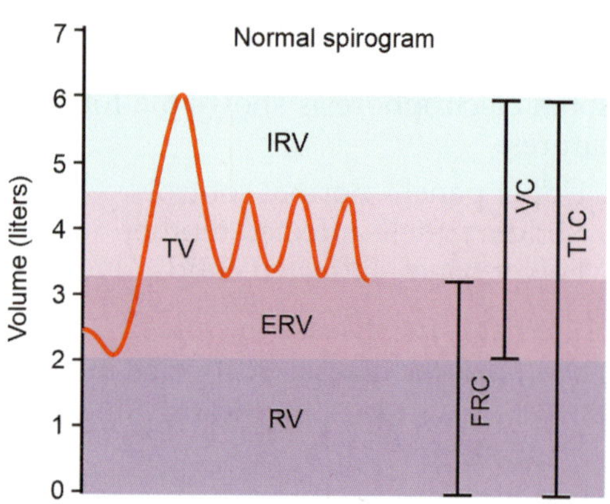

Fig. 18.26A

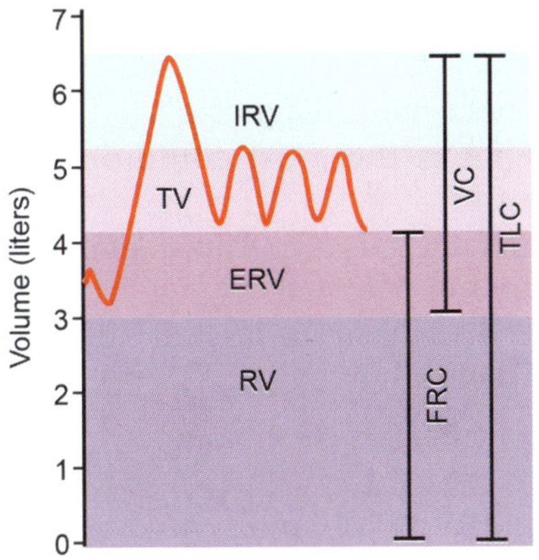

Fig. 18.26B

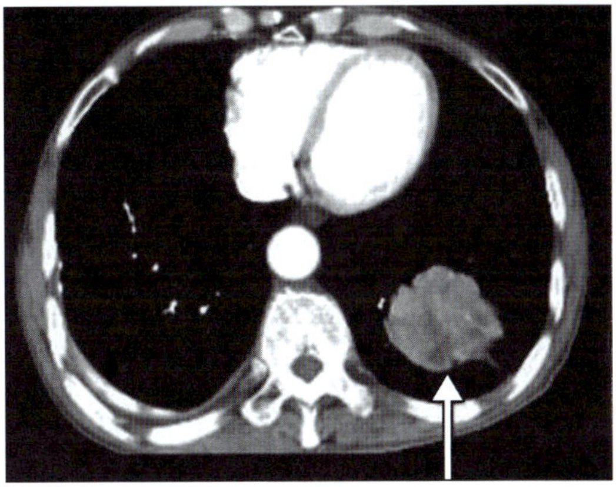

Fig. 18.27

Q1. What is your diagnosis? 1
Q2. Why these patients are called pink puffers? 1
Q3. Which hypothesis explains the pathogenesis? 1
Q4. What are the causes of death? 1

PC 29

A patient presented with chest tightness, dyspnoea and wheezing. Peripheral blood shows eosinophilia. Sputum reveals Curschmann spirals and Charcot-Leyden crystals.

Q1. What is your diagnosis? 1
Q2. If the attack remains for a prolonged time (days or week) instead of a few minutes to hour; what is that condition known as? 1
Q3. Which constituent of eosinophils causes epithelial damage? 1
Q4. What is Charcot-Leyden crystals? 1

PC 30

A 75-year-old man presented with weight loss, cough, chest pain and dyspnoea. Contrast-enhanced CT scan of lung shows a 5.5 cm, round, completely enhanced mass in left lobe of lung (arrow).

Q1. What is your provisional diagnosis? 1
O2. How would you confirm the diagnosis? 1
Q3. What are the histologic types? 2

PC 31

An elderly woman is suffering from hypertension for years. Now she develops oedema over ankle (pedal) and pretibial. USG reveals hepatosplenomegaly and ascites. Echocardiography reveals left ventricular hypertrophy (LVH).

Q1. What is your diagnosis? 1
Q2. If there were pulmonary congestion and edema along with LVH and hypertension, then what was your diagnosis? What particular cells may be found in this case? 1+1 = 2
Q3. What particular colour change may be observed in liver? 1

PC 32

A 56-year-old man (smoker and diabetic) suddenly developed acute chest pain and presented with rapid, weak pulse, profound sweating (diaphoresis) and dyspnoea.

Q1. What is your diagnosis?
Q2. What are the most sensitive and specific biomarkers? 1
Q3. What gross features and light microscopic features will be seen in the affected organ(s) after 1–3 days? 2

PC 33

A child has mitral valve prolapse and bicuspid aortic valve. He develops fever.

Echocardiography shows irregular masses on the valve cusps. Blood culture reveals a pathogenic organism.

Q1. What is your diagnosis? 1

Q2. What is the causative organism most likely? 1

Q3. What are that irregular masses known as and what is the composition? 1

Q4. How the masses on valve differ in rheumatic heart disease (RHD)? 1

PC 34

A 38-year-old female presented with epigastric burning or aching pain. The pain tends to occur 1 to 3 hours after meals during the day and is worse in night. Pain relieves by alkali or food.

Q1. What is your diagnosis? 1

Q2. What is common organism associated in the pathogenesis? 1

Q3. What are the common locations? 2

PC 35

A 48-year-old male presented with bloody diarrhoea with stringy, mucoid material lower abdominal pain and cramps. On colonoscopy, pseudopolyps and mucosal bridges found.

Q1. What is your diagnosis? 1

Q2. What are the histologic features? 2

Q3. What are the extraintestinal manifestations? 1

PC 36

A young child suddenly develops malaise, fever, nausea and oliguria. 1–2 weeks after a sore throat. Urine is smoky or cola-coloured.

Q1. What is your diagnosis? 1

Q2. What biochemical markers you will advise for? 1

Q3. What are the light microscopic features of kidney biopsy? 2

PC 37

A 52-year-old man presented with generalised oedema. Urinary findings show massive proteinuria (>3.5 g/day) and lipiduria.

Q1. What is your diagnosis? 1

Q2. What is the most common primary cause? 1

Q3. Why there is hyperlipidaemia in these types of patients? 1

Q4. What do you understand by selective proteinuria? 1

PC 38

A 7-year-old child presented with fever, chills, neutrophilia and marked to intense throbbing pain near upper end of femur (neck region) of right side. X-ray shows a lytic focus of bone destruction surrounded by a zone of sclerosis. Biopsy of the affected bone shows the following features:

Q1. What is your diagnosis? 1

Q2. What is the commonest organism? 1

Q3. Which area of bone is affected in neonate and children? 1

Q4. In sickle cell disease, which organism cause such lesion? 1

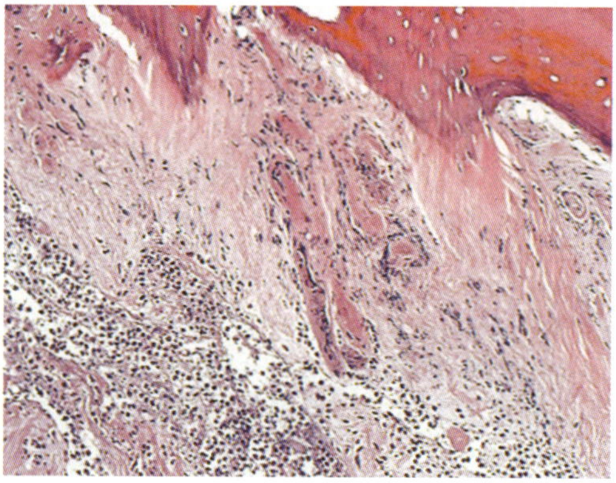

Fig. 18.28

PC 39

A 12-year-old girl child presented with painful enlarging masses at mid of left thigh and the affected site is tender, warm and swollen. X-ray shows mottled, destructive osteolytic lesion with poorly marginated edges in the diaphysis of left femur (blue circle). Sunburst periosteal reaction (red circle) and lamellated periosteal reaction in an onion-skin reaction (white arrows) also seen.

Q1. What is your diagnosis? 1

Q2. Where from does the tumour originate? 1

Q3. What are the light microscopic features? 2

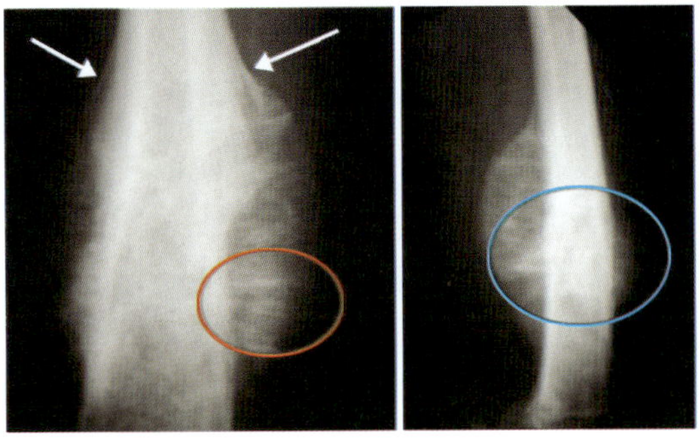

Fig. 18.29

PC 40

70-year-old man presented with urinary symptoms such as difficulty in starting or stopping the stream, dysuria. On rectal examination, a suspected nodule was found. Serum PSA level was high.

Q1. What is your diagnosis? 1

Q2. Which grading system is used for this tumour? 1

Q3. What is the cut-off value of serum PSA in normal men? 1

Q4. Name one IHC marker for this tumour? 1

PC 41

A 68-year-old female complains of tender hepatomegaly, weight loss, fatigue and upper abdominal pain. CT scan shows a large mass (red arrow).

Q1. What is your provisional diagnosis? 1

Q2. Which biochemical marker you will advise for? 1

Q3. What are the etiologic factors of this tumour? 1

Q4. How does this tumour appear grossly? 1

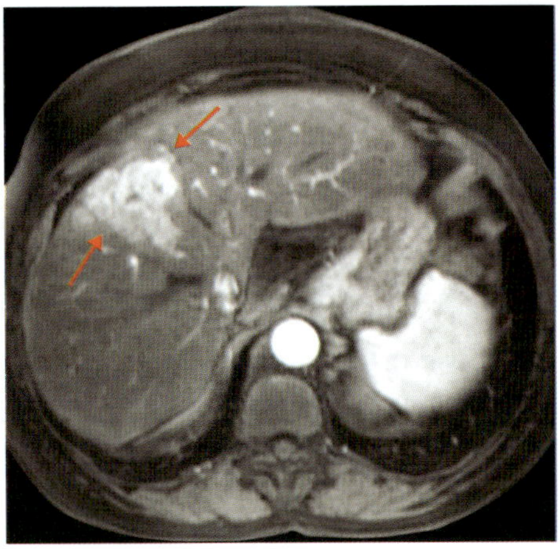

Fig. 18.30

PC 42

36-year-old female sex worker presented with low grade fever, weight loss, persistent diarrhoea and cervical lymphadenopathy for 4 months.

Q1. What is your clinical diagnosis? 1

Q2. Which one is the commonest type in India? 1

Q3. Which antigen and antibody most commonly used for detecting the disease? 1

Q4. What is the most common fungal infection associated with this disease? 1

PC 43

A 28-year-old male worker presents with raised itchy superficial chest lesion slowly developing over an old scar.

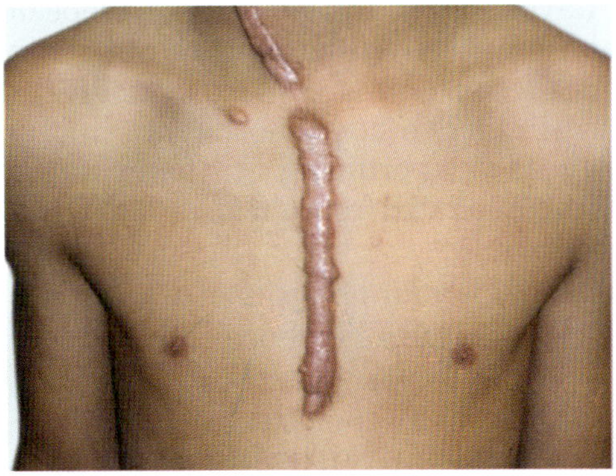

Fig. 18.31

Q1. What is this lesion? 1

Q2. What is the basic defect? 1

Q3. Name another closely related pathologic lesion? 1

Q4. How these two lesions can be differentiated? 1

PC 44

A 55-year-old female presented with irregular vaginal bleeding for 3 months.

Cervical cytology (Pap smear) shows highly dysplastic cells with degenerated round and oval nuclei and dense eosinophilic cytoplasm.

Q1. What is your provisional diagnosis? 1

Q2. Which virus is an important factor? 1

Q3. What are the histologic subtypes? 2

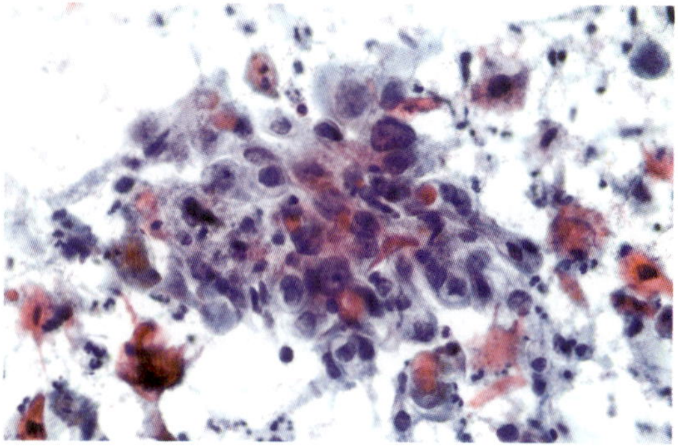

Fig. 18.32

PC 45

A 12-year-old boy presented with repeated painful knee swelling after minor trauma which leads to progressive deformities and crippling. The boy also has a tendency towards easy bruising but petechiae are absent. Aspirated from left knee joint yielded blood.

Q1. What is your provisional diagnosis? 1

Q2. What is the inheritance of the disease? 1

Q3. What are the molecular defects? 1

Q4. What will be BT, PT and PTT in this case? 1

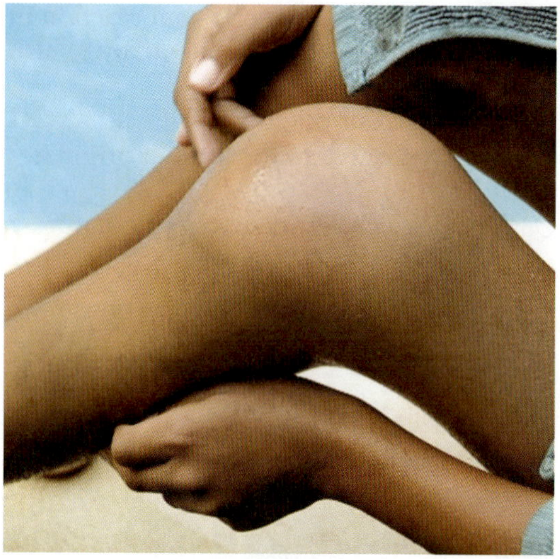

Fig. 18.33

PC 46

A 23-year-old male presented with splenomegaly, thrombocytopenia, bone pain and pathologic fractures. Bone marrow aspirates show the following features:

Q1. What is your provisional diagnosis? 1

Q2. What is the genetic defect? 1

Q3. In which organ(s), the particular cell can be found? 1

Q4. What are the different subtypes of the disease? 1

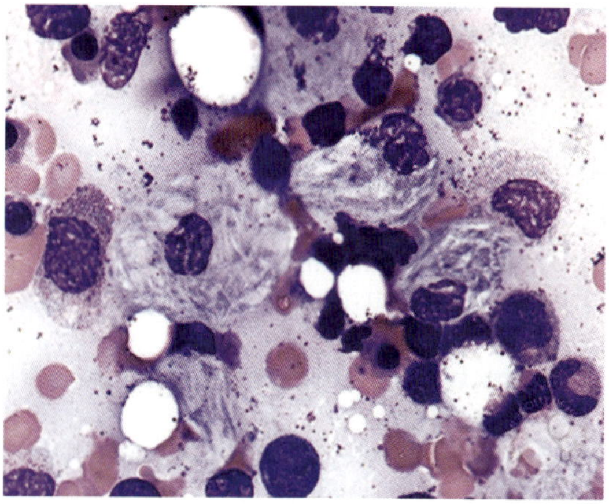

Fig. 18.34

PC 47

A female patient complains of fever, dysuria and frequency of urine.

Name: Mrs S. Tarafdar
Age: 22 years
Sex: Female
Address: 32/1 AJC Bose Road, Kolkata-14

Report on examination of urine
Physical: Appearance: Hazy
Sp. gravity: Q. I.
Odour: Fishy
Sediment: Present
Chemical: Reducing substance: Nil
Protein: Present
Ketone bodies: Nil
Microscopical: Epithelial cells: 3–4 cells/HPF
Pus cells: 10–15 cell/HPF
RBC: 2–3 cells/HPF
Casts: Nil
Crystals: Nil

Q1. What is the patient likely to be suffering from? 1
Q2. What would be the specific gravity of urine in this case and why? 1
Q3. How will you confirm the cause leading to this condition? 1
Q4. What is the appearance of the kidney, if the patient suffers for a prolonged time? 1

PC 48

Name: P. Mudi
Age: 12 years
Sex: Female

Report of examination of blood
Haemoglobin: 9 g/dl
ESR: 12 mm at 1 hr.
TLC: 8600/cu mm
DLC: Neutrophil: 53%
Lymphocyte: 39%
Monocyte: 03%
Eosinophil: 05%
RBC: Microcytic hypochromic
Anisocytosis +
Poikilocytosis +
Platelets: Adequate

Q1. What is the clinical condition of this patient? 1
Q2. Mention two common causes that may lead to such blood picture. 1
Q3. Enumerate further test you would like to come to a definite diagnosis. 1
Q4. If you examine the stool of this patient what pertinent findings may be present? 1

PC 49

Name: Hafiz Mondal
Age: 15 years
Sex: Male

Patient is referred from the ENT OPD of NRS Medical College for FNAC of neck glands

Report on examination of FNAC of cervical lymph node

Smears show necrotic material and epithelioid cells in aggregate

Q1. What is the provisional diagnosis? 1
Q2. How will you confirm the diagnosis? 1
Q3. Draw a labelled diagram of microscopic features of such lymph node. 2

PC 50

Name: T. Ali
Age: 24 years
Sex: Male

Report on examination of CSF
Physical: Appearance: Hazy
Pressure: Coming out in jet flow
Chemical: Glucose: 20 mg/dl
Protein: 75 mg/dl
Microscopic: Total cell count: 350 cells/cu mm

Q1. What is the condition of this patient is suffering from? 1
Q2. What type of cells do you expect in microscopical examination of CSF? 1

Q3. What are the clinical features of this condition? 1

Q4. What further examination would you find out the cause? 1

Answers to Problem Cards

PC 1

1. This is dry gangrene, a type of necrosis.
2. Necrosis is a localised area of death in living tissue and is accompanied by inflammatory reaction. This cell death is irreversible.
3. Causes are hypoxia, ischaemia and toxins (poisoning).
4. Coagulative necrosis, liquefactive necrosis, caseous necrosis, fat necrosis, fibrinoid necrosis and gangrenous necrosis (dry and wet gangrene).

PC 2

1. Apoptotic body.
2. Programmed cell death during embryogenesis and endometrial cell breakdown during menstruation.
3. Councilman bodies in viral hepatitis and graft-versus-host disease (GVHD).
4. Chromatin condensation.

PC 3

1. Tuberculosis
2. Langhans giant cells
3. i. IL-1 and IL-2: Stimulate proliferation of more T cells
   ii. IFN-γ activates macrophages.
   iii. TNF-α promotes fibroblast proliferation and activates endothelium.
   iv. Growth factors (TGF-β, PDGF) stimulate fibroblast growth.

PC 4

1. Deep vein thrombosis
2. **Virchow's triad:** Endothelial injury, alteration in the normal blood flow and blood hypercoagulability
3. • Mutation of factor V (most common)
   • Antithrombin III deficiency
   • Protein C or protein S deficiency
4. Fibrin, more enmeshed red cells and few platelets (therefore called red or stasis thrombi). Also, **lines of Zahn,** which represent pale platelet and fibrin deposits alternating with red cell layers (hence apparent laminations).

PC 5

1. Splenic infarction (white infarct)
2. Solid organs (like spleen, kidney or heart) have increased tissue density and it limits the seepage of blood from adjoining capillary beds into the necrotic area.
3. Organs with loose tissues like lung and small intestine (arterial occlusion). Organs with dual blood supply like ovary and testis (venous occlusion).
4. Red infarcts: Ill-defined haemorrhagic margins which change in colour to brown.

   White infarcts: Well defined margins and progressively pallor with time.

PC 6

1. Down syndrome
2. • In 95% of cases, there is trisomy 21 (extra copy of chromosome of 21, so total chromosome 47).
   • In 4% of cases, robertsonian translocation
   • In 1% of cases, mosaic pattern (both 46, XY and 47 chromosomes)
3. Most common cause is maternal meiotic non-disjunction.

   Meiotic non-disjunction occurs in chromosome 21 in ovum.
4. These children have 10–20-fold increased risk of developing acute leukaemia (more commonly ALL and specifically acute megakaryoblastic leukaemia, AML-M7).
   • Reduced fertility in females (males are totally infertile)
   • Increased risk of respiratory infections (RTI).

PC 7

1. Immediate (type 1) hypersensitivity; Anaphylaxis
2. Mast cell mainly. Also, TH_2 (T helper cells) play some role.
3. Histamine is responsible for early clinical features because it is preformed mediator.

   PAF is the major mediator of the late phase reaction.
4. IgE.

PC 8

1. Acquired immunodeficiency syndrome (AIDS) with human immunodeficiency virus (HIV) infection.
2. According to the Centers for Disease Control (CDC) and Prevention, US in 1993, irrespective of presence of symptoms, any HIV-infected person having CD4+ T cell count of <200/µl is labelled as AIDS.
3. Kaposi's sarcoma, primary CNS lymphoma, NHL and Hodgkin lymphoma, HPV-associated carcinoma (cervix, vagina, anus) and bacillary angiomatosis.
4. ELISA (enzyme-linked immunosorbent assay) is the most sensitive test, and Western blot is the most specific test.

PC 9

1. Amyloidosis
2. Kidney, spleen (sago spleen and lardaceous spleen), heart and oral cavity (gingiva and tongue)
3. Congo red: Pink or red colour to amyloid deposits in tissue.

   Metachromatic stains like crystal violet or methyl violet: Rose pink.
4. Biopsy from renal tissue, rectum, abdominal fat and gingiva. The rectum is the best site for taking the biopsy. The staining of abdominal fat aspirate is quite specific but has low sensitivity.

PC 10

1. Benign tumour
2. Some microscopical features are present in malignant tumour which is lacking or absent in benign tumour:
   - Pleomorphism: Both the cells and nuclei display this
   - Nuclear atypia: Hyperchromatism, irregular nuclear membrane
   - A typical, bizarre mitoses: Increased in number
   - Loss of polarity and lack of differentiation
3. i. Carcinoma arises from epithelial cells, whereas sarcomas arise from mesenchymal cells.

   ii. Carcinoma metastasizes by lymphatic route, while sarcomas prefer haematogenous route.

PC 11

1. Jaundice
2. Normal value of serum bilirubin is 0.3–1.2 mg/dl, about 80% of which is unconjugated bilirubin.
3. Physiological jaundice of newborn, haemolytic anaemia, diffuse hepatocellular disease (viral hepatitis), Criggler-Najjar syndrome, Gilbert syndrome
4. Biliary tract obstruction, primary biliary cirrhosis, Dubin-Johnson syndrome, Rotor syndrome.

PC 12

1. Left-sided pleural effusion due to accumulation of exudate.
2. Glucose content of the effusion fluid will be low (<60 mg/dl) and protein content will be high (2.5–3.5 g/dl).
3. LDH content will be high compared to transudate and ratio will be >0.6.
4. Anasarca or dropsy is a severe and generalised oedema with widespread subcutaneous tissue swelling.

   Causes: Renal oedema, cardiac oedema and nutritional edema.

PC 13

1. Acute lymphoblastic leukaemia (ALL).
2. The bone marrow is hypercellular and shows 20–95% lymphoblasts of B or T cell origin. Megakaryocytes are reduced or absent.
3. CD34 and CD19 are positive
4. PAS +ve and acid phosphatase (focal) +ve

PC 14

1. Acute myeloid leukaemia (AML)
2. Auer rods
3. Thrombocytopenia cause spontaneous bleeding in AML patients. Also, procoagulants and fibrinolytic factors released by the leukaemic cells exacerbate the bleeding tendency.
4. CD34 and CD22 in the first panel.
   TdT and CD19 in the second panel.

PC 15

1. Chronic myeloid leukaemia (CML).
2. It is caused by splenomegaly. Splenomegaly occurs as a result of extensive extramedullary haematopoiesis.
3. Philadelphia chromosome (Ph). Ph chromosome is formed by reciprocal balanced translocation between part of long arm of chromosome 22 arm with part of long arm of chromosome 9 {t (9;22) (q34; q11)}.
4. NAP score will be reduced. (Remember, NAP score will be high in myeloid leukaemoid reactions. Also, NAP score in CML returns to normal with successful treatment, in infections and corticosteroid administration.)

PC 16

1. Chronic lymphocytic leukaemia (CLL).
2. This happens because of production of autoantibodies by non-neoplastic B cells.
3. There may be prolymphocytic transformation (15–30% of patients) or a transformation to diffuse large B cell lymphoma (DLBCL), so-called Richter syndrome (5–10% of patients).
4. CD23, CD20 and CD19 (pan B cell markers).

PC 17

1. Hodgkin lymphoma or Hodgkin disease
2. Classic form of Hodgkin lymphoma, mixed cellularity type.
3. CD30 positive in 98% of cases
   CD15 positive in 80% of cases
   CD20 positive in small subset
4. Classic form of Hodgkin lymphoma, nodular sclerosis type.

PC 18

1. Multiple myeloma (plasma cell dyscrasia).
2. Presence of M band (M protein) due to presence of **monoclonal** (hence the name M) immunoglobulin. This Ig is usually IgG (55%), followed by IgA (25% of cases).
3. Sharply punched out bone lesions.
4. Present of Bence-Jones protein (light chains of immunoglobulin). Also, increased urinary protein 6 g/dl.

PC 19

1. Chronic immune thrombocytopenic purpura (ITP).
2. Decreased platelet count and presence of abnormally large platelets (mega thrombocytes).
3. Bone marrow reveals a modestly increased number of megakaryocytes. Some of them are immature with large, non-lobulated, single nuclei.
4. Autoantibodies directed against platelet membrane glycoprotein IIb–IIIa or Ib–IX may be found in plasma and bound to platelet surface near about 80% of patients.

Note

Usually spleen is of normal size. Typically, there is congestion of splenic sinusoids and enlargement of the splenic follicles, often associated with reactive germinal centres.

PC 20

1. Iron deficiency anaemia.
2. Mild to moderate increase in the erythroid progenitors (normoblasts). Perls'-Prussian blue reveals disappearance of stainable iron from macrophages (sideroblasts) in the bone marrow.
3. Serum iron and ferritin level are low, whereas total iron binding capacity (TIBC) is high (which is a reflection of elevated transferrin level). This results in a reduction of transferrin saturation to <15%.

PC 21

1. Megaloblastic anaemia
2. Red blood cells (RBCs) are macrocytic and oval (macro-ovalocytes). Neutrophils are larger than normal (macropolymorphonuclear) and some hypersegmented, having ≥5 lobes (normally 3–4 lobes) neutrophils.
3. The characteristic large cells are megaloblasts. These cells are large with a deeply basophilic cytoplasm, prominent nucleoli and a distinctive, fine nuclear chromatin pattern.

PC 22

1. Sickle cell anaemia.
2. Point mutation in the sixth codon of β-globin chain that leads to the replacement of a glutamine residue with a valine residue.
3. These crises are episodes of hypoxic injury and infarction which cause severe pain. The affected organs are bones, lungs, liver, brain, spleen and penis.
4. Mixing of blood sample with an oxygen-consuming reagent such as metabisulphite induces sickling of red cells. This is known as **sickling test**. It can be done with 2% metabisulfite or dithionite.

PC 23

1. Hereditary spherocytosis
2. There are intrinsic defects in the red cell due to diverse mutations which lead to an insufficiency of membrane skeletal components. The pathogenic mutations commonly seen in ankyrin, spectrin, band 3 and band 4.2.
3. Aplastic crises are usually triggered by acute parvovirus infection. This virus infects and kills red cell progenitors (normoblasts), causing red cell production to cease.
4. Osmotic fragility test which is increased in hereditary spherocytosis.

Note

Spherocytes on peripheral blood smear are not pathognomonic of hereditary spherocytosis (HS) as it may be found in autoimmune haemolytic anaemia, ABO haemolytic disease (but not with RH haemolytic disease) of newborn, G6PD deficiency and infections/burns.

PC 24

1. β-Thalassemia major
2. β-Thalassemia minor (trait)
3. Anisopoikilocytosis, target cell, microcytes, basophilic stippling, and fragmented red cells.
4. The marrow is hypercellular and active. The expanding marrow erodes existing cortical bone and induces new bone formation, giving rise to a "crew-cut" appearance.

PC 25

1. β-Thalassemia minor (thalassemia trait).
2. The person will be heterozygous β-thalassemia (β^0/β, or β^+/β). One β globin chain will be normal, other is defective.
3. Anaemia will be either absent or if present mild.

4. It will reveal increase in HbA_2 ($\alpha_2\delta_2$) to 5.4% of the total haemoglobin (normal 2.5 + 0.3%). Adult haemoglobin or HbA will be 84% of total haemoglobin (normal 96%).

PC 26

1. Lung (pulmonary) infection, bronchopneumonia type.
2. Focal opacities due to consolidation in right lung.
3. *Staphylococcus aureus*
4. There will be suppurative, neutrophil-rich exudate which fills the bronchi, bronchioles and adjacent alveolar spaces.

PC 27

1. Bilateral 'fluffy or wooly' opacities predominantly in the upper zones with fibrotic infiltration. Diagnosis is pulmonary tuberculosis (Koch).
2. Erosion of blood vessels by the active pulmonary lesion, particulary bronchial artery is the source of haemoptysis.
3. Ziehl-Neelsen or ZN stain (acid-fast stain) is used to detect the organism, i.e. tubercle bacilli. The acid fastness of tubercle bacilli is due to mycolic acids, cross-linked fatty acids and other lipids in the cell wall of the bacilli. The bacilli take up stain by heated carbolfuchsin and resist decolourisation by weak acids and alcohol unlike other organisms, which cannot resist decolourisation. So, tubercle bacilli are acid fast as well as alcohol (ethanol) fast.

Note

False positive AFB (acid-fast bacilli) staining in ZN stain may be seen due to *Nocardia*, *Legionella*, *Cryptosporidium*, *Isospora*, *Rhodococcus* and some protozoa.

PC 28

1. Emphysaema of lung, a type of COPD (chronic obstructive pulmonary disease)
2. These patients over ventilate and remain well oxygenated as well as tachypnoea.
3. Protease-antiprotease imbalance hypothesis. There is destructive effect of high protease coupled with low antiprotease lead to tissue damage.
4. Death is due to:
   i. Respiratory acidosis and coma
   ii. Right-sided heart failure, and
   iii. Massive collapse of the lungs secondary to pneumothorax.

PC 29

1. Bronchial asthma
2. Status asthmaticus
3. Major basic protein of eosinophils.
4. These are collections of crystalloids, made up an eosinophil lysophospholipase binding protein called galectin.

PC 30

1. Lung cancer (carcinoma).
2. Initially FNAC may be done to determine the malignant nature of the neoplasm. But final diagnosis should be made after lung biopsy and histopathologic examination.
3. There are five main histologic types:
   i. Adenocarcinoma
   ii. Squamous cell carcinoma or epidermoid carcinoma
   iii. Small cell carcinoma
   iv. Large cell carcinoma
   v. Combined carcinoma, e.g. adenosquamous carcinoma (combination of adenocarcinoma and squamous cell carcinoma).

PC 31

1. Congestive heart failure (CHF) due to right-sided heart failure.
2. Congestive heart failure (CHF) due to left sided-heart failure.

   In the lung, some RBCs extravasate into pulmonary oedema fluid within the alveolar spaces, where they are phagocytosed and digested by macrophages, which store iron of haemoglobin in the form of haemosiderin. These haemosiderin laden macrophages are known as **heart failure cells**.

3. In the liver, congestion is most prominent around central veins within hepatic lobules, which show red-brown centrilobular discolouration. But the peripheral region becomes paler. This combination of dark and pale colour produces **nutmeg liver**.

PC 32

1. Myocardial infarction.
2. Cardiac-specific proteins, particularly troponin T and troponin I.
3. Gross features: Mottling with yellow-tan infarct centre.

   Microscopic features: Coagulation necrosis with loss of nuclei and muscle striations, dense neutrophilic infiltration into the infarcted area (interstitial).

PC 33

1. Infective endocarditis (subacute bacterial endocarditis).
2. *Streptococcus viridans* in case of previously damaged valves. *Staphylococcus aureus* in both normal and abnormal valves. But *S. viridans* is more common organism and less virulent.
3. There are vegetations which contain fibrin (thrombotic debris), inflammatory cells and bacteria or other organisms.
4. In RHD, vegetations are small, warty and present along the lines of closure of valve leaflets. In infective endocarditis they are large, irregular and present on the valve-cusps that can extend onto the chordae.

PC 34

1. Peptic ulcer disease.
2. *Helicobacter pylori* or *H. pylori* (spiral-shaped or curved bacilli).
3. • Duodenum (first part)
   • Stomach (lesser curvature near the junction of body and antrum).
   • Margins of jejunostomy
   • Gastro-oesophageal junction in GERD or Barrett's oesophagus.
   • In ileal Meckel's diverticulum containing ectopic gastric mucosa.
   • Stomach, duodenum and/or jejunum (multiple ulcers) in Zollinger-Ellison syndrome.

PC 35

1. Ulcerative colitis, a type of inflammatory bowl disease (IBD).
2. There are diffuse inflammatory infiltrates which are limited to the mucosa and superficial submucosa. There are cryptitis, crypt abscess, architectural crypt distortion and epithelial metaplasia. But noncaseating granuloma is absent unlike Crohn's disease.
3. Migratory polyarthritis, sacroiliitis, ankylosing spondylitis, uveitis, skin lesions, pericholangitis and primary sclerosing cholangitis.

PC 36

1. Acute proliferative (poststreptococal/postinfectious) glomerulonephritis or nephritic syndrome.
2. • Anti-streptolysin O (ASO)
   • Anti-deoxyribonuclease B (anti-DNAse B)
   • Anti-streptokinase (ASKase)
   • Anti-nicotinyl adenine dinucleotidase (anti-NADase)
3. The glomeruli are enlarged and hypercellular with diffuse involvement. The diffuse hypercellularity of glomerular tuft is due to proliferation of mesangial, endothelial and occasionally epithelial cells (acute proliferative lesions). Also, there are infiltration of leukocytes, mainly neutrophils and sometimes monocytes (acute exudative lesions).

There may be interstitial oedema and inflammation and the tubules often contain red cell casts.

PC 37

1. Nephrotic syndrome
2. In children, most common cause is minimal change glomerulonephritis. In adults, most common cause is membranous glomerulonephritis and focal segmental glomerulosclerosis.
3. A highly selective proteinuria consists mostly of low-molecular weight proteins (albumin 70 kD; transferrin 76 kD molecular weight). In non-selective or poorly selective proteinuria there are other proteins like high molecular weight globulins in addition to albumin.

PC 38

1. Pyogenic osteomyelitis (bacterial osteomyelitis).
2. *Staphylococcus aureus* is the commonest pathogen (80–90% of the cases).
3. In the neonate, the metaphyseal vessels penetrate the growth plate, resulting in frequent infection of the metaphysis, epiphysis, or both.

   But in children, pathogenic organism typically affects the metaphysis as metaphyseal vessels do not penetrate growth plate.

   Again, in adults, bacteria infect epiphyses and subchondral regions due to closure of growth plate and the metaphyseal vessels reunite with their epiphyseal counterparts.
4. In sickle cell disease, Salmonella bacteria are the causative organism.

PC 39

1. Ewing's sarcoma
2. The tumour arises from medullary cavity in diaphysis and usually affects long tubular bones, especially the femur and the flat bones of pelvis.
3. The tumour is composed of sheets of uniform small, round cells which are slightly larger than lymphocytes having scant cytoplasm, that may appear clear because it is rich in glycogen. There may be presence of **Homer-Wright rosettes** (where the tumour cells are arranged in a circle about a central fibrillary space) which are indicative of neural differentiation. The tumour contains fibrous septae and a little stroma. Necrosis may be present. Mitotic figures are a few in number.

PC 40

1. Prostatic adenocarcinoma
2. Gleason system is used for prostatic adenocarcinoma. According to this system, prostate cancers are divided into 5 grades on the basis of glandular patterns of differentiation.
3. In most laboratories, serum PSA level of 8 ng/ml is used as a cut-off.

   However, upper age specific reference range is better:
   - For men 40–49 years: 2.5 ng/ml
   - For men 50–59 years: 3.5 ng/ml
   - For men 60–69 years: 4.5 ng/ml
   - For men 70–79 years: 6.5 ng/ml
4. AMACR (alpha-methyl-coenzyme A-racemase), which is positive in 82–100% of prostatic adenocarcinoma.

PC 41

1. Hepatocellular carcinoma (HCC)
2. Serum α-fetoprotein (AFP).
3. Four major etiologic factors:
   i. Chronic viral infection (HBV, HCV)
   ii. Chronic alcoholism
   iii. Non-alcoholic steatohepatitis (NASH)
   iv. Food contaminants (primarily aflatoxins)
4. HCC appears grossly as (1) a unifocal large mass, (2) multifocal (widely distributed variable size nodules), (3) a diffusely infiltrative cancer.

✍ **Note**

False positive AFP may be seen due to yolk sac tumours, embryonal carcinoma, and many non-neoplastic like cirrhosis, massive liver necrosis, chronic hepatitis (specially HCV infection), normal pregnancy, fetal distress or death and fetal neural tube defects such as anencephaly and spina bifida.

PC 42

1. Human immunodeficiency virus (HIV) infection causing AIDS (acquired immunodeficiency syndrome).
2. HIV 1 group M subtype C is the commonest type.
3. p24 is the most readily detected viral antigen and is the target for the antibodies, used to diagnose HIV infection.
4. Candidiasis is the most common fungal infection in AIDS in India. *Pneumocystis jiroveci* (previously *carini*) is most common fungal infection in AIDS in world.

PC 43

1. Keloid scar.
2. There is excessive formation of the repair components (here collagen) leading to abnormality of the repair process and leads to complication of would healing.
3. Hypertrophic scar.
4. In hypertrophic scar, the scar tissue is restricted to the original wound and regress.

   In keloid, the scar tissue grows beyond the boundaries of the original wound and does not regress.

PC 44

1. Squamous cell carcinoma (keratinizing type)
2. Human papillomavirus, strain HPV 16 and HPV 18 (also HPV 31 and HPV 33).
3. • Squamous cell carcinoma (arise from ectocervix)
     - Keratinizing or nonkeratinizing type
     - Verrucous
     - Papillary transitional
     - Lymphoepthelioma-like
   • Adenocarcinoma (arise from endocervical glands)
     - Mucinous
     - Endometrioid
     - Clear cell
     - Serous
     - Mesonephric
     - Well differentiated villoglandular
     - Minimal deviation (adenoma malignum)
   • Other tumours/carcinomas
     - Adenosquamous
     - Glassy cell
     - Carcinoid tumour
     - Neuroendocrine
     - Small cell
     - Undifferentiated

PC 45

1. Haemophilia A (factor VIII deficiency)
2. X-linked recessive trait. So, it mainly affects males and homozygous females.
3. Mutations in factor VIII, which is an essential cofactor for factor IX in the coagulation cascade. The genetic lesions include deletions, nonsense mutations that create stop codons and mutations that cause errors in mRNA splicing.
4. Bleeding time (BT) and prothrombin time (PT) will be normal, whereas partial thromboplastin time (PTT) will be prolonged.

PC 46

1. Gaucher disease showing Gaucher cells in marrow.
2. It is autosomal recessive disorder resulting from mutations in the gene encoding glucocerebrosidase. So, glucocerebrosides accumulate in massive amounts within phagocytic cells.
3. Gaucher cells are found in spleen, liver, bone marrow, lymph nodes, tonsils, thymus are Peyer's patches.

4. There are 3 subtypes:
   Type I: Chronic non-neuropathic form
   Type II: Acute neuropathic form
   Type III: Intermediate between type I and type II.

PC 47

1. Urinary tract infection or UTI.
2. The specific gravity of urine will be increase (normal specific gravity of urine 1.016–1.025).
3. Urine culture test. More than 85% cases of UTI, causative organisms are gram-negative bacilli (*E. coli*, Proteus, Klebsiella)
4. Patient will develop chronic pyelonephritis. Grossly, the kidneys are usually irregularly scarred. If bilateral involvement, then they are asymmetric. The characteristic findings are coarse, discrete, corticomedullary scars overlying dilated, blunted or deformed calyces and flattening of the papillae.

PC 48

1. Iron deficiency anaemia
2. i. Increased blood loss: Menstruation in reproductive females
   ii. Increased requirements: Pregnancy, lactation and adolescence
3. i. Red cell indices: MCV↓, MCH↓, MCHC↓
   ii. Biochemical:
      - Total iron binding capacity (TIBC) is high (normal 250–450 µg/dl).
      - Serum ferritin is very low (normal 30–250 ng/ml).
      - Serum iron level is low (normal 40–140 µg/dl).
4. Parasitic worms (helminths), specifically hookworms, which include:
   1. *Ancylostoma duodenale*
   2. *Necator americanus*
   3. *Ancylostoma ceylanicum*.

> **Note**
>
> Other parasites which cause anaemia are:
> - *P. falciparum* (malaria): Normochromic anaemia
> - *L. donovani* (kala-azar): Normochromic anaemia
> - *Schistosoma haematobium*: Normochromic anemia
> - *Trichuris trichiura*: Normochromic anaemia
> - *T. gambiense* (sleeping sickness): Normochromic anaemia
> - *Diphyllobthrium* latum (*D. latum*): Megaloblastic and pernicious anaemia.

PC 49

1. Caseating granulomatous lymphadenitis, possibly due to tuberculosis.
2. Tuberculosis is caused by *Mycobacterium tuberculosis* bacilli. The diagnosis can be confirmed by:
   i. Culture of the aspirate: In LJ media and BACTEC media, gives positive culture.

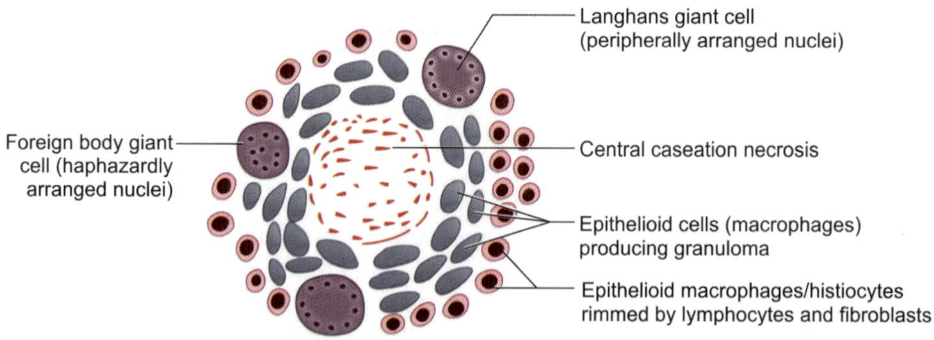

ii. ZN stain: Red-coloured tuberculous bacilli seen.

iii. Other: ESR will be high, Mantoux test may be positive. TB PCR may detect DNA of bacteria (insertion sequence IS 1081).

PC 50

1. Pyogenic (bacterial) meningitis. Because CSF pressure is highly increased (coming injet flow), CSF is hazy, glucose low (normal 40–80 mg%), protein content high (normal 15–45 mg/dl) and cell count is high (normal 1–4/mm^3).
2. Mostly neutrophils (>90%).
3. Severe headache, fever, vomiting, drowsiness, stupor, coma and occasionally convulsions. The most important clinical sign is stiffness of neck on forward bending (Kernig's sign) which is due to increased neck muscle tone and stiffness.
4. To find out the exact pathogen (bacteria), blood culture is needed followed by Gram stain (Gram +ve or Gram –ve bacteria).

Section

VI

OSPE (Objective Structured Practical Examination)

Chapter

19

OSPE: Discussion of 100 Cases

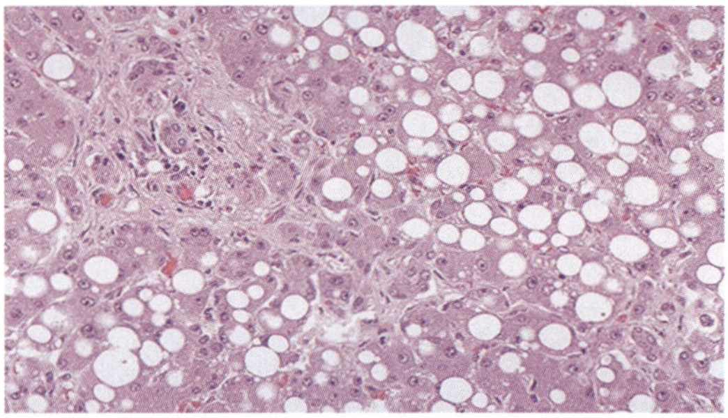

Q1. Examine the microscopic photograph of the lesion involving the liver and answer the following:

A. Identify the lesion? (1)

B. Name any two causes of lesion? (1)

C. Is it reversible lesion? Can it be malignant? (1)

D. What are essential criteria for histologic diagnosis of its malignant form? (1)

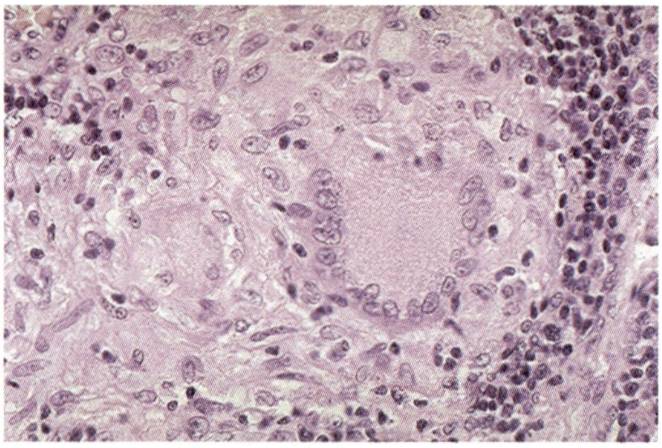

Q2. A 46 years old woman goes to the clinician for routine check-up. On examination there are enlarged lymph node. Tuberculin skin test was positive. Lymph nodes were removed and sent to Lab for HPE.

A. Examine the focused microscopic slide and identify the lesion. (1)

B. Define it. (1)

C. Name the type of necrosis seen. (1)

D. Name 2 other types of necrosis. (1)

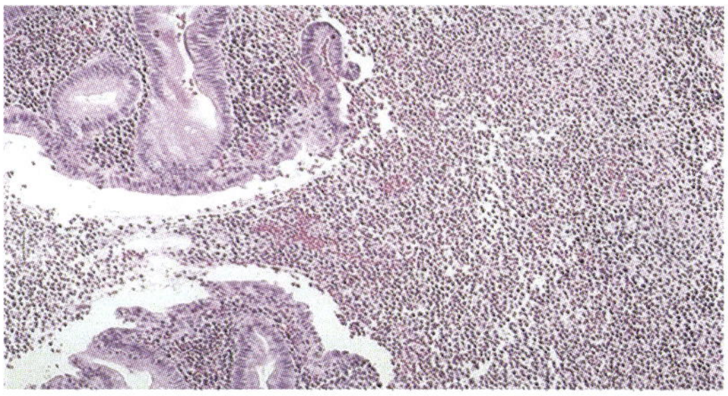

Q3. A 10 years old boy admitted in emergency with fever, nausea, loss of appetite and pain in right iliac fossa. On examination rebound tenderness was present. On Lab investigation WBC 12 × 10^3/μl, Hb-12.8 g/dl, platelets 250 × 10^3/μl. Patient was operated and specimen sent to lab. Histopathology slides are prepared and one slide is provided to you for microscopic examination.

A. Examine the focused slide and identify the lesion. (1)
B. Name the cell characteristics of this type. (1)
C. Give 2 outcomes. (1)
D. Enumerate the cardinal signs and chemical mediators for pain. (1)

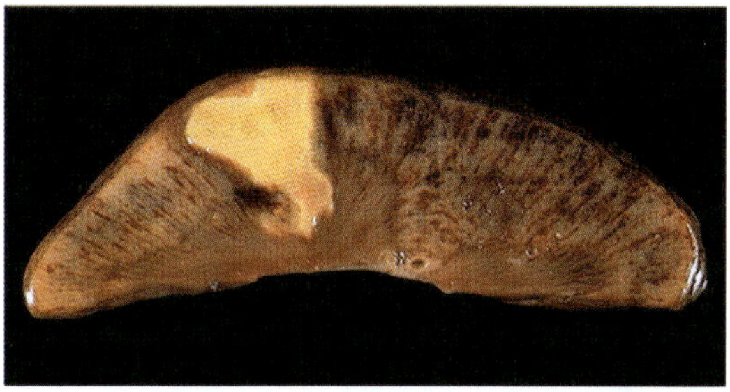

Q4. Yellowish wedge-shaped area is seen in the nephrectomy specimen of a 33 years old female. This area has demarcated borders and can be differentiated from the surrounding viable structures.

A. Identify the pattern of necrosis. (1)
B. What is the possible cause of this pattern of necrosis? (1)
C. Give its microscopic features. Any 2. (2)

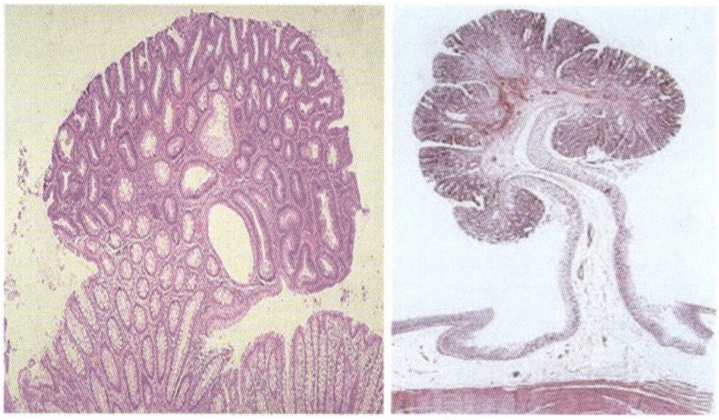

Q5. Observe the above photomicrograph and answer the following questions:

A. Name this tumour. Name the tumour suppressor gene which mutation may lead to such tumour. (1)
B. What are the differences between right-sided and left-sided carcinoma? (2)
C. What is the relative malignant potential of different types of adenomas. (1)

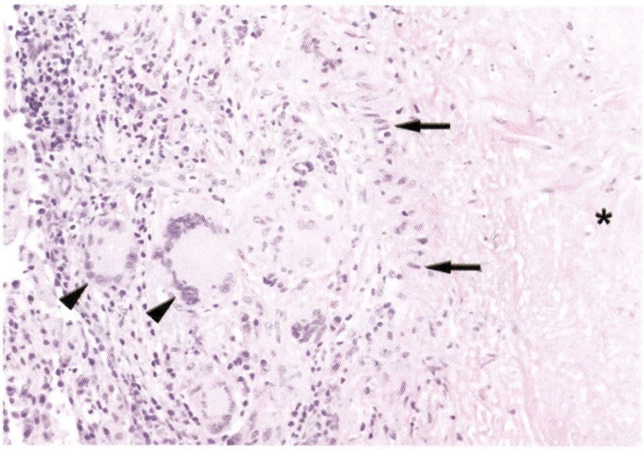

Q6. A 62 years old lady presented with weight loss and chronic cough and was diagnosed as suffering from pulmonary Tuberculosis. Her lung biopsy was performed which showed the following pictures.

A. What is the type of inflammation? (1)
B. What type of necrosis? (1)
C. Give 2 identifications points (arrow mark)? (1)
D. What is necrosis? (1)

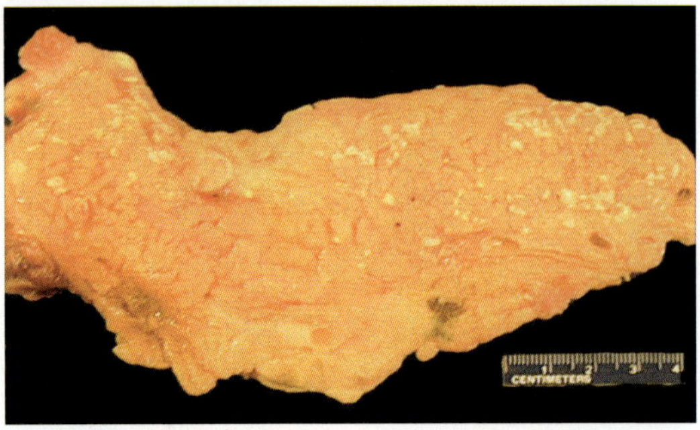

Q7. Laparotomy was done in a 32 years old lady with the provisional diagnosis of acute pancreatitis. Mesentery showed discrete white chalky deposits as shown in image.

A. Identify the pattern of necrosis. (1)
B. What would be the possible cause of this pattern of necrosis in a patient of acute pancreatitis? (1)
C. Name any other organ in which this pattern of necrosis can be seen. (1)
D. Which type of calcification will be seen in this patient? (1)

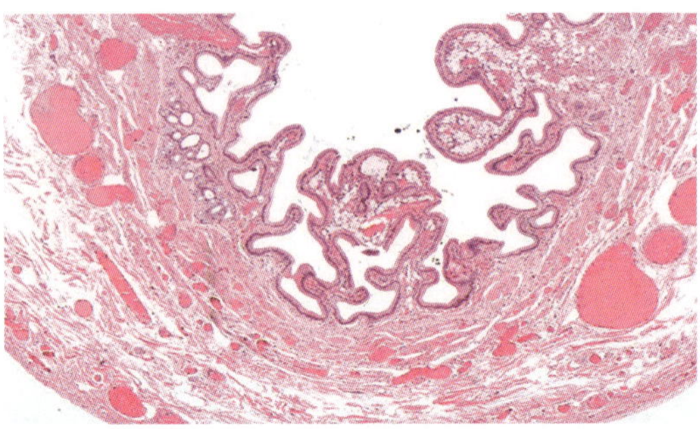

Q8. An obese lady of 40 years of age is suffering from recurrent dull boring, sometimes colicky pain in right hypochondrium. The pain increases on taking food especially fatty food. She was operated and HP slides are prepared.

A. Examine the focus slide and identify it. Write microscopic findings (2 diagnostic points) (1)
B. Name the cell characteristic of this type of inflammation. (1)
C. Enumerate 4 complications of this lesion. (2)

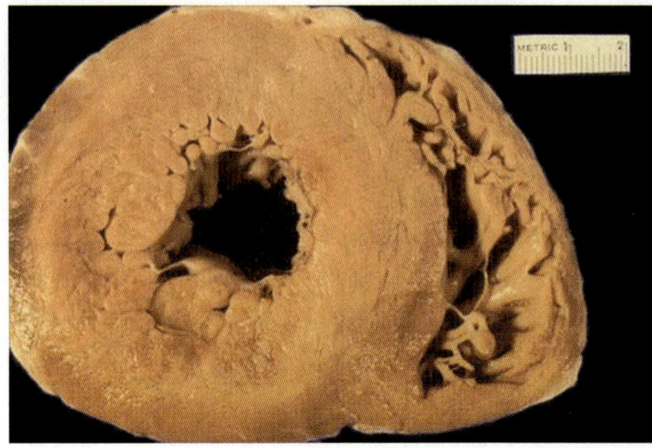

Q9. Examine the specimen and answer the following questions.

A. Is the heart enlarged? Name the process of Cellular adaptation that has occurred and define it. (1)
B. Name 2 other types of cellular adaptation. (1)
C. Give examples of each? (2)

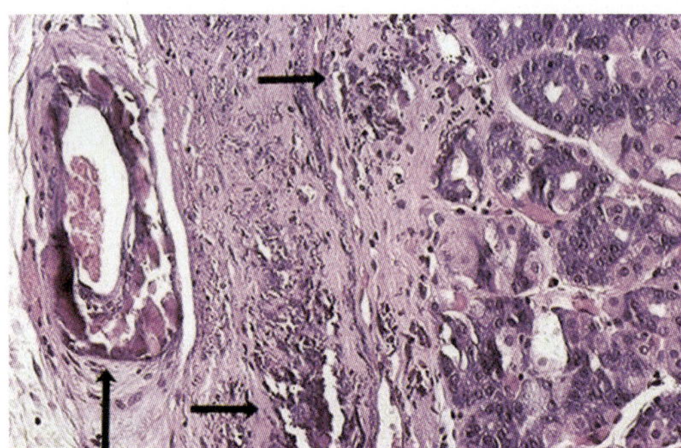

Q10. Observe the above photomicrograph and answer the following questions:

1. Examine the focused slide (arrow) and identify. (1)
2. Name two organs where it commonly occurs. (1)
3. What is the common cause? (1)
4. Different types of this kind of deposits? (1)

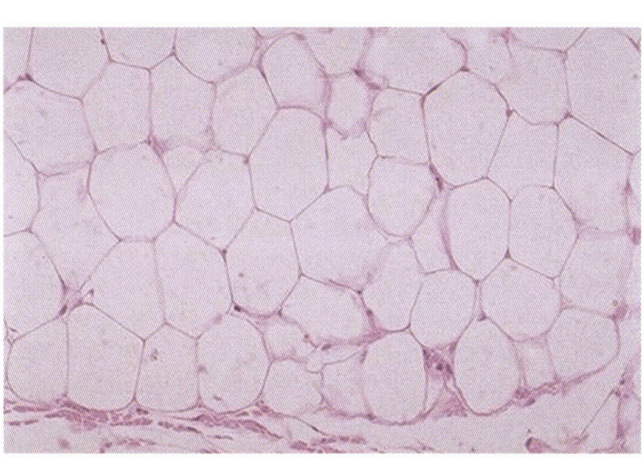

Q11. Observe the above photomicrograph and answer the following questions:

1. Examine the focused microscope slide and identify (2 microscopic findings). Name the malignant form of this lesion? (2)
2. Name the ONE other painless soft tissue swelling. (1)
3. Name any hereditary condition which may be seen associated with this lesion. (1)

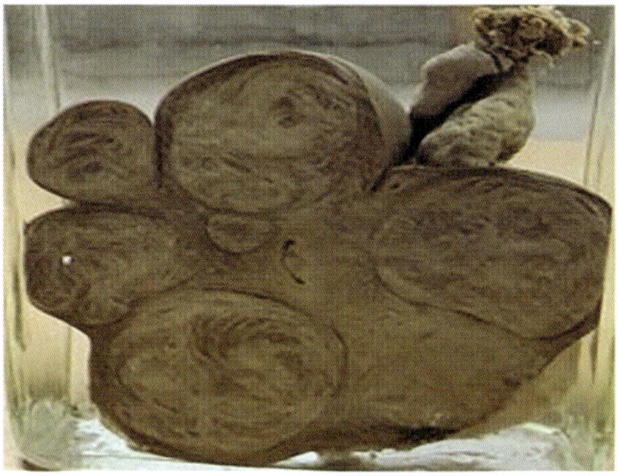

Q12. A 28-year-old female married for last 2 years present to emergency with spontaneous abortion. Her routine clinical and lab tests are within normal limit except USG revealed multiple sharply circumscribed nodule myometrium ranging from 2 to 5 cm in diameter.

A. Macroscopic (Gross) identifying points. Where can it occur in the uterus? (1)
B. What is the composition of this tumour? (1)
C. What will you find on microscopic examination? Enlist two points of differentiation between the above benign and malignant lesion microscopically? (2)

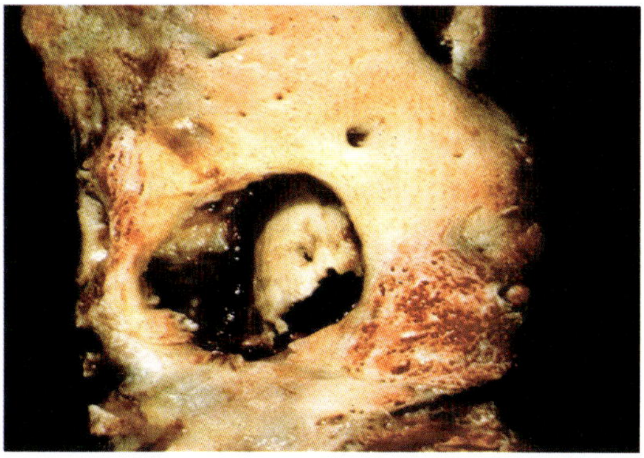

Q13. A 22-year-old male presented with localized pain above his right knee joint with recurrent fever. Later on, he developed discharging sinuses from the skin overlying the right knee.

A. What is the most likely diagnosis? (1)
B. Name any 2 causative agents. (1)
C. Macroscopic (2 gross) identifying points. (2)

to a trauma.

Involucrum: The proliferation of bone surrounding the sequestrum and the cavity where it sits are called the involucrum.

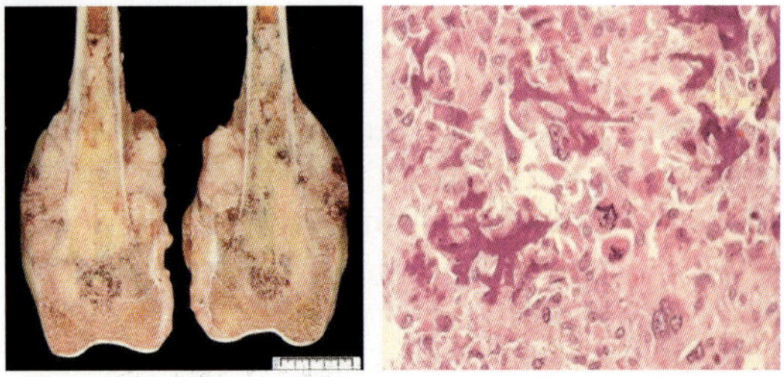

Q14. An 18-year-old female presented to the rheumatology clinic with 2 months history of pain and swelling in her upper thigh with weight loss.

A. What is the most likely diagnosis? (1)
B. Most common bone and site involved. (1)
C. What will you find on microscopic examination? Any two. (2)

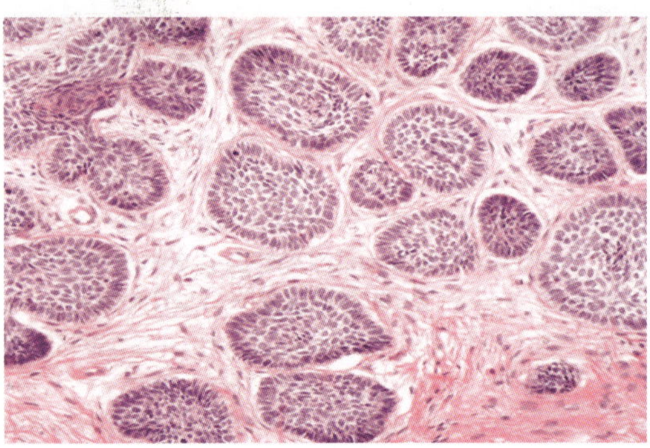

Q15. A non-healing ulcer on face with raised margins was detected in an old lady. Which was biopsied and slide was prepared.

A. What is likely diagnosis? (1)
B. Write 4 diagnostic points of this lesion. (1)
C. What is the biologic behaviour of this tumour? (1)
D. What is the clinical location and type of growth pattern seen in this tumour. (1)

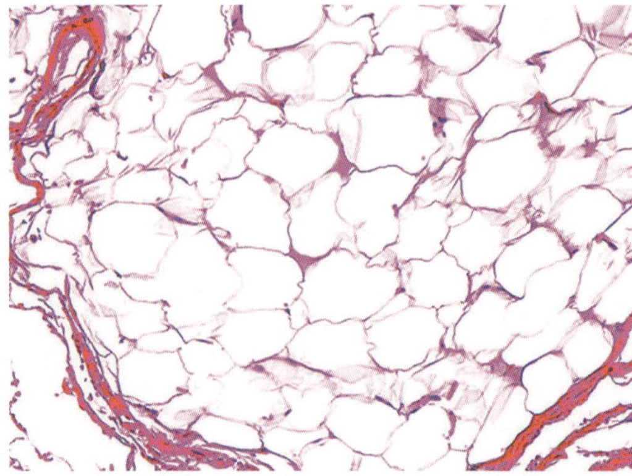

Q16. A 35-year-old lady presents to the surgical OPD with a painless lump over the shoulder on examination it is freely mobile. On excision, it is well encapsulated. Examine the HP slide prepared.

A. What is the diagnosis? Name the malignant variant of this lesion. (1)
B. Write 2 microscopic identification features of this lesion. (2)
D. Name 2 other variants of this tumour? (1)

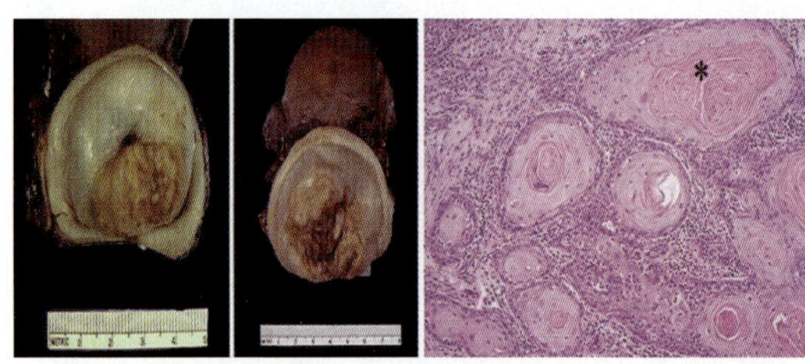

Q17. A 50-year-old patient, Para 5 was referred to gynaecologic oncology service after an evaluation for abnormal vaginal bleeding. Cervical biopsies was taken. She was operated and HP slides were prepared.

A. What is your diagnosis (1)
B. Write any 2 gross features (1)
C. Write any 2 microscopic findings (2)

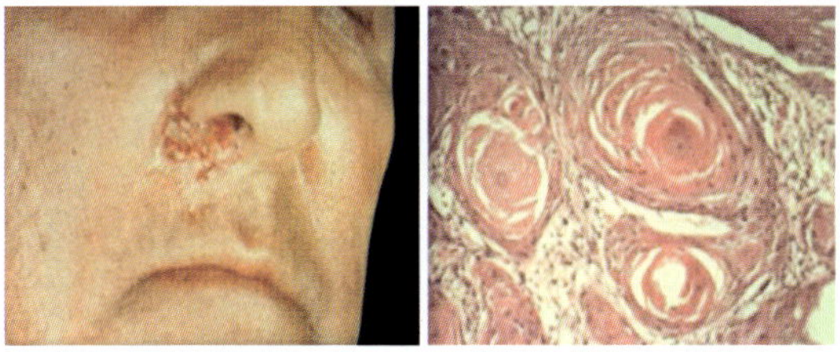

Q18. This 57-year-old man gave history of a lesion of the face which was removed and irradiated. Recently he noted a recurrent lesion which was firm and nodular with an area of ulceration at the angle of left nares.

A. What is your diagnosis? (1)
B. Two microscopic features? (2)
C. Name any 2 etiological factors? (1)

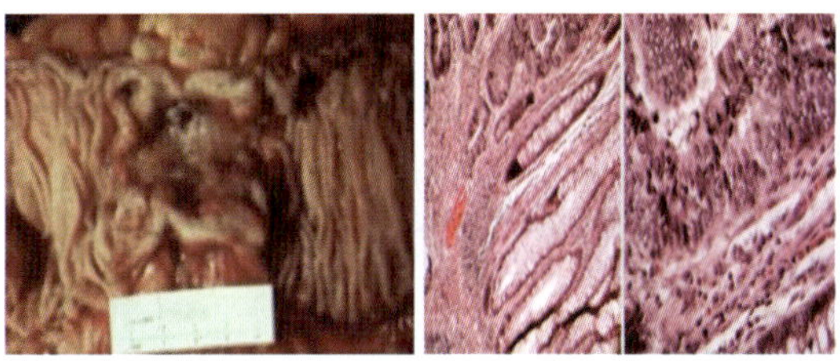

Q19. This 54-year-old woman was admitted for the acute onset of abdominal pain, nausea and vomiting for 24 hours. A mass was felt in the lower abdomen and the abdomen was tender. At operation a fistula was found between the transverse and sigmoid colon. A biopsy was taken.

A. What is your diagnosis? (1)
B. What is the etiology. (2)
C. What are its complications. (1)

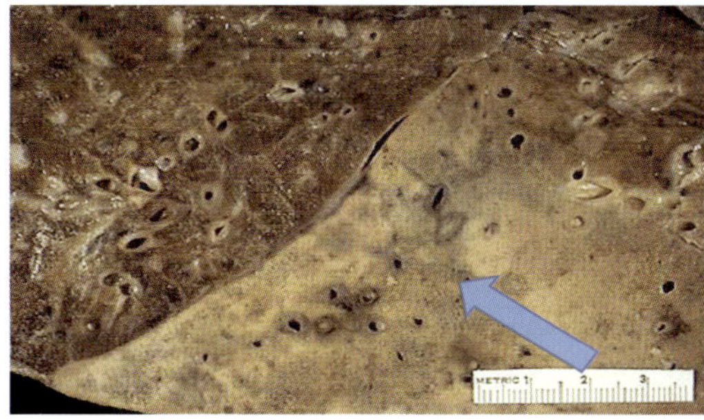

Q20. Clinical history of a male patient aged 40 years old complaining of high-grade fever, cough, dyspnoea and chest pain.

A. What is your diagnosis (1)
B. What are the microscopic findings? (2)
C. What are the different stages? (1)

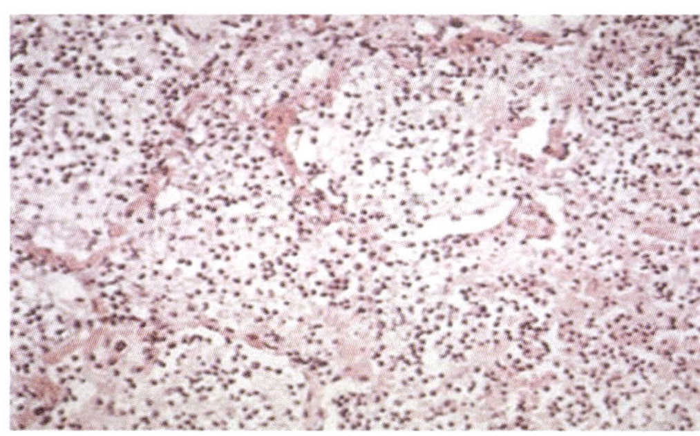

Q21. Microphotograph of a lesion in the lung from a 45-year-old male, with high grade fever, chills, pleuritic pain and shortness of breath.

A. What is your diagnosis? Define the lesion. (1)
B. Give 2 points in favour of diagnosis. (2)
C. What is most common microorganism causing the lesion? (1)

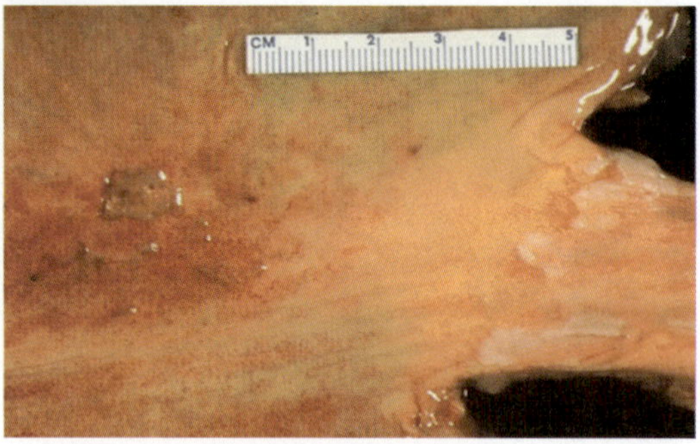

Q22. A 40-year-old woman with h/o intake of NSAIDs presented in the emergency with acute pain in the epigastric region. On upper GI endoscopy, a 1 cm diameter acute gastric ulcer was seen as shown in given photograph.

A. Describe the ulcer. Give 2 common sites of peptic ulcer. (1)

B. Name the infection that plays an important role in pathogenesis of peptic ulcer. (1)

C. What is the initial pathology. (2)

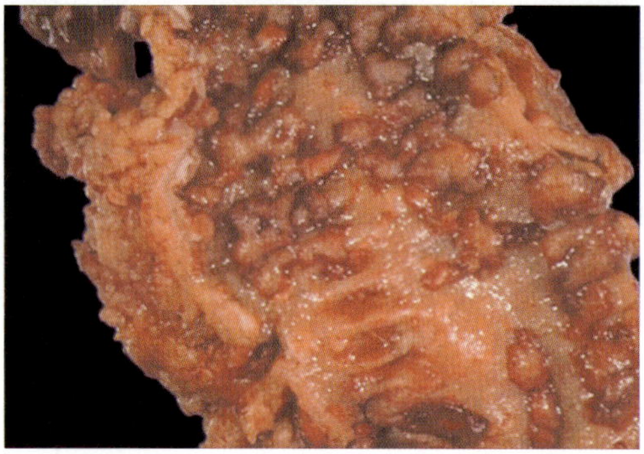

Q23. Given photograph shows the gross appearance of the colon of a patient who presented with h/o recurring attacks of bloody mucoid diarrhoea for last 6 months. The symptoms persisted for weeks and then subsided.

A. Give the diagnosis. (1)

B. What are pseudopolyps? Skip lesions are seen in which disease? (1)

C. Enumerate 4 extraintestinal manifestations? (2)

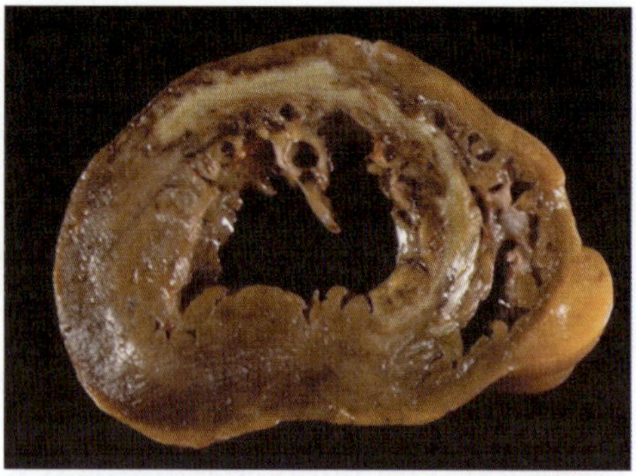

Q24. Photograph of gross section through heart of a patient who died of acute MI (Myocardial Infarction). (Autopsy specimen).

A. Describe the appearance of infarct. (1)

B. What is transmural infarct? (1)

C. Give any 4 complications of acute MI. (2)

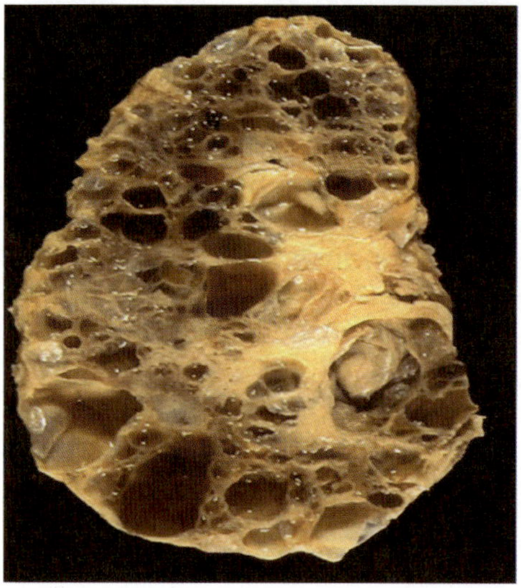

Q25. Carefully examine the gross specimen (or photograph) of kidney in a patient with progressive renal insufficiency and answer the following questions.

A. Give your diagnosis. (1)

B. Give any 2 features seen on gross examination. (2)

C. What is the pattern of inheritance of this disorder? (1)

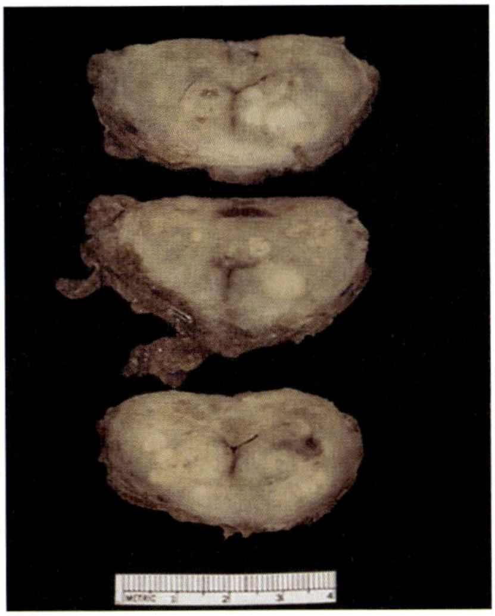

Q26. Carefully examine the given photograph/ gross specimen of prostate which is enlarged and the patient had increased PSA levels. Answer the following question.

A. Give your diagnosis. (1)

B. Give the gross appearance. Can this condition coexist with hyperplasia? (1)

D. Write microscopic findings? (2)

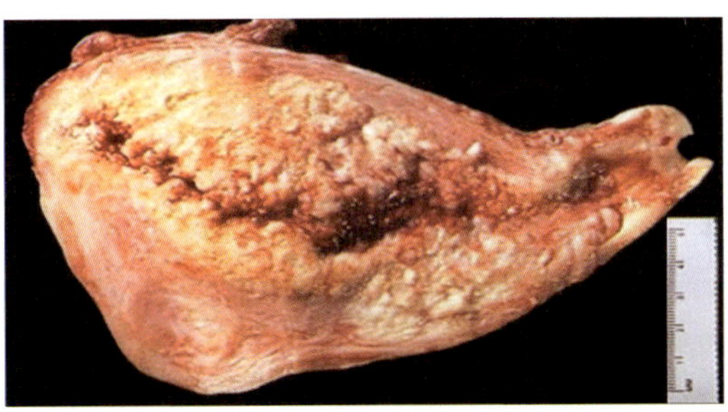

Q27. Specimen of uterus (cut section) from a patient with history of postmenopausal bleeding diagnosed as endometrial carcinoma. Answer the following:

A. Describe the gross morphology of lesion. (2)

B. What are risk factors for the development of endometrial adenocarcinoma. (1)

C. What will be gland: Stroma ratio to call it endometrial hyperplasia? (1)

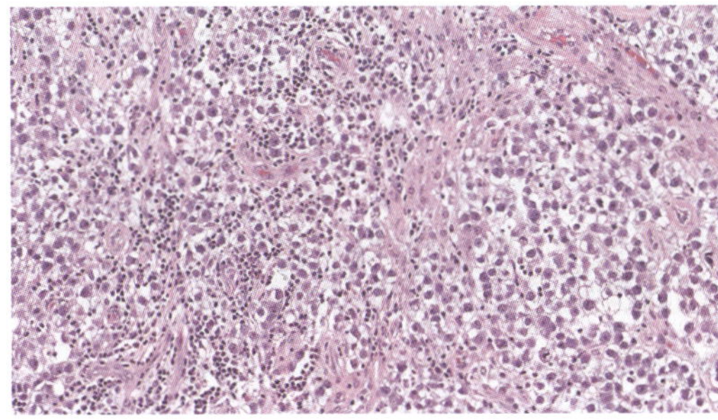

Q28. Microphotograph of a biopsy from a 45-year-old male, with scrotal swelling. It was diagnosed as a case of seminoma. Answer the following:

A. Is it benign or a malignant tumour? (1)

B. Name any 4 other germ cell tumours of the testis. (2)

C. In addition to surgery what is the primary mode of therapy for pure classic seminoma? (1)

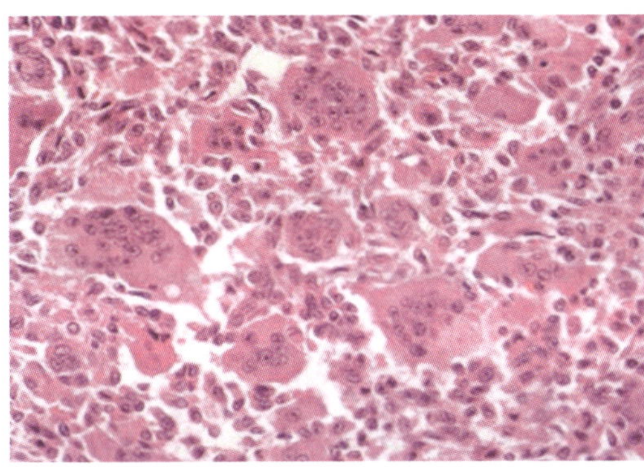

Q29. Microscopic slide of a tissue from bone of a 20 years old female with h/o painful swelling of the knee joint which shows lytic lesion eroding the subchondral bone plate on radiological examination. Answer the following.

A. Give your diagnosis. (1)

B. Give important features of identification (Gross and microscopy) (2)

C. Is it benign or a malignant tumour. (1)

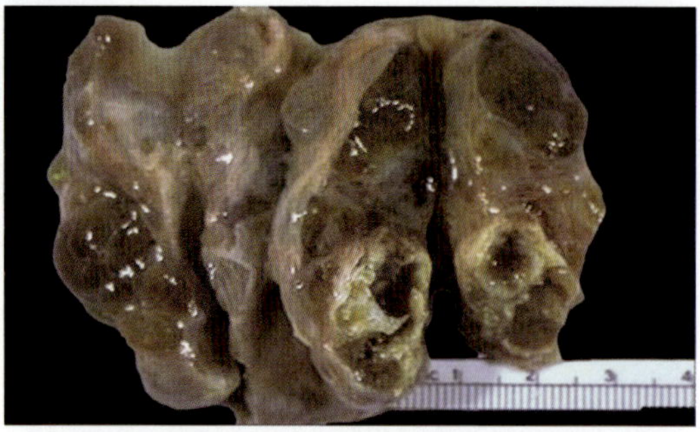

Q30. Specimen of thyroid gland removed after surgery in a 30-year-old female showing multiple nodules.

A. Give your diagnosis. (1)

B. Describe the gross morphology of the lesion. (2)

C. How would radioactive iodine scan look in a thyroid gland such as the one picturized here? (1)

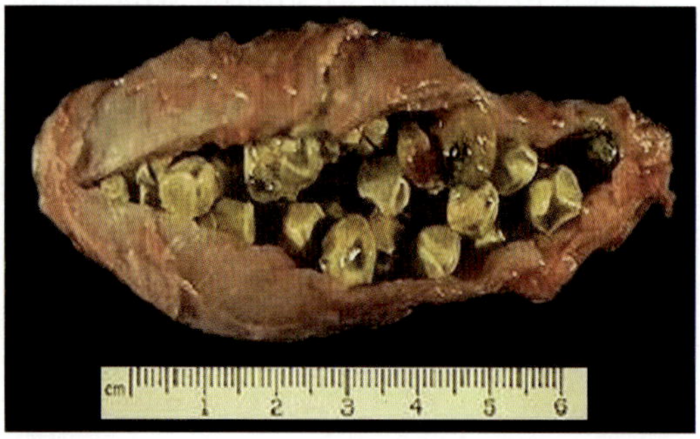

Q31. A 57 years old female complained of abdominal pain in right upper quadrant, abdominal USG indicates acute cholecystic and multiple stones in the lumen. Emergency cholecystectomy was carried at and specimen was preserved.

A. What are the risk factors and complications of gallstones? (1)

B. Gross and Microscopic finding of acute cholecystitis. (2)

C. What are the types of stones? (1)

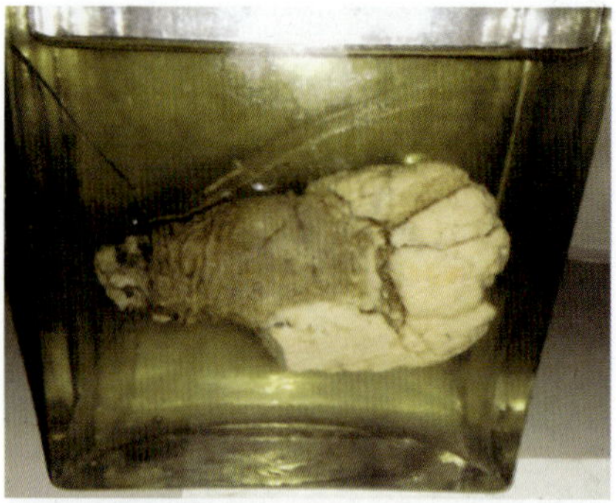

Q32. Gross specimen of penis in jar has following features:

A. What is your diagnosis? (1)

B. What are risk factors of this tumour? (1)

C. What is verrucous carcinoma? (1)

D. What are the histologic subtypes of Squamous cell carcinoma? (1)

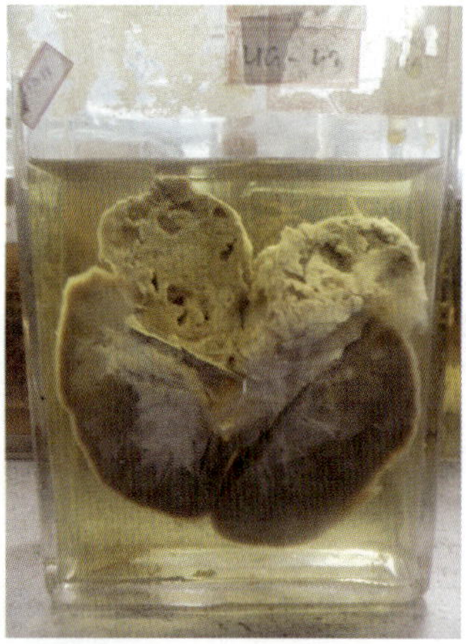

Q33. Observe the above museum specimen and answer the following questions:

A. What is the diagnosis of this mounted specimen? (1)

B. What are the light microscopic features? (1)

C. What special stain is used to demonstrate constitutes in clear cytoplasm? (1)

D. What are the classic diagnostic features? (1)

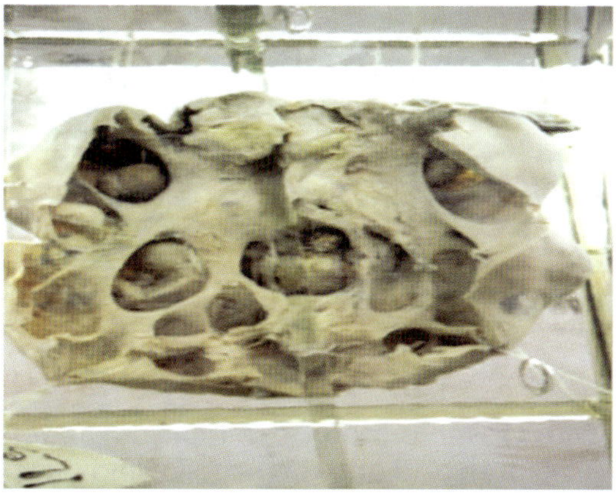

Q34. Observe the above museum specimen and answer the following questions:

A. What is the diagnosis of this mounted specimen? (1)

B. enumerate the causes. (1)

C. What is flea beaten kidney? What are the causes? (2)

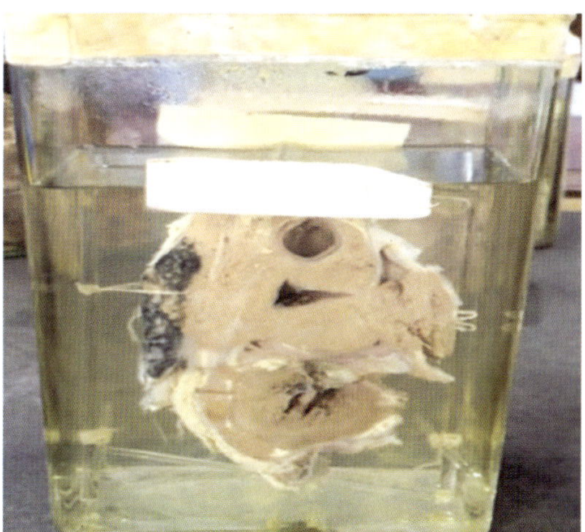

Q35. Observe the above museum specimen and answer the following questions:

A. What is the diagnosis of this mounted specimen? (1)

B. Classify the tumour? (1)

C. What are the risk factors? (1)

D. What are the precursor lesions? (1)

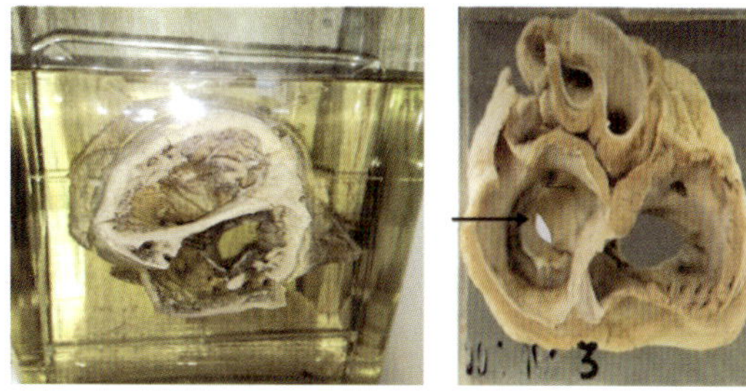

Q36. Observe the above museum specimen and answer the following questions:

A. What is the diagnosis of this mounted specimen? (1)

B. What are the clinical features and most common cause? (1)

C. What are the complications and consequences? (2)

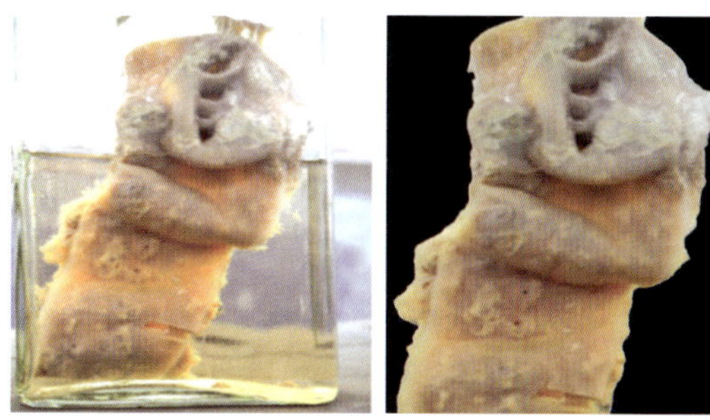

Q37. Observe the above museum specimen and answer the following questions:

A. What is the diagnosis of this mounted specimen? (1)

B. What are the different stages in the evolution? (1)

C. What are the components? (1)

D. Which vessels are spared by this? (1)

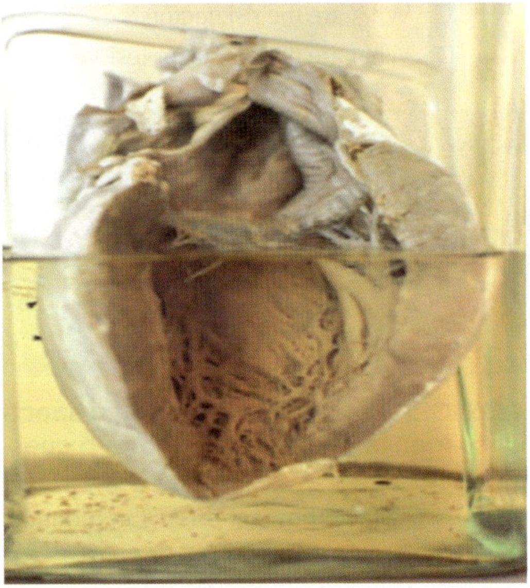

Q38. Observe the above museum specimen and answer the following questions:

A. What is your diagnosis of this mounted specimen? (1)

B. What are common causes? (1)

C. What are the light microscopic features? (2)

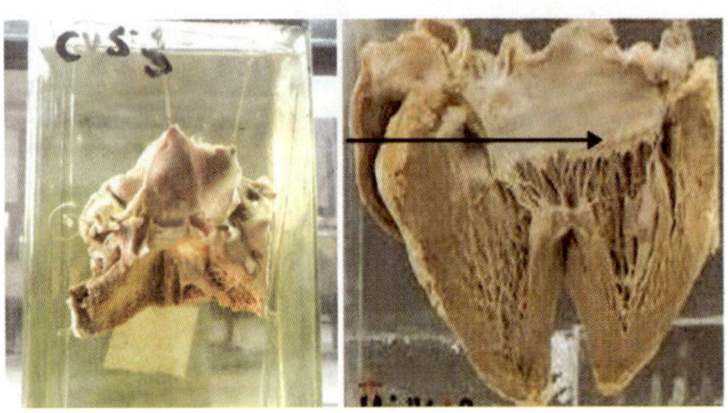

Q39. Observe the above museum specimen and answer the following questions:

A. What is your diagnosis of this mounted specimen? (1)

B. What are the different types of vegetations? (2)

C. Which valve is most commonly involved? (1)

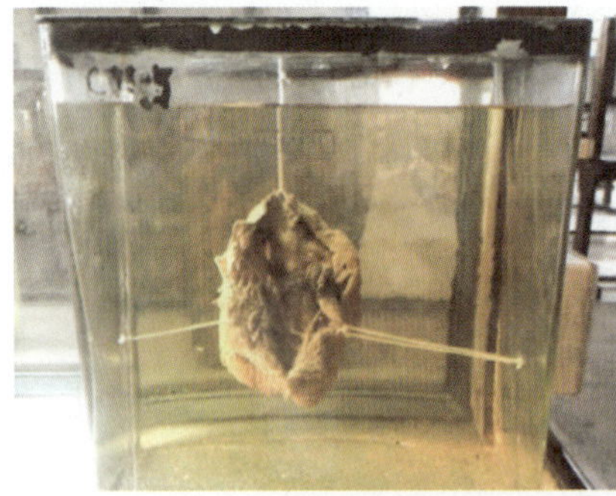

Q40. Observe the above museum specimen and answer the following questions:

A. What is your diagnosis of this mounted specimen?

B. What are the causes? (1)

C. What are the clinical features? (1)

D. What are the components of fluid in this? (1)

HAEMATOLOGY

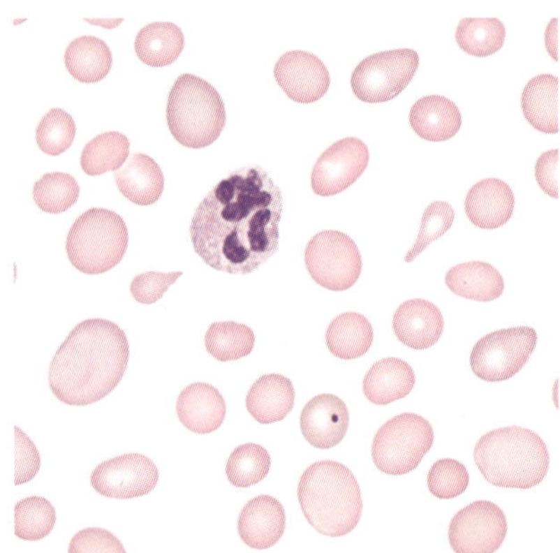

Q41. A 45-years-old male presents with progressively increasing weakness and pallor. He gives history of on-and-off diarrhoea, numbness in hands and feet for the last 6 months. Blood picture shows pancytopenia. Blood film provided.

A. Write down your findings? (2)

B. Name 2 sets you should advise (1)

C. What will be the Red cell indices in this case. (1)

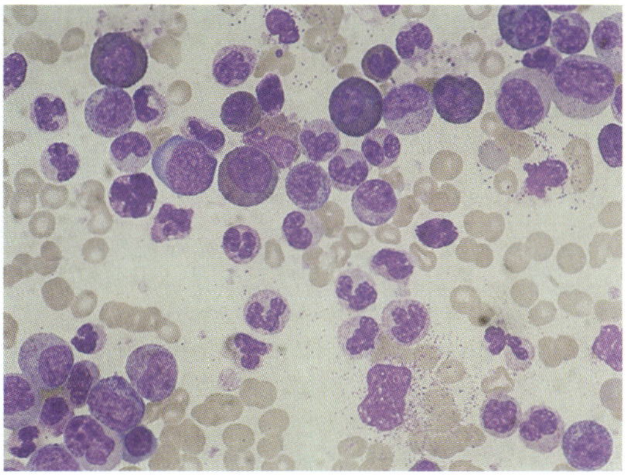

Q42. A 55-year-old male presented with fever, weakness and massive splenomegaly.

Labs:

Hb	9 g/dl
WBC	165×10^9/L
Platelets	765×10^9/L
Promyelocytes	08%
Myelocyte	22%
Metamyelocyte	12%
Basophil	02%
Stabs	7%
Neutrophils	37%
Blast cells	2%
Eosinophils	10%

A. What is the diagnosis? (1)
B. Which chromosomal abnormality is consistently seen in this disorder? (1)
C. Give 2 etiological factors of this disorder. (1)
D. What type of blast crisis is seen in this type of leukaemia? (1)

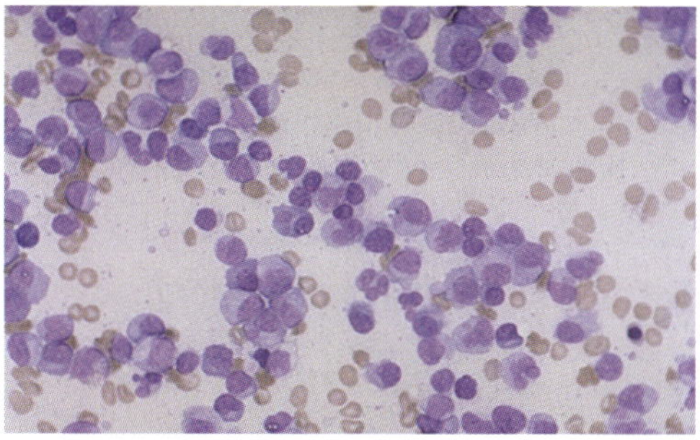

Q43. A 55-year-old male presents with fever, weight loss and bone pains. X-Ray shows lytic lesions in skull and vertebral bones.

Laboratory findings (hematology):

Hb	8 g/dl
TLC	7×10^9/L
Platelet	150×10^9/L
ESR	100 mm/hr

A. Give one change in serum electrophoresis pattern. (1)
B. What is the diagnosis? (1)
C. What is Bence Jones protein? (1)
D. What are different types of immunoglobulin? (1)

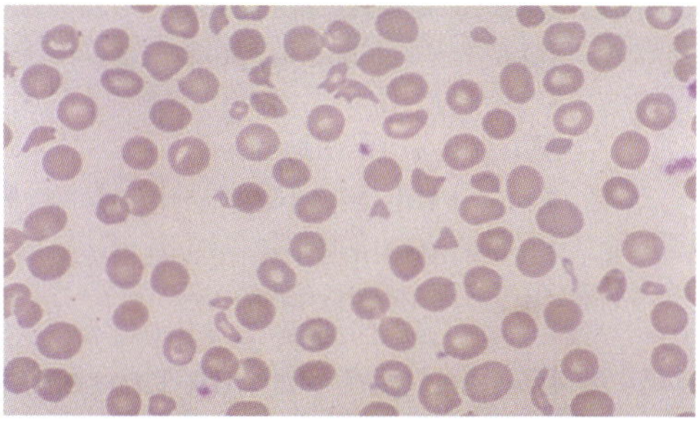

Q44. A 35-year-old female gave history of induced abortion by a Dai. She presented with massive bleeding per vagina and gangrene of left toe.

Laboratory findings show PT—prolonged, APTT—prolonged, Fibrinogen—increased and Platelet—reduced.

A. What is the morphology of red blood cells? (1)

B. Give the most likely diagnosis. (1)
C. Name the type of anaemia associated with this condition. (1)
D. What tests will confirm the diagnosis? (1)

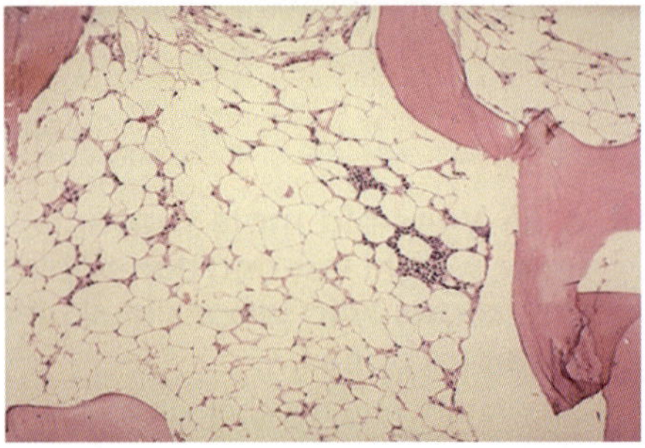

Q45. A 25-year-old male presented in emergency department with marked ulceration of mouth and multiple tray transition abscesses. He had no hepato-splenomegaly. His laboratory findings were WNL (within normal limits) 6 months back.

Present investigations are:

WBC	1.8 × 10^9/L	MCH	28 pg
RBC	2 ×10^9/L	MCHC	33 g/dl
Platelets	×10^9/L	RDW	13.6
Hct	0.33/L	Lymphocytes	92%
MCV	89/L	Neutrophil	68%

A. What is your diagnosis? (1)
B. How is this disease classified? (2)
C. Describe the findings in the given slides of bone marrow. (1)

Q46. A 40-year-old woman presented with jaundice. There was no history of contact with hepatitis, foreign travel, injections and transfusion. She was not an alcoholic. She had been well in the past but suffered from increasingly intense pruritis during the last 1 year.

Laboratory findings: Bilirubin 5.6 mg/dl, AST 98U/L, ALT 1200 U/L, Alkaline phosphate 522 U, Total protein 7.5 g/L, Albumin-3.8 g/L, Gamma-glutamyl transpeptidase 242 I/L.

Answer the following:

A. What is the diagnosis? (1)
B. Which biochemical finding suggests the jaundice? (1)
C. Name the enzymatic markers of hepatocytic injury. (1)
D. What protein kind bilirubin in plasma? (1)

Q47. 10-year-old boy was admitted in the nephrology ward with generalized oedema. On initial investigation his urine revealed proteinuria. After detailed investigations he was diagnosed as a case of nephrotic syndrome.

A. How will you differentiate between nephritic and nephrotic syndrome on the basis of 24-hour urinary proteins? What plasma albumin levels will you expect in a patient of nephritic syndrome? (1)
B. Which 3 features constitute the nephrotic syndrome? (1)
C. What are the primary and secondary causes of nephrotic syndrome? (2)

Q48. A 24-year-old woman with history of excessive moistness of palms. She also noticed that her eyes have become more prominent as she has lost weight. On examination her pulse was 92/min at rest and she had a slightly enlarged thyroid glands.

Laboratory findings: Serum TSH <0.1 mU/L, fT_3 (FreeT_3): 12 pmol/L

Isotope scan of thyroid showed an enlarged gland with uniformly increased uptake.

Autoantibodies to thyroid microsome and thyroglobulin present.

A. What is the diagnosis? (1)
B. Which one test will you order in a suspected hyper/hypothyroid patient? What result will you expect? (2)

C. In a patient developing tetany after thyroid surgery with low serum calcium levels. What is the cause? (1)

Q49. A 10 years old boy had following glucose levels:

i. Fasting blood glucose = 145 mg/dl

ii. 2 hours PP blood glucose = 218 mg/dl

HbA1c = 11.5%

Urinary glucose = +++

Ketone bodies = Present

Answer the following questions:

A. What is your diagnosis? What are the 3 main types of glucose measurements performed in laboratory? (1)

C. What is the effect of insulin deficiency on fat and protein metabolism? From what are ketone bodies formed? (1)

D. Classify diabetes. (2)

Q50. A patient in emergency with complaints of chest pain. His investigation was carried out with following results.

Laboratory findings:

CPK	12500 U/L
AST	69 U/L
LDH	578 U/L
CKMB	208 U/L

A. What is your diagnosis? (1)

B. In a patient of myocardial infarction (MI) would you expect to find raised levels of LDL or HDL? Why? (1)

C. What is the first test you will order to confirm an MI? (1)

D. What is the best possible alternative? (1)

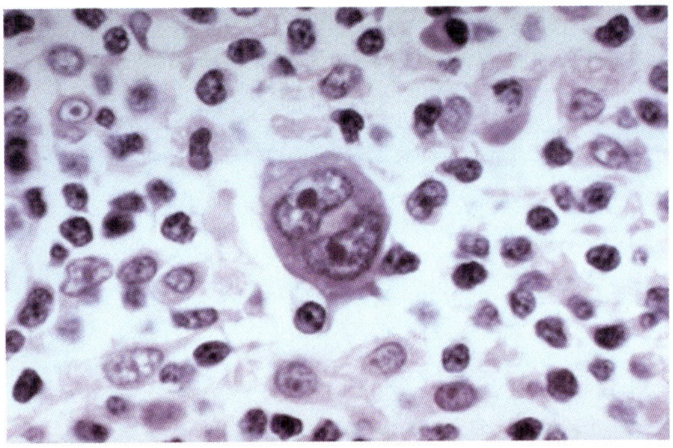

Q51. A 60-year-old female admitted with fever, weight loss. She had massive matted cervical Lymph node (6 cm in diameter). She also had axillary lymph node (LN) enlargement.

(1) Hb 12 g/dl (2) WBC-15 × 10^9/L with 8% eosinophils (3) Platelet 475 × 10^9/L. LN biopsy showed effacement of architecture.

A. What is your diagnosis? (1)

B. What is the characteristic cell in the centre of slide? (1)

C. What is the nature of the lymphocytes? (1)

D. Name relevant CD markers (1)

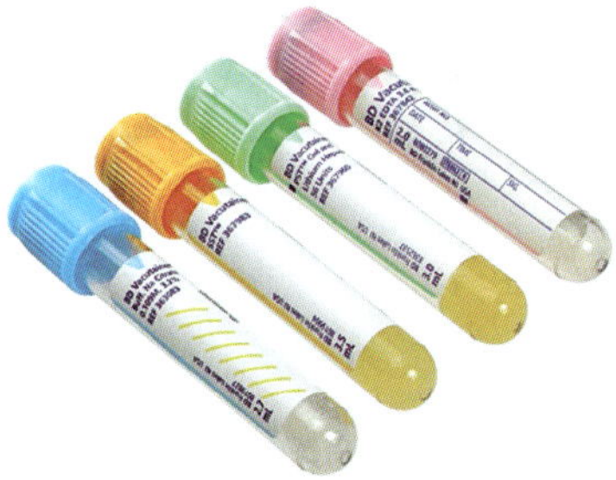

Q52.

A. Identify the instrument. (1)

B. Mention different Vacutainer tubes and their uses. (1)

C. What is the ratio of sodium citrate used in coagulation studies? (1)

D. What is the ratio of sodium citrate used in ESR studies? (1)

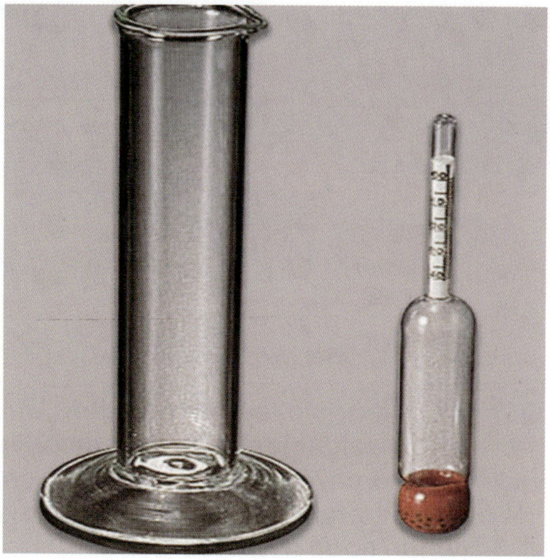

Q53.

A. Identify the instrument. What are the different parts? (1)

B. What is the principle behind its application and normal value of specific gravity? (1)

C. What is the temperature, protein and glucose correction done to measure the specific gravity? (1)

D. What is isosthenuria? (1)

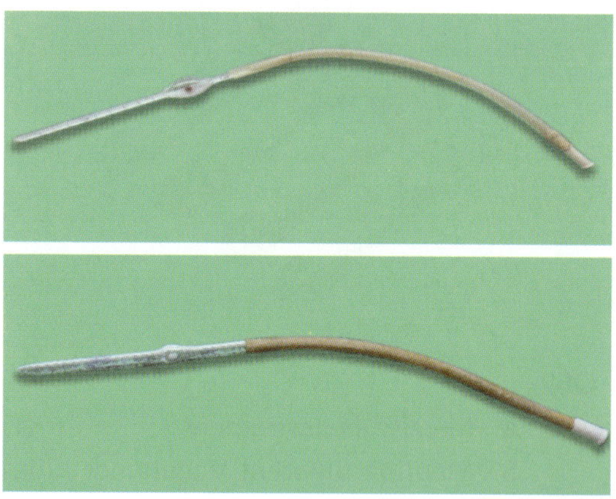

Q54.

A. Identify the Instruments. (1)

B. Name any 2-diluting fluid for RBC count and dilution used. (2)

C. What is the composition of this fluid? (1)

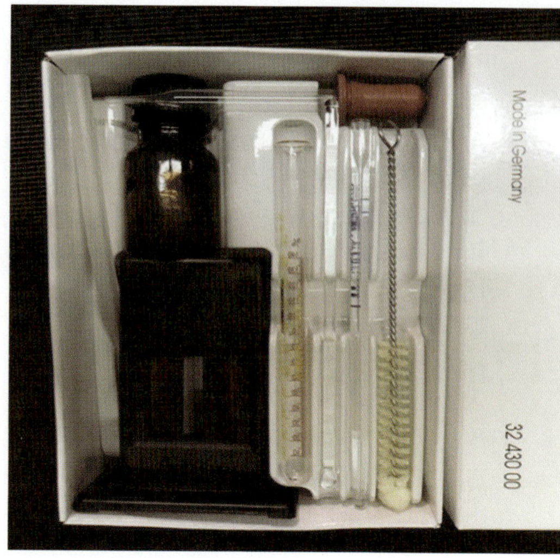

Q55.

A. What is the instrument and describe its parts? (1)

B. What are the other different methods? (1)

C. What is the principle? (1)

D. Components of Drabkins solution? (1)

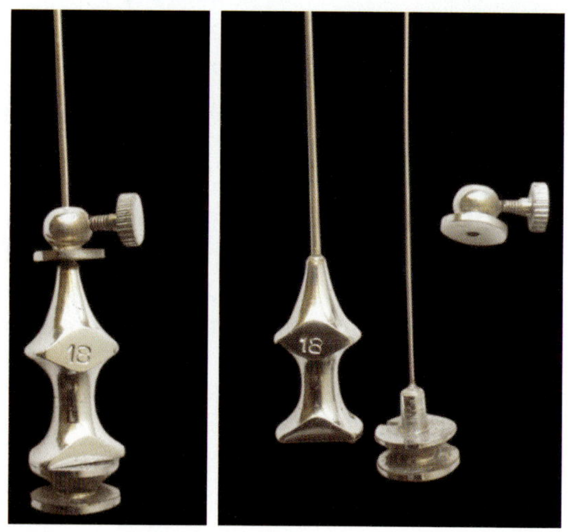

Q56.

A. Identify the instrument. (1)

B. Indications of its use. (2)

C. Name 2 other BMA needles. (1)

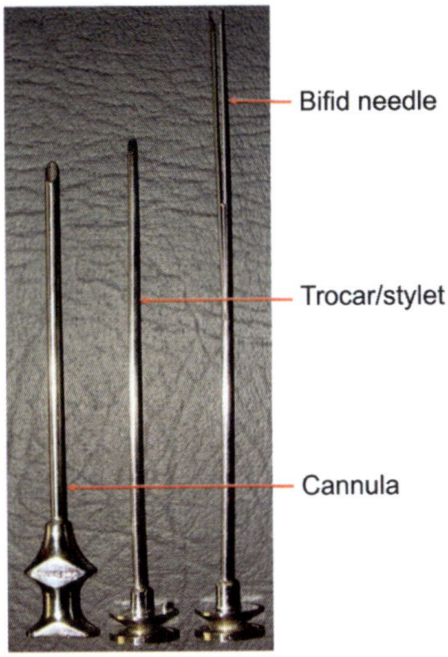

Q57.

A. Identify the instrument? (1)
B. What are the Indications of its use? (2)
C. What are the contraindications? (1)

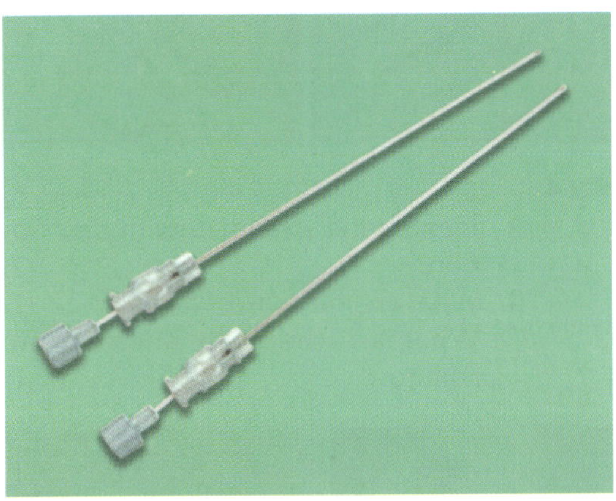

Q58.

A. Identify the instrument? (1)
B. Indication of its uses? (2)
C. Most common site. (1)

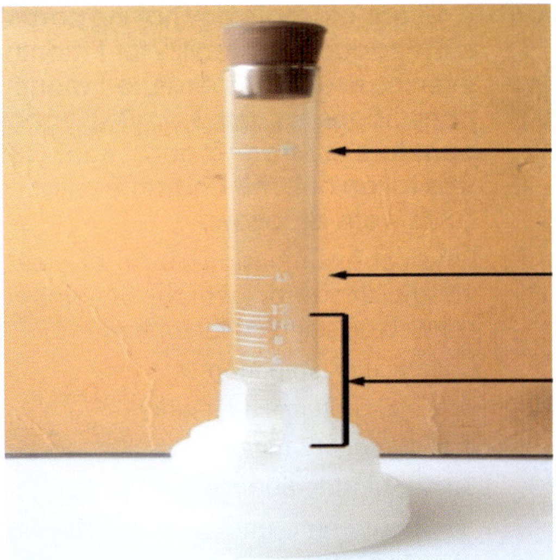

Q59.

A. Identify the instrument? (1)
B. Write its use? (1)
C. Name and composition of reagent used? (1)
D. What is microalbuminuria? (1)

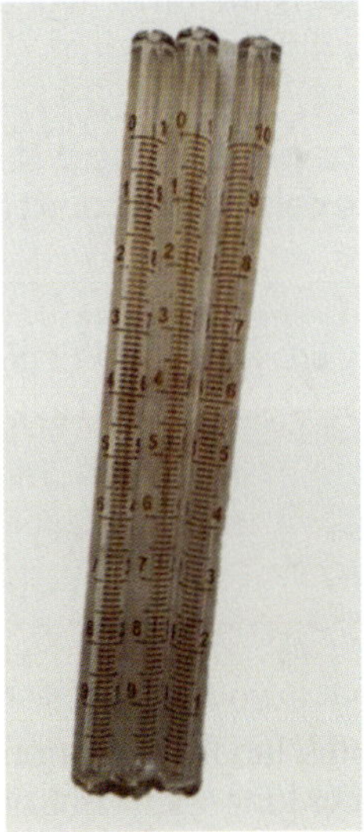

Q60.

A. Identify the instrument? (1)
B. Its uses? (1)
C. What are the normal values? (1)
D. What are the causes of increase value. (1)

Q61. A 4-year-old male boy having persistent headache, irritability for 1 month, evening rise of temperature 1 month, convulsions for last 3 days. Lumbar puncture was done and 10 ml CSF was taken out. The characteristics of fluids were as follows:

Physical examination-10 ml of clear, yellowish fluid, which developed cobweb on standing for 24 hrs.

Chemical examination:

1. Total protein-180 mg/dl
2. Glucose-42 mg/dl
3. S. Chloride-600 meq/l

   Microscopic finding-total cells-144 cells/cumm

   Differential count

   a. Lymphocytes-70%

   b. Neutrophils-30%

A. What is your diagnosis? (1)

B. What are the points favouring your diagnosis? (1)

C. What is the other type and how will you differentiate it? (2)

Q62. 10-year-old boy had following glucose levels, what could be the diagnosis

Fasting blood glucose	145 mg/dl
2 hrs PP blood glucose	218 mg/dl
Hba1c	11.5%
Urinary glucose	+++
Ketone bodies	Present

A. What is your diagnosis? (1)

B. Which lab investigation in the above shows long-term control? Write down the criteria for diagnosis. (2)

C. What is the macro vascular complication? (1)

Q63. A patient presented in emergency with complaint of chest pain. His investigation was carried out with following results

Random Blood Sugar	200 mg/dl
Urea	50 mg/dl
CPK	1280 u/L
AST	69 u/L
LDH	578 u/L
CK MB	208 u/L

A. Give your diagnosis? (1)

B. Which one of the above biochemical investigations supports your diagnosis? (1)

C. Name one investigation which you would like to perform to support your diagnosis at this stage of attack. (1)

D. Write gross and microscopic findings. (1)

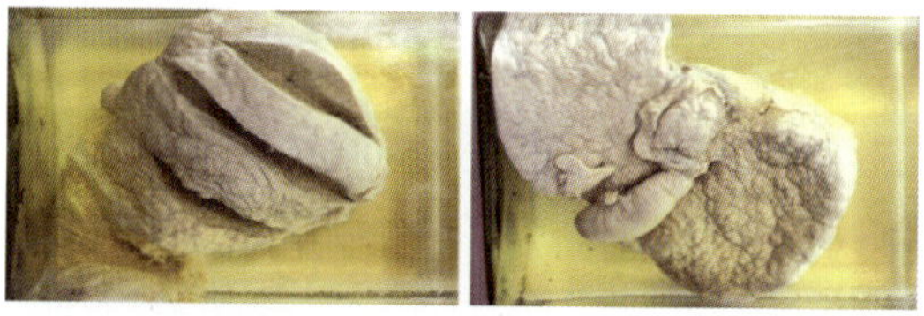

Q64.

A. Identify the specimen with description? (2)

B. What are the causes? (any 4) (1)

C. What are the light microscopic features? (1)

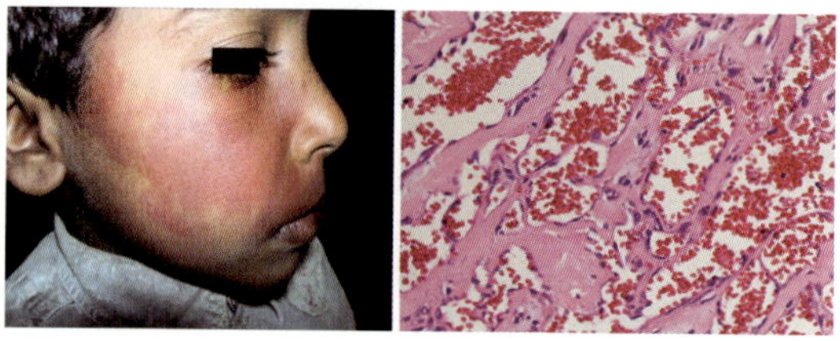

Q65.

A. Identify the slide. Name the malignant counterpart? (1)

B. What will be the microscopic finding? (1)

C. What are the different histologic types. Mention any four. (2)

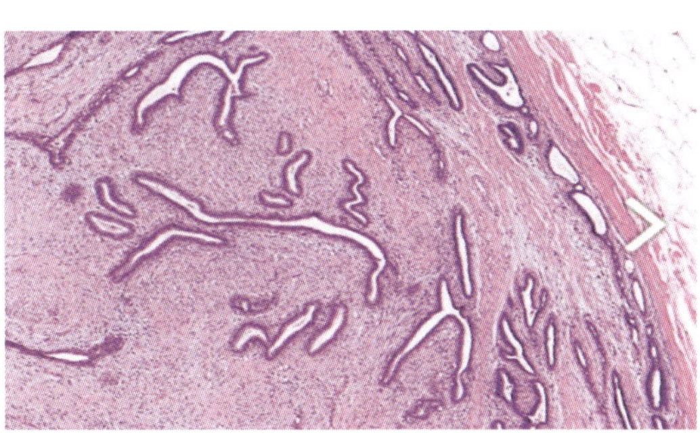

Q66. Image shows a section from a mildly painful breast lesion in a 24-year-old female. Carefully examine the cut section of the given photograph/slide and answer the following.

A. Is this lesion benign or malignant? (1)

B. List 4 important histological features of these types of breast lesion. (2)

C. Does the lesion increase the risk of cancer/carcinoma in this patient? (1)

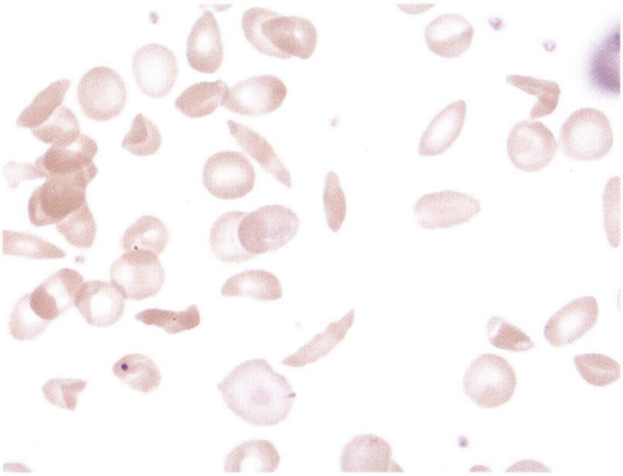

Q67. Photograph is provided to you is a PBS of an 8-year-old African child who presented with severe anaemia and splenomegaly. His full blood counts are:

Hb	5 g/dl
MCV	80 fl
MCH	28 pg
MCHC	32%

Hb electrophoresis showed increased HbS.

Carefully examine the slide/Photomicrograph and answer the following:

A. What is the diagnosis? (1)

B. What is the pathology of this anaemia? (2)

C. What is the mutation seen? (1)

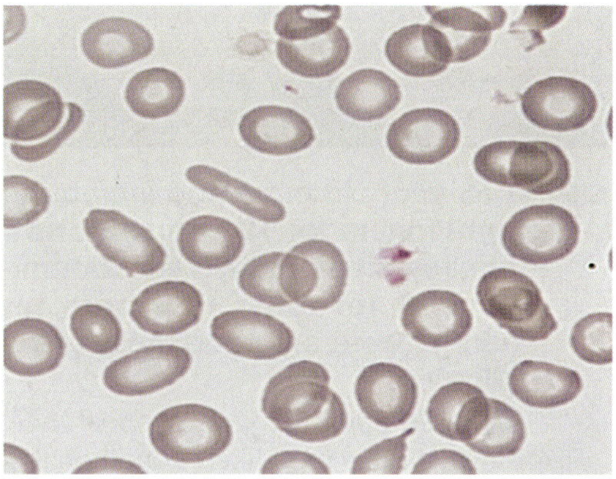

Q68. A 45-year-old female presented with excessive menstrual bleeding for the one year, she looked pale, her blood counts are Hb = 8 g/dl, MCV = 60 fl, MCH = 19, RDW = 26 fl. Serum ferritin was reduced and a peripheral smear was taken. Carefully examine the given photograph and answer the following:

A. Describe the RBC morphology in one line. (1)

B. What type of anaemia is it? (1)

C. Name 3 other causes of microcytic hypochromic anaemia. (2)

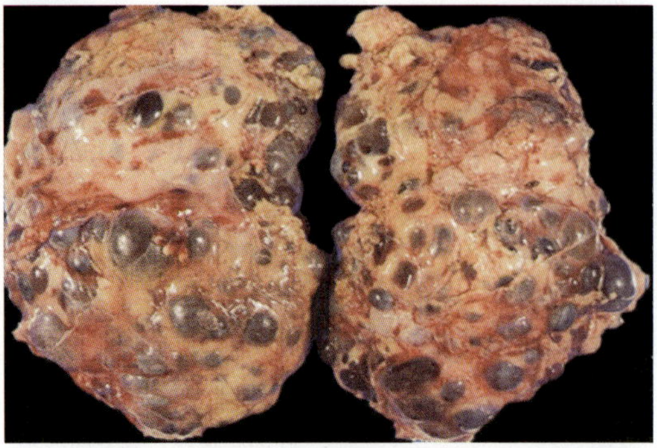

Q69. A 65-year-old male had increasing renal failure for 10 years. He now requires haemodialysis. An abdominal USG revealed that both his kidneys were enlarged. Answer the following:

A. Based upon this gross appearance, what is the most likely condition that is (+) in this patient. (1)
B. Is it unilateral or bilateral? (1)
C. Which gene is mutated? (1)
D. What are different types of cysts in kidney? (1)

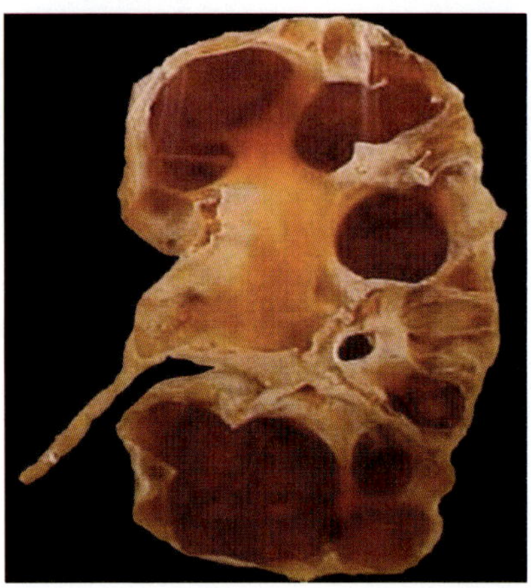

Q70. This is picture of a non-functional kidney from a 35-year-old male. Carefully examine the photograph and answer the following:

A. Describe the cut surface. (1)
B. What are the causes (any 4)? (2)
C. What are the microscopic and gross features in chronic cases?

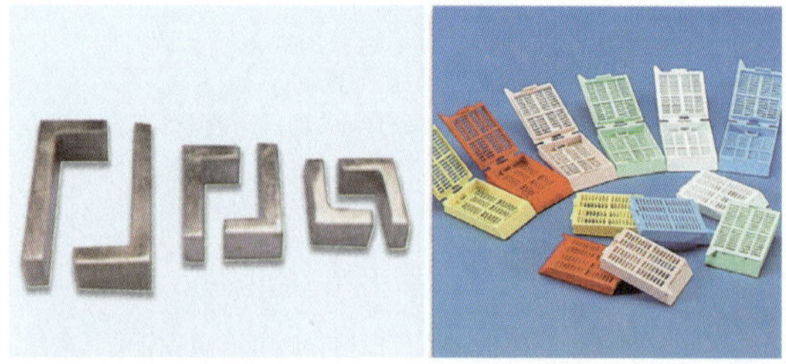

Q71.

A. Name the first instrument? (1)
B. What is its use? (1)
C. What is the second instrument? (1)
D. What is its use and why? (1)

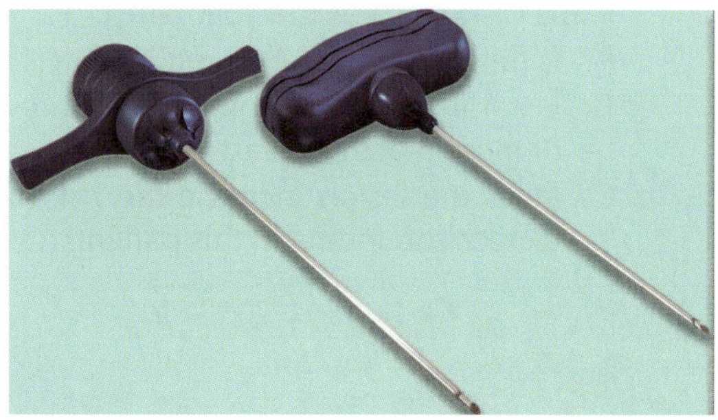

Q72.

A. Identify the instrument. (1)
B. Name 2 other needle. (2)
C. Name any 2-fixatives used. (1)

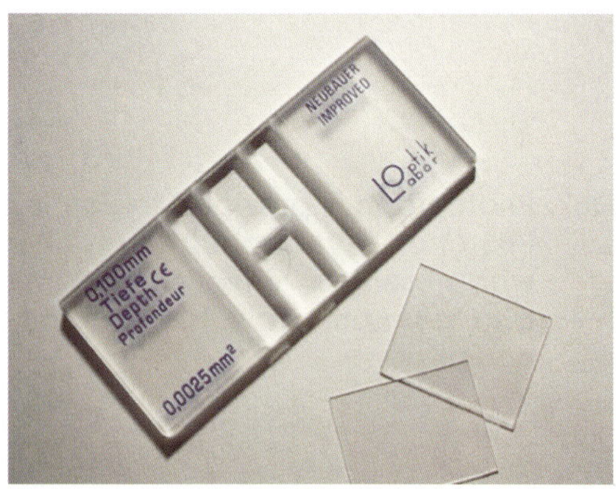

Q73.

A. Identify the instrument. (1)
B. What are its uses? (1)
C. What is the difference between old and modified version? (2)

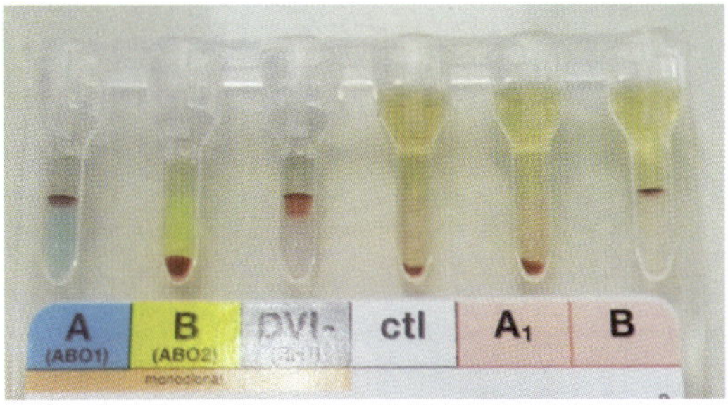

Q74.

A. Interpret the blood group and identify the method. D. What are the subtypes of blood group A? (1)

B. What is Bombay blood group? (1)

C. What is Thomson Friedenreich phenomenon? (1)

D. What are the advantages of this method? (1)

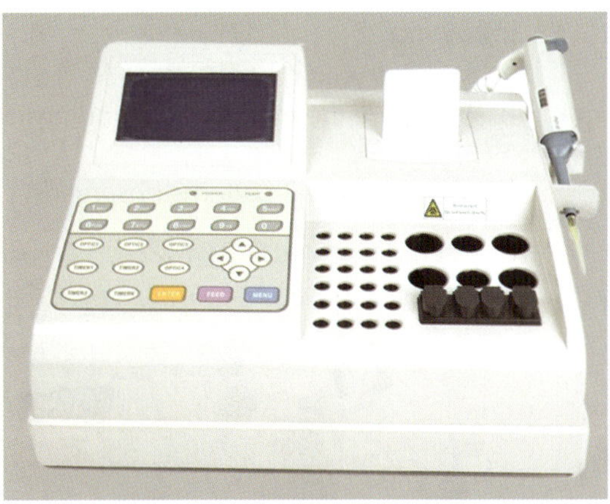

Q75.

A. Identify the instrument and write its 2 uses. (1)

B. What is clot retraction study? (1)

C. If patient has prolonged PT and normal APTT then what are the possibilities? (1)

D. If patient has prolongation of both PT and APTT then what are the possibilities? (1)

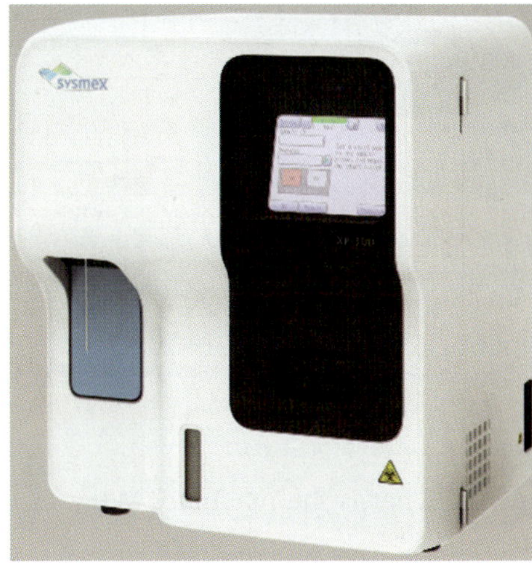

Q76.

A. Identify the instrument. (1)

B. What is the electronic method for counting WBC? (1)

C. What is the electronic method for counting platelets? Is it advantageous or disadvantageous? (2)

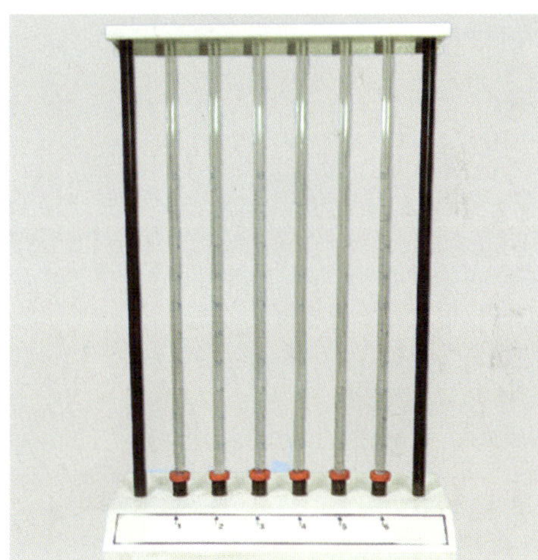

Q77.

A. Identify the instrument and write length and diameter of tube. (2)

B. What is the other instrument which can be used instead of this and why this instrument is preferred? (1)

C. Enumerate causes of increased and decreased in value. (1)

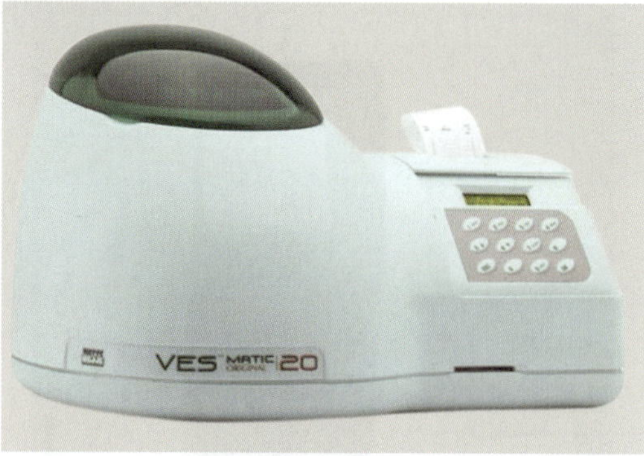

Q78.

A. What is the machine? What are its uses? (1)
B. What is the method and what are the other methods? (2)
C. Enumerate red cell indices? (1)

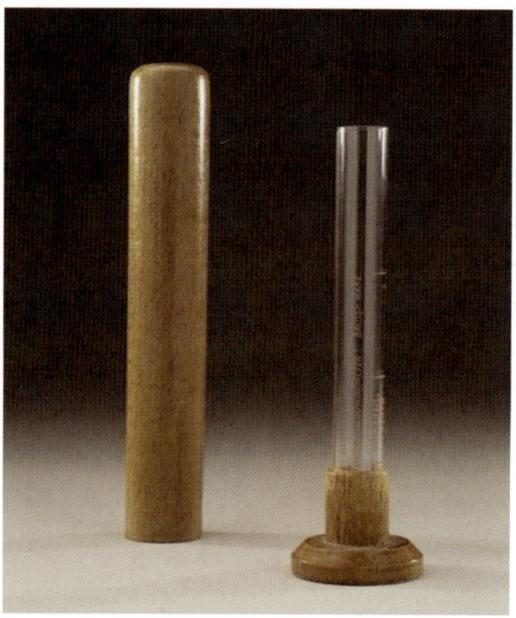

Q79.

A. What is the instrument? (1)
B. What are the 3 qualitative methods? (2)
C. Constituent of reagent. (1)

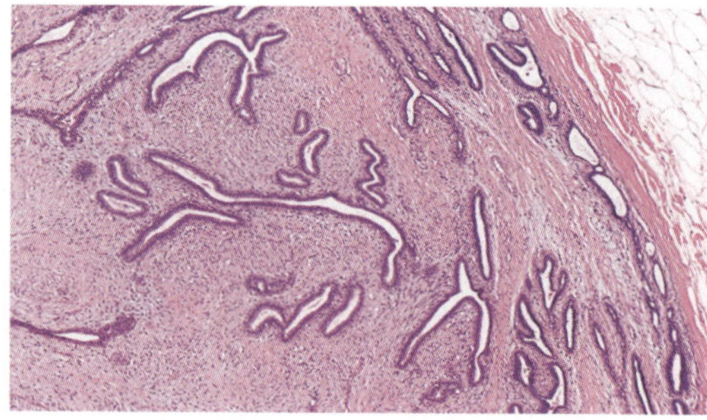

Q80. A 15-year-old female patient was admitted in the hospital with mass in left breast for 1 year, no pain, no discharge, no redness, no fever, and no weight loss. Size is increasing gradually. On examination, a round 2 x 2 cm lump with well-defined border, mobile and firm to rubbery consistency was found. Biopsy was done and HP slides were prepared. Examine the slide and answer the following.

A. What is your diagnosis? (1)
B. What are the microscopic findings? (2)
C. What are the 2 patterns observed? (1)

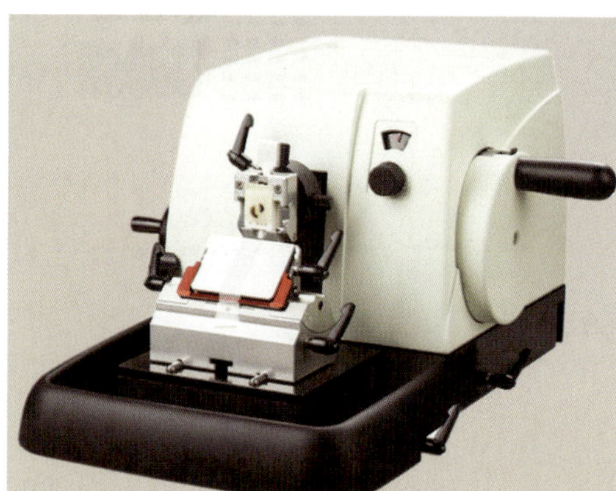

Q81.

A. Identify the instrument. (1)
B. What is the role of clearing agent? (1)
C. What is frozen section? (1)
D. What is decalcification? (1)

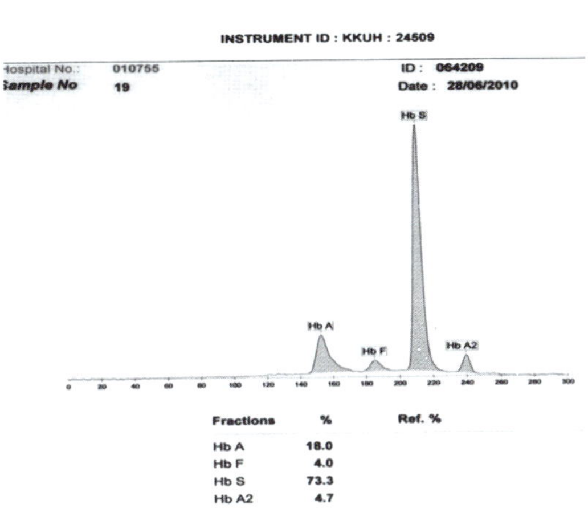

Q82.

A. Name the test performed. (1)
B. What are the findings? (1)
C. What is the most likely diagnosis? (1)
D. Name two investigations further needed. (1)

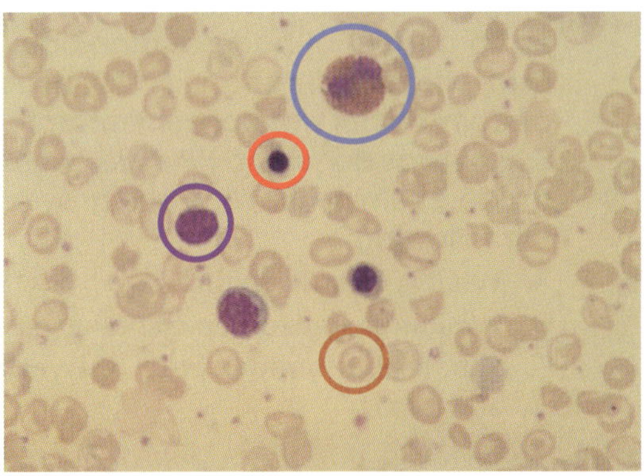

Q83.

A. What are the findings? (1)
B. What are the most likely causes? (1)
C. What further investigations will you order? (2)

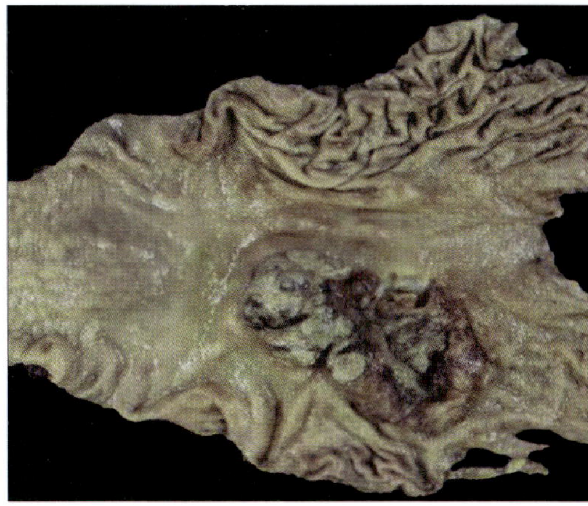

Q84.

A. Identify the specimen. (1)
B. What are the common sites? (1)
C. What are the different types? (2)

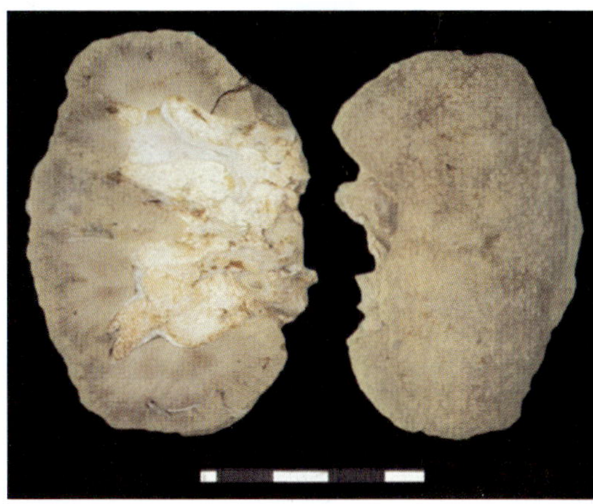

Q85.

A. Identify the specimen. (1)
B. What are the causes? (1)
C. Difference between chronic glomerulonephritis and chronic pyelonephritis. (2)

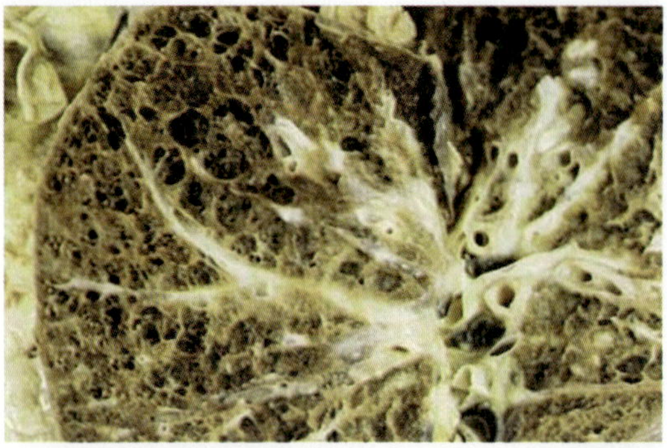

Q86.

A. Identify the specimen. (1)

B. What are the light microscopic findings? (2)

C. What are the different types? (1)

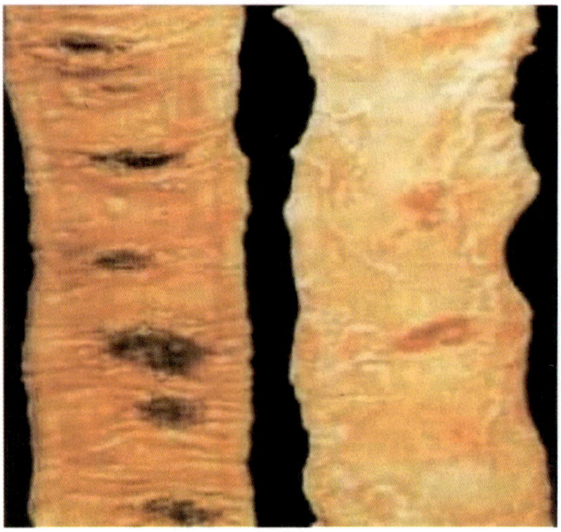

Q87.

A. Identify the specimen. (1)

B. What are the different ulcerative lesions of small intestine? (1)

C. What is hyperplastic ileocecal tuberculosis? (2)

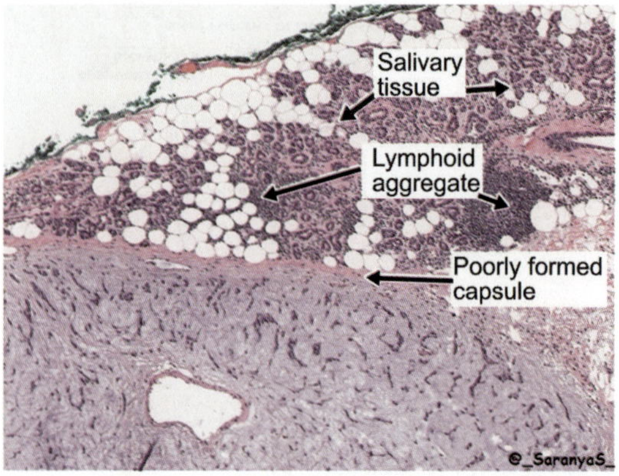

Q88. A 62-year-old female reported to pathology department with complaint of slow growing swelling of right side of face. Swelling was noticed 6 months back and is slowly increasing. On examination swelling was noticed extending over the angle of mouth, superiorly lifting pinna of ear, downwards cervically up to middle of body of mandible, firm with no fixation. FNAC was performed but was not confirmatory. Biopsy was done and HP slides were made. Examine the slide and answer the following:

A. What is your diagnosis? (1)

B. What is the microscopic finding? (2)

C. What is monomorphic salivary adenoma? (1)

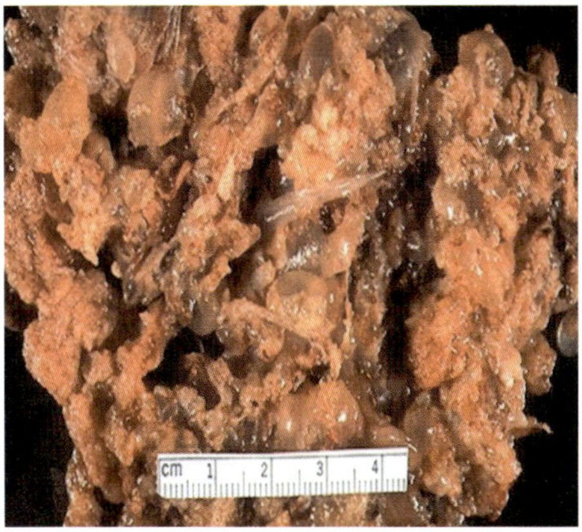

Q89.

A. Identify the specimen. (1)
B. What is the microscopy? (1)
C. Is it benign or malignant lesion? (1)
D. pathophysiology of complete mole. (1)

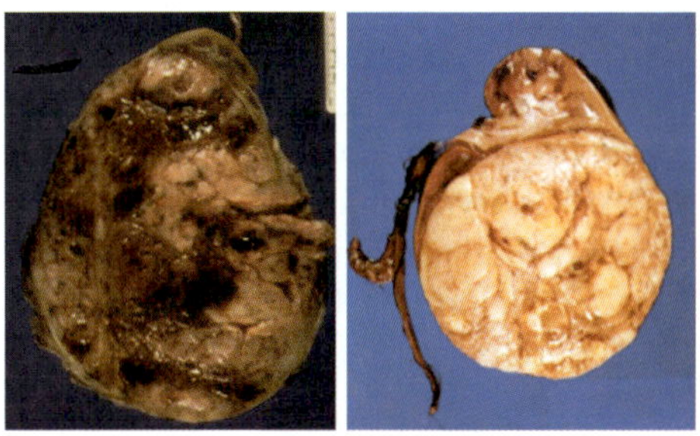

Gross

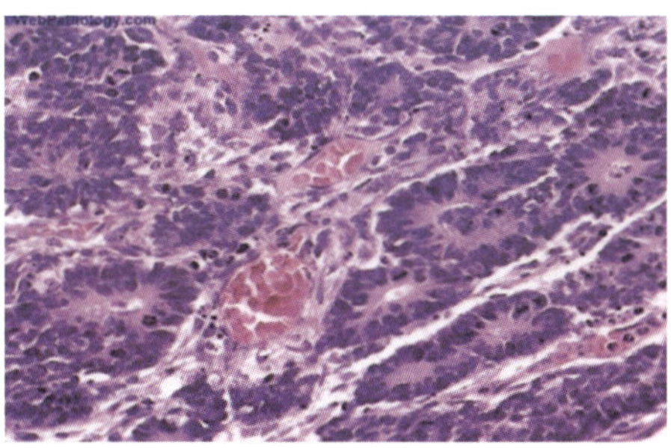

Microscopic

Q90. Look at the bisected specimen of kidney and microphotograph (histology). Answer the following:

A. Identify the specimen. (1)
B. What is the mutation? (1)
C. What are the 3 elements formed? (2)

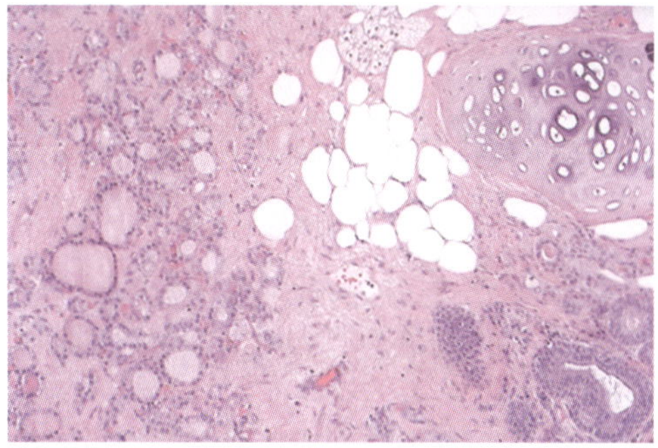

Q91. Carefully examine the given specimen (photograph) and answer the following question.

A. Identify the lesion of ovary. (1)
B. What are the identification points? (1)
C. What is the most common risk factor for this lesion? (1)
D. Benign or malignant (1)

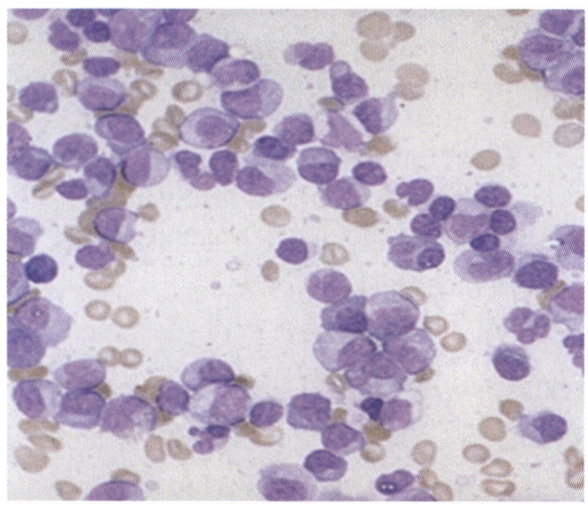

Q92. Carefully examine the given specimen (photograph) with clinical scenario and answer the following questions. A 50 years old male presented with fever, weight loss and bone pain: Radiological examination reveals, sharply punched out defects in bone. Electrophoresis analysis reveals: M Band

A. What is your diagnosis? (1)
B. What are morphological features? (1)
C. What is Bence Jones protein? (1)
D. Name one biochemical parameter for its prognosis. (1)

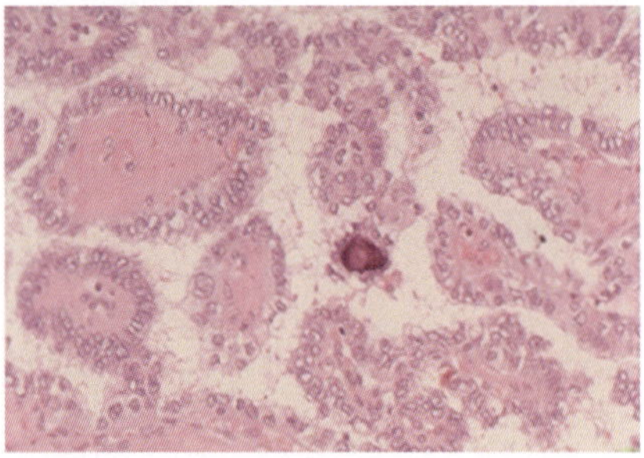

Q93. A 23-year-old female had a history slowly enlarging neck mass. Examination revealed a single firm non-tender nodule within right lobe of thyroid. Lab data revealed a T4 of 7.2 ug/dl (N= 4.8–11.2). Serum calcitonin was not elevated. An Ultrasound examination suggested a solid mass while a thyroid scan revealed decrease uptake within the nodule. She was taken for surgery.

A. What is diagnosis? (1)
B. What are 4 major types of carcinomas? (1)
C. What is the probable biological behaviour of this lesion? (1)
D. Write the nuclear features? (1)

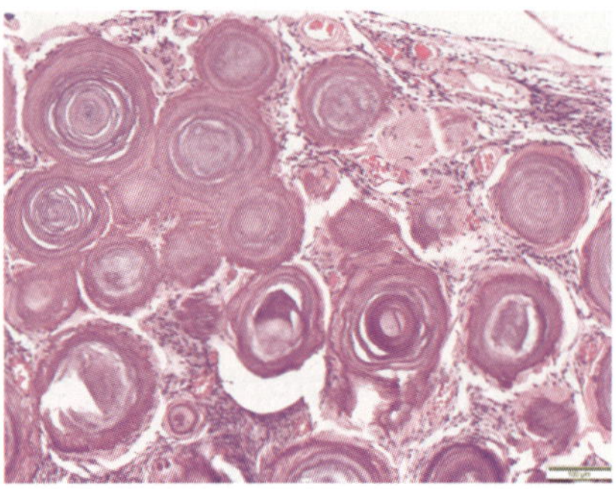

Q94. Carefully examine the focused microscopic slide of tissue obtained from a space-occupying lesion in the brain of a 20-year-old male with history of headache and fits/seizures.

A. Give your diagnosis. (1)
B. Give 2 points to support your diagnosis. (1)
C. Name its different histologic pattern. (2)

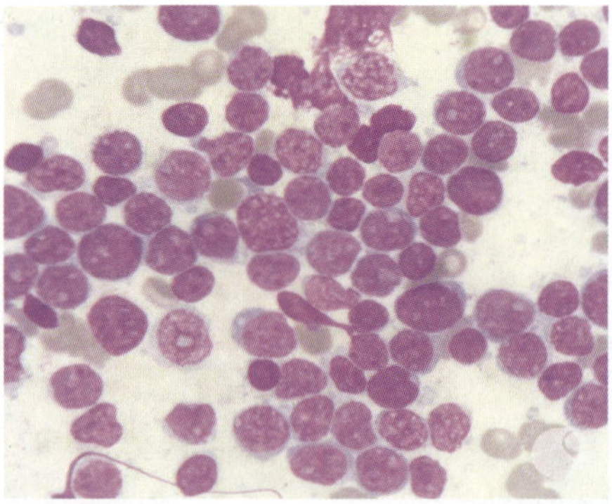

Q95. 5-year-old child presents with fever, lymphadenopathy and bone pains.

Lab picture

Hb	8 g/dl
TLC	18,000 × 10^9/L
Platelets	80 × 10^9/L
Blast cells	15%

Carefully read the clinical scenario and examine the Giemsa-stained bone marrow slide. Answer the following.

A. Give your finding and diagnosis. (1)
B. What stain is indicated to differentiate ALL form AML? (2)
C. Enumerate the CD markers? (1)

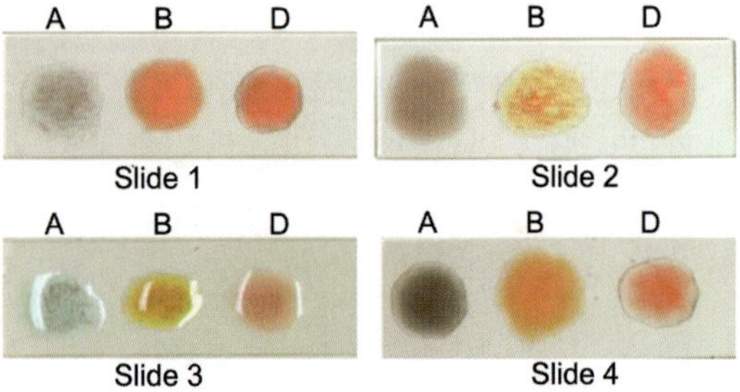

Q96. Provided are four tests. Examine carefully and answer the given questions.

A. What is the blood group in Slides 1, 2, 3 and 4? (1)
B. What is Rh blood group? (1)
C. Give the class of antibody formed against ABO blood group antigen.(1)
D. Give the class of antibody formed against Rh blood group antigen. (1)

Q97. A medical student presents with symptom of fever, nausea, vomiting and pain in right hypochondrium. There is history of passing dark coloured urine with liver function test levels

Bilirubin	8.5 mg/dl
AST	800 U/L
ALT	1200 U/L
Alkaline phosphate	150 U/L
Total protein	7.5 g/dl
Albumin	3.8 g/dl

A. What is the diagnosis? (1)
B. Give 2 points that suggest the diagnosis? (1)
C. Which serological viral marker would you like to perform in this case? (2)

Q98. A young man sustained multiple injuries in a motorcycle accident. He received multiple blood transfusions and underwent surgery. 24 hours after admission, he had only passed 400 ml of urine was clinically dehydrated and his blood pressure was 90/50 mmHg.

Laboratory investigations:

Urea	160 mg/dl (normal 10–50 mg/dl)
Creatinine	1.9 mg/dl (normal 0.4–1.4 mg/dl)
Potassium	5.7 mmol/L (normal 3.4–5.2 mmol/L)
Sodium	130 mmol/L (normal 134–154 mmol/L)

A. What is your diagnosis? (1)
B. Why are urea and creatinine level raised in the patients? What laboratory investigations would you prefer to monitor treatment in this patient? (1)
C. Criteria and staging for diagnosis. (2)

Q99. A 10-year-old boy was referred to hospital for investigations of short stature. He had only grown 2 cm in height since last 2 years. On examination, there was no abnormality apart from his short stature.

Lab investigations:

S. growth hormone-4 mU/L (after vigorous exercise)

4 mU/L (during documented hypoglycaemia induced in insulin)

Following stress, the level of growth hormones should be more than 20 mU/L.

A. What is your diagnosis? (1)
B. Name 3 other causes of short stature. (1)
C. Enumerate the regulating mediators? (2)

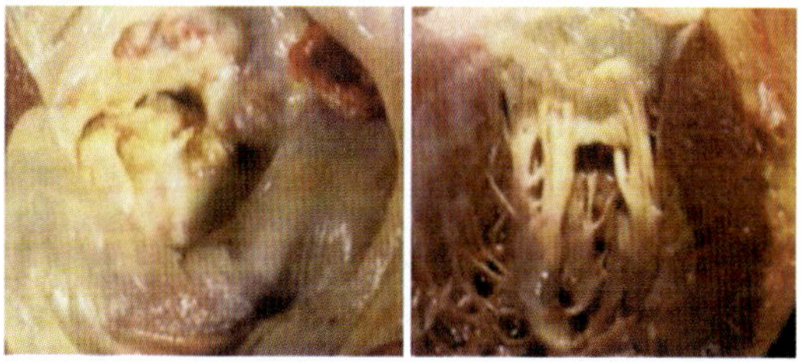

Q100. Carefully examine the given gross specimen/macroscopic photograph and answer the following questions:

A. Based on the appearance of the heart shown here, the most likely underlying cause of her illness is. (1)
B. What is Aschoff bodies? (1)
C. What is a MacCallum plaque? (1)

Answer Keys

Ans 1. A. Fatty liver

B. (a) Alcohol (b) Viral hepatitis (c) Obesity (d) Diabetes mellitus (e) Malnutrition. Yes

C. Yes, this is reversible. No, it is not malignant.

D. Liposarcoma. Microscopic identification of lipoblasts containing multiple vacuoles in the cytoplasm which impinge upon nucleus. There are scalloped nuclei and nuclei show anisonucleosis, prominent nucleoli.

Ans 2. A. Granuloma

B. Granuloma is a **focal area of granulomatous inflammation**. It consists of a microscopic aggregation of macrophages that are transformed into epithelium like cells surrounded by a collar of mononuclear leukocytes, principally lymphocytes and occasionally plasma cells.

C. Caseous necrosis

D. Coagulative necrosis, liquefactive necrosis, fat necrosis.

Ans 3. A. Acute inflammation (acute appendicitis)

B. Polymorphonuclear neutrophils. It involves the mucosa and infiltrates the muscle layer (which is characteristic for diagnosis).

C. Complete resolution, fibrosis, chronic inflammation.

D. Signs: Calor, rubor, tumor, dolor, and functio laesa. Chemical mediators of pain: histamine, bradykinin, prostaglandins, serotonin.

Ans 4. A. Coagulative necrosis.

B. Obstruction of the artery will lead to ischemia.

C. (a) Loss of cell nuclei, cell border/cytoplasm not recognizable (b) Dilated and congested blood vessels at the haemorrhagic zone (c) Cellular infiltration by neutrophils, RBC and lymphocytes.

Ans 5. A. Colon polyp/adenomatous polyp. FAP/APC gene

B. *See* the Table below.

C. Villous adenoma have more propensity for atypical changes (malignant potentiality) followed by tubulovillous adenomas and then tubular adenomas.

Parameters	Right-sided colorectal carcinoma	Left-sided colorectal carcinoma
• Site	Caecum and ascending colon	Rectosigmoid area and descending colon
• Growth pattern	Ulceroproliferative, exophytic, polypoid soft to firm mass	Circumferential, napkin-ring firm mass
• Invasiveness	More invasive	Less invasive
• Involvement of other structures	Common like mesentery, lymph nodes, distant metastasis	Less common
• Clinical presentation	Silent and diagnosed late	Obstructive features, so diagnosed early
• Prognosis	Poor	Good

Ans 6. A. Chronic inflammation
B. Caseous necrosis
C. (a) Presence of giant cell (Langhans giant cell) (B) Epithelioid histiocytes (macrophages)
D. Necrosis is a localised area of death in living tissue and is accompanied by inflammatory reaction. This death is irreversible.

Ans 7. A. Fat necrosis
B. Fatty tissue necrosis is probably caused by lipase (one of the few pancreatic enzymes that need no activation) after an abrupt effusion of zymogens from peripheral acinar cells into the interstitial space.
C. Breast
D. Dystrophic calcification.

Ans 8. A. Chronic cholecystitis, irregular mucosal folds and ulceration in mucosa, all layers show chronic inflammatory cells infiltration and fibrosis.
B. Lymphocytes.
C. (a) Pancreatitis (b) CBD obstruction (c) cholangitis (d) Perforation (e) Empyema GB.

Ans 9. A. Yes, hypertrophy: An increase in size of cells, resulting in an increase in size of the organ.
B. Hyperplasia, atrophy, metaplasia.
C. 1. Hyperplasia—increase in the size of the breasts during pregnancy, increase in thickness of endometrium during menstrual cycle, and liver growth after partial resection.
2. Atrophy—disuse and neurogenic atrophy.
3. Metaplasia—*see* the Table below.

Ans 10. A. Calcification (dystrophic)
B. Kidney, blood vessels.
C. Abnormal calcium metabolism
D. Dystrophic and metastatic calcification.

Ans 11. A. Lipoma, capsulated lobule of mature adipose tissue separated by thin fibrous septa. Liposarcoma.
B. Fibroma
C. Lipomas can sometimes, though rare, be associated with certain disorders such as multiple hereditary lipomatosis, Gardner syndrome, adiposis dolorosa, and Madelung disease.

Ans 12. A. Cut section shows well circumscribed homogenously white tumour with whorling pattern. Intramural, submucosal, subserosal fibroid or leiomyoma.
B. Benign smooth muscle tumour.
C. i. Section shows bundles of smooth muscular cells intermingled with fibrous tissue in whorling pattern.
ii. Necrosis and mitosis.

Ans 13. A. Osteomyelitis
B. *Staphylococcus aureus*, *Salmonella*, sickle cell disease, tuberculosis (TB).
C. Sequestrum: A sequestrum is a piece of necrotic bone detached from the healthy tissue, usually secondary to a trauma.

Tissue	Normal	Metaplasia
Airways	Pseudostratified columnar epithelium	Squamous epithelium
Urinary bladder	Transitional epithelium	Squamous epithelium
Esophagus	Squamous epithelium	Columnar epithelium (Barrett's esophagus)
Cervix	Glandular epithelium	Squamous epithelium

Involucrum: The proliferation of bone surrounding the sequestrum and the cavity where it sits are called the involucrum.

Ans 14. A. Osteosarcoma

B. Long bones and weight-bearing bones around knee site, i.e. lower end of femur and upper end of tibia. Metaphyseal growth plates.

C. Anaplastic spindle shaped cells producing lace like osteoid matrix, necrosis, atypical mitosis, tumour giant cells.

Ans 15. A. Basal cell carcinoma.

B. i. Irregular nests of basaloid cells present in dermis

ii. Peripheral palisade arrangement

iii. Variability of basophilic cells with hyperchromatic nuclei

iv. Stroma shrinks away from epithelioid tumour nests creating cleft.

C. Locally invasive, slow growing malignant tumour which does not metastasise.

D. Occurs most often on the face above a line drawn from angle of mouth to the lobe of the ear. Clinically it appears as an ulcer with pearly, rolled up margin also called as rodent ulcer.

Ans 16. A. Lipoma. Liposarcoma

B. i. Sheets of mature adipocytes.

ii. Scanty fibrovascular storm.

C. Unconventional forms of lipomas include the following: angiolipoma, chondroid lipoma, lipoblastoma, myolipoma, pleomorphic lipoma/ spindle cell lipoma, intramuscular and intermuscular lipoma, lipomatosis of nerve, lipoma of the tendon sheath and joint, lipoma arborescens, multiple symmetric lipomatosis, diffuse lipomatosis, adiposis dolorosa, and hibernoma.

Ans 17. A. Carcinoma cervix

B. i. Abnormal growth in the cervix

ii. Tumour is a fungating red to tan yellow mass.

C. i. Nests of neoplastic squamous cells are invaded through chronically inflamed stroma.

ii. Keratin pearls within nest of tumour cells.

Ans 18. A. Squamous cell carcinoma.

B. i. Nests of well differentiated squamous cells.

ii. Keratin pearls.

C. i. Prolong exposure of UV radiation.

ii. Chemical-Asbestos, Nickel.

Ans 19. A. Adenocarcinoma

B. i. Genetic (FAP, HNPCC, colorectal adenoma/polyp)

ii. Inflammatory bowel disease (IBD)

iii. Diet (Low fibre/Ca/vit D/high fat/smoking/alcohol)

C. Complications: Intestinal obstruction, perforation (peritonitis, pericolic abscess, fistulae), metastasis to liver.

Ans 20. A. Lobar pneumonia, stages of grey hepatisation.

B. i. Red cells disintegrate with persistence of neutrophil and fibrin and macrophage.

ii. Consolidate alveoli

iii. Organizing pneumonia with transformation of exudate to fibrin myxoid mass.

C. i. Congestion

ii. Red hepatisation

iii. Grey hepatization

iv. Resolution.

Ans 21. A. Lobar pneumonia. Lobar pneumonia affects one or more sections (lobes) of the lungs. Bronchial pneumonia (also known as bronchopneumonia. affects patches throughout both lungs.

B. i. Lung parenchyma, normally empty alveolar spaces are filled with leucocytes and pink fibrin.
   ii. Fibrinous (grey hepatization) and haemorrhage (red), inflammation.

C. Streptococcus pneumonia.

Ans 22. A. Shallow, sharply demarcated with surrounding hyperaemia.
Duodenum first part, stomach usually antrum gastroesophageal junction

B. *H. pylori* infection

C. Excessive gastric acid secretion is only one factor in the pathogenesis of peptic ulcer disease. Decreased mucosal defence against gastric acid is another cause. The integrity of the upper gastrointestinal tract is dependent upon the balance between "hostile" factors such as gastric acid, and Pylori.

Ans 23. A. Ulcerative colitis

B. Isolated islands of regenerating mucosa bulge upwards to create pseudopolyps in ulcerative colitis. Skip lesions are seen in Chron's disease.

C. Extraintestinal manifestations:
- Peripheral arthritis, seronegative
- Ankylosing spondylitis or sacroiliitis
- Erythema nodosum
- Pyoderma granulosum
- Primary sclerosing cholangitis (PSC)

Ans 24. A. Centre is tan with surrounding hyperemia.

B. An infarct that extends through full thickness of ventricular wall.

C. Pericarditis, Arrhythmias, contractile dysfunction, infarct expansion, myocardial rupture, mural thrombus, ventricular aneurysm.

Ans 25. A. Adult polycystic kidney disease

B. i. Enlarged kidney.
   ii. Masses of cysts with no intervening parenchyma.
   iii. Fluids in cysts.

C. Autosomal dominant.

Ans 26. A. Prostatic adenocarcinoma.

B. i. Irregular yellowish nodules.
   ii. Mostly in the posterior portion.
   Yes, it can coexist.

C. M/E:
- Glandular crowding and infiltrative growth pattern
- Nuclear enlargement, nucleolar prominence
- Round generally monomorphic nuclei
- Amphophilic cytoplasm
- Mitoses
- Apoptotic bodies
- Stromal desmoplasia
- Intraluminal contents: Crystalloids, pink amorphous secretions, blue mucin
- Glomerulations, collagenous micronodules (mucinous fibroplasia)
- Absence of basal cell layer (generally requires immunohistochemical confirmation).

Ans 27. A. Uterus: (i) Dilated uterine cavity.
Present as (ii) irregular mass involving endometrium and projects through endometrial cavity.
Or as a (iii) diffuse tumour involving the entire endometrial surface.

B. Obesity, diabetes, hypertension, infertility with anovulatory cycles unopposed estrogenic stimulation.

C. > 3:1

Ans 28. A. Malignant

B. Embryonal carcinoma, Yolk sac tumour, choriocarcinoma, teratoma, spermatocytic seminoma.

C. Radiotherapy

Ans 29. A. Giant cell tumour (GCT) of bone (osteoclastoma).

B. Gross: Typical gross lesion is a soft, friable, slightly brownish or red-tan, somewhat poorly defined neoplasm in the end of a long bone

Microscopy: Sheets of round to oval shaped stromal neoplastic mononuclear cells admixed with numerous osteoclast-type of giant cells (containing 100 or more nuclei). Nuclei of giant cells are similar to nuclei of stromal neoplastic cells.

C. Benign but locally aggressive.

Ans 30. A. Thyroid gland, Multinodular goitre

B. i. Gland shows multiple nodules on cut surface.

ii. Some nodules show cystic degeneration, haemorrhage, fibrosis and calcification.

C. Heterogeneous uptakes, patchy warm and cold nodules.

Ans 31. A. Old age, female gender, obesity, multiparity, family history, rapid weight loss, physical inactivity, dietary habit, oral contraceptives.

(a) Pancreatitis (B) Bile duct Obstruction (C) Cholangitis (D) Perforation (E) Empyema GB

B. *Gross*: Gallbladder is usually enlarged and tense. It may have red or blotchy discolouration due to subserosal haemorrhage. The serosa is usually covered by fibrinous exudate.

Microscopy: In the early phase, there will be oedema, congestion and mucosal erosion. There will be inflammatory cell infiltration in the mucosa and muscularis layer.

C. Cholesterol, pigment and mixed.

Ans 32. A. Carcinoma penis

B. HPV types 16 and 18, cigarette smoking and males with bad genital hygiene and without circumcision.

C. This is an exophytic well differentiated variant of squamous cell carcinoma which has low malignant potential. These tumours are locally invasive but they rarely metastasize.

D. Keratinising squamous cell carcinoma (SCC), Non-keratinising SCC, basaloid SCC, warty carcinoma, papillary variants of SCC.

Ans 33. A. Renal cell carcinoma (RCC)

B. The most common variant is clear cell variant RCC (70–80%). Other variants are RCC papillary (chromophil) type (10–15%), RCC chromophobe type (5%), Bellini duct carcinoma (rare) and Xp11 translocation RCC (rare).

C. PAS (Periodic acid-Schiff) which demonstrates glycogen in the cytoplasm of tumour cells. Frozen section techniques by applying fat stains (Sudan III, Sudan IV, Sudan Black or Oil red O), which demonstrates fat/lipid in the cytoplasm of tumour cells.

D. Triad of painless haematuria (usually intermittent), palpable renal mass and costovertebral pain.

Ans 34. A. Hydronephrosis

B. i. Renal pelvis: Calculi, tumours, uretero-pelvic stricture

ii. Intrinsic ureter: Calculi, tumours, blood clot, inflammation

iii. Extrinsic ureter: Tumour compression (e.g. carcinoma cervix), pregnancy, retroperitoneal fibrosis

iv. Urinary bladder: vesicoureteral reflux, calculi, tumours, neurogenic.

v. Prostate: Hyperplasia (BHP), carcinoma, prostratitis

vi. Uretha: Posterior valve stricture, rarely tumours.

C. i. Kidney is enlarged. The cortex shows tiny petechial haemorrhage visible through capsule giving the characteristic appearance of flea-bitten kidney. Cut surface also shows this haemorrhage.

ii. Causes are: Acute post-streptococcal glomerulonephritis, malignant nephrosclerosis, rapidly progressive GN (RPGN), haemolytic-uraemic syndrome, thrombotic thrombocytopenic purpura and Henoch–Schonlein purpura.

Ans 35. A. Bronchogenic carcinoma

B. i. Adenocarcinoma (males 37%, females 47%)

ii. Squamous cell carcinoma (males 32%, females 25%)

iii. Small cell carcinoma (males 14%, females 18%)

iv. Large cell carcinoma (males 18%, females 10%)

C. Tobacco smoking accounts from 80 to 90% of lung cancers. High-dose ionizing radiation, uranium, asbestos and air-pollutants are other risk factors. Genetic predisposition and p53 mutation also play an important role.

D. Four types of epithelial precursor lesion:

i. Squamous dysplasia and carcinoma *in situ*.

ii. Atypical adenomatous hyperplasia.

iii. Adenocarcinoma *in situ*.

iv. Diffuse idiopathic pulmonary neuroendocrine hyperplasia.

Ans 36. A. Mitral stenosis of heart.

B. Rheumatic fever is the most common cause. Clinical features are pulmonary hypertension, left atrial and left ventricular hypertrophy, opening snap and diastolic murmur.

C. i. Congestive cardiac failure, atrial fibrillation, recurrent haemoptysis, subacute bacterial endocarditis and embolism.

ii. Mitral valve stenosis hampers normal blood flow from left atrium to left ventricle during diastolic period. This leads to hypertrophy of left atrium, pulmonary congestive, brown induration of lungs and right ventricle hypertrophy (cor pulmonale).

Ans 37. A. Atheroma of aorta.

B. Fatty streaks are the earliest lesions in atherosclerosis. Then formation of atheromatous plaques occurs in which there are intimal thickening and lipid accumulation. Complications like erosion, ulceration and rupture may occur which may lead to thrombosis.

C. They have three layers or zones. Inner layer contains necrotic core (lipid, cholesterol clefts, fibrin, foam cells, cell debris). Outer layer is fibrous cap composed of smooth muscle and collagen. In-between is the cellular layer (smooth muscle, lymphocytes, macrophages with less connective tissue).

D. Internal mammary arteries and arteries of upper extremities are spared. As internal mammary arteries are not affected, these are used as graft in coronary bypass surgery.

Ans 38. A. Left ventricular hypertrophy

B. It occurs due to systemic hypertension and aortic valvular disease. The overall weight of heart increases >375 g in males and >350 g in females. Congestive heart failure is the most common cause of death in untreated patients.

C. i. Hypertrophic myocardial cells
ii. Hyperchromatic
iii. Myofiber degeneration.

Ans 39. A. Rheumatic heart disease (Verrucous lesions)

B. i. In rheumatic heart disease (RHD), vegetations are small (1–2 mm), warty and seen along lines of closure of the valve leaflets.

ii. In infective endocarditis, vegetations are large, irregular masses.

iii. In nonbacterial thrombotic endocarditis, vegetations are small, bland and attached at the line of closure of valve leaflets.

iv. In SLE, vegetations are small or medium-sized which are seen on both sides of valve leaflets.

C. The mitral valve is affected most commonly (65–70%) followed by aortic valve involvement (25% of cases). Tricuspid valve involvement is uncommon and involvement of pulmonary valve is very rare.

Ans 40. A. Fibrinous pericarditis

B. Chronic renal failure (uraemia), Myocardial infraction, acute rheumatic fever, SLE, post-infraction (Dressler) syndrome, chest radiation and trauma.

C. Development of a loud pericardial friction rub is very characteristic of fibrinous pericarditis. Also, there are pain, systemic febrile reactions and signs of cardiac failure.

D. Accumulation of larger amounts of yellow to brown turbid fluid, which is made brown and cloudy by the presence of leukocytes and red cells and fibrin. Overtime, fibrin may be lysed with resolution or it may be organized.

HAEMATOLOGY

Ans 41. A. 1. Macro-ovalocytes
2. Hypersegmented neutrophils.
3. Evidence of dyserythropoiesis: Basophilic stippling, Cabot ring, Howell Jolly bodies.

Diagnosis: Megaloblastic anemia.

B. 1. Vitamin B_{12} level
2. Folic acid level

C. Increased mean corpuscular volume (MCV, >100 fl) and mean corpuscular hemoglobin (MCH) but MCH (mean Corpuscular hemoglobin)is normal.

- Normal value of MCV is 82–98 fl, MCHC, 31–36 g/dl and MCH 27–32 pg.

Ans 42. A. Chronic myeloid leukaemia (CML)

B. Philadelphia chromosome; balanced or reciprocal translocation, [t (9;22) (q34; q11)].

C. Radiation, chemical carcinogens

D. Acute myeloid leukaemia (AML) in more than 70% cases and rest ALL (acute lymphoblastic anaemia).

Ans 43. A. Monoclonal spike (M spike) in gamma region, which is known as M band, seen in 60–70% of patients.

B. Multiple myeloma

C. Kappa light chain in urine

D. Normal immunoglobulins are IgM, IgD, IgG, IgE, IgA. In multiple myeloma there is increase of IgG most commonly (55%), followed by IgA (25%). Myeloma expressing IgM, IgD, or IgE may occur but rare.

Ans 44. A. Fragmented red cells

B. Disseminated Intravascular coagulation (DIC)

C. Microangiopathic haemolytic anaemia

D. D-dimer and fibrinogen degradation products.

Ans 45. A. Aplastic anaemia

B. Primary-(due to drugs, chemicals, radial) and secondary.

C. i. Fat spaces

ii. Hematopoietic tissue.

Ans 46. A. Cholestatic jaundice

B. Very high alkaline phosphate

C. AST, ALT, LDH

D. Albumin.

Ans 47. A. Nephrotic > 3.5 g/day/1.73 m^2 body surface area, Nephritic <3.5 g/day. Low levels.

Heavy proteinuria (protein to creatinine ratio >3–3.5-or 24-hour urine collection protein >3–3.5 g/ 24 hours)

- hypoproteinaemia (serum albumin <2.5 g per dl)
- oedema
- hyperlipidaemia

C. Diseases that affect only the kidneys and lead to nephrotic syndrome are called primary causes of nephrotic syndrome. The most common primary causes of nephrotic syndrome are:

Focal segmental glomerulosclerosis (FSGS). This disease affects the kidney's glomeruli, causing some of these filters to become scarred. FSGS is the most common cause of nephrotic syndrome in Black adults.

Membranous nephropathy. This disease causes protein to build up in a part of the kidney called the glomerular basement membrane. It is the most common cause of nephrotic syndrome in white adults.

Minimal change disease. Also called nil disease, this disease is the main cause of nephrotic syndrome in children. Among adults, nephrotic syndrome is more common in older age.

Other causes

Other causes of nephrotic syndrome, also called secondary causes, include

Diabetes, lupus (SLE), amyloidosis, infections, such as HIV/AIDS, hepatitis B, and hepatitis C, some allergic reactions, some medicines, such as nonsteroidal anti-inflammatory drugs, genetic disorders that affect the kidneys.

Ans 48. A. Thyrotoxicosis-Graves' disease.

B. TSH assay-Low in hyperthyroidism, high in hypothyroidism.

C. Hypoparathyroidism caused by removal of parathyroid glands during surgery.

Ans 49. A. Uncontrolled juvenile diabetes. After a loading oral carbohydrate dose, we do

i. Fasting glucose tolerance test.

ii. Random glucose tolerance test.

iii. Oral glucose tolerance test.

B. Catabolism. Unrestricted fatty acid oxidation in liver.

C.

I. Type 1 diabetes
   a. Immunologically mediated
   b. Idiopathic
II. Type 2 diabetes
III. Other specific types
   - Genetic disorder of β-cell function (MODY, mitochondrial DNA)
   - Genetic disorders in insulin action (lipoatrophic diabetes)
   - Exocrine pancreas diseases (pancreatitis, hemochromatosis)
   - Endocrinopathies (acromegaly, Cushing's syndrome)
   - Drug-induced (*glucocorticoids*, tiazidics)
   - Infections (cytomegalovirus, congenital rubeola)
   - Uncommon immunological forms (insulin receptor antibodies)
   - Other genetic syndrome (Down, Tumer, Prader-Willi syndrome)
IV. Gestational diabetes

Source: Adapted from American Diabetes Association.

Ans 50. A. Acute myocardial infarction.
B. LDL. It is the LDL that promotes atheroma formation.
C. Troponin T and Troponin I. These are proteins which regulate Ca^{++} mediated contractility of heart. They have complete tissue specificity and high sensitivity.
D. CK-MB which is the MB fraction of creatinine kinase derived principally from the myocardium but also in small amounts from skeletal muscle.

Ans 51. A. Hodgkin's lymphoma
B. Reed–Stenberg or RS cells
C. T cells
D. CD 15, 20, 30

Ans 52. A. Vacutainer
B. *See* the Table below.
C. 1:9
D. 1:4

Ans 53. A. Urinometer. The float, weight, stem
B. (a) Buoyancy (b) specific gravity of urine is usually 1.016–1.025 (range 1.005–1.035) in normal persons.
C. i. 0.001 for each 3°C above/below standard temperature (20°C)
ii. 0.003 for every 1 g/100 ml of protein
iii. 0.004 for every 1 g/100 ml of glucose.
D. Fixed special gravity at 1.010 regardless of volume of water consumption by the person.

Ans 54. A. (1) RBC Pipette (2) WBC Pipette
B. Hayem's, Dacie's and dilution 1:200.
C. i. Hayem's fluid (sodium sulphate, mercuric chloride, distilled water)
ii. Dacie's fluid (trisodium citrate, formalin, distilled water).

Ans 55. A. Sahli's hemoglobinometer
i. Sahli's graduated Hb tube.
ii. Comparator
iii. Sahli's pipette or Hb pipette
iv. Stirrer
B. Spectrophotometric method, gasometric method, automated hemoglobinometry
C. Blood is mixed with an acid solution so that Hb is converted to brown

Tube	Colour	Name	Anticoagulant	Test
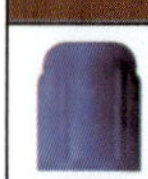	Light blue	Sodium citrate	3.8% or 3.2% sodium citrate	Blood clotting factor PT/INR (plasma)
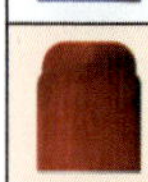	Red	Red or plain	No additive	Immunology, drug, serology
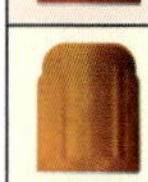	Gold	SST (serum separating tube)	Clot activator with gel	All biochemistry test (LFT, KFT, TFT.....)
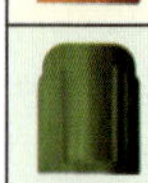	Green	Heparin tube	Sodium or lithium heparin	Special test, trace elements
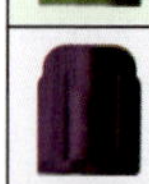	Lavender	EDTA	EDTA	CBC'ESR, blood bank (whole blood)
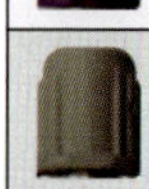	Gray	Sodium fluoride	Sodium fluoride or potassium oxalate	Blood sugar (plasma)

colored acid hematin. This is then diluted with water till the brown colour matches that of the brown glass standard.

D. Potassium cyanide 50 mg, Pot. Ferricyanide 200 mg, Pot. Dihydrogen phosphate 140 mg, non-ionic detergent 1 ml, distilled water 1L.

Ans 56. A. Salah's bone marrow aspiration needle.

B. 1. Red cell disorders—Megaloblastic anemia, pure red cell aplasia
2. WBC cell disorders—Leukemia and subleukemic leukemias
3. Platelet—ITP
4. Myeloproliferative disorder and myelodysplastic syndrome
5. Storage disorders like Gaucher disease and Niemann–Picks disease
6. Pyrexia of unknown origin
7. Assessment of Iron stores
8. Metastasis

C. 1. Klima's bone marrow aspiration needle.
2. Illionois sternal needle
3. Jamshidi BMA.

Ans 57. A. Vim Silverman liver biopsy needle.

B. (a) Evaluation of Jaundice
(b) Liver cirrhosis.
(c) Storage disorders—glycogen storage disorder, hemochromatosis, Wilson's disease.

C. Bleeding diathesis, haemangioma, Hydatid cyst.

Ans 58. A. Lumbar puncture needle

B. Diagnostic indications:
i. Meningitis
ii. Pyrexia of unknown origin (PUO)
iii. Subarachnoid haemorrhage
iv. Myelography

Therapeutic indications
i. Raised intracranial tension
ii. Spine deformity
iii. Local infection
iv. Bleeding diathesis

C. In adults and older children-usually between L3 and L4
In infants, usually between L4 and L5.

Ans 59. A. Eshbach's albuminometer

B. Quantitative estimation of albumin in urine

C. Picric acid and citric acid in water

D. Urinary excretion of albumin in the range 30–300 mg/24 hours.

Ans 60. A. Wintrobe tube

B. i. PCV estimation
ii. ESR estimation
iii. Preparation of buffy coat smear

C. i. PCV in adult male: (40–50%)
ii. PCV in female: (38–45%)
iii. PCV in newborn (44–68%)

D. i. Anemia and leukemia
ii. Secondary to bleeding
iii. Pregnancy
iv. Renal disease.

Ans 61. A. Tuberculous meningitis

B. Raised protein, decrease glucose, raised chloride, lymphocytosis, formation of cobweb coagulum after standing.

C. *See* the Table in next page.

Ans 62. A. a. Uncontrolled juvenile diabetes type1.

b. HbA1c.
Fasting glucose test: ≥126 mg per dl (7.0 mmol per L)
Two-hour OGTT (75-g load): ≥200 mg per dL (11.1 mmol per L)
Random glucose test: ≥200 mg per dL with symptoms
A1c measurement: ≥6.5%

c. Ischemic heart disease, peripheral vascular disease, cerebrovascular disease.

CSF analysis	Bacterial	Tuberculosis	Viral	Fungal	Aseptic
Pressure	Increased	Increased	Normal to elevated	Normal to mild increase	Increased
Color	Turbid	Turbid	Clear	Clear	Clear to turbid
Glucose	<40 mg%	Low	Normal to mild less	Low to normal	Low
Proteins	Elevated	Greatly elevated	Normal to mild elevation	Normal to mild increase	Elevated
Lactate	Elevated (>6 mmol/L)	Elevated	0–6 mmol/L	Normal	Normal
RBCs	Elevated	Elevated	Normal	Normal	Elevated
WBCs	10–2000 mm^3	Elevated, but <500	>100 mm^3	10–50 mm^3	Mildly elevated
WBC types	Neutrophils	Lymphocytes	Lymphocytes	Lymphocytes	Neutrophils
Gram's stain	Positive	Acid fast bacilli	Negative	Positive	Negative
Microbial culture	Positive	Positive (yield is high early stages)	Negative	Positive	Negative
Biomarkers	Elevated C-reactive proteins	Antibodies in CSF (detection of anti-M37Ra, anti-antigen 5, and anti-M37Rv)			
		Elevated CSF procalcitonin, Adenosine deaminase	Low CRP and adenosine deaminase		Seen following neurosurgery or antibiotic use
PCR test		Help in identification of organisms even after antibiotics are started	Helps in identification of the organisms		

Ans 63. A. Acute MI in a diabetic patient

B. Raised CPK, LDH, CK-MB

C. Troponin T.

D. Gross-mottling with yellow tan infarct canter

Microscopy: Coagulation necrosis with loss of nuclei and muscle striations, dense neutrophilic infiltration into the infarcted area.

Ans 64. A. Micronodular cirrhosis

- Liver is shrunken and atrophic
- Surface is irregular and multiple small nodules of <3 mm in size are seen
- Colour is yellowish orange
- Consistency is firm
- Gallbladder is seen in gallbladder fossa of liver.

B. Alcoholic cirrhosis, primary biliary cirrhosis, hereditary hemochromatosis, hepatic venous outflow obstruction,large bile duct obstruction,Indian childhood cirrhosis.

C. Liver architecture is disrupted. Initially developing fibrous septa are delicate and extend through sinusoids from central to portal tract or portal to portal tract

- Regenerative activity of entrapped parenchyma hepatocytes generate uniform micronodules. Later these micronodules become larger and produce macronodules creating a hobnail appearance.
- Hepatocytes look normal in some nodules while may be irregular with dysplastic changes in other.

Ans 65. A. Hemangioma, angiosarcoma.

B. Shows dilated blood vessels filled with RBC and liked by benign endothelial cells.

C. Cavernous hemangioma

- Congenital hemangioma
- Epithelioid hemangioma
- Glomeruloid hemangioma
- Hobnail hemangioma
- Infantile hemangioma
- Intramuscular angioma
- Lobular capillary hemangioma/ pyogenic granuloma
- Microvenular hemangioma
- Sinusoidal hemangioma
- Spindle cell hemangioma
- Verrucous hemangioma.

Ans 66. A. Benign lesion.

B. They are: Biphasic tumour, proliferation of both glandular and stromal elements:

- Two recognized growth patterns-intracanalicular, peri canalicular
- Glandular elements have intact myoepithelial cell layer.

C. Usually there is no increased risk of cancer/carcinoma. But very rarely it may progress to carcinoma.

Ans 67. A. Sickle cell disease.

B. Chronic haemolysis, microvascular occlusion, tissue damage, sickle shaped RBCS.

C. Point mutation in the 6th codon of beta-globin chain that leads to the replacement of a glutamine residue with a valine residue.

Ans 68. A. Microcytic, hypochromic RBC with control pallor, poikilocytosis.

B. Microcytic hypochromic anaemia/ iron deficiency.

C. They are:

i. Iron deficiency anaemia.
ii. Anaemia diluting chronic blood loss.
iii. Anaemia of chronic disease.
iv. Thalassemia.

Ans 69. A. Adult polycystic kidney disease (autosomal dominant).

B. Bilateral

C. PKD 1 on chronic 16, most common. Also, PKD3, PKD3

D. Polycystic kidney disease, renal dysplasia, medullary cystic disease, simple renal cyst, renal cysts in hereditary malformation syndrome, glomerulocystic disease.

Ans 70. A. Kidney demonstrating marked hydronephrosis (dilated cystic spaces) with nearly complete loss of cortex.

- Multiple cystic cavities seen in renal pelvis and calyces. Wall of these cystic spaces communicate with renal pelvis.

B. Renal pelvis: Calculi, tumours, uteropelvic stricture

- Intrinsic ureter: calculi, tumours, blood clot, inflammation
- Extrinsic ureter: Tumour, compression, pregnancy, retroperitoneal fibrosis
- Urinary bladder: VUR, tumours, neurogenic

- Prostate: BHP, carcinoma, prostatitis
- Urethra: Posterior valve stricture, rarely tumours.

C. In chronic cases, there is tubular atrophy with marked diffuse interstitial fibrosis. Progressive blunting of the apices of the pyramids occurs, and these eventually become cupped.

Ans 71. A. L mold
B. Tissue embedding used to prepare paraffin blocks.
C. Plastic tissue cassettes.
D. Tissue processing these cassettes are totally resistant to most reagents and their slots offer maximum flow through for good fluid exchange and proper drainage.

Ans 72. A. Jamshidi trephine biopsy needle.
B. Islam's needle, Westerman Jensen, drills.
C. Zenkers acetic solution, B-5 fixative.

Ans 73. A. Improved Neubauer chamber
B. Cell Counting-RBC, WBC, platelet, sperm, bacteria, etc.
C. i. In old Neubauer chamber, the gap between triple lines was very wide and the rectangular space between them looks as similar as the squares in which cells are to be counted. Chances of error were very high.
ii. In new Neubauer chamber, central square is divided into 25 squares as compare to 16 in old.

Ans 74. A. A +ve, Gel card method. There are 2 subtypes-A1 (80%) and A2 (20%) based on presence of A1 antigen and A2 on RBC.
B. Both antigens A and B or RBCs are formed from H substance (H antigen). Rarely, persons do not inherit H gene (very rare HH genotype) and they are unable to produce H substance (H antigen). So, they cannot produce A and B blood group antigens on RBC membrane. This rare blood group is called Bombay blood group or Oh group.
C. Polyagglutination or pan agglutination: If RBCs are contaminated by certain bacteria like Pseudomonas aeruginosa, then RBCs may be agglutinated by all blood group sera (antibody) or even by normal human serum. This phenomenon is known as Thomson–Friedenreich phenomenon.
D. Monoclonal antibodies are used. So, it is very sensitive and weak antigen can also be detected.

Ans 75. A. Coagulometer to determine PT and APTT.
B. A clot forms at the end of blood coagulation. In normal circumstances, the clot undergoes contraction. When serum is expressed from the clot, the clot becomes denser. The platelets release one substance (called thromboplastin) which is responsible for clot retraction. Normal clot retraction begins within 30 seconds after the blood has clotted, and at one hour it is about 30% normally.

Clot retraction test is done when there is suspicion of haemorrhagic disorder related to platelets. Poor clot retraction is seen if platelet count is low (thrombocytopenia or in poor platelet function with normal platelet count (Thrombasthenia).

C. i. Congenital deficiency of factor VII, which is very rare.
ii. Initiation of oral anticoagulant therapy (warfarin).
D. In this case, both tests are replaced with 1:1 mixture of patient's

plasma and normal plasma (control) as substrate. Of both PT and APTT now become normal, then the patient has deficiency of one or many of these factors; factors I, II, V and X (common for PT and APPTT). After that, individual specific assay is done to find out deficiency of particular factor.

Ans 76. A. Automated blood cell counter.

B. Electronic counter is based on aperture impedance method, or light scattering technology, or both. In this method, particles (WBCs) passing through a chamber in single file scatter the light and convert by a chamber in single file scatter the light and convert by a detector into pulses proportionate to the size of the cells, which are counted electronically. During, counting of WBCs, a lysate is used to lyse RBCs.

C. The principal is electrical impedance like counting RBCs. Platelet counting by electronic method is disadvantageous.

Disadvantages are:

- Debris and fragments of blood cells (small size) are counted as platelets.
- Howell–Jolly bodies and Heinz bodies are also counted as platelets.
- Equipment is costly and calibration error may occur.

Ans 77. A. Westergren Pipette with ESR stand (pipette is 30 cm in length and 2.5 mm in diameter).

B. Wintrobe's tube

This instrument is preferred because:

i. When ESR becomes high Westergren method gives more accurate result.

ii. It is more sensitive because the pipette is longer and there are more markings (graduations).

C. Causes of high ESR:

i. Chronic infection: Tuberculosis, chronic osteomyelitis, chronic bronchiectasis, chronic lung abscess.

ii. Autoimmune disease: SLE, rheumatoid arthritis, acute rheumatic fever.

iii. Acute inflammation: Acute MI, extensive inflammation

iv. Neoplasm: Hodgkin's disease, leukaemia, multiple myeloma.

Causes of Low ESR:

i. Congestive heart failure, polycythaemia, hypofibrinogenaemia and abnormal red cell disorders.

Ans 78. A. Automated ESR machine for ESR estimation.

B. Electronic method by automated analysers.

The other methods used are:

i. Westergren method.

ii. Wintrobe method.

iii. Landau method.

C. MCV (mean corpuscular volume)

MCH (mean corpuscular haemoglobin)

MCHC (mean corpuscular haemoglobin concentration).

Ans 79. A. Esbach albuminometer

B. i. Heat coagulation test

ii. Heller's test

iii. Sulphosalicylic acid

C. Esbach's reagents

i. Picric acid-05 g

ii. Citric acid-10 g

iii. Distilled water-500 ml.

Ans 80. A. Fibroadenoma

B. i. Fibrous capsule

ii. Fibrous tissue

iii. Benign stroma and epithelial component

iv. Myxoid changes.

C. i. Intracanalicular pattern

ii. Pericanalicular pattern.

Ans 81. A. Rotary microtome

B. Clearing agent (xylene or toluene) is a solvent of wax; helps to replace alcohol in dehydrated tissue and thus it facilitates paraffin wax penetration into tissue. Clearing agent must be miscible with alcohol. It usually makes the tissue transparent, hence the name. But some clearing agents do not make tissue transparent, so better terminology would be 'de-alcoholising agent'.

C. The basic principle in frozen section is to freeze the tissue (–5° to –25° C commonly-23°C), so that the water within the tissue transform into ice. The tissue becomes firm. The ice acts as embedding medium (like paraffin wax in routine tissue processing and sections are cute by a special microtome known as cryostat.

D. The presence of calcium salts and other minerals in bone and ither tissue prevents the preparation of good histologic sections by routine methods. Incomplete removal of these minerals results in ragged and torn sections and in damage to the cutting edge of the microtome knife.

Ans 82. A. Hb electrophoresis

B. HbA-very low
HbF-normal
Hb S—very high

C. Sickle cell anaemia

D. Solubility test, blood smear.

Ans 83. A. i. Nucleated RBCs
ii. Marked microcytosis
iii. Hypochromasia with severe anemia
iv. Eosinophils
v. Target cells

B. β thalassemia major

C. i. Iron (Fe) profile
ii. Hb Electrophoresis
iii. Genetic Study(DNA analysis for α and β globin mutations).

Ans 84. A. Gastric carcinoma

B. i. Pyloric-antrum region (lesser curvature): 50–60%
ii. Cardiac region of stomach: 25%
iii. Body and fundus: 25%
iv. Greater curvature of stomach: 12%

C. i. Depth of Invasion (early and advanced carcinoma)
ii. Macroscopic growth pattern (flat mucosal lesions, exophytic, ulcerative and diffuse infiltrative type)
iii. Histologic types (intestinal types and diffuse type as per Lauren's classification).

Ans 85. A. Granular contracted kidney.

B. i. Chronic glomerulonephritis
ii. Chronic pyelonephritis (U-shaped scar)
iii. Benign nephrosclerosis (benign hypertension, V-shaped scar)
iv. Diabetic nephropathy, myeloma kidney, amyloid kidney.

C. *See* the Table below.

Parameters	Chronic glomerulonephritis	Chronic pyelonephritis
• Causes	Different types of glomerulonephritis	Reflux nephropathy or chronic obstructive pyelonephritis
• Pathogenesis	End stage glomerular disease due to specific glomerulonephritis	Chronic tubolointerstitial inflammation and fibrosis associated with renal disease.

(Contd.)

(*Contd.*)

Parameters	Chronic glomerulonephritis	Chronic pyelonephritis
• Gross appearance of kidney surface	Diffusely, granular, cortical surfaces	Depressed area on dilated and blunted calyx
• Nature of scar	Fine and symmetrical	Coarse and asymmetrical
• Glomeruli	Reduces in number and atrophic	Normal; may show periglomerular fibrosis
• Tubules	Atrophied	Atrophy in some hypertrophy in others.
• Interstitial and periglomerular fibrosis	Mild	More severe
• Renal calyx and pelvis	Normal	Dilated
• Clinical features	Onset is insidious. Proteinuria, oedema, azotemia, hypertension	May be asymptomatic. Some present with back pain, fever, pyuria, polyuria, nocturia, bacteria, with gradual onset of hypertension and renal insufficiency.

Ans 86. A. Emphysema of lung.

B. i. Abnormally large alveoli separated by thin septa.
   ii. Adjacent alveoli become confluent, creating large airspaces.
   iii. As alveolar walls are destroyed, there is decrease in the capillary bed.

C. i. Centriacinar (centrilobular) emphysema
   ii. Panacinar (panlobular) emphysema
   iii. Paraseptal (distal acinar) emphysema
   iv. Irregular emphysema
   v. Interstitial emphysema

Ans 87. A. Tuberculosis ulcer of small intestine.

B. Peptic ulcer in duodenum, typhoid ulcer, tubercular ulcer, Crohn's disease and bacillary dysentery ulcers.

C. It is variant of intestinal tuberculosis characterized by thickening of terminal ileum, caecum and ascending colon along with mucosal ulceration. Clinically, a mass is palpable and may be misdiagnosed as ileocecal carcinoma.

Ans 88. A. Pleomorphic adenoma

B. This is a biphasic tumour composed of epithelial component and stromal component.
   i. Well stained benign acini and ducts of salivary gland. The glandular epithelial cells do not show anisonulcleosis or features of malignancy.
   ii. Pale blue loose connective myxomatous tissue stroma
   iii. Thin capsule

C. If tumour is entirely made of glandular component without any myxomatous stromal component.

Ans 89. A. Partial hydatidiform mole

B. Chorionic villi markedly swollen and expandable due to hydropic swelling of villous stromal core.

C. Benign

D. A complete mole occurs when an empty ovum is fertilised by a sperm (46XX/ 46XY).

Ans 90. A. Wilms tumour

B. WT1 Gene

C. i. Blastemal
   ii. Stroma
   iii. Epithelial.

Ans 91. A. Struma ovarii (Teratoma)
B. i. Thyroid tissue
ii. Cartilage, adipose tissue and intestinal glands.
C. Nulliparity
D. majority benign.

Ans 92. A. Multiple myeloma
B. A marrow reveals diffuse infiltration of sheets like masses of plasma cells with prominent Golgi apparatus and eccentrically placed nucleus.
C. Kappa light chains in urine.
D. beta 2 microglobulin

Ans 93. A. Papillary thyroid carcinoma (PTC)
B. Papillary, medullary, follicular, Anaplastic
C. PTC tend to be indolent.
D. Nuclear grooving/inclusion.

Ans 94. A. Meningioma
B. Clusters or whorls of meningothelial cells and scanty vascular stroma.
C. i. Psammomatous
ii. Secretary
iii. Microcystic

Ans 95. A. i. Replacement of marrow by blast cells.
ii. Acute Leukaemia
a. Sudan Black, MPO
b. CD45, TdT, CD3, CD10, CD33.

Ans 96. A. A+ve, B+ve, AB+ve, O+ve
B. Rh Blood group is positive (Rh+)
C. IgM
D. IgG.

Ans 97. A. Acute viral hepatitis
B. Increased bilirubin and transaminase (AST, ALT) level
C. Anti HAV IgM, Anti HEV IgM, HBsAg, Anti HCV.

Ans 98. A. Acute renal failure
B. Due to hypovolemia and tissue injury. Renal function test (serum urea, creatinine, serum electrolytes).
C. Criteria and staging for acute kidney injury.

Stage	Serum creatinine	Urine output
1.	1.5–1.9 times baseline OR ≥0.3 mg/dl (>26.5 μmol/L) increase	<0.5 ml/kg/h for 6–12 hours
2.	2.0–2.9 times baseline	<0.5 ml/kg/h for ≥12 hours
3.	3.0 times baseline OR Increase in serum creatinine to ≥4.0 mg/dl (353.6 μmol/L) OR Initiation of renal replacement therapy OR, In patients <18 years, decrease in eGFR to <35 ml/min per 1.73 m^2	<0.3 ml/kg/h for ≥24 hours OR Anuria for ≥12 hours

Minimum criteria for Acute Kidney Injury include an Increase in serum creatinine by ≥0.3 mg/dl (>26.5 μmol/L) observed within 48 hours; or an Increase in serum creatinine to ≥1.5 times baseline, which is known or presumed to have occurred within the prior 7 days; or Urine volume <0.5 ml/kg/h for 6 hours.

Ans 99. A. Dwarfism due to growth hormone deficiency low serum growth hormone level did not increase after induced stress.
B. Cretinism, malnutrition, achondroplasia
C. Growth hormone secretion is regulated by the hypothalamus and the mediators of GH actions. Regulatory factors include GH releasing hormone (GHRH), somatostatin, GH releasing peptide (Ghrelin), and IGF1.

Ans 100. A. Mitral valve stenosis due to RHD (rheumatic heart disease)
B. Aschoff bodies are fibrinoid necrosis surrounded by macrophages, lymphocytes and plasma cells in myocardium due to myocarditis in RHD.
C. It is left artrial endocardial thickening due to endocarditis in RHD.
D. Congestive cardiac failure, atrial fibrillation, SABE, embolism.

Chapter

20

DOPS (Direct Observation of Procedural Skills)

DOPS (Direct Observation of Procedural Skills)

Task 1: Measure blood pressure of the Mrs Ranjana Mukherjee, 48 years old lady in sitting posture and write it in the answer sheet provided.

S. No.	Criteria	Marks	Candidate number
1.	Asks if the patient exercised, smoked, consumed alcohol 30 minutes prior (If yes, refrains) and was sitting calm for 5 minutes	0.5	
2.	Makes the patient seated on a chair, back supported, feet flat on floor, and arm on a firm surface at the level of heart	0.5	
3.	Checks cuff tubing and bulb for obstruction/leakage	0.5	
4.	Wraps cuff smoothly and snugly around patients' arm with lower edge one inch above elbow, centered over branchial artery	1	
5.	Palpates radial artery	0.5	
6.	Inflates the cuff steadily, releases it slowly and notes reading when pulse reappears	1	
7.	Places the bell of stethoscope over the brachial artery	0.5	
8.	Inflates cuff 40 mm Hg above that estimated by palpatory method and releases slowly	0.5	
9.	When the sound is heard, notes the reading as systolic and at absence as diastolic	1	
10.	Documents the patient details, position, arm used and the blood pressure correctly	1	
11.	Global score	3	
12.	**Total Marks**	**10**	

Guidelines for Global Score

Score 0: Made critical error (measured the blood pressure with cuff loosely tied or measured in standing posture);

Score 1.5: Expected standard (Systemically measured without stressing the patient);

Score 2: Better than expected (Expected standard plus documented correctly and thanked the patient after the procedure);

Score 3: Exceptional performance (Better than expected plus kept the cuff inside apparatus, closed the mercury tank and sphygmomanometer after measurement).

Task 2: Elicit relevant history from Mr Nirmal Maji, a 55-year-old gentleman with peripheral vascular disease.

S. No.	Criteria	Marks	Candidate number
1.	Clarifies the identity and asks the age of the patient	1	
2.	Enquires about the presenting symptoms and duration of each	1	
3.	Asks about the nature of pain	1	
4.	Enquires about intermittent claudication and claudication distance	1	
5.	Asks about the aggravating factors	0.5	
6.	Asks about the relieving factors	0.5	
7.	Enquires about coexisting chest pain/intestinal angina	0.5	
8.	Enquires about coexisting medical disorders (hypertension/diabetes)	0.5	
9.	Enquires about smoking (duration and no. of cigarettes/beedies per day)	1	
10.	Global score	3	
11.	**Total Marks**	**10**	

Guidelines for Global Score

Score 0: Made critical error (Failed to clarify identity or failed to elicit history about presenting symptoms, e.g. patient complained of pain but candidate did not ask any detail about pain);

Score 1.5: Expected standard (Systemically elicits history about all the presenting complaints, enquires about smoking and communicates without use of medical jargon);

Score 2: Better than expected (Expected standard plus enquires for other coexisting symptom/medical disorders);

Score 3: Exceptional performance (Better than expected plus compassionate to patients).

Task 3: Perform an appropriate test to detect the presence/absence of reducing substances in the given sample of urine. Record your findings and inference in the answer sheet provided.

S. No.	Criteria	Marks	Candidate number
1.	Takes exactly 5 ml of Benedict's solution using a pipette	1	
2.	Boils solution to check for autoreduction	1	
3.	Adds exactly 8 drops of urine	1	
4.	Boils for two minutes	0.5	
5.	Sees the colour of the precipitate and writes down the observation	1	
6.	Records the inference correctly	1	
7.	Closes the reagent bottle and leaves the test tube in the stand	0.5	
8.	Cleans up the place of work or kept the place clean	1	
9.	Global score	3	
10.	**Total Marks**	**10**	

Guidelines for Global Score

Score 0: Made critical error (Failed to add required quantity of urine or failed to identify Benedict's solution);

Score 1.5: Expected standard (Performed all the steps correctly in the same order);

Score 2: Better than expected (Expected standard plus able to correctly infer the color obtained);

Score 3: Exceptional performance (Better than expected plus did not spill reagent/urine).

Chapter

21

Museum Specimens OSPE

Q1.

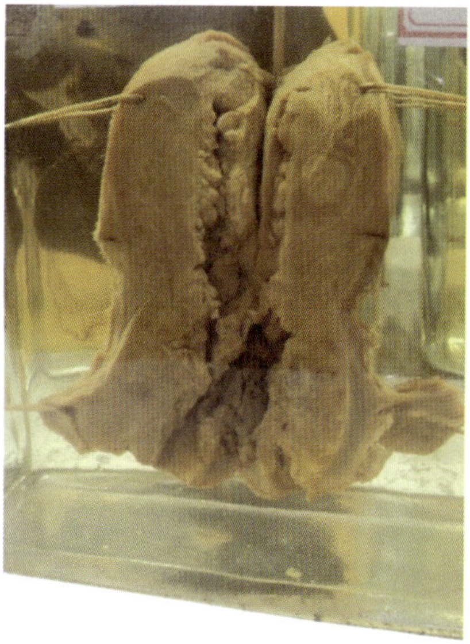

A. Describe the specimen. (1)

B. What is your clinical diagnosis of this museum specimen? (1)

Q2.

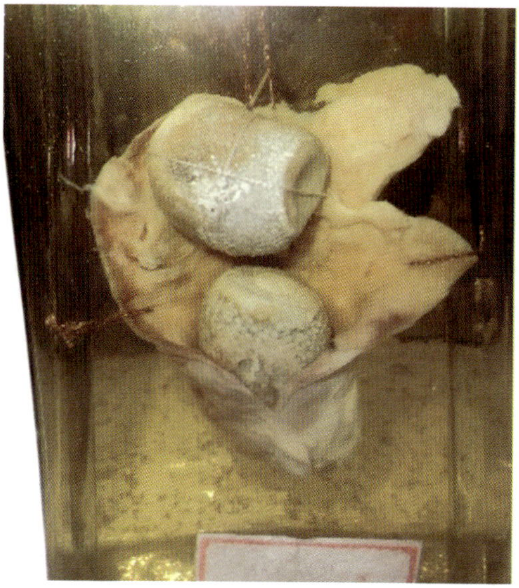

A. Describe the specimen. (1)

B. What is your clinical diagnosis of this museum specimen? (1)

Q3.

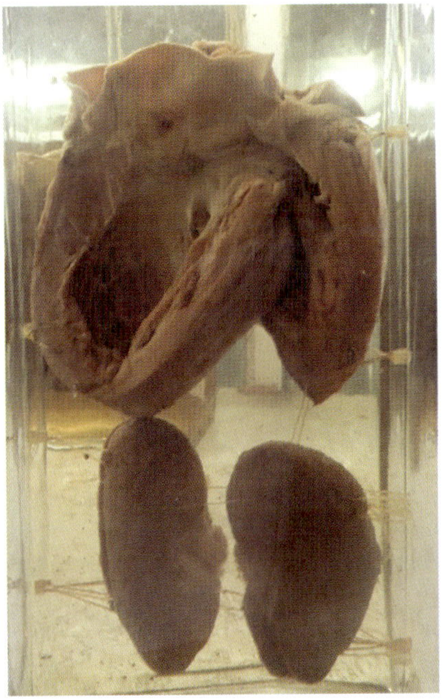

What is your clinical diagnoses of these two museum specimens?

(1 + 1 = 2)

Q4.

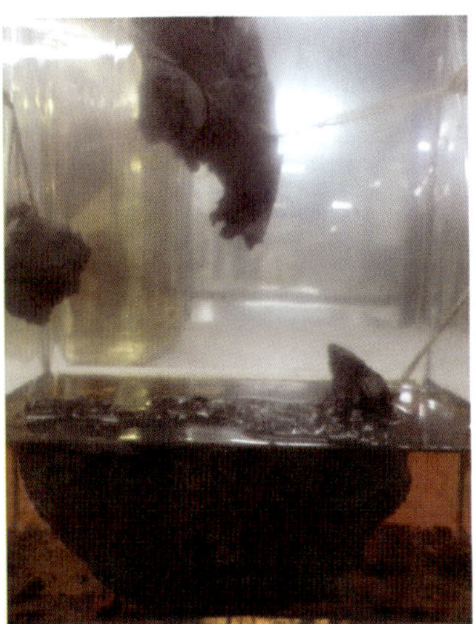

A. Describe the specimen. (1)

B. What is your clinical diagnosis of this museum specimen? (1)

Q5.

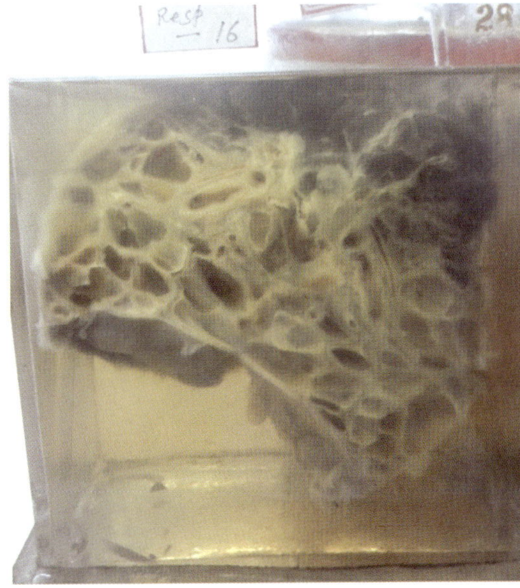

A. Describe the specimen. (1)

B. What is your clinical diagnosis of this museum specimen? (1)

Q6.

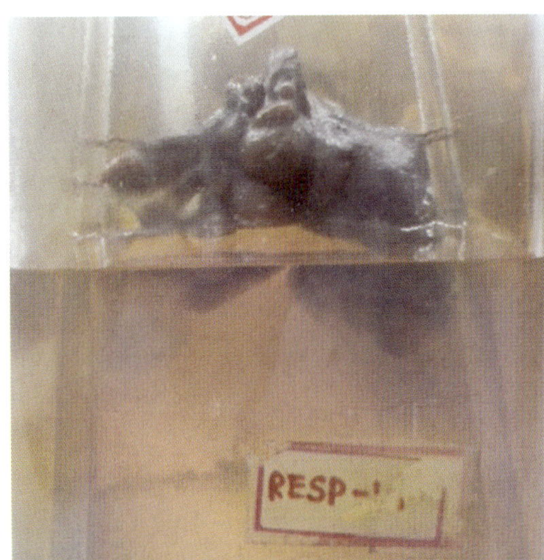

A. Describe the specimen. (1)

B. What is your clinical diagnosis of this museum specimen? (1)

Q7.

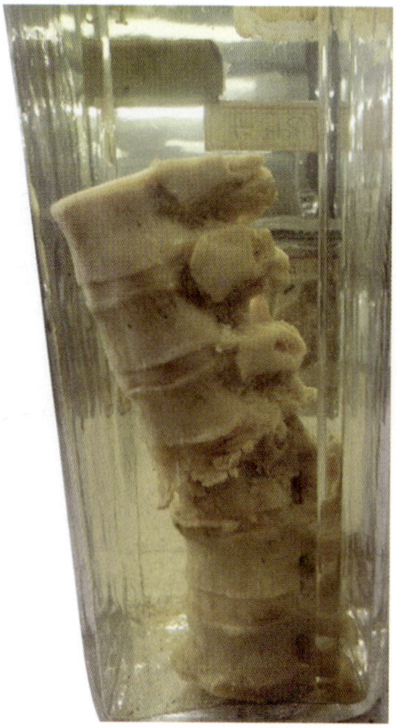

A. Describe the specimen. (1)

B. What is your clinical diagnosis of this museum specimen? (1)

Q8.

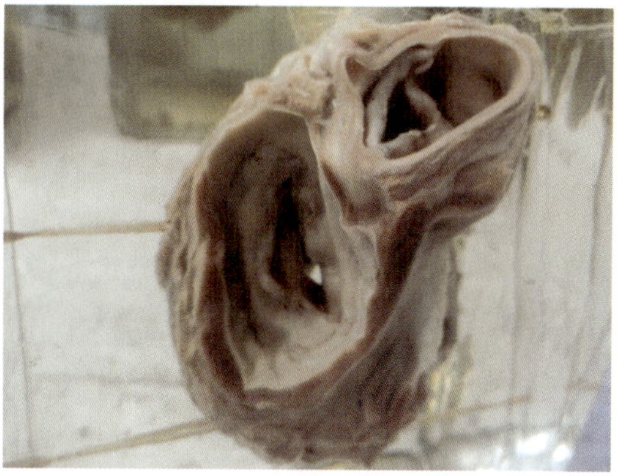

A. Describe the specimen. (1)

B. What is your clinical diagnosis of this museum specimen? (1)

Q9.

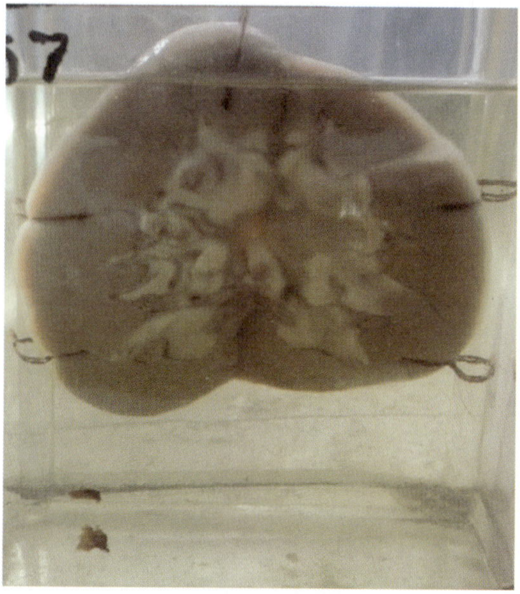

A. Describe the specimen. (1)

B. What is your clinical diagnosis of this museum specimen? (1)

Q10.

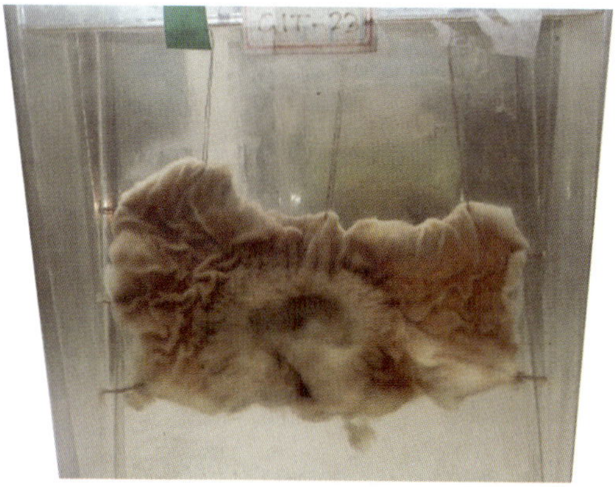

A. Describe the specimen. (1)

B. What is your clinical diagnosis of this museum specimen? (1)

Q11.

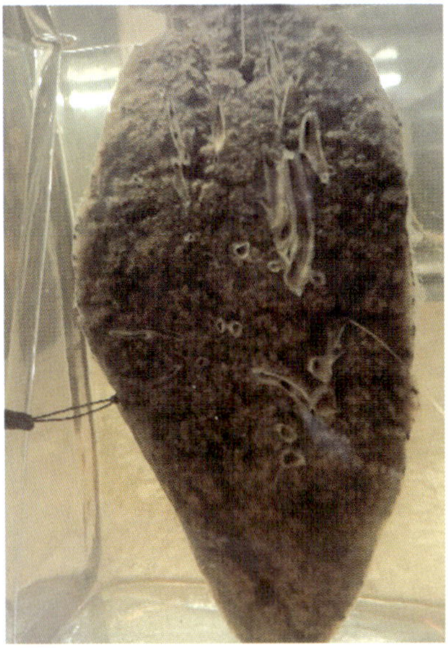

A. Describe the specimen. (1)
B. What is your clinical diagnosis of this museum specimen? (1)

Q12.

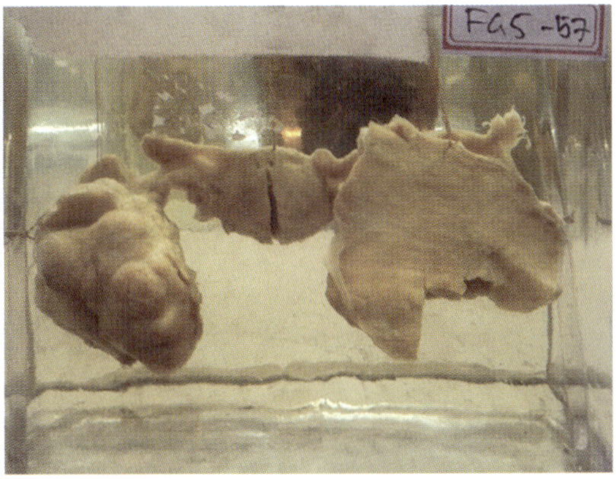

A. Describe the specimen. (1)
B. What is your clinical diagnosis of this museum specimen? (1)

Q13.

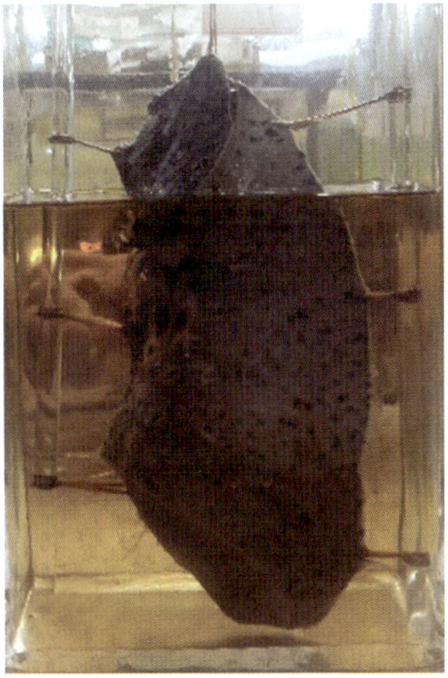

A. Describe the specimen. (1)
B. What is your clinical diagnosis of this museum specimen? (1)

Q14.

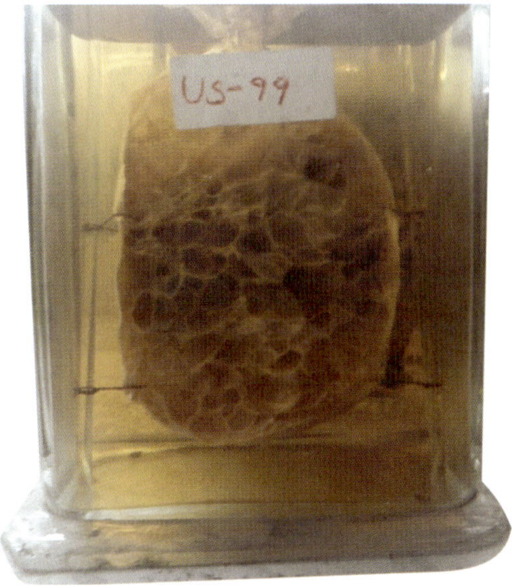

A. Describe the specimen. (1)
B. What is your clinical diagnosis of this museum specimen? (1)

Q15.

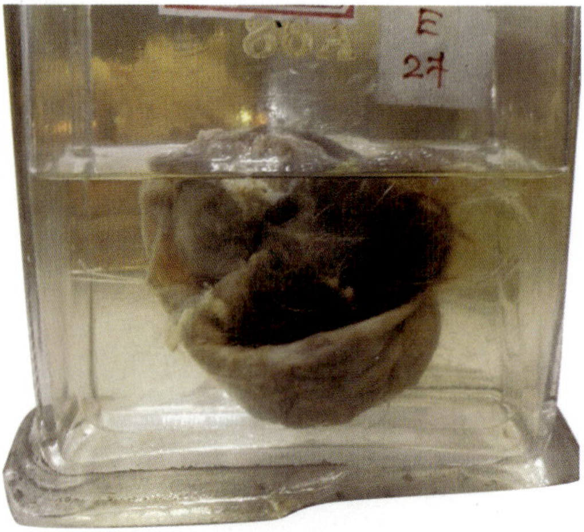

A. Describe the specimen. (1)
B. What is your clinical diagnosis of this museum specimen? (1)

Q16.

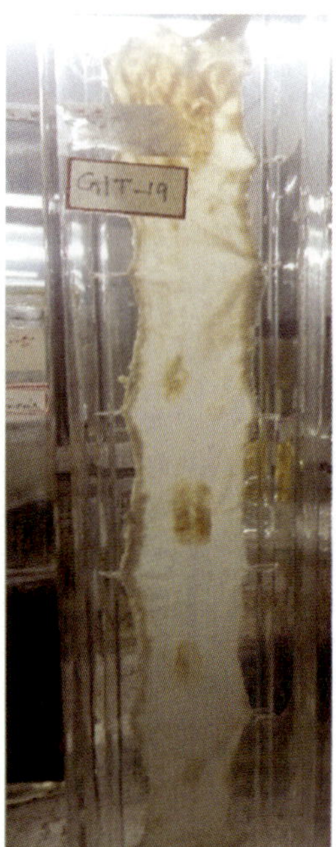

A. Describe the specimen. (1)
B. What is your clinical diagnosis of this museum specimen? (1)

Q17.

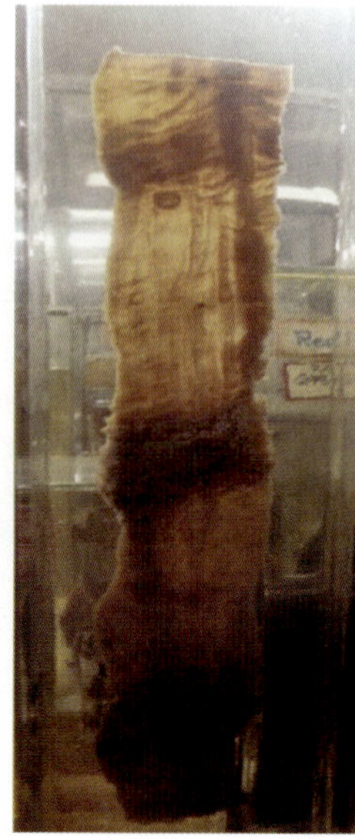

A. Describe the specimen. (1)
B. What is your clinical diagnosis of this museum specimen? (1)

Q18.

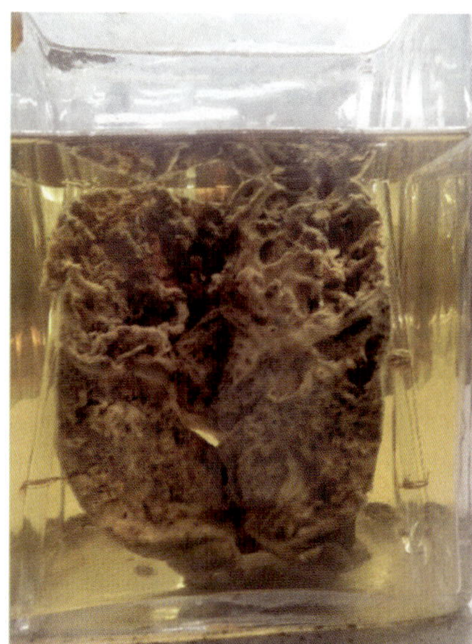

A. Describe the specimen. (1)
B. What is your clinical diagnosis of this museum specimen? (1)

Q19.

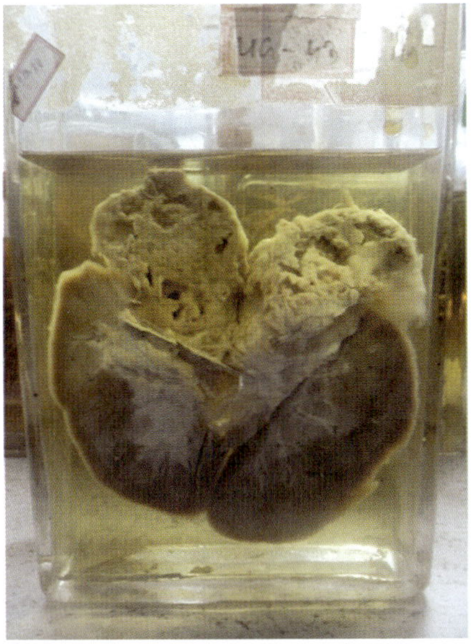

A. Describe the specimen. (1)
B. What is your clinical diagnosis of this museum specimen? (1)

Q20.

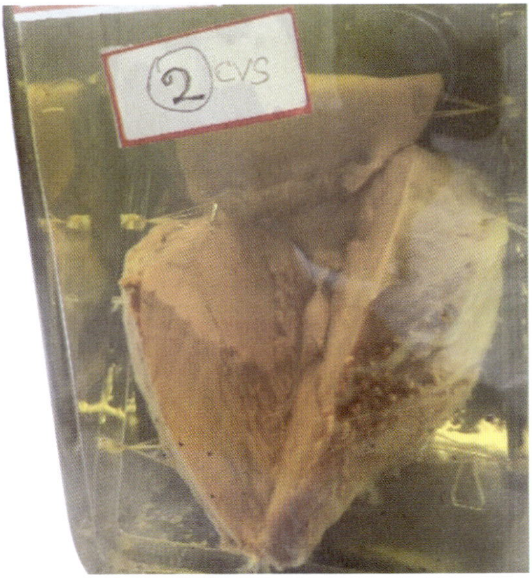

A. Describe the specimen. (1)
B. What is your clinical diagnosis of this museum specimen? (1)

Q21.

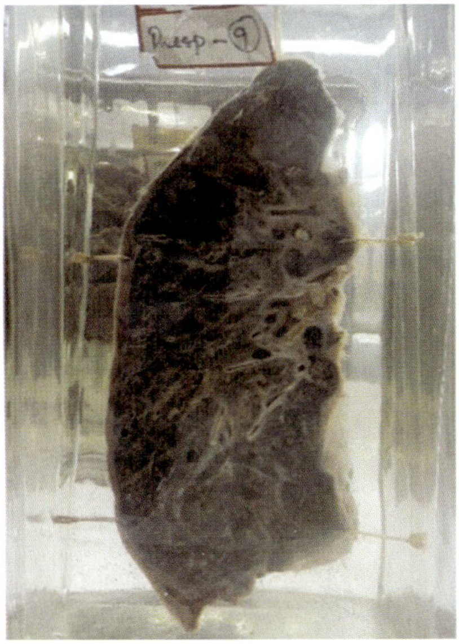

A. Describe the specimen. (1)
B. What is your clinical diagnosis of this museum specimen? (1)

Q22.

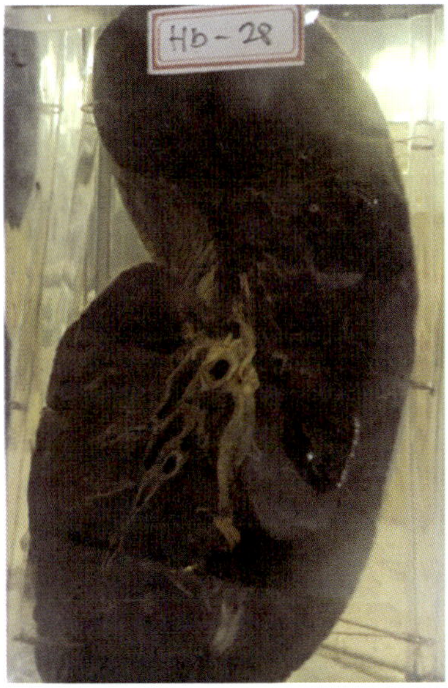

A. Describe the specimen. (1)
B. What is your clinical diagnosis of this museum specimen? (1)

Q23.

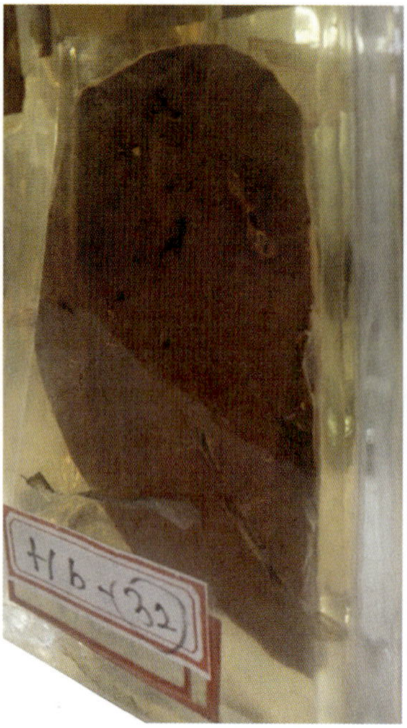

A. Describe the specimen. (1)
B. What is your clinical diagnosis of this museum specimen? (1)

Q24.

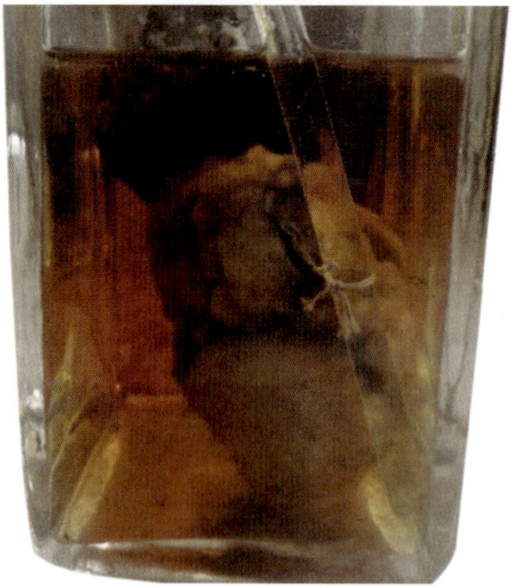

A. Describe the specimen. (1)
B. What is your clinical diagnosis of this museum specimen? (1)

Q25.

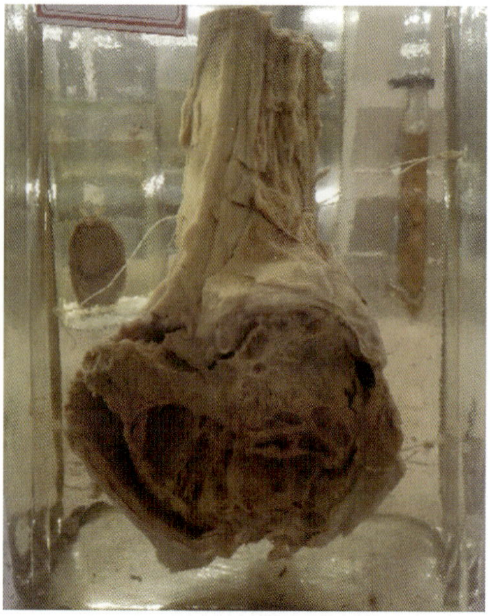

A. Describe the specimen. (1)
B. What is your clinical diagnosis of this museum specimen? (1)

Q26.

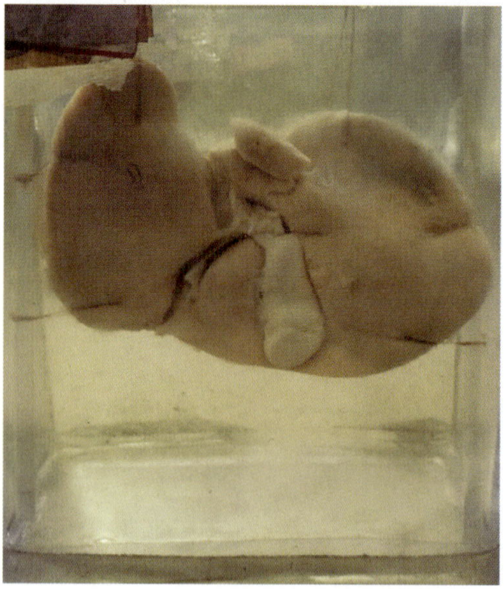

A. Describe the specimen. (1)
B. What is your clinical diagnosis of this museum specimen? (1)

Q27.

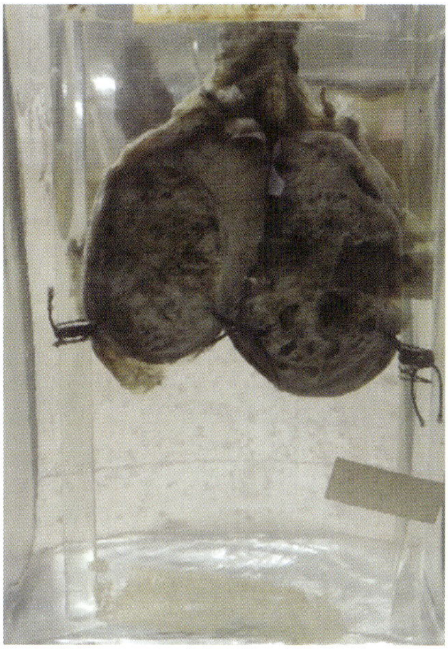

A. Describe the specimen. (1)
B. What is your clinical diagnosis of this museum specimen? (1)

Q28.

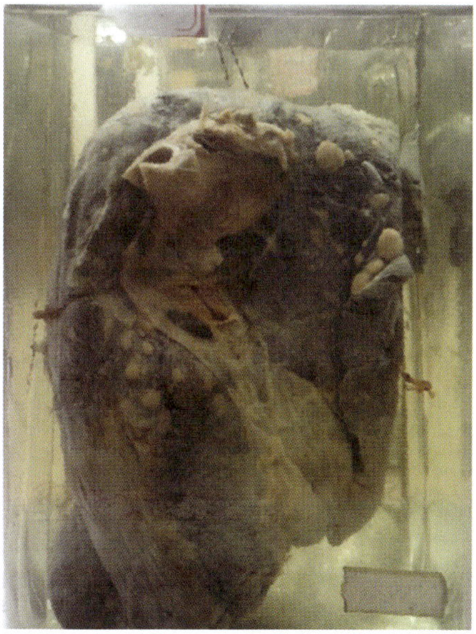

A. Describe the specimen. (1)
B. What is your clinical diagnosis of this museum specimen? (1)

Q29.

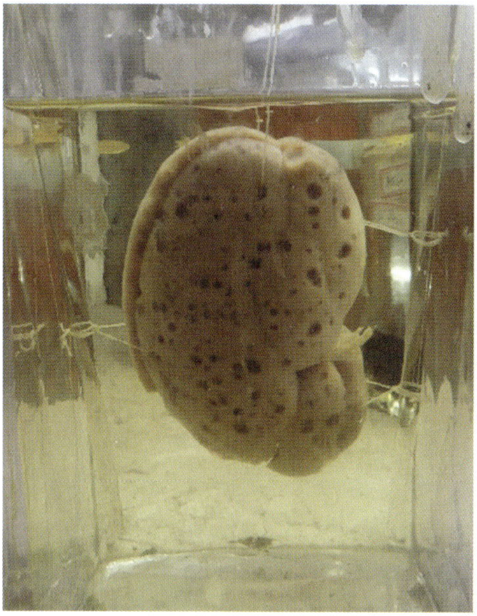

A. Describe the specimen. (1)
B. What is your clinical diagnosis of this museum specimen? (1)

Q30.

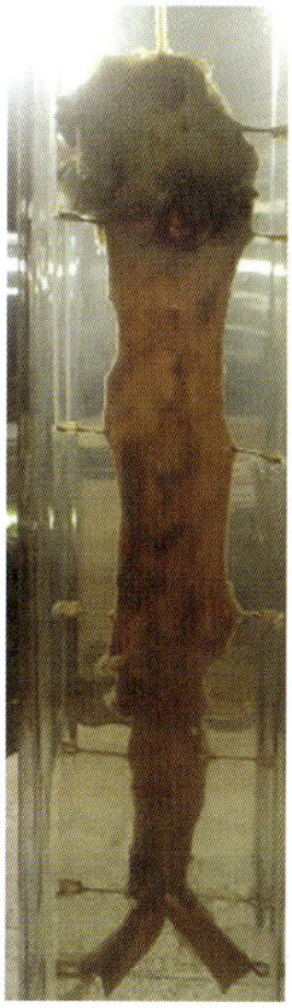

A. Describe the specimen. (1)
B. What is your clinical diagnosis of this museum specimen? (1)

Q31.

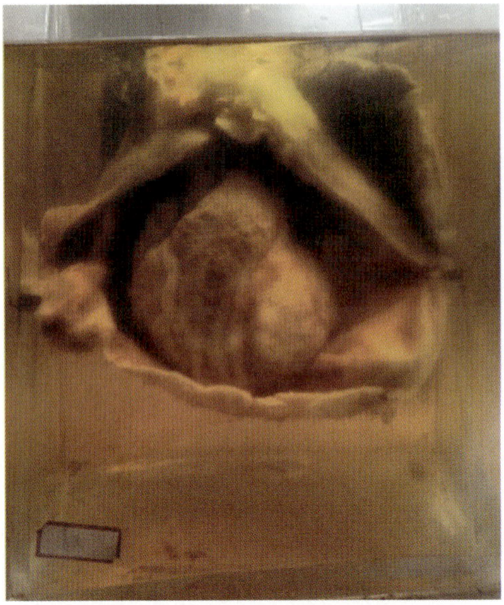

A. Describe the specimen. (1)
B. What is your clinical diagnosis of this museum specimen? (1)

Q32.

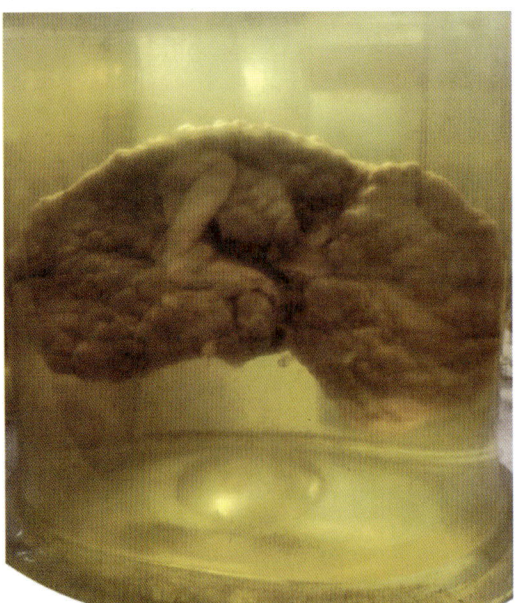

A. Describe the specimen. (1)
B. What is your clinical diagnosis of this museum specimen? (1)

Q33.

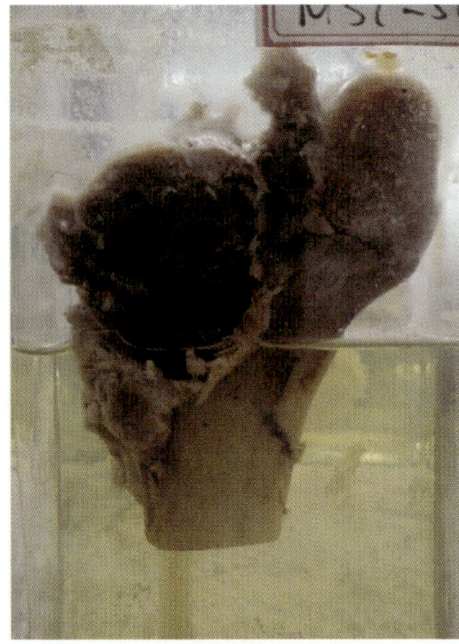

A. Describe the specimen. (1)
B. What is your clinical diagnosis of this museum specimen? (1)

Q34.

A. Describe the specimen. (1)
B. What is your clinical diagnosis of this museum specimen? (1)

Q35.

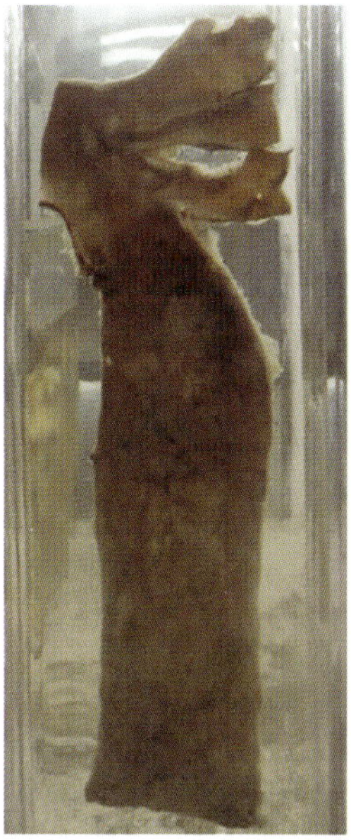

A. Describe the specimen. (1)
B. What is your clinical diagnosis of this museum specimen? (1)

Q36.

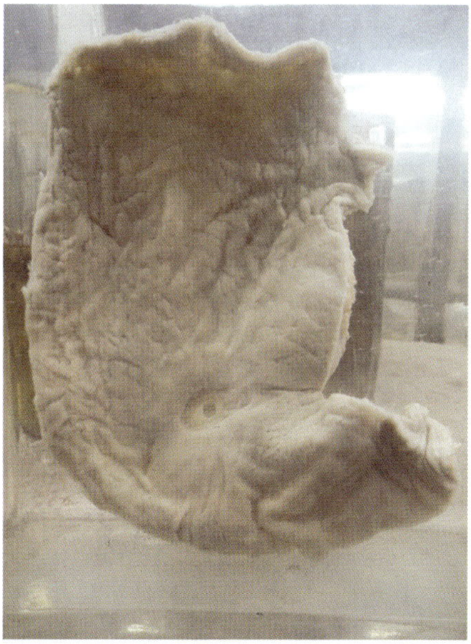

A. Describe the specimen. (1)
B. What is your clinical diagnosis of this museum specimen? (1)

Q37.

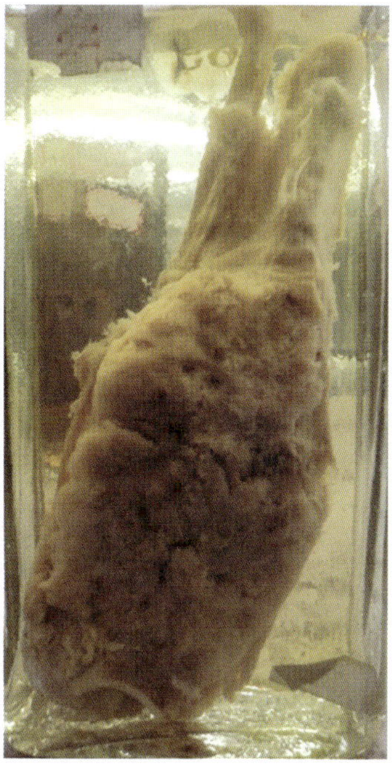

A. Describe the specimen. (1)
B. What is your clinical diagnosis of this museum specimen? (1)

Q38.

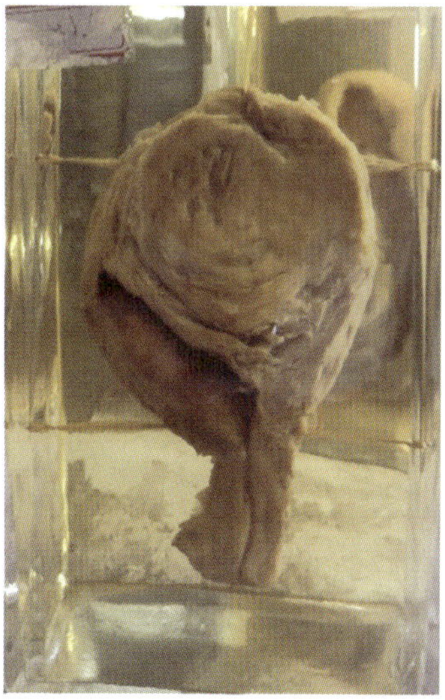

A. Describe the specimen. (1)
B. What is your clinical diagnosis of this museum specimen? (1)

Q39.

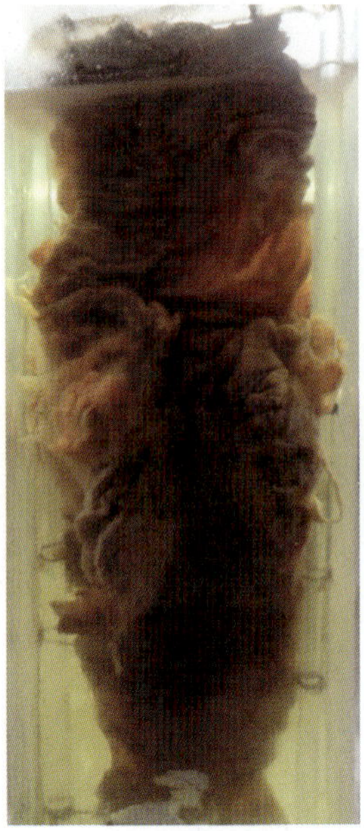

A. Describe the specimen. (1)
B. What is your clinical diagnosis of this museum specimen? (1)

Q40.

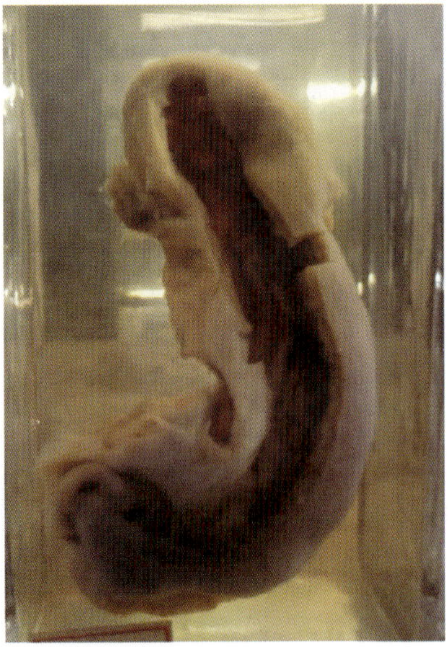

A. Describe the specimen. (1)
B. What is your clinical diagnosis of this museum specimen? (1)

Q41.

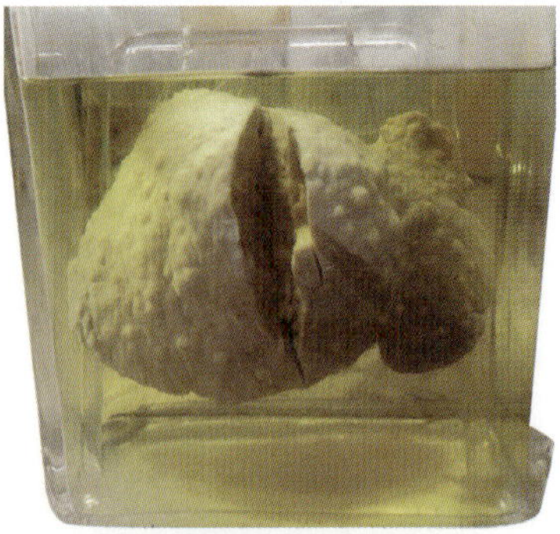

A. Describe the specimen. (1)
B. What is your clinical diagnosis of this museum specimen? (1)

Q42.

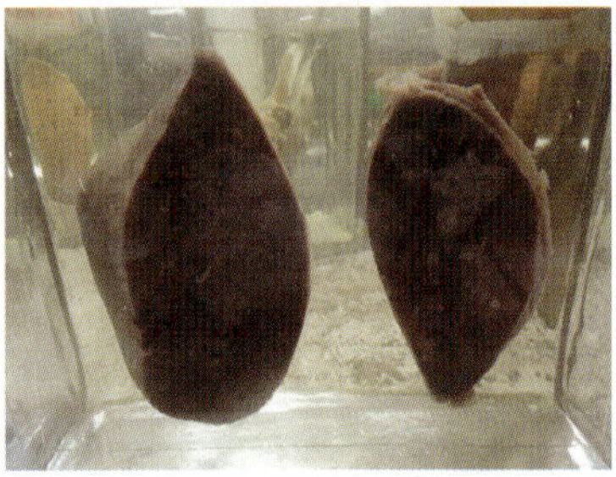

A. Describe the specimen. (1)
B. What is your clinical diagnosis of this museum specimen? (1)

Q43.

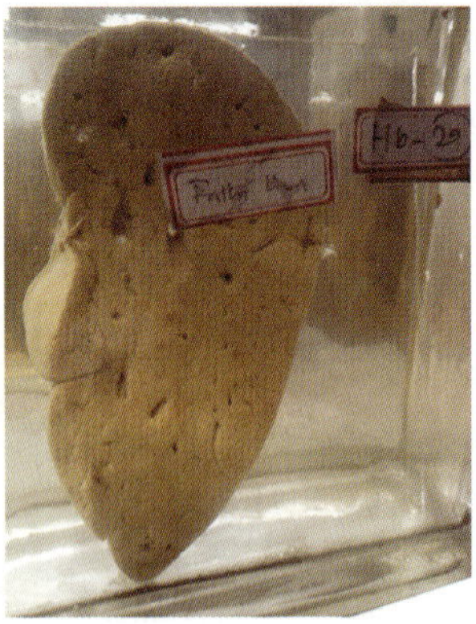

A. Describe the specimen. (1)
B. What is your clinical diagnosis of this museum specimen? (1)

Q44.

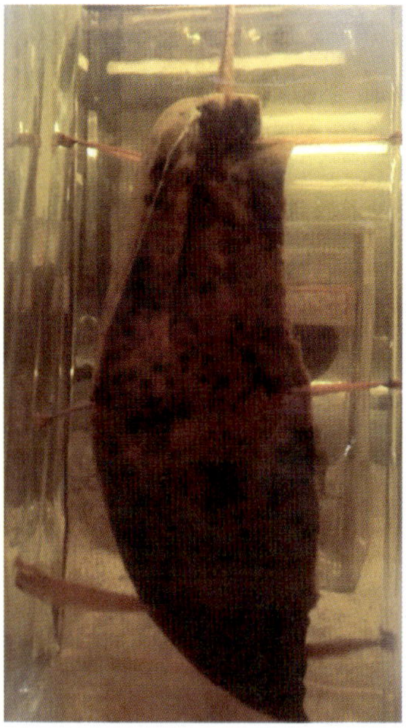

A. Describe the specimen. (1)
B. What is your clinical diagnosis of this museum specimen? (1)

Q45.

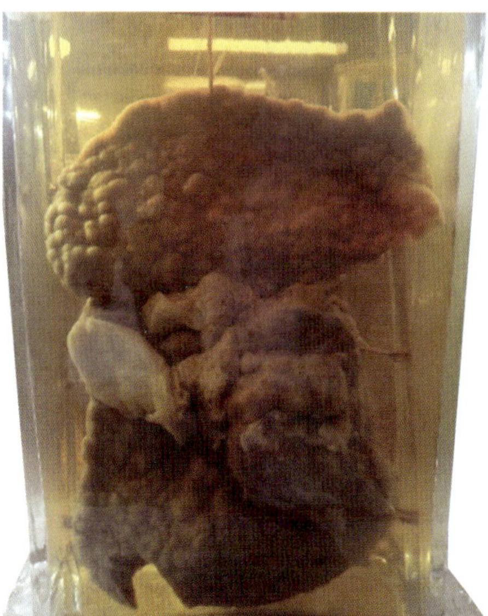

A. Describe the specimen. (1)
B. What is your clinical diagnosis of this museum specimen? (1)

Q46.

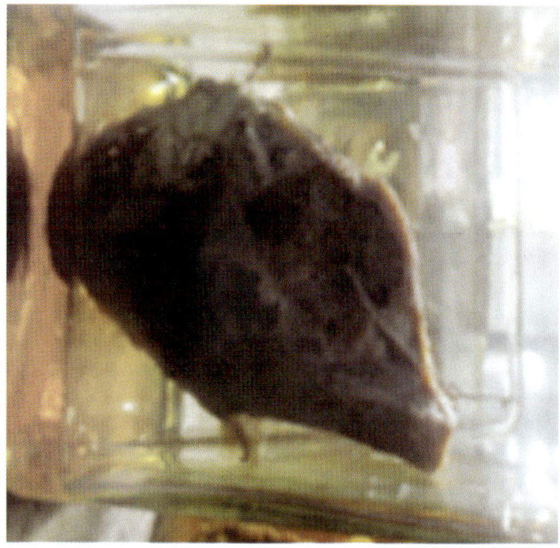

A. Describe the specimen. (1)
B. What is your clinical diagnosis of this museum specimen? (1)

Q47.

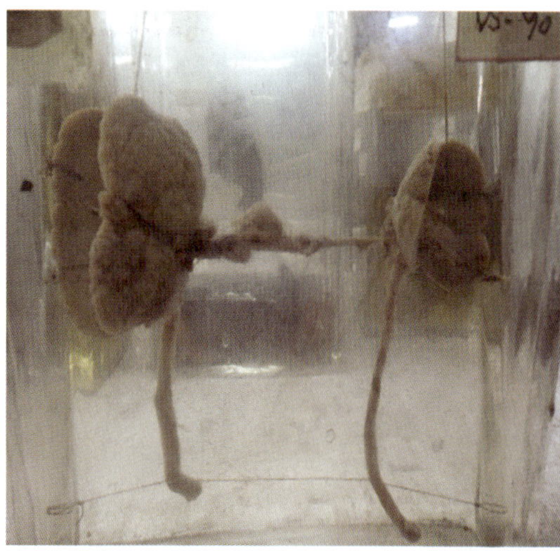

A. Describe the specimen. (1)
B. What is your clinical diagnosis of this museum specimen? (1)

Q48.

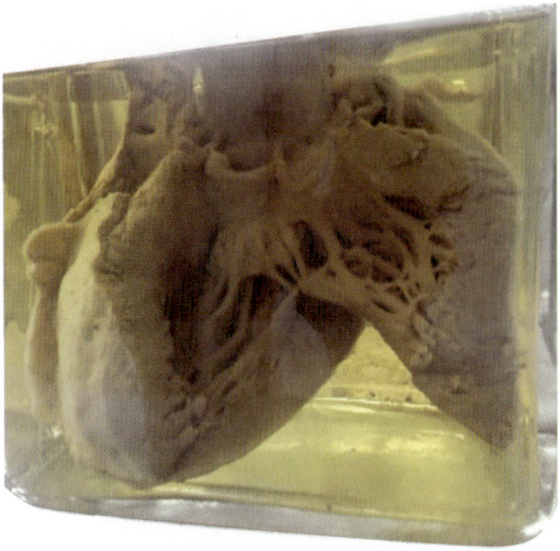

A. Describe the specimen. (1)
B. What is your clinical diagnosis of this museum specimen? (1)

Q49.

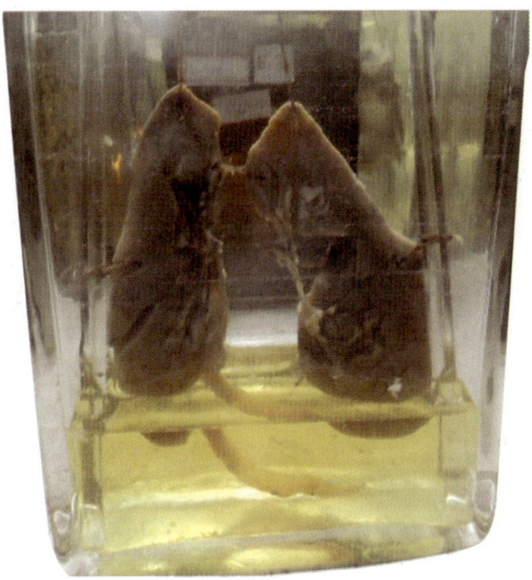

A. Describe the specimen. (1)
B. What is your clinical diagnosis of this museum specimen? (1)

Q50.

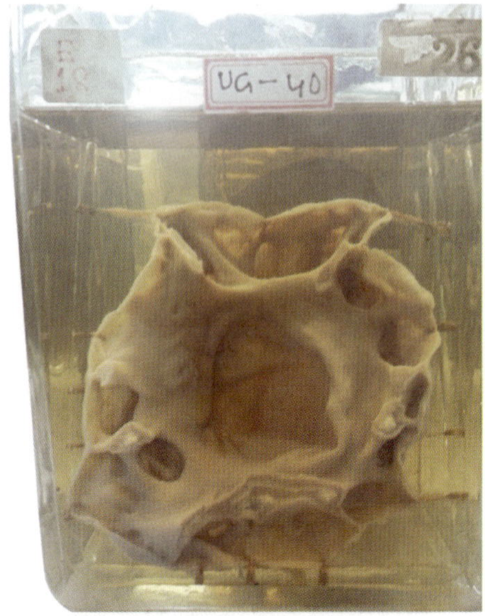

A. Describe the specimen. (1)
B. What is your clinical diagnosis of this museum specimen? (1)

Q51.

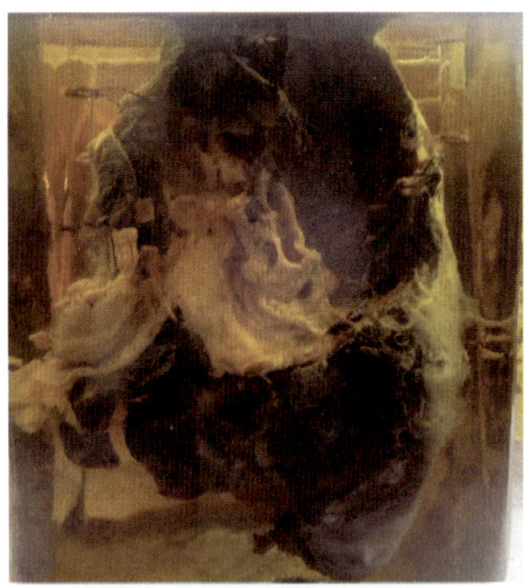

A. Describe the specimen. (1)
B. What is your clinical diagnosis of this museum specimen? (1)

Answers of Museum Specimens (OSPE)

Ans 1. A. Mounted specimen o uterus and cervix in a jar showing following features:
A gray-white exophytic solid mass in the cervix. The surface is irregular. The tumour involves the ectocervix, endocervix and reaches endometrial cavity. A small fibroid (leiomyoma is also seen in the myometrium.
B. Carcinoma of Cervix.

Ans 2. A. Mounted specimen of gallbladder in a jar showing following features:
Partially cut open specimen of gallbladder showing two large stones in the lumen. Gallbladder wall is thick and mucosa is reddened.
B. Chronic calculous cholecystitis.

Ans 3. (i) Endocarditis; (ii) Flea beaten kidney.

Ans 4. A. Mounted specimen of bisected lung in a jar showing following features:
Multiple black colored nodules involving the lung parenchyma.
B. Malignant melanoma of lung.

Ans 5. A. Mounted specimen of bisected lung in a jar showing following features:
Marked dilatation of bronchi and bronchioles with fibrosis of the adjoining areas. Dilated airways take various shapes, i.e. cylindrical, fusiform, and saccular. But it is predominantly cylindrical.
B. Bronchiectasis of lung.

Ans 6. A. Mounted specimen of part of lung tissue in a jar showing following features:
Many medium to large sized bullous lesion involving the lung parenchyma.
B. Emphysema of lung.

Ans 7. A. Mounted specimen of a portion of spine (vertebrae) in a jar showing following features: Destruction of part of vertebral body and intervertebral disc. The affected vertebrae are weak and tend to collapse, producing an acute anteflexion or angular kyphosis. Intervertebral space is diminished.
B. Tuberculosis (TB) of spine.

Ans 8. A. Mounted specimen of heart in a jar which is cut transversely showing following features: Ventricles, atrium and valves of the heart. Left ventricle is recognized by its thick wall compared to right ventricle. Mitral valve is seen in-between left ventricle and left atrium which has become thickened, puckered, fibrosed and deformed. Commisures are fused resulting in stenosis and having **'fish-mouth' appearance**.
B. Mitral stenosis.

Ans 9. A. Mounted bisected specimen of kidney in a jar showing following features:
Kidney is enlarged, pale and soft. Surface is smooth and capsule is intact. Renal parenchyma is edematous.
B. Large white kidney

Ans 10. A. Mounted specimen of a portion of stomach in a jar showing following features:
A large ulcero-proliferative mass/ growth with a large central ulcer (>3 cm diameter). The growth is situated in the body of stomach. Margin of the ulcer is heaped up, base of the ulcer is haemorrhagic and necrotic. Perforation in the ulcer is also noted.

B. Carcinoma of stomach (gastric carcinoma.

Ans 11. A. Mounted specimen of a portion of lung in a jar showing following features:

The lung is studded with numerous uniform small **millet-sized white spots (tubercles)** surrounded by intense congestion. These millet-sized white spots (tubercles) (1–3 mm in diameter) are seen both in subpleural location and in parenchyma.

B. Miliary tuberculosis of lung.

Ans 12. A. Mounted specimen of uterus with bilateral ovaries in a jar showing following features:

Body of uterus (without cervix) is normal sized. Both the ovaries are enlarged and bosselated. One ovary is cut and it shows yellowish-white solid mass.

B. Krukenkenberg tumour (bilateral metastatic deposits in ovaries).

Ans 13. A. Mounted specimen of a lobe of lung showing in a jar following features:

Diffuse inflammation affecting the entire lobe which looks gray. Cut surface shows gray, dry and granular appearance.

B. Lobar pneumonia (in gray hepatization stage).

Ans 14. A. Mounted specimen of kidney in a jar showing following features:

Multiple smooth walled dilated cysts are seen in the kidney. Both small and large cysts are seen resembling bunches of grapes.

B. Polycystic kidney.

Ans 15. A. Mounted specimen of already cut open ovarian cyst in a jar showing following features: External surface is smooth and ovary is enlarged. Already cut open ovary showing a multilocular cyst containing sebaceous, greasy pultaceous/cheesy material and tufts of hairs.

B. Dermoid cyst (Mature cystic teratoma.

Ans 16. A. Mounted specimen of part of small intestine in a jar showing following features:

Multiple small ulcers on the mucosa small intestine. Long axis of ulcers oriented parallel to the long axis of the intestine. Margins are regular and well circumscribed. Edges are of undermined. Ulcers are round to oval with foci of hemorrhage.

B. Typhoid ulcer of small intestine.

Ans 17. A. Mounted specimen of part of small intestine in a jar showing following features:

Multiple large ulcers on the mucosa of small intestine. Long axis of ulcers oriented transversely to the intestinal axis. Margins are irregular and may encircle the intestine (circumferential).

B. Tubercular ulcer of small intestine

Ans 18. A. Mounted specimen of lung in a jar showing following features:

Yellowish caseous necrosis of variable size. Foci of caseous necrosis accompanied by fibrosis. Some of the cavities have irregular, ragged yellowish-gray walls.

B. Fibrocaseous (cavitating) tuberculosis of lung.

Ans 19. A. Mounted specimen of bisected kidney in a jar showing following features:

A large well circumscribed rounded tumour is seen in the upper pole. The tumour has a variegated appearance due to areas of haemorrhage, necrosis and cystic spaces (solid-cystic). Cut surface of the tumour is yellowish-gray or golden yellow in colour.

B. Renal cell carcinoma (hypernephroma, Grawtiz's tumour).

Ans 20. A. Mounted specimen of cut open heart in a jar showing following features:

Thickness of left ventricular wall is increased (>1.5 cm, normal is 1.2–1.5 cm) and decreased in size of left ventricular wall. Papillary muscles and trabeculae carneae are prominent.

B. Left ventricular hypertrophy (LVH).

Ans 21. A. Mounted specimen of lung in a jar showing following features:

Fibrocaseous TB of lung. *See* Q18 for description.

Ans 22. A. Mounted specimen of spleen in a jar showing following features:

There is marked enlargement of spleen. The organ is firm, and the capsule is thickened and fibrosis.

B. Congestive splenomegaly.

Ans 23. A. Mounted specimen of liver in a jar showing following features:

The centrilobular regions are grossly red-brown and slightly depressed (because of cell death) and are accentuated against the surrounding zones of uncongested tan liver. So, there is alternative dark and light areas.The liver takes on a variegated mottled appearance reflecting hemorrhage and necrosis.

B. Nutmeg liver

Ans 24. A. Mounted specimen of liver in a jar showing following features:

A large cauliflower-like fungating mass having rolled out and everted margin. The mass arises from the inner surface of prepuce and glans penis. The surface of the mass is ulcerated. Resected margin of penis (opposite side of growth) is grossly unremarkable.

B. Carcinoma of penis.

Ans 25. A. Mounted specimen of humerus (lower end) in a jar showing following features:

A fusiform growth involving lower end of humerus (epiphysis). The growth is red-brown, friable mass with areas of cystic degeneration due to necrosis. Due to presence of small cystic spaces (degeneration), it has a honey-comb appearance.

B. Giant cell tumour of bone (osteoclastoma).

Ans 26. A. Mounted specimen of liver in a jar showing following features:

The liver is enlarged and soft in consistency. It is yellow in colour and greasy.

B. Fatty liver

Ans 27. A. Mounted specimen of bisected testis (orchidectomy) in a jar showing following features: Large gray-white variegated mass involving testis. Foci of hemorrahage and necrosis are noted. Spermatic cord is unremarkable.

B. Non-seminomatous germ cell tumour (NSGCT) of testis.

Ans 28. A. Mounted specimen of lung in a jar showing following features:

Multiple small to intermediate sized nodules involving the lung parenchyma. Some of them are projecting through surface.

B. Metastatic deposits (metastatic carcinoma in lung).

Ans 29. A. Mounted specimen of kidney in a jar showing following features:

Small, pinpoint petechial hemorrhages are seen on cortical surface due to rupture of arterioles or glomerular capillaries. The kidney looks pale otherwise.

B. Flea-beaten kidney (due to malignant hypertension).

Ans 30. A. Mounted specimen of large vessel (abdominal aorta in a jar showing following features: Elevated white to yellowish fibrous or fibrofatty patches or plaques (0.3–1.5 cm long) are seen close /surrounding to the opening of ostia of branch vessels. Intimal surface is identified by many small holes which are actually ostia of branch vessels.

B. Atheroma of abdominal aorta

Ans 31. A. Mounted specimen of cut open heart in a jar showing following features:

There is deposition of fibrin over the pericardium. Fibrin deposited in-between two layers of pericardium (visceral and parietal) exhibits bread and butter appearance. The surface is dry, with a fine granular roughening.

B. Fibrinous pericarditis.

Ans 32. A. Mounted specimen of liver in a jar showing following features:

Liver is shrunken and colour is yellowish-orange. Many small (<3 mm in diameter) and large (> 3 mm in diameter) nodules are seen all over the liver surface. Consistency of the liver is firm. Gallbladder is seen in the gallbladder fossa.

B. Cirrhosis of liver (mixed micro- and macronodular type).

Ans 33. A. Mounted specimen of upper end of femur in a jar showing following features:

A fusiform growth involving lower end of humerus (epiphysis). The growth is red-brown, friable mass with areas of cystic degeneration due to necrosis. Due to presence of small cystic spaces (degeneration), it has a honey-comb appearance.

B. Giant cell tumour of bone (osteoclastoma.

Ans 34. A. Mounted specimen of upper end of tibia in a jar showing following features:

Tubular tibial bone with fragile bone and a large hole (cloaca). Dry, irregular piece of dead bone with granular surface **(sequestrum)** is seen through cloaca. Also seen sheath of living reactive oven or lamellar bone deposited around sequestrum. This is **involucrum**.

B. Osteomyelitis with involucrum

Ans 35. A. Mounted specimen of abdominal aorta in a jar showing following features:

Elevated white to yellowish fibrous or fibrofatty patches or plaques (0.3–1.5 cm long) are seen close/ surrounding to the opening of ostia of branch vessels. Intimal surface is identified by many small holes which are actually ostia of branch vessels.

B. Atheroma (atherosclerosis) of abdominal aorta

Ans 36. A. Mounted specimen of stomach in a jar showing following features:

A single deep ulcer is present in the body of stomach which is round in shape. The gastric rugal folds are essentially normal, and the margins and base of the ulcers are not indurated. Perforation is noted in the central area of the ulcer.

B. Gastric ulcer with perforation.

Ans 37. A. Mounted specimen of tibia and fibula (long bone) in a jar showing following features:

A bulky gray-white solid mass involving the lower end of tibia. The tumour looks fleshy with irregular fusiform shape and located at the end of long bone (tibia and gives the lesion so called **'leg of mutton' appearance**. Areas of hemorrhage and necrosis are found.

B. Osteosarcoma

Ans 38. A. Mounted specimen of uterus and cervix in a jar showing following features:

Hemisection of uterus and cervix showing one large globular mass in the myometrium(intramural). This growth is well-circumscribed, whitish, glistening and encircled by fibrous capsule. This growth has a typical whorled or so-called **"watered silk"** appearance.

B. Fibroid (leiomyoma. of uterus.

Ans 39. A. Mounted specimen of part of large intestine (cut open) in a jar showing following features: An ulceroproliferative, exophytic polypoid mass in the colon. The mass is cauliflower like, soft and friable projecting in the lumen. Crater like ulcerations with raised margins are noted.

B. Carcinoma of colon.

Ans 40. A. Mounted specimen of part of large intestine (cut open) in a jar showing following features: The stomach is shrunken and wall is very thick. A diffuse infiltrative gastric adenocarcinoma makes markedly thickened gastric wall. Extensive mucosal ulceration is noted.

B. Linitis plastica or leather bottle stomach (Brinton's disease).

Ans 41. A. Mounted specimen of liver (partially cut open) in a jar showing following features:

Liver is shrunken and colour is yellowish-orange. Many small (<3 mm in diameter) and large (>3 mm in diameter) nodules are seen all over the liver surface. Consistency of the liver is firm. Gallbladder is seen in the gallbladder fossa.

B. Cirrhosis of liver (mixed micro- and macronodular type).

Ans 42. A. Mounted specimen of liver (cut open) in a jar showing following features: Liver is enlarged and cut surface contain pale, waxy areas corresponding to the abundant amorphous, lightly eosinophilic amyloid deposits.

B. Amyloidosis of Liver.

Ans 43. Mounted specimen of liver (partially cut open) in a jar showing following features:

A. Liver is yellow, tan fatty, greasy and enlarged. It is soft in consistency.

B. Fatty liver (Hepatic Steatosis).

Ans 44. Mounted specimen of liver (partially cut open) in a jar showing following features:

A. The liver takes on a variegated mottled appearance, reflecting hemorrhage and necrosis in the centrilobular region.

B. Nutmeg liver.

Ans 45. Mounted specimen of liver in a jar showing following features:

A. The liver is diffusely nodular and firm. The nodules are of different sizes and both micronodules (<3 mm in diameter) and macronodules (>3 mm in diameter) are present. Gallbladder is also present under the liver.

B. Mixed or micro-macronodular cirrhosis.

Ans 46. Mounted specimen of liver (partially cut open) in a jar showing following features:

A. Multiples mass involving the liver. These masses are of different sizes (2–5 cm in diameter).

B. Metastatic deposits in liver (multicentric hepatocellular carcinoma is also a possibility. But multicentric HCC is uncommon than metastatic deposits. Final diagnosis to be confirmed by history, biopsy/histopathological examination and other investigations.

Ans 47. Mounted specimen of kidney (bisected and cut open) in a jar showing following features:

A. Both kidneys are symmetrically contracted. Surface is finely granular. Consistency seems to be firm.

B. Granular contracted kidney (due to chronic glomerulonephritis).

Ans 48. Mounted specimen of heart (partially cut open) in a jar showing following features:

A. Thickness of left ventricular wall is increased (>1.5 cm, normal is 1.2–1.5 cm) and decreased in size of left ventricular chamber. Papillary muscles and trabeculae carneae are prominent.

B. Left ventricular hypertrophy (LVH).

Ans 49. Mounted specimen of kidney (bisected and cut open) in a jar showing following features:

A. Kidney is enlarged, pale and soft. Surface is smooth and capsule is thin.

B. Large white kidney.

Ans 50. Mounted specimen of kidney (cut open) in a jar showing following features:

A. Kidney is enlarged and multiple cystic cavities are noted. Many of these cystic spaces contain white stones.

B. Hydronephrosis.

Ans 51. Mounted specimen of lung (cut open) in a jar showing following features:

A. Yellowish caseous necrosis area of variable size. Foci of caseous necrosis accompanied by fibrosis. Cavities are also noted having irregular, ragged yellowish-gray walls.

B. Fibro-caseous tuberculosis of lung.

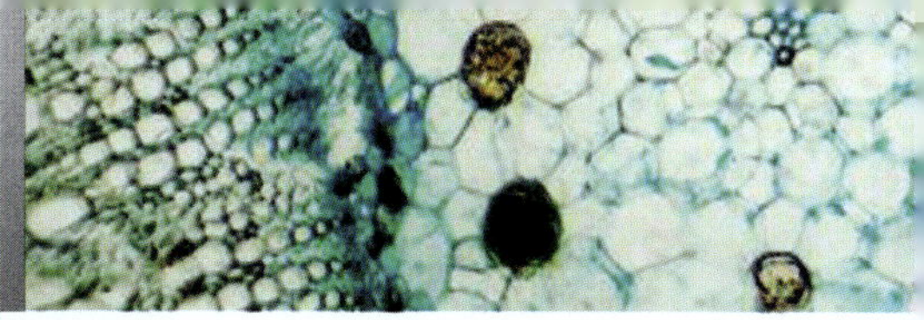

Section

VII

Schematic Diagrams (HP Slides) and Definitions of General Pathology

Chapter

22

Schematic Diagram (Hand Drawn) of Histopathology (HP) Slides

COAGULATIVE NECROSIS

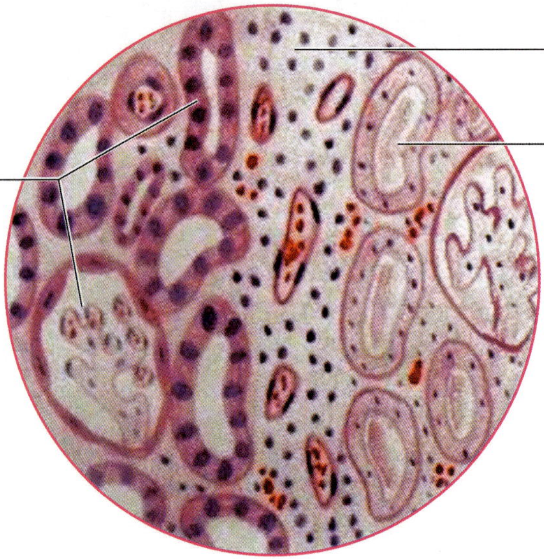

Gross

Area of necrosis is a pale segment of tissue and is dry on cut surface.

Microscopic Examination

i. The hallmark of coagulative necrosis is that architectural outlines of cells and structures are identified but without intact nuclei and cytoplasmic details.
ii. The margin of infarct shows inflammatory reaction, initially by polymorphonuclear cells (acute) but later macrophages, lymphocytes and fibrous tissue predominate (chronic).

CASEOUS NECROSIS

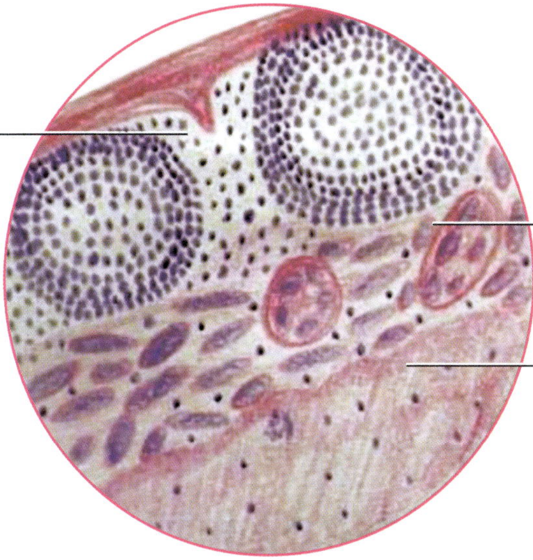

Gross

The lymph nodes are matted together. The cut surface shows characteristic map like areas of yellowish, granular, soft necrotic material resembling dry cheese elsewhere is grey brown.

Microscopic Examination

i. The caseous areas are composed of structureless, eosinophilic, and granular debris which may contain foci of dystrophic calcification.
ii. The periphery of caseous foci shows granulomatous inflammation consisting of slipper-shaped epithelioid cells with interspersed giant cells of Langhan's type and peripheral mantle/collar of lymphocytes.

FATTY LIVER

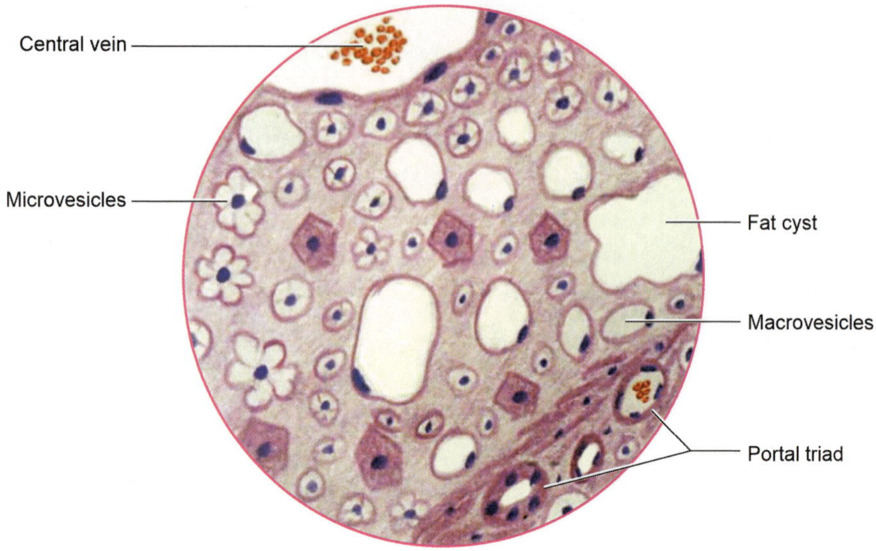

Gross

The liver is enlarged and yellow with tense, glistening capsule and rounded margins. The cut surface bulges slightly and is pale-yellow and greasy to touch.

Microscopic Examination

i. The liver is enlarged and yellow with tense, glistening capsule and rounded margins. The cut surface bulges slightly and is pale-yellow and greasy to touch.
ii. Fat in the cytoplasm of the hepatocytes is seen as clear area which may vary from minute droplets in the cytoplasm of a few hepatocytes (microvesicular) to distention of the entire cytoplasm of most cells by coalesced droplets (macrovesicular) pushing the nucleus to periphery of the cell.
iii. When the steatosis is mild, centrilobular hepatocytes are mainly affected, while the progressive accumulation of fat involves the entire lobule.
iv. Occasionally, the adjacent cells containing fat rupture producing fatty cysts.
v. Infrequently, lipogranulomas may appear consisting of collection of macrophages, lymphocytes and multinucleate giant cells.
vi. Special stains such as Sudan III, Sudan IV, Sudan black and oil red O can't be employed to demonstrate fat in the paraffin embedded tissue.

KIDNEY AMYLOIDOSIS

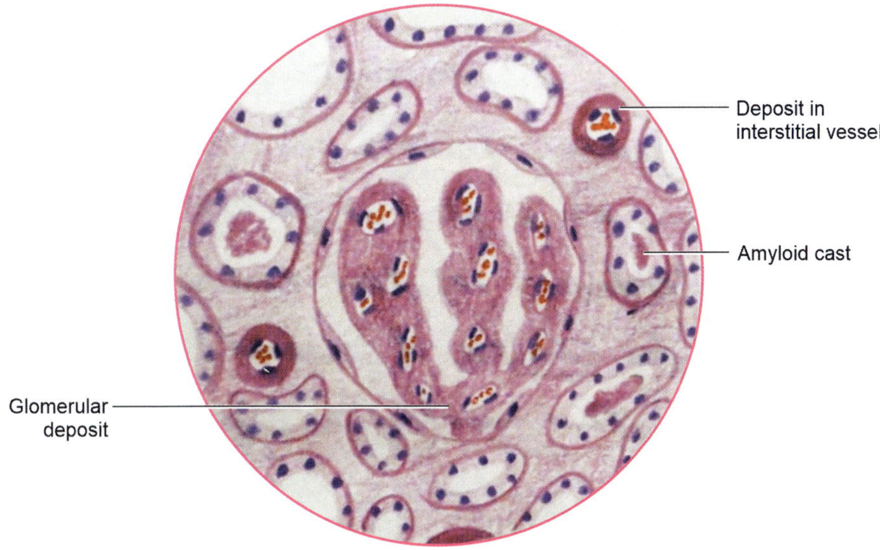

Gross

The kidneys may appear normal, enlarged or terminally contracted due to ischaemic effect of narrowing of vascular lumina. The cut surface is pale, waxy and translucent.

Microscopic Examination

i. The amyloid is seen as amorphous, eosinophilic, hyaline extracellular material. It is deposited mainly in the glomeruli, initially on the glomerular basement membrane but later extends to produce luminal narrowing and distortion of the glomerular capillary tuft.

ii. The amyloid deposits in the tubules begin close to the tubular epithelial basement membrane. Subsequently, the deposits may produce degenerative changes in the tubular epithelial and amyloid casts tubular lumina.

iii. The walls of small arteries and arterioles in the interstitium of the kidney are narrowed due to amyloid deposit.

iv. Congo red staining imparts pink or red color to the amyloid when seen in ordinary light but demonstrates green birefringence when viewed under polarizing microscopy.

LIPOMA

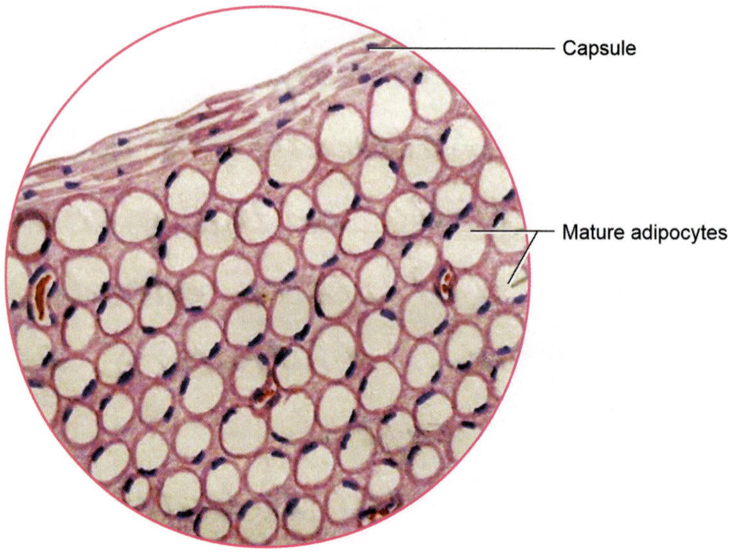

Gross

The tumor is small, encapsulated, round to oval.

The cut surface is soft, lobulated, yellowish and greasy.

Microscopic Examination

i. A thin fibrous capsule surrounds the periphery.
ii. The tumor is composed of lobules of mature adipose cells separated by thin fibrous septa.

ACUTE APPENDICITIS

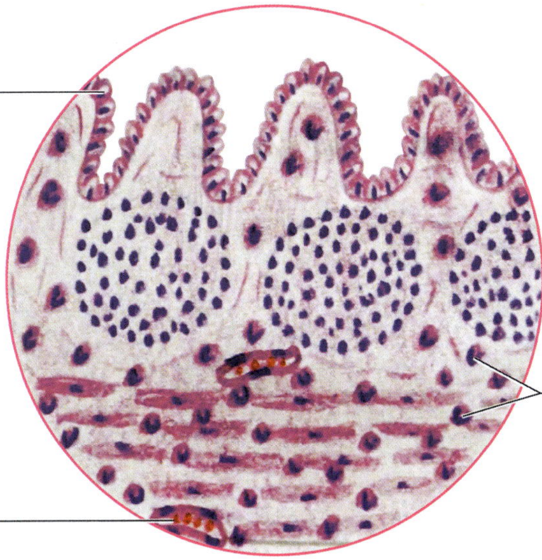

Gross

The appendix is swollen and serosa is hyperaemic and coated with fibrinopurulent exudate. The mucosa is ulcerated and sloughed.

Microscopic Examination

i. Most important diagnostic feature is neutrophilic infiltration of the muscularis.
ii. Mucosa is sloughed and blood vessels in the wall are thrombosed.
iii. Peri-appendiceal inflammation is seen in advanced cases.

CVC LUNG

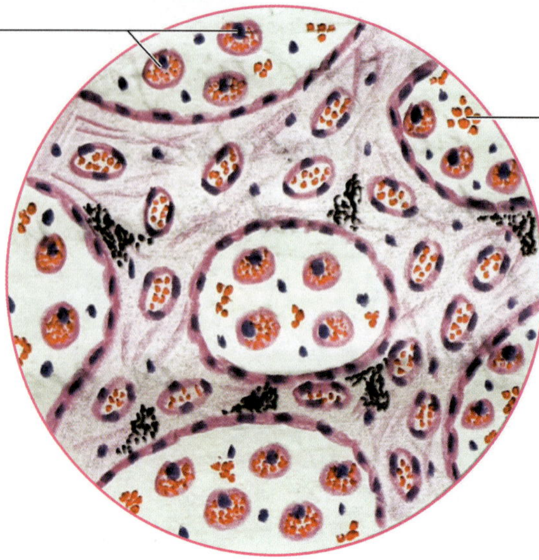

Gross

Both lungs are dark brown in color, heavy and firm. Cut surface shows brown coloration referred to as brown induration.

Microscopic Examination

i. Vessels in the alveolar septa are dilated and congested.
ii. Rupture of dilated and congested capillaries may result in minute intra-alveolar haemorrage.
iii. The characteristics finding is the presence of large number of alveolar macrophages filled with yellow brown hemosiderin pigment so called heart failure cells in the alveoli.

CVC LIVER

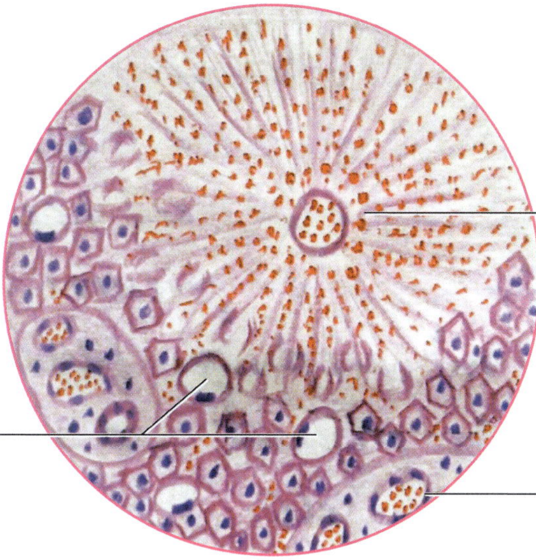

Gross

The liver is enlarged. The cut surface shows characteristic alternate dark areas representing congested centre of each lobule and light areas being the fatty peripheral part so called nutmeg liver.

Microscopic Examination

i. The central vein and the sinusoids in the centrilobular region and are distanced and dilated with blood.
ii. The hepatocyte in the centrilobular region undergo degeneration and atrophy, probably as a result of anoxia.
iii. Eventually, the centrilobular zone shows central haemorrhagic necrosis.
iv. The peripheral hepatocytes are either normal or may show fatty change.

CVC SPLEEN

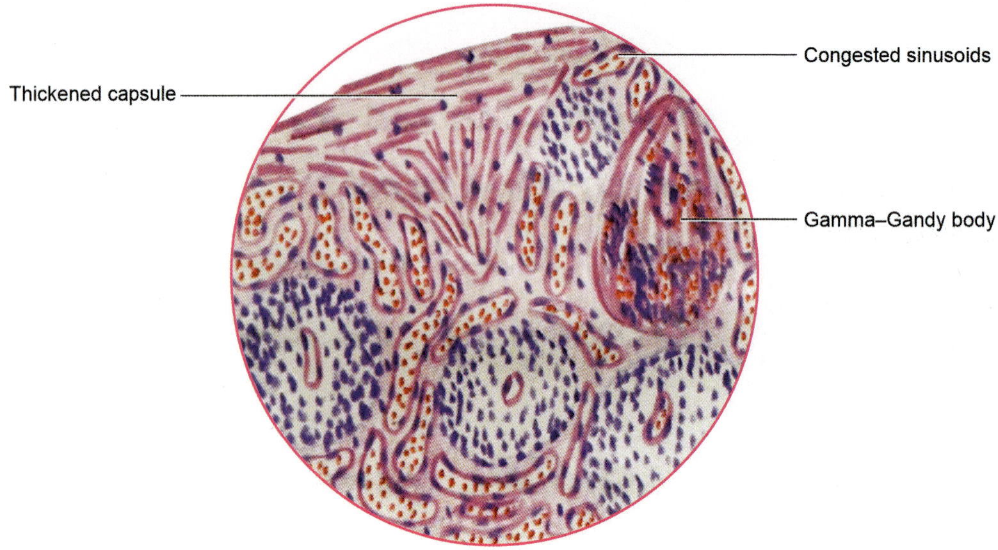

Gross

The spleen becomes enlarged, firm and tense. The weight of the organ is increased to (250 g and more). The capsule may get thickened and fibrous. The cut surface shows fibrosis and is nasty in appearance with indistinct Malpighian corpuscles.

Microscopic Examination

i. The red pulp shows marked congestion and dilation of sinusoids with area of recent and old haemorrage.
ii. The haemorrhages may get organised and show diffuse fibrosis together with iron pigments and calcium deposits so called siderotic nodules or Gamma–Gandy bodies.
iii. In the late stages, there is hyperplasia of pigment laden macrophages and thickening of fibrous tissue framework of the organ, termed fibrocongestive splenomegaly.

CHRONIC CHOLECYSTITIS WITH CHOLELITHIASIS

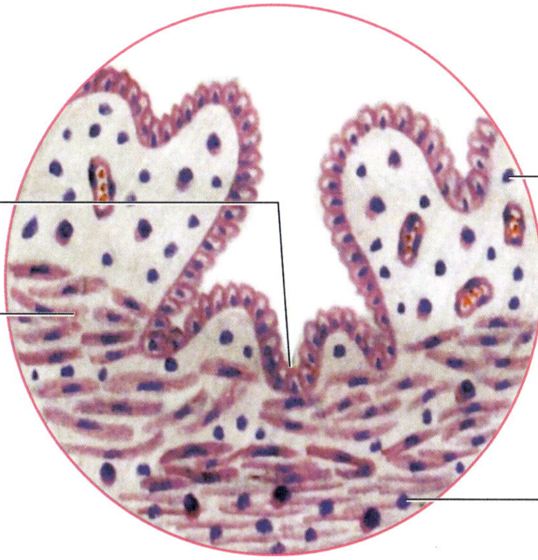

Gross

The gallbladder is generally contracted and the wall is thickened. Cut section of wall of gallbladder is grey-white due to dense fibrosis. The mucosal folds may be thickened, atrophied or flattened. The lumen commonly contains gallstones, most often multiple multifaceted mixed type; others are pure gallstones (cholesterol, pigment and calcium containing) and combined type gallstones.

Microscopic Examination

i. Penetration of mucosa deep into the wall of the gallbladder up to the muscularis layer to form Rokitansky–Aschoff sinuses.
ii. Variable degree of chronic inflammatory cells (lymphocytes, plasma cells and macrophages) in the lamina propria and subserosal layer.
iii. Variable degree of fibrosis and thickening of perimuscular layer.

OSTEOSARCOMA

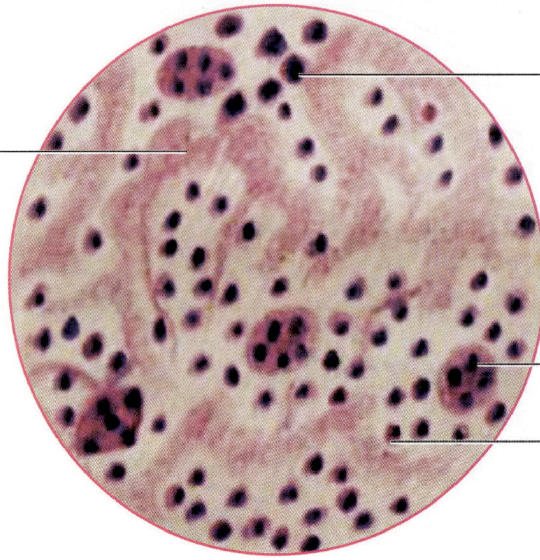

Gross

The tumour appears as a grey-white, bulky mass at the metaphyseal end of a long bone of the extremity, generally sparing the articular end of the bone. Codman's triangle formed by the angle between lifting of periosteum and underlying surface of the cortex may be grossly identified. Cut surface of the tumour is grey-white with areas of haemorrhages and necrotic bone.

Microscopic Examination

i. **Sarcoma cells:** The tumour cells are anaplastic mesenchymal stromal cells which show marked pleomorphism and polymorphism. variation in size as well as shape. The tumour cells may be spindled, round, oval, polygonal or bizarre tumour giant cells. They show hyperchromatism and atypical mitoses.
ii. **Osteogenesis:** The anaplastic sarcoma cells form osteoid matrix and bone directly, which lies interspersed in the areas of tumour cells.

OSTEOCLASTOMA

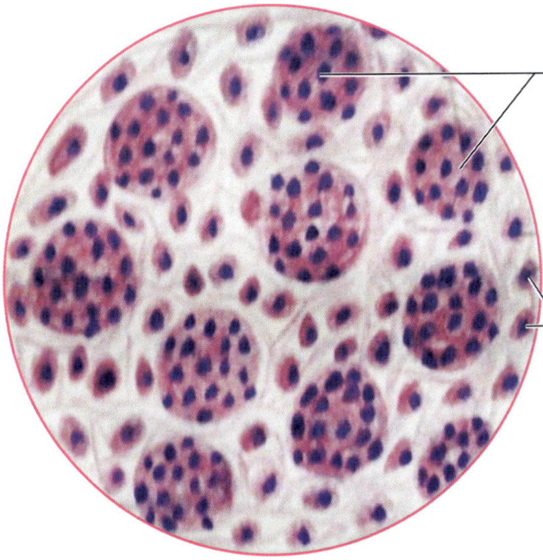

Gross

Giant cell tumuor is eccentrically located in the epiphyseal end of a long bones, which is expanded. The tumour is well-circumscribed, dark-tan and covered by thin shell of subperiosteal bone. Cut surface of the tumour is characteristically haemorrhagic necrotic and heavy-combed.

Microscopic Examination

i. Large number of osteoclast-like giant cells which are regularly scattered throughout the stroma.
ii. Giant cells may contain as many as 100 benign nuclei and are similar to normal osteoclasts.
iii. Stromal cells are mononuclear cells and are the tumour cells and determine the behaviour of the tumour. They are uniform, plump, spindle-shaped or round to oval but may have varying degree of atypia and mitosis.

SQUAMOUS CELL CARCINOMA

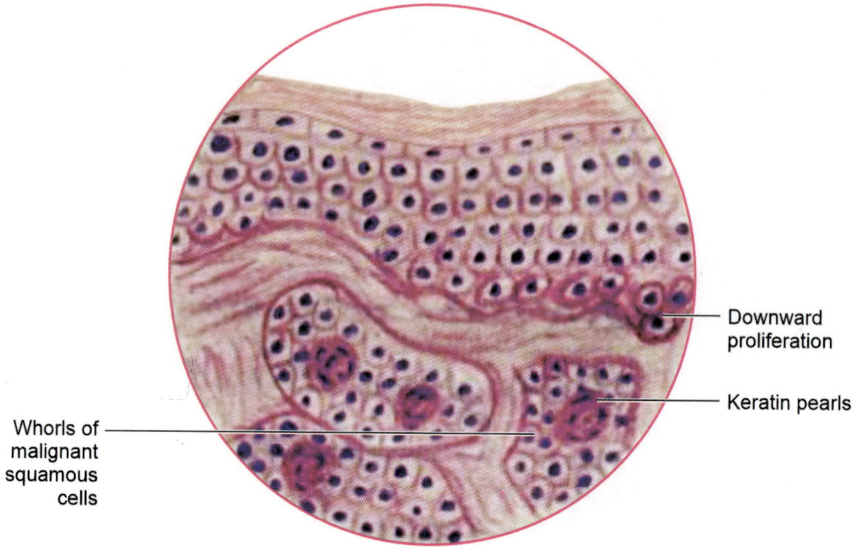

Gross

The tumour is either in the form of nodular and ulcerative growth, or fungating and polypoid mass with without ulceration. The margin of the growth is elevation and induration. Cut section of the growth shows grey white, endophytic, tumour as well as exophytic tumour.

Microscopic Examination

i. There is downward as well as outward proliferation of squamous epithelium with increased number of layers which shows loss of orderly maturation.
ii. The mass of tumour cell invades through the basement membrane into subepithelium on dermis.
iii. In better differentiated tumours, the tumour cells are arranged in concentric layer or whorls and contain concentric layer of keratin material in the centre of the cell whorls.

MALIGNANT MELANOMA

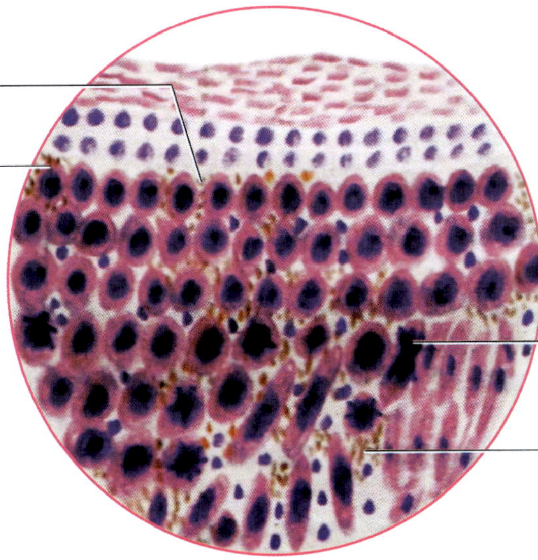

Gross

Malignant melanoma may appear as flat, macular or slightly elevated, nodular lesion. The lesion exhibits variation in pigmentation appearing in shades of black, brown, grey, blue or red. The borders are irregular.

Microscopic Examination

i. The tumour has marked junctional activity at the epidermo-dermal junction and grows horizontally as well as downwards into the dermis.

ii. The invading tumour cells are arranged in a variety of patterns-solid masses, sheets, islands, nests, etc.

iii. The individual tumour cell is usually larger than the nervous cells, contain large vesicular nuclei with peripherally condensed chromatin and having prominent eosinophilic nucleoli. The cytoplasm is amphophilic.

iv. Melanin pigment is present in the cytoplasm in the form of uniform fine granules (unlike coarse pigment granules at the periphery of the lesion in benign nerves).

BASAL CELL CARCINOMA

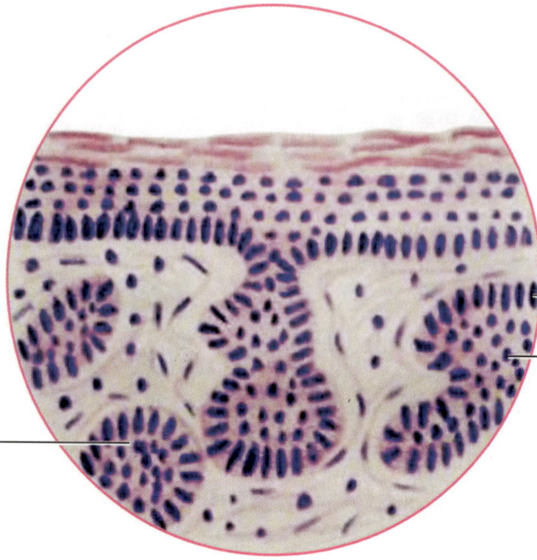

Gross

The tumour is commonly a nodular growth with central ulceration(nodulo-ulcerative). The margins of the tumours are pearly white and rolled while the base shows ulceration. The tumour burrows into the underlying tissues like a rodent and destroys them.

Microscopic Examination

i. The tumour cells resemble normal basal cell layer of the skin and grow downwards from the epidermis in a variety of patterns-solid masses, nests, islands, strands, keratotic masses, adenoid, etc.
ii. All patterns of tumour cells have one common characteristic feature-the cells forming the periphery of tumour have parallel alignment or show palisading (basaloid cells).
iii. The tumour cells are basophilic with hyperchromatic nuclei.
iv. Stroma shrinks away from epithelial tumour nests, creating clefts which help in differentiating it from the adrenal tumours.

FIBROADENOMA

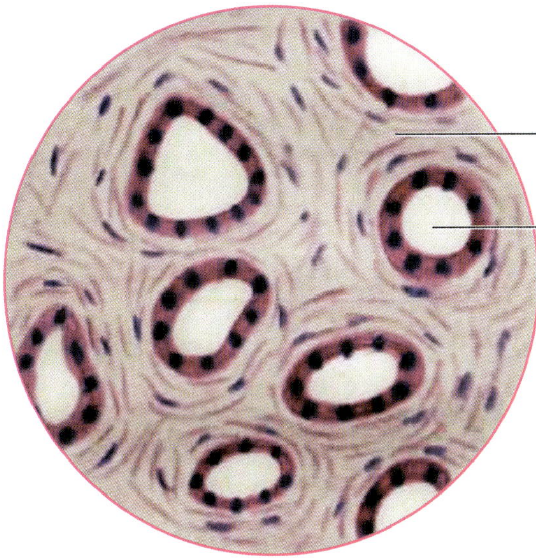

Gross

Typically, fibroadenoma is a small (2–4 cm diameter), solitary, well-encapsulated, spherical or discoid mass. The cut surface is firm, grey-white, slightly myxoid and may show slit-like spaces.

Microscopic Examination

The arrangement between fibrous overgrowth and ducts may produce 2 types of patterns: Intracanalicular and pericanalicular.

i. Intracanalicular pattern is one in which the stroma compresses the ducts so that they are reduced to slit-like clefts lined by ductal epithelium and may appear as cords of epithelial elements surrounding masses of fibrous tissue.
ii. Pericanalicular pattern is characterised by encircling masses of fibrous tissue around the patent or dilated ducts.

INFILTRATING DUCT CARCINOMA (NOS) (BREAST CANCER)

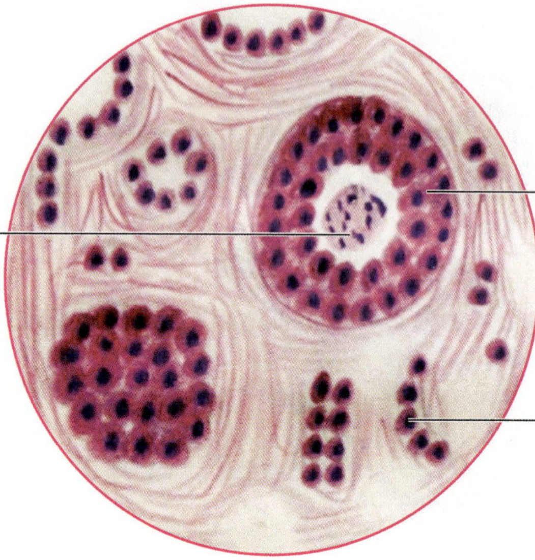

Gross

The tumour is irregular, 1–5 cm in diameter, hard, cartilage-like mass that cuts with a grating sound. Sectioned surface of the tumour is grey-white to yellowish with chalky streaks and often extends irregularly into the surrounding fat.

Microscopic Examination

i. Anaplastic tumour cells form various patterns-solid nests, cords, poorly-formed glandular structures and some intraductal foci.
ii. Infiltration by these patterns of tumour cells into diffuse fibrous stroma and fat.
iii. Invasion by the tumour cells into peri-vascular and perineural space, besides lymphatics and vascular emboli.

PLEOMORPHIC ADENOMA

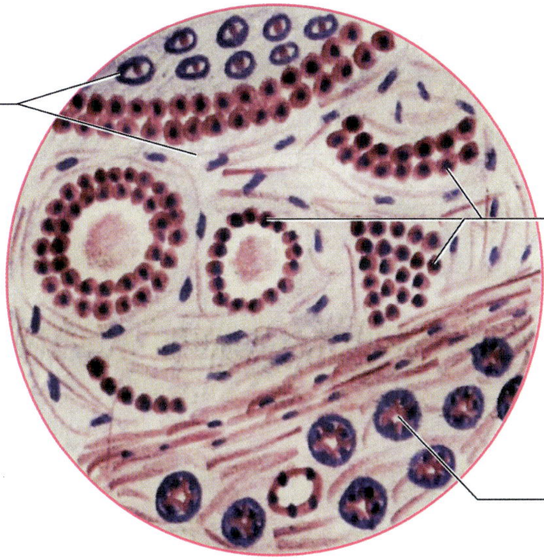

Gross

The tumour is circumscribed, pseudo-encapsulated, rounded and multilobulated, firm mass, 2–5 cm in diameter. The cut surface is grey-white and bluish, variegated, with soft to mucoid consistency.

Microscopic Examination

i. The pleomorphic adenoma has two components:
ii. Epithelial and mesenchymal.
iii. Epithelial component consists of various patterns like ducts, acini, tubules, sheets and strands of monomorphic cells of ductal or myoepithelial origin. These ductal cells are cuboidal or columnar while myoepithelial cells are polygonal or spindle-shaped.
iv. Mesenchymal component present in loose connective tissue includes myxoid, nucleoid and chondroid matrix which stimulates cartilage (pseudocartilage).

ADENOCARCINOMA STOMACH

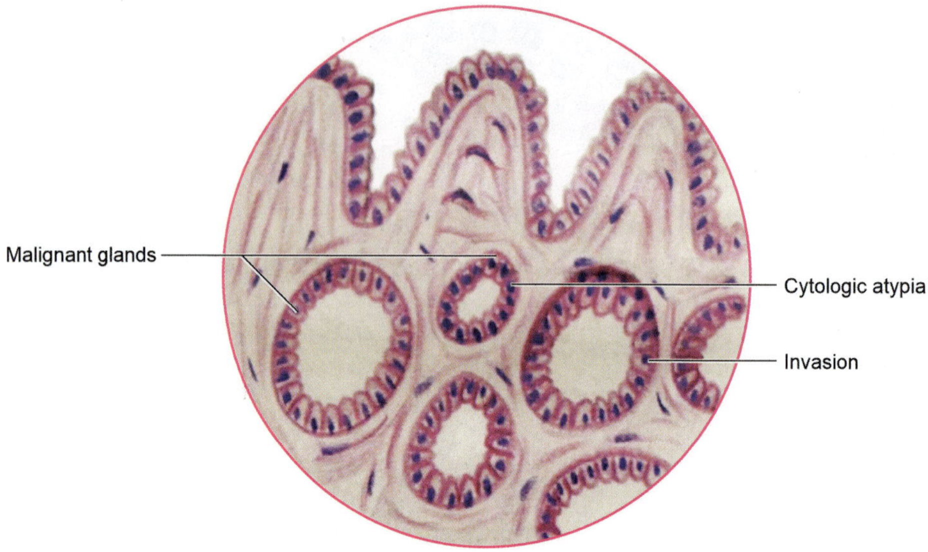

Gross

Most common pattern is flat, infiltrating and ulcerative growth with irregular necrotic base and raised margin. Other gross patterns include fungating (polypoid), scirrhous (linitis plastica), colloid (mucoid) and ulcer cancer.

Microscopic Examination

i. Tubular and acinar pattern of growth is seen infiltrating the stomach wall.
ii. The tumour inside the walls of stomach for variable depth.
iii. The tumour cells show varying degree of anaplasia but is more often poorly-differentiated with high degree of anaplasia.

LEIOMYOMA

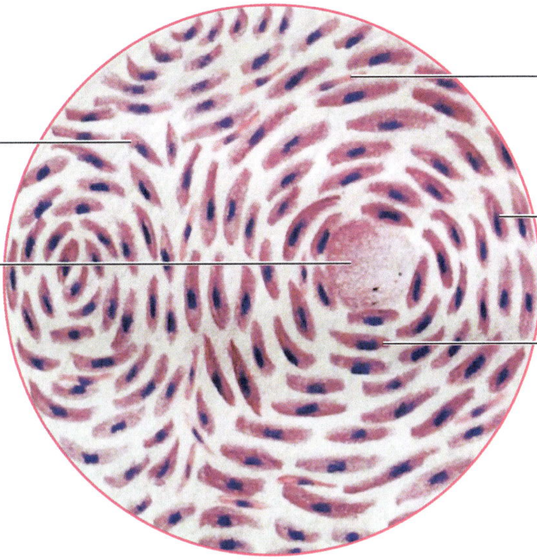

Gross

Uterine leiomyomas, depending upon location, maybe subserosal, intramural or submucosal, leiomyoma is a circumscribed, firm to hard tumour. Cut surface presents a whorled appearance. Hyaline change in leiomyoma is common and appears glassy and homogenous.

Microscopic Examination

i. There is a mixture of smooth muscle muscle fibers and fibrous tissue in varying proportions. Some of the muscle fibres may be cut longitudinally and some transversely.
ii. Smooth muscle fibres admired with fibrous tissue are arranged in a whorled pattern at many places.
iii. The cytoplasm of smooth muscle fibres is pinker and their nuclei are short, plump and fusiform while the cytoplasm of fibroblasts is light pink in colour and nuclei are longer, slender and have painted ends.
iv. Areas of hyaline change appear as pink, homogenous and acellular lying in the centre of the whorls or between them.

SQUAMOUS CELL PAPILLOMA

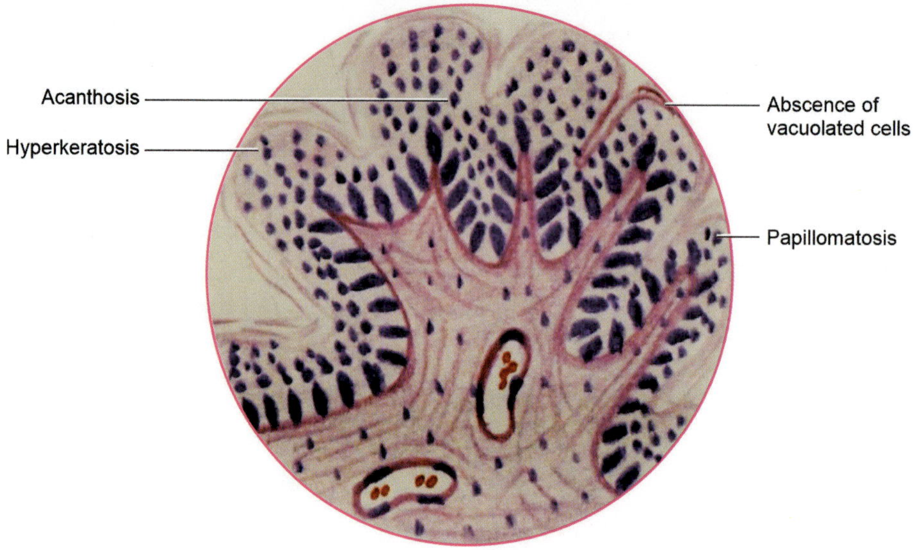

Gross

Surface of the tumour shows finger-like process.

Microscopic Examination

i. The epidermis is thickened but orderly and is thrown into finger-like process or papillae.
ii. The central core of the papillae is composed of loose fibrovascular tissue.

NODULAR HYPERPLASIA PROSTATE (BPH)

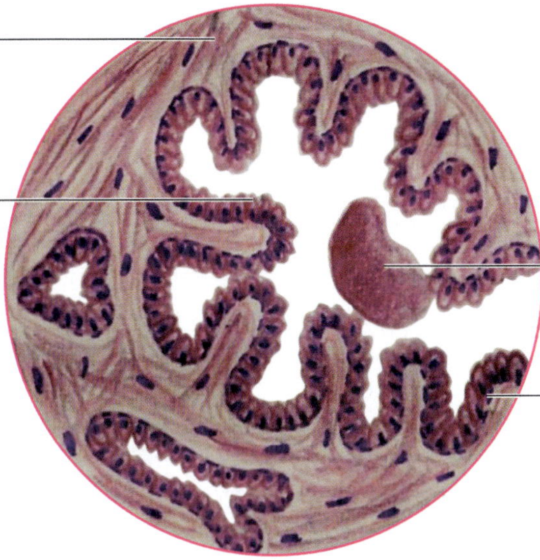

Gross

The enlarged prostate is nodular, smooth and firm and weighs 2–4 times its normal weight (normal average weight 20 g). The appearance on cut section shows nodularity having varying admixture of yellowish-pink, soft, honey-combed appearance (glandular hyperplasia) and firm homogenous appearance (fibromuscular hyperplasia).

Microscopic Examination

i. There is hyperplasia of all three tissue elements in varying proportions-glandular, fibrous and muscular.
ii. Glandular hyperplasia predominates in most cases and is characterised by exaggerated intra-acinar papillary in folding with delicate fibrovascular cores. Glands are lined by two layers of epithelium.
iii. Fibromuscular hyperplasia appears as aggregates of spindle cells giving and appearance similar to fibromyoma of the uterus.

LOBAR PNEUMONIA (RED HEPATISATION STATE)

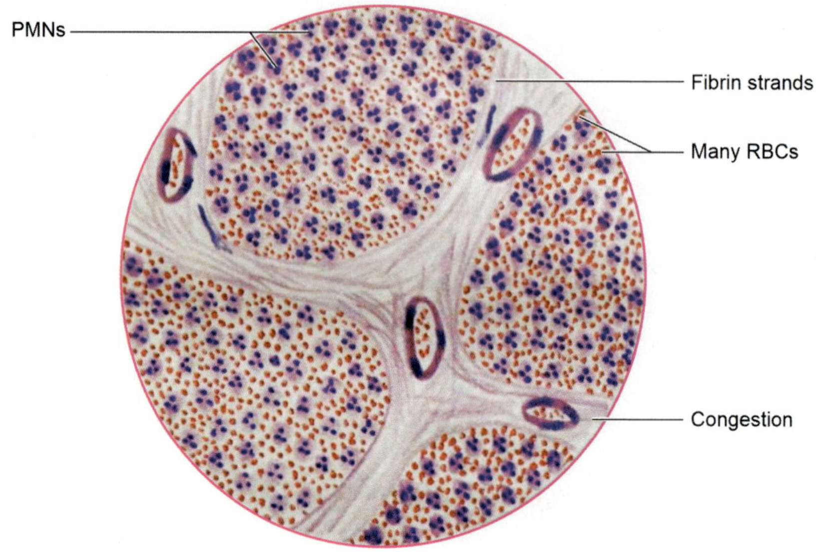

Gross

The affected lobe is red, firm and consolidated. Cut surface of the involved lobe is airless, red-pink, dry, granular and has liver-like consistency.

Microscopic Examination

i. Air space contain strands of fibrin.
ii. There is marked cellular exudate of neutrophils and extravasation of red cells.
iii. Neutrophils may show ingested bacteria.

TERATOMA

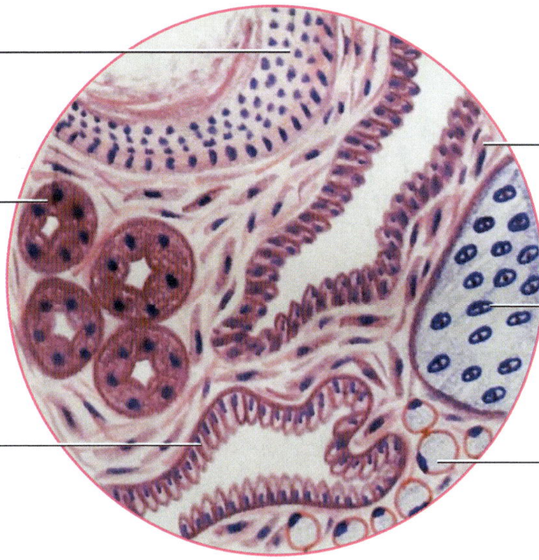

Gross

Benign cystic teratoma is characteristically a unilocular cyst, 10–15 cm in diameter. On sectioning the cyst is filled with paste-like sebaceous secretions and desquamated Keratin admired with masses of hair. The cyst wall is thin and opaque grey-white. Quite often, the cyst wall shows a solid a solid prominence where tissue elements such as tooth, bone, cartilage and other tissues are present.

Microscopic Examination

i. Viewing a benign cystic teratoma in different microscopic fields reveals a variety of mature differentiated tissues, producing kaleidoscope appearance.

ii. Ectodermal derivatives are most prominent. The lining of the cyst wall is by stratified squamous epithelium and its adrenal structures such as sebaceous glands, sweat glands and hair follicles.

iii. Tissues of mesodermal and endodermal origin are commonly present and include bronchus, intestinal epithelium, cartilage, bone, smooth muscle, neural tissue, salivary gland, retina, pancreas and thyroid tissue.

THROMBUS ARTERY

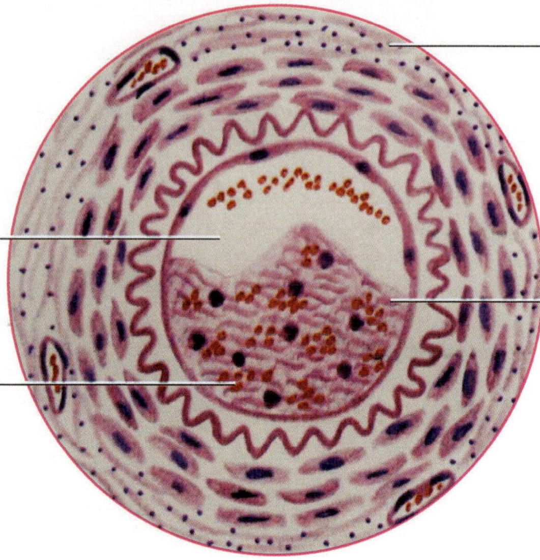

Gross

Coronary artery thrombi are generally:

- mural and occlusive
- overlies an atherosclerotic lesion
- grey-white and friable
- cut surface shows laminations called lines of Zahn.

Microscopic Examination

i. The internal elastic lamina is degenerated and disrupted at the site of attachment of thrombus to the vessel wall.

ii. The residual lumen of the original artery is slit-like and shows flowing blood.

iii. The structure of thrombus shows lines of Zahn composed of layers of light-staining fibrin strands and platelets enriched in dark-staining red cells.

iv. Organised thrombus shows ingrowth of granulation tissue at the base having spindle cells and capillary channels.

MONCKEBERG'S ARTERIOSCLEROSIS

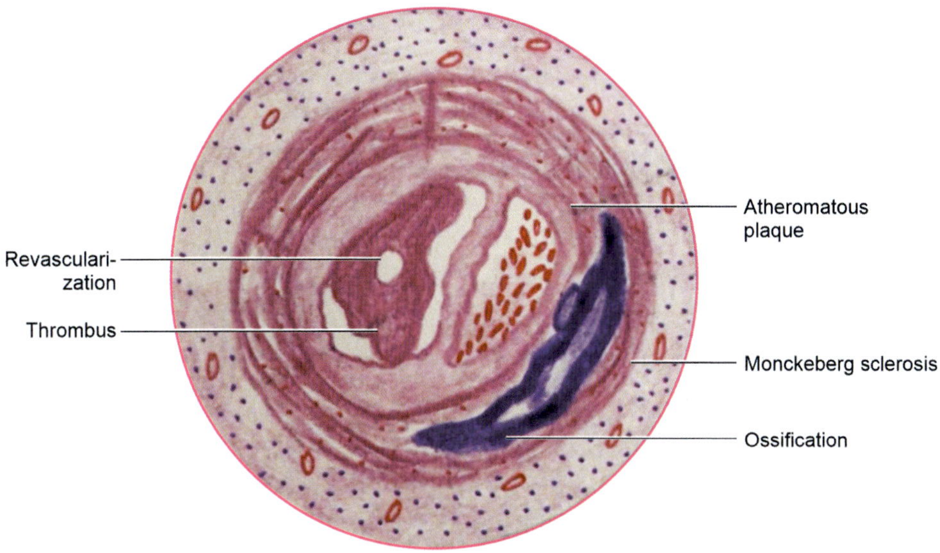

Gross

Medial dystrophic calcification produces pipestem like rigidity of affected artery(large and medium-sized muscular arteries, especially of extremities and of the genital tract in the elderly) without significant luminal narrowing.

Coexistent changes of atherosclerosis may be present.

Microscopic Examination

i. Smooth muscle of media is replaced by a cellular hyaline fibrous tissue.
ii. Foci of dystrophic calcification are seen in the media as basophilic coarse granules.
iii. Inflammation is conspicuously absent.

SQUAMOUS METAPLASIA CERVIX

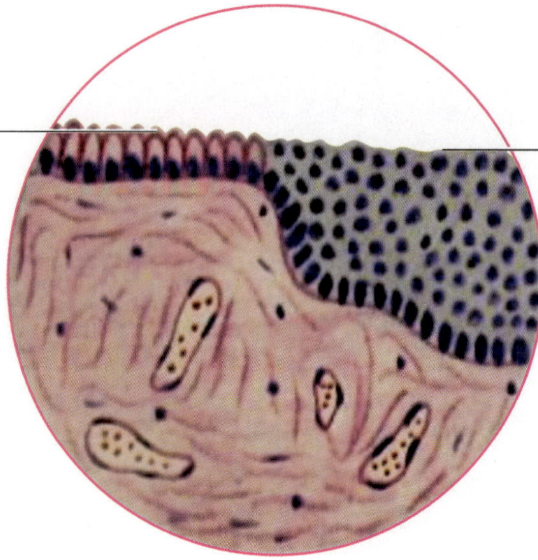

Gross

Cervix is pearly white and isthmus is elongated. Commonly encountered in prolapsed uterus.

Microscopic Examination

i. Columnar lined mucosa as well as cervical glands show foci of squamous cell change.
ii. Surface of the cervix may show keratinization and hyperkeratosis.
iii. There is generally some degree of subepithelial chronic inflammatory cell infiltrate.

ENDOMETRIAL HYPERPLASIA

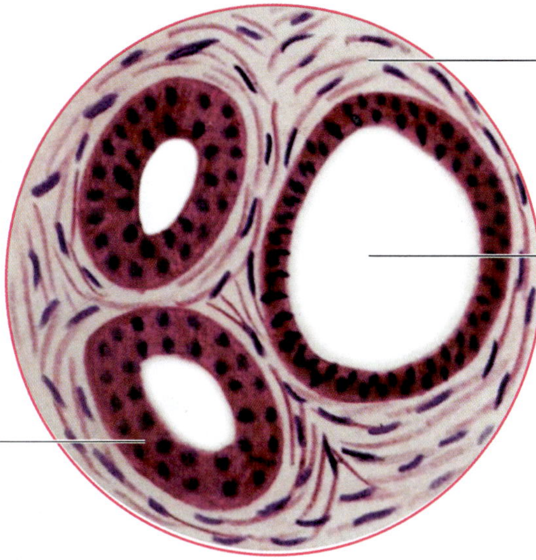

Gross

Florid to pseudopolypoid endometrium (thickened protruded endometrium line secretary phase).

Microscopic Examination

i. Presence of varying-sized glands, many of which are large and cystically dilated and are lined by atrophic epithelium.
ii. The stroma is sparsely cellular and edematous.

ULCER WITH GRANULATION TISSUE

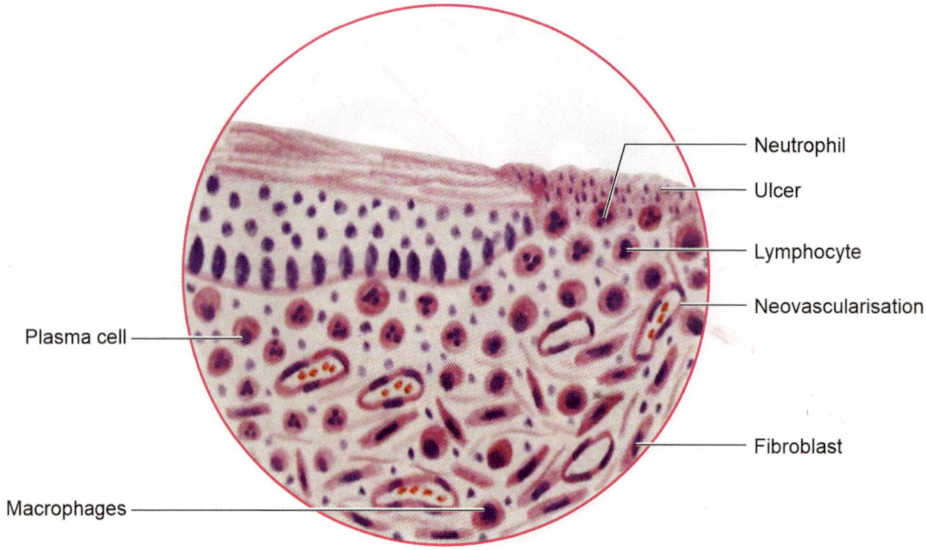

Gross

During the migratory phase of wound healing, granulation tissue is =>

- light red or dark pink in colour (neovascularization)
- soft to tough; pulsatile on palpation.
- moist; bumpy (granular) in appearance due to punctate haemorrhages.

Microscopic Examination

i. Composed of tissue matrix having =>
ii. Fibroblasts, i.e. keratinocytes
iii. Macrophages, i.e. endothelial cells.
iv. Neutrophils

Vascularisation is also seen (new thin-walled capillaries). Inflammatory cell infiltration of extracellular matrix.

PSAMMOMATUS MENINGIOMA

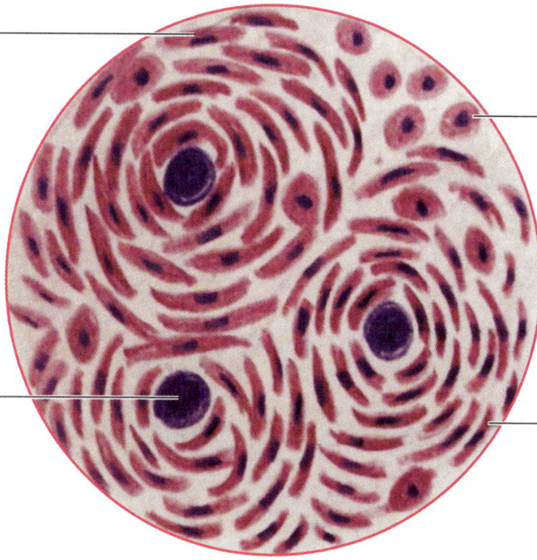

Gross

Meningioma is well circumscribed, solid, spherical or hemispherical mass of variable size (1–10 cm in diameter). The tumour is generally firmly attached to the dura while the overlying bone may show hyperotosis. Cut surface of the tumour is firm and fibrous, sometimes with foci of calcification.

Microscopic Examination

i. There is conspicuous whorled pattern of tumour cells, often around central capillary-sized blood vessels.
ii. Many of the whorls may show psammoma bodies.
iii. There is combination of cells with syncytial and fibroblastic features.

METASTATIC CARCINOMA OF LYMPH NODE

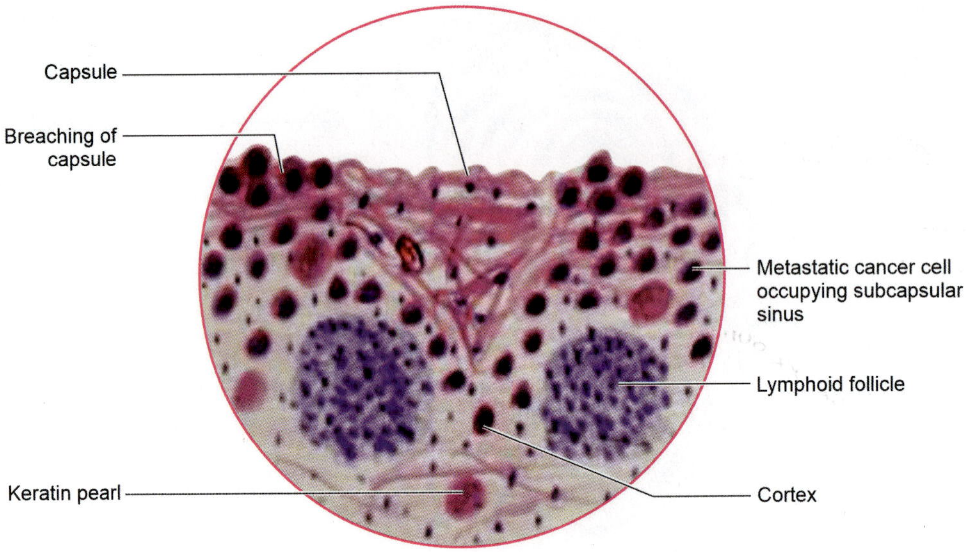

Gross

The affected lymph nodes are enlarged and matted. Cut surface shows homogenous, grey-white deposits with areas of necrosis.

Microscopic Examination

i. The tumour is seen as solid nests, cords and poorly-formed glandular structures.
ii. The tumour cells show varying degrees of anaplasia and mitotic activity.
iii. Part of cortex and capsule of the lymph node are intact.

REACTIVE HYPERPLASIA LYMPH NODE

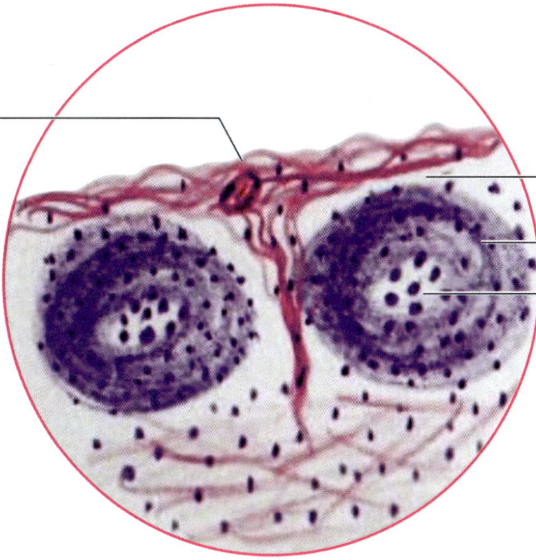

Gross

The affected lymph nodes are enlarged, firm and non-tender.

Microscopic Examination

i. Follicular hyperplasia: Most common and is characterised by enlargement and prominence of germinal centres of lymphoid follicles.
ii. Paracortical lymphoid hyperplasia and enlargement of paracortex so that lymphoid follicles are effaced.
iii. Sinus histiocytosis: Distension and engorgement of the sinusiods of the lymph node with chistiocyctosis and endothelial cells.

Chapter

23

Definitions and Other Important Aspects of General Pathology in Viva

- **Pathology** is the study (logos) of disease (pathos). More specifically, it is devoted to the study of structural, biochemical and functional changes in cells, and organs that underlie disease.
- **Hypertrophy** refers to an increase in the size of cells, resulting in an increase in the size of the organ.
- **Hyperplasia** is an increase in the number of cells in an organ or tissue, usually resulting in increased mass of the organ or tissue.
- **Atrophy** is reduced size of an organ or tissue resulting from a decrease in cell size and number.
- **Metaplasia** is a reversible change in which one differentiated cell type (epithelial or mesenchymal) is replaced by another cell type.
- **Necrosis** is always a pathologic process of cellular death which results from denaturation of intracellular proteins and enzymatic digestion of the lethally injured cell. Necrotic cells are unable to maintain membrane integrity and their contents often leak out, a process that may elicit inflammation in the surrounding tissue.
- **Apoptosis** is a pathway of cell death that is induced by a tightly regulated suicide program in which cells destined to die by activating enzymes that degrade the cells' own nuclear DNA and nuclear and cytoplasmic proteins. Apoptotic cells break up into fragments, called apoptotic bodies, which contain portions of the cytoplasm and nucleus.
- **Steatosis (fatty change):** The terms steatosis and fatty change describe abnormal accumulations of triglycerides with parenchymal cells.
- **Hyaline:** The term hyaline usually refers to an alteration within cells or in the extracellular space that gives a homogeneous, glassy, pink appearance in routine histologic sections.
- **Lipofusin:** It is an insoluble pigment, also known as lipochrome or wear-and-tear pigment. It is composed of polymers of lipids and phospholipids in complex with protein. Suggesting that it is derived through lipid peroxidation of polyunsaturated lipids of subcellular membranes.
- **Melanin:** It derives from the Greek (*melas*, black), is an endogeneous, non-hemoglobin-derived, brown-black pigment formed when the enzyme tyrosinase catalyzes the oxidation of tyrosine to dihdroxyphenylalanine in melanocytes. It is the only endogenous brown-black pigment.
- **Dystrophic calcification** occurs in dead tissues at sites of necrosis and serum

calcium level is normal. It often causes organ dysfunction.

- **Metastatic calcification** may be seen in living tissue also and serum calcium level is high. It usually does not cause clinical dysfunction. It is found in organs which loose acid and have alkaline environment inside them, like lungs (most commonly), kidney, stomach, systemic artery, pulmonary veins, etc. [Remember, calcification begins in mitochondria of all organs except kidney which begins in basement membrane].
- **Telomerase** is a specialized RNA-protein complex that uses its own RNA as a template for adding nucleotides to the ends of chromosomes.
- **Housekeeping functions of different intracellular organelles:**
  a. *Mitochondria*: Synthesize ATP through oxidative phosphorylation and synthesize metabolic intermediates needed for anabolic metabolism , apoptosis
  b. *Golgi apparatus*: Assembles proteins physically
  c. *Smooth endoplasmic reticulum*: Hormone and lipoprotein synthesis, modification of hydrophobic compounds into water-soluble molecules.
  d. *Rough endoplasmic reticulum*: Synthesize new proteins for the plasma membrane.
  e. *Lysosomes*: Digestion of proteins, polysaccharides, lipids, nucleic acids.
  f. *Peroxisomes*: Breakdown of fatty acids, generating hydrogen peroxide
  g. *Proteosomes*: Selectively chews up denatured proteins, releasing peptides
  h. *Endosomal vesicles*: Shuttle internalized material to appropriate intracellular sites.
  i. *Cytosol*: Metabolism, transport, protein translation.
  j. *Nucleus*: Cell regulation, proliferation, DNA transcription.
- **Intermediate filaments:** These are 10-nm diameter fibrils which impart tensile strength to tolerate mechanical stress. Examples are:
  i. *Lamin A, B, and C*: Nuclear lamina of all cells
  ii. *Desmin*: Muscle cells, forming the scaffold on which actin and myosin contract
  iii. *Vimentin*: Mesenchymal cells (fibroblasts, endothelium)
  iv. *Neurofilaments*: Axon of neurons, imparting strength and rigidity
  v. *Glial fibrillary acidic protein*: Glial cells around neurons
  vi. *Cytokeratins*: Acidic (type I) and neutral/basic (type II); 30 different types are present in different cells: used as cell marker.
- **Pro-apoptotic genes:** Bax, Bad, Bak, Bim, Puma, Noxa, P53.
- **Anti-apoptotic genes:** Bcl-2, Bcl-XL< Mcl-1; also FLPI<IAP, and Bcl-x.

Parameter	Necrosis	Apoptosis
Self-induced	No. Always pathological	Yes. Both physiological and pathological
Nature	Passive	Active (requires energy)
Cell size	Increased	Decreased
Inflammatory reaction	Present	Absent
Plasma membrane	Disrupted	Intact
Cell involvement	Affects contiguous (adjacent) group cells	Affect large cell
Electrophoresis	Smear pattern	Step ladder pattern

- **Necroptosis:** It resembles necrosis morphologically and apoptosis mechanistically as a form of programmed cell death. It is triggered by ligation of TNFR1, and viral proteins of RNA and DNA viruses. Necroptosis is casapase-independent but dependent on signalling by the RIP1 and RIP3 complex. The release of cellular contents evokes an inflammatory reaction as in necrosis.

- **Pyroptosis:** It occurs in cells infected by microbes. It involves activation of caspase-1, which cleaves the precursor form of IL-1 to generate biologically active IL-1. Here inflammasome is formed and NLRP3 (Nod-like receptor 3) activate caspase-1. Caspase-1 along with closely related caspase-11 also lead to death of the infected cell.
- **Antioxidants:** They act by inhibiting the generation of free radicals or scavenging the already present free radicals. They are of two types:
  a. Enzymatic: Superoxide dismutase, catalase, glutathione peroxidase
  b. *Non-enzymatic*: Vitamin E, A, and C; Sulfhydryl containing compounds like cysteine and glutathione; serum proteins like albumin, ceruloplasmin and transferrin.
- **Commonly used stains:**
  a. *Glycogen*: PAS stain with diastase, Carmine (best)
  b. *Lipid*: Oil red 'O', Sudan Black
  c. *Amyloid*: Congo red, thioflavin T and S
  d. *Calcium*: von Kossa, alzarine red
  e. *Hemosiderin and Ferric iron*: Perls' Prussian blue stain
  f. *Trichrome stain*: It stains different components with three colors, hence the name Trichrome.
     1. Black: cell nuclei, 2. Red: muscle, cell cytoplasm, 3. Blue: collagen, mucus
- **Criteria for Systemic Inflammatory Response Syndrome (SIRS):** 2 or more of the following conditions must be present:
  i. Fever (oral temperature >38°C) or Hypothermia (<36°C)
  ii. Tachypnea (>24 breaths/minute)
  iii. Tachycardia (>90 beats/minute)
  iv. Leukocytosis (>12,000/µl), Leukopenia (<4000/µl) or >10% bands.

Feature	Arterial thrombus	Venous thrombus
Pathogenesis	Endothelial injury or site of tuberculosis	Stasis of blood
Blood Flow	Associated with active blood flow	Associated with sluggish blood flow
Sites	Coronary, cerebral, and femoral arteries	Superficial and deep leg veins, ovarian veins
Propagation	Retrograde manner from point of attachment	Antegrade manner (towards heart)
Gross	Lines of Zahn present	Lines of Zahn absent
Microscopic	White thrombi (pale platelet layer alternating with dark RBC layer)	Red thrombi (red cells mixed with relatively less platelets)
Occlusion	Incomplete lumen occlusion	Complete vessel occlusion
Complications	Ischemic and Infarction of organs	Embolism, edema, and ulceration

INFLAMMATION

- **Cardinal signs of inflammation:** Four cardinal signs of inflammation are (i) Rubor (redness), (ii) Tumor, (iii) Calor (heat), (iv) Dolor (pain), and (v) Functio laesa (loss of function). The fifth sign was added by Rudolf Virchow.
- **Acute inflammation:** It is a rapid host response that serves to deliver leukocytes and plasma proteins, such as antibodies, to sites of infection or tissue injury. Acute inflammation has three major components: (i) alterations in vascular calibre that lead to an increase in blood flow, (ii) structural changes in the microvasculture that permit plasma proteins and leukocytes to leave the circulation, and (iii) emigration of the leukocytes from the microcirculation, their accumulation in the focus of injury, and their activation to eliminate the offending agent.

- **Diapedesis (transmigration):** It is the migration of the leukocytes through the endothelium during inflammation. It occurs mainly in the post-capillary venules.
- **Chemotaxis:** After exiting the microcirculation, leukocytes emigrate in tissues toward the site of injury by a process called chemotaxis, which is defined as locomotion oriented along a chemical gradient. Both exogenous and endogenous substances can act as chemoattractants. The most common exogenous agents are bacterial products. Endogenous chemoattractants include cytokines, complement C5a and LTB4.
- **Phagocytosis:** Phagocytes (i.e. neutrophils, monocytes, and macrophages) require an enzyme to produce reactive oxygen species to destroy bacteria after they ingest the bacteria in a process called phagocytosis. This enzyme is calve "phagocyte NADPH oxidase" (PHOX).
- **Cytokines:** These are proteins produced by many cell types (principally activated lymphocytes and macrophages, but also endothelial , epithelial and connective tissue cells) that modulate the functions of other cell types. Cytokines include interleukins, interferons and tumor necrosis factor alpha (TNF-α). These produce local and systemic effects. Most important cytokine responsible for systemic effects of inflammation are interleukin-1 (IL-1) and tumor necrosis factor-alpha (TNF-α).
- **Chemokines:** Family of cytokines that act primarily as chemoattractants for specific types of leukocytes. They are classified accordingly to the arrangement of conserved cystine residue in mature proteins. (i) α-chemokine (CXC): e.g. IL-8, IL-1, TNF, (ii) β-chemokines (C-C): MCP-1, RANTES < Eotoxin, (iii) γ-chemokines (C chemokines): lymphotactin; and (iv) CX3C: Fractalkaline.
- **Lysomal granules:** Neutrophils and monocytes contain lysosomal granule that contribute to microbial killing. Neutrophils have 2 main types of granules.

Primary (azurophilic) granules	Secondary (specific) granules
• Require high level of agonists to be released extracellularly • Potentially more destructive • Secrete – Myeloperoxidase (MPO) – Acid hydrolase – Cathepsin G – Proteinase 3 – Elastase – Defensin – Nonspecific collagenase	• Secreted at lower concentration of agonists • Secrete extracellularly more readily • Secrete: – Lysozyme – Collagenase type IV – Phospholipase A2 – Lysozyme – Lactoferin – Alkaline phosphatise – Gelatinase – Plasminogen activator – Histaminase

- **Complement system:** It consists of more than 20 proteins and constitute 5–10% of plasma proteins. These are numbered C1 to C9. This system functions in both innate and adaptive immunity for defence against microbial pathogens. Breakdown (cleavage) products of complement proteins are elaborated that cause increased vascular permeability, chemotaxis, and opsonisation. There are 3 pathways: Classic pathway, Alternative pathway and Lectin (mannose binding lectin) pathway.
- **Serous inflammation:** It is marked by the outpouring of a thin fluid that may be derived from the plasma or from the secretions of mesothelial cells lining the peritoneal, pleural and pericardial cavities. Accumulation of fluid in these cavities is called an effusion.
- **Catarrhal inflammation:** It is the commonest type of inflammation wherein increased mucus secretion is present. *Example*: common cold.
- **Fibrinous inflammation:** There is deposition of fibrin in extracellular space. It is due to large vascular leaks or local procoagulant stimuli (cancer).
- **Purulent (suppurative) inflammation:** Purulent exudates are characterized by

pus made of neutrophils, liquefied debris of necrotic cells, and edema fluid. Most common cause is bacteria which causes liquefactive necrosis.

- **Abscess:** Abscess is localized collections of purulent inflammatory tissue caused by suppuration buried in a tissue, an organ, or confined space. They are produced by deep seeding of pyogenic bacteria into a tissue.
- **Ulcer:** An ulcer is a local defect, or excavation of the surface of an organ or tissue that is produced by the sloughing (shedding) of inflamed necrotic tissue.
- **Chronic inflammation:** It is inflammation of prolonged duration (weeks or months) in which inflammation, tissue injury, and attempts at repair coexists, in varying combinations.
- **Granuloma:** It is a focus of chronic inflammation consisting of a microscopic aggregation of macrophages that are transformed into epithelium-like cells, surrounded by a collar of mononuclear leukocytes, principally lymphocytes and occasionally plasma cells. In usual H&E section, the epithelioid cells have pale pink granular cytoplasm with indistinct cell boundaries, often appearing to merge into one another. The nucleus is less dense than that of a lymphocyte, is oval or elongate and may show folding of the nuclear membrane.
- **Regeneration:** It refers to the proliferation of cells and tissues to replace lost structures, such as growth of an amputated limb in amphibians.
- **Repair:** Most often consists of a combination of regeneration and scar formation by the deposition of collagen.
- **Permanent cells:** Cells of the body which never divide, e.g. neurons, skeletal muscle fibres and cardiac myocytes.
- **Stable cells:** These cells have a low rate of multiplication and are usually present in the G0 phase. When stimulated, they enter the G1 phase and multiply. *Example*: Cells of proximal tubule of kidney, hepatocytes, pancreatic cells, fibroblasts, etc.
- **Labile cells:** These cells can generate throughout life, e.g. hematopoietic cells, cells of skin, gastrointestinal mucosa, etc.
- **Granulation tissue:** Fibroblasts and vascular endothelial cells proliferate in the first 24–72 hours of the repair process to form a specialized type of tissue called granulation tissue. The term derives from its pink, soft, granular appearance on the surface of wounds. So, granulation tissue = fibroblasts + small blood vessels (angiogenesis) + chronic inflammatory cells (macrophages and lymphocytes).
- **Stem cell:** It is a cell with a unique capacity to produce unaltered daughter cells (self-renewal) and to generate specialized cell types (potency).

Role of Mediators in Inflammation

- **Vasodilation:** Prostaglandins (PGD2, PGE2, PGI2), nitric oxide, histamine
- **Increased vascular permeability:** Histamine, Serotonin, C3a and C5a, Bradykinin, Leukotriens C4, D4 and E4, PAF, Substance P
- **Chemotaxis:** TNF, IL-1, Chemokines, C3a, C5a, Leukotriens B4
- **Fever:** Il-1, TNF, Prostaglandins
- **Pain:** Prostaglandins. Bradykinin
- **Tissue damage:** Lysosomal enzymes of leukocytes, reactive oxygen species, NO
- **Positive acute phase proteins/reactants:** CRP, Ferritin, Ceruloplasmin, Haptoglobin, Complement factors, Mannose binding protein, Serum amyloid A, Fibrinogen, Alpha 2, macroglobulin, Procalcitonin
- **Negative acute phase proteins/reactants:** Albumin, Transferrin, Retinol-binding protein, Antithrombin, Transcortin, Transthyretin.

Hemodynamic Disorders

- **Virchow's triad:** Related to thrombus. It includes (1) vascular (endothelial) injury, (2) abnormal blood flow (stasis or turbulence) and (3) hypercoagubility.

- **Haemostasis:** It is defined as a sequence of events leading to cessation of bleeding by the formation of a stable fibrin-platelet haemostatic plug. The process involves the vascular endothelium, platelets and the coagulation system.
- **Edema:** If the movement of water into tissues (or body cavities) exceeds lymphatic drainage, then fluid accumulates. An abnormal increase in intestinal fluid within tissues is called edema.
- **Anasarca:** It is a severe and generalized edema with widespread subcutaneous tissue swelling.
- **Dependent edema:** When edema is influenced by gravity and distribution of edema fluid occurs due to gravity, it is called dependent edema (e.g. the legs when standing, the sacrum when recumbent).
- **Pitting edema:** Finger pressure over substantially edematous subcutaneous tissue displaces the interstitial fluid and leaves a depression, making it a sign.
- **Transudate:** A transudate is a fluid with low protein content (most of which is albumin) and a specific gravity of < 1.012. It is essentially an ultrafiltrate of blood plasma that results from osmotic or hydrostatic imbalance across the vessel wall without an increase in vascular permeability.
- **Exudate:** An exudate is an extravascular fluid that has a high protein concentration, cellular debris and a specific gravity >1.020. It is formed mainly due to alteration in the normal permeability of small blood vessels in the area of injury.
- **Hyperemia:** It is an active process in which arteriolar dilation (e.g. at sites of inflammation or in skeletal muscle during exercise) leads to increased blood flow. Affected tissues turn red (erythema) because of the engorgement of vessels with oxygenated blood.
- **Congestion:** It is a passive process resulting from reduced outflow of blood from a tissue. It can be systemic, as in cardiac failure, or local, as in isolated venous obstruction. Congested tissue take on a dusky reddish-blue color (cyanosis) due to red cell stasis and the accumulation of deoxygenated hemoglobin.
- **Nutmeg liver:** In chronic hepatic congestion, central region of lobule shows loss of cells and have red brown color which is accentuated against surrounding normal liver.
- **Petechiae:** Minute 1–2 mm haemorrhages into skin, mucous membranes, or serosal surfaces. These are most commonly associated with locally increased intravascular pressure, low platelet counts (thrombocytopenia), or increase vascular fragility (e.g. in amyloidosis).
- **Purpura:** Slightly larger (≥ 3 mm) haemorrhages are called purpura. These may be associated with many of the same disorders that cause petechiae or can be secondary to trauma, vascular inflammation (vasculitis), or increase vascular fragility (e.g. amyloidosis).
- **Ecchymoses:** Larger (>1–2 cm) subcutaneous hematomas (i.e. bruise) are called ecchymoses.
- **Thrombosis:** It is the process of blood clot formation within intact vessels, and this blood clot within intact vessel is known as thrombus.
- **Infarction:** An infarct is an area of ischemic necrosis caused by occlusion of either the arterial supply or the venous drainage.
- **Embolism:** An embolus is detached intravascular solid, liquid, or gaseous mass that is carried by the blood to a site distant from its point of origin.
- **Thromboembolism:** Most of the emboli originate from a dislodged thrombus, hence called thromboembolism.
- **Paradoxical embolism:** Rarely, an embolus can pass through an inter-atrial or interventricular defect and gain access to the systemic circulation (paradoxical embolism).

- **Red infarct:** It occurs due to arterial occlusion in loose tissues or organs having dual blood supply. *Example*: Lung, liver, small intestine. It may also be due to venous occlusion (testis, ovary).
- **White infarct:** It occurs due to arterial occlusions in solid organs with an arterial occlusion. *Example*: Heart, spleen, kidney, brain.
- **Shock:** It is defined as systemic hypotension due to either to reduced cardiac output or to reduced effective circulating blood volume.
- **Lines of Zahn:** Thrombi often have grossly and microscopically apparent laminations called lines of Zahn. These represent pale platelet and fibrin deposits alternating with darker red-cell rich layers.

Genetic Disorders

- **Gene:** The gene is the basic physical and functional unit of heredity. It consists of a specific sequence of nucleotides at a given portion on a given chromosome that synthesizes/codes for a specific protein (or, in some cases, an RNA molecule).
- **Mutation:** A mutation is defined as a permanent change in the DNA.
- **Locus:** The portion of gene on a chromosome is called a locus.
- **Point mutation:** It is a genetic mutation where a single nucleotide base is changed, inserted or detected from a DNA or RNA sequence of an organism's genome.
- **Frameshift mutation:** It is a genetic mutation involving the insertion or deletion of nucleotide in which the number of inserted or deleted base pairs is not divisible by three. Due to the triplet nature of gene expression by codons, the insertion or deletion can change the reading frame, resulting in a completely different translation from the original. *Example*: Single base deletion at ABO locus, to form O allele. Four base insertion in Tay–Sachs disease.
- **Missense mutation:** It is a point mutation in which a single nucleotide changes results in a codon that codes for a different amino acid in the resulting protein. It is a type of nonsynonymous substitution. *Example*: Sickle cell mutation.
- **Nonsense (stop codon) mutation:** It is a mutation in a base in the DNA that prematurely stops the translation (reading) of messenger RNA (m RNA) resulting in a polypeptide chain that ends prematurely and a protein product that is truncated (abbreviated) and incomplete and usually non-functional. *Example*: β-thalassemia.
- **Hereditary disorders:** These are derived from one's parents and are transmitted in the germ line through the generations and are therefore also **familial**.
- **Congenital disorders:** Congenital simply implies "born with". Some congenital diseases are not genetic; for example, congenital syphilis. Not all genetic diseases are congenital; individuals with Huntington disease, for example, begin to manifest their condition only after their 20s or 30s.
- **Incomplete inheritance:** Some individuals inherit the mutant gene but are phenotypically normal. Thus 50% penetrance indicates that 50% of those who carry the gene express the trait.
- **Variable expressivity:** In contrast to penetrance, if a trait is seen in all individuals carrying the mutant gene but is expressed differently among individuals, the phenomenon is called variable expressivity.
- **Gain of function mutation:** Protein product of the mutant allele has properties not normally associated with the natural/wild/-type protein. It is less common and affects normal proteins with toxic properties. *Example*: Huntington's disease.
- **Loss of function mutation:** It leads to reduced production of a gene product or give rise to inactive protein. It is more common and affects regulatory proteins

and subunits of multimeric proteins. *Example*: Marfan syndrome, Ehler Danlos syndrome.

- **Uniparental disomy:** It is suspected when in an individual manifesting a recessive disorder but only one parent is a carrier. *Example*: Prader–Willi syndrome, Angelman syndrome, Russel–Silver syndrome.
- **Mitochondrial inheritance:** Mutation in the mitochondrial DNA has the characteristic feature of maternal inheritance because the ovum contains the mitochondria with their abundant cytoplasm whereas sperms contain minimal number of mitochondria. *Example*: Leber's optic neuropathy, Leigh's disease, MELAS (mitochondrial encephalopathy, lactic acidosis, and stroke like syndrome), NARP syndrome (neuropathy, ataxia, and retinitis pigmentosa), Pearson syndrome, Kearns–Sayre syndrome.
- **Genetic imprinting:** It is defined as differential expression of a gene based on chromosomal inheritance from maternal or paternal origin. *Example*: Microdeletion of chromosome 15q11-13. If microdeletion occurs in maternal chromosome; **Angleman syndrome** occurs. But paternal chromosomal microdeletion may cause **Prader–Willi syndrome**. It is also seen in Beckwith–Wiedmann syndrome and Albright's hereditary osteodystrophy.
- **Triplet repeat mutations:** The mutation in these disease group is characterized by a long repeating sequence of three nucleotides. It is characteristically different from other because it is dynamic in nature (degree of amplification of a sequence of three nucleotides increases during gametogenesis). *Example*: (a) In coding region expansion (Gain of function type mutation): Huntington's disease, Spinocerebellar ataxia type 1, 2, 3, 6, 7 and Spinobulbar muscular atrophy (Kennedy's disease). (b) In non-coding region expansion (Loss of function type mutations): Fragile X syndrome, Friedrich's ataxia, myotonic dystrophy.
- **Gonadal (Germline) Mosaicism:** Normally, autosomal dominant disorders have affected parents but in some patients with autosomal dominant disorders, the parents are not involved. In such patients, it results from a new mutation in the in the egg or the sperm from which they were derived. But the siblings are usually not affected. *Example*: Osteogenesis imperfacta, tuberous sclerosis. Gonadal mosaicism results from a mutation that occurs postzygotically during early (embryonic) development.
- **Karyotype and karyotyping:** A karyotype is a standard arrangement of a photographed or image stained chromosome pairs in metaphase stage in order of decreasing length.

  Study of chromosomes is called karyotyping.
- **Epigenetics:** It is defined as the study of heritable chemical modification of DNA or chromatin that does alter the DNA sequence itself. *Example*: Methylation of DNA, and the methylation and acetylation of histones.
- **Isochromosome:** It is formed when one arm of chromosome is lost and the remaining arm is duplicated, resulting in a chromosome consisting of two short arms or two long arms.
- **Deletion:** Loss of a portion of a chromosome. *Example*: 46, XY, del(15).
- **Ring chromosome:** Due to break at both ends of a chromosome with fusion of the damaged ends. *Example*: 46, XY, r(10).
- **Inversion:** Rearrangement which involves two breaks within a single chromosome with re-insertion of the inverted, intervening segment.
  a. *Pericentric*: If the breaks are on opposite sides of the centromere.
  b *Paracentric*: Inversion involving only one arm of the chromosome.
- **Translocation:** Segment of one chromosome is transferred to another.
  a. *Balanced or reciprocal translocation*: Break occurs in either short or long arms of

two chromosomes and genetic material of almost same quantity is transferred between these two chromosomes.

b. *Robertsonian or unbalanced translocation*: A translocation between two acrocentric chromosomes, leading to one very large chromosome and one extremely small one, along with small product being lost.

IMMUNITY

- **Innate immunity (also known as natural or native immunity):** It refers to defence mechanisms that are present since birth and have evolved to recognize microbes. It is the first line of defence. It is non-specific and has no memory.
- **Adaptive immunity (also called acquired or specific immunity):** It consists of mechanisms that are stimulated by microbes and are capable of recognizing non-microbial substances also. Adaptive immunity after exposure to antigens. It is more specific and has memory.
- **Pattern recognition receptors (PRR):** These are peptides molecules on the leukocytes which recognize particular structural pattern on a microorganism called pathogen associated molecular pattern (PAMPS).
- **Toll-like receptors (TLR):** These are pattern recognition receptors that are homologous to the Drossophila protein Toll. Different TLRs are specific for components of different bacteria and viruses. TLRs are located on the cell surface and in endosomes, so they are able to recognize and initiate cellular responses to extracellular and ingested microbes.
- **Anergy:** It is diminished reactivity to one or more specific antigens.
- **Regulatory T cells:** Regulatory T cells are CD 4+ T cells that constituvely express CD25, the α-chain of the IL-2 receptors, and a transcription factor of the forkhead family, called Fox p3. Mutation in Fox p3 result in severe autoimmunity in humans and mice.
- **All leukocytes:** CD45 (LCA or leukocyte common antigen), and CD 45B.
- **Medullary thymocytes (naïve T-cells):** CD 45RA and CD45 RC.
- **Cortical thymocytes (memory T cells):** CD 45 R0.
- **Helper T cell (CD 4+ T cell):** It is known as the master regulator of the immune system. They bind only to antigens presented with class II MHC molecules. So, they are called as MHC-II restricted. These recognize exogenous peptides.
- **Cytotoxic T cells (or CD8+ T cells):** Bind only to antigens presented with class I MHC molecules. So, they are called as MHC-I restricted. These recognize exogenous peptides.
- **Antigen presenting cells:** When antigen presenting cells phagocytose the antigen, they process it inside themselves and present on their surface in association with MHC molecule. This processed antigen is now presented to the T cells.
  a. *Professional APC*: They express MHC II molecules. They capture and present antigen routinely. *Examples*: Dendritic cell (including Langerhans cell, B cell, macrophage).
  b. *Non professional APC*: They express MHC I molecule. They can be induced to present antigen by cytokines like IFN-γ. *Examples*: Endothelial cells, fibroblasts, thymic epithelial cells, glial cells and pancreatic cells.
- **Agretope:** The part of the antigen associated with MHC molecules on the APC (antigen presenting cell).
- **Epitope:** The antigenic part in contact with T cell Receptor (TCR).
- **Dendritic cells:** They have numerous fine cytoplasmic processes that resemble dendrites. There are two types:
  a. *Interdigitating dendritic cells* (*or dendritic cells*): They are most important antigen-presenting cells for initiating primary immune responses against protein antigens. Langerhans cells are immature dendritic cells within the epidermis.

b. *Follicular dendritic cells*: They are present in the germinal centres of lymphoid follicles in the spleen and lymph nodes. These cells bear Fc receptors for IgG and receptors for C3b. They can trap antigen bound to antibodies or complement proteins.

- **Microorganisms free in plasma:** Polio virus, HBV, most bacteria and fungi, some protozoa (African trypanosomes) and all helminths.
- **In WBCs:** Herpes virus, HIV, mycobacteria, *Leishmania*, *Toxoplasma gondii*.
- **In RBCs:** Tick fever virus, parasites (*Plasmodium* and *Babesia*)
- **Intracellular organisms:**
  a. *Bacteria*: Mycobacteria, *Listeria*, *Legionella*
  b. *Fungi*: *Cryptococcus neoformans*
  c. *Protozoa*: *Leishmania*, *Trypanosomes*, *Toxoplasmas*.
- **NK or natural killer cells:** NK cells are also called Large granular lymphocytes as they are morphologically larger than both T and B lymphocytes). It represents 5–10% of peripheral lymphocytes. They derive from bone marrow and thymic microenvironments. NK cells are activated in presence of IL-2 to lymphocyte activated killer (LAK) cells. They express CD16 and CD 56.
- **MHC (major histocompatibility complex):** It is a cluster of genes located on short arm of chromosome 6(6p) whose main physiologic function is to bind peptide fragments of foreign proteins for presentation to antigen specific T cells. It is also known as human leukocyte antigen. There are 3 types, class I, II, and III gene (*see* Table below).
- **MHC class I:** (a) HLA (A, B, and C): recognized by CD+8 lymphocytes, (b) HLA-E: Self recognition, inhibitory receptors, target for NK cells, (c) HLA-G: expressed selectively in extravillous trophoblasts; maintains materno-foetal tolerance, (d) HLA-F: unknown role.
- **MHC class II:** HLA-D, (P, Q, R)
- **MHC class III:** Complement and other proteins.
- **Type I hypersensitivity:** It is defined as a rapidly developing immunologic reaction occurring within minutes after the combination of an antigen with antibody bound to mast cells in individuals previously sensitized to the antigen. It is commonly referred to as allergy. *Example*:
  a. Localized hypersensitivity: Urticaria, angioedema, allergic rhinitis (hay fever), bronchial asthma, eczema, food allergies
  b. Systemic hypersensitivity: Anaphylactic shock, (antibiotic like penicillin),

Class I Gene	Class II Gene	Class III Gene
• Code for MHC I molecule • Comprises HLA A, B, C, E, F and G loci • Present on all nucleated cells and platelets • Detected by alloantisera • Present antigen to CD8 T cells • Required for virus infected cells, cancer cells • Major role in graft rejection	• Codes for MHC II molecule • Comprises HLA-D locus (viz. HLA-DP, HLA-DQ, HLA-DR) • Present on antigen presenting cells like B cells, dendritic cells, endothelial cells and fibroblasts • Detected by mixed lymphocyte reaction • Present antigen to CD4+ T cells • It is required for graft-versus-host disease	• Codes for complement proteins, C2, C4, properdin, factor B, TNF, HSP-70, tyrosine hydroxylase • No direct role in immune system. But involves in autoimmune disorders

bee stings, insect bites, others (Casoni's test, Schultz–Dale phenomenon, Prausnitz–Kusnter reaction, Theobald Smith phenomenon).

- **Type II hypersensitivity reaction:** It is mediated by antibodies directed towards endogenous or exogenous specific antigens present on cell surfaces or extracellular matrix. *Examples* are:
  a. *Opsonization and complement and Fc receptor mediated phagocytosis*: Transfusion reactions, erythroblastosis fetalis, Autoimmune hemolytic anemia, autoimmune thrombocytopenic purpura.
  b. *Complement and Fc receptor mediated inflammation*: Goodpasture syndrome, acute rheumatic fever, vasculitis due to ANCA, vascular rejection in organ grafts.
  c. *Antibody mediated cellular dysfunction*: Myasthenia gravis, Graves' disease, pernicious anemia, insulin-resistant diabetes.
- **Type III hypersensitivity reaction (immune complex disease):** Antigen–antibody complexes produce tissue damage mainly by eliciting inflammation at the sites of deposition. The antigen can be exogenous or endogenous. The formed immune complexes may be present in the circulation (circulating immune complexes) or may get deposited inside the vessels or extravascular sites (*in situ* immune complex). *Examples*:
  a. *Infections*: Post-streptococcal glomerulonephritis, subacute infective endocarditis.
  b. *Autoimmune diseases*: SLE, Rheumatoid arthritis, polyarteritis nodosa (PAN), Hashimoto's thyroiditis.
  c. *Malignancy*: Hodgkin lymphoma, Leukemias.
  d. *Drug reactions*: Arthus reaction, serum sickness, penicillamine toxicity.
  e. *Others*: Farmer's lung, Schick test, type II lepra reaction.

  Type III hypersensitivity reaction can be divided into localized and Systemic also.
  i. *Localized type III hypersensitivity*: Arthus reaction, polyarteritis nodosa, Farmer's lung, Schik test.
  ii. *Systemic hypersensitivity*: SLE, Henoch–Schonlein purpura, reactive arthritis, serum sickness, post-streptococcal glomerulonephritis, type II lepra reaction.
- **Type IV hypersensitivity (cell mediated hypersensitivity):** It is initiated by antigen-activated (sensitized) T lymphocytes. It includes the delayed type hypersensitivity reactions mediated by CD4+ T cells, and direct cell cytotoxicity mediated by CD8+ T cells.
  Examples: Chronic graft rejection, Tuberculin reaction, type I lepra reaction, temporal arteritis, type I diabetes, Lepromin test, contact dermatitis, primary biliary cirrhosis, inflammatory bowel disease, Crohn's disease, multiple sclerosis, sarcoidosis, rheumatoid arthritis.
- **Immunological tolerance:** It is the phenomenon of unresponsiveness to an antigen as a result of exposure of lymphocytes to that antigen.
- **Self-tolerance:** It refers to lack of responsiveness to an individual's own antigen, and it underlies our ability to live in harmony with our tissues and cells.
- **Central tolerance:** In this process, immature self-reactive T- and B-lymphocyte clones that recognize self-antigens during their maturation in the central (or generative) lymphoid organs (the thymus for T cells and the bone marrow for B cells) are killed or rendered harmless.
- **Peripheral tolerance:** It means silencing of potentially auto-reactive T and B cells in peripheral tissues (mainly for T cells). Suppression is done by regulatory T cells or Treg. regulatory T cells are CD4+ cells which express:
  a. CD25: α chain of the IL-2 receptor
  b. FOX P3: transcription factor of the forkhead family.

These CD25 and FOX P3 are required for development and maintenance of functional CD4+ regulatory T cells.

- **Anergy:** This refers to prolonged or irreversible functional inactivation of lymphocytes induced by encounter with antigens under certain conditions.
- **Autoimmunity:** It arises from a combination of the inheritance of susceptibility genes, which may contribute to the breakdown of self-tolerance, and environmental triggers, such as infections and tissue damage, which promote the activation of self-reactive lymphocytes.
- **Hyperacute rejection:** It takes place in persons with preformed antibodies usually within minutes to hours of transcription. The preformed antibodies result in immune complex disease with the presence of neutrophils within arterioles, glomeruli, and peritubular capillaries and fibrin-platelet thrombi in vessel wall. There is presence of necrosis of the renal cortex. It is type II hypersensitivity reaction.
- **Acute rejection:** It occurs after days to months after transplantation. It can be acute humoral rejection or acute cellular rejection. It is type II+ type IV hypersensitivity reaction.
  a. *Acute cellular rejection*: It is seen within few months after transplantation. There is presence of endothelitis with the presence of CD4 and CD8 T cells in the interstitium along with the mononuclear cells in the glomerular and peritubular capillaries.
  b. *Acute humoral rejection* (*rejection vasculitis*): It is mediated mainly by anti-donor antibodies and it manifests mainly as damage to the blood vessels in the form of necrotizing vasculitis with endothelial cell necrosis, neutrophilic infiltration, deposition of immunoglobulins, complement, fibrin and thrombosis. There is associated necrosis of the renal parenchyma. C4d deposition is an indicator of antibody mediated (humoral) graft rejection.
- **Chronic rejection:** It occurs months to years after transplantation. Vascular changes consist of dense, obliterative intimal fibrosis in the cortical arteries resulting in glomerular loss, interstitial fibrosis and tubular atrophy, duplication of basement membranes of the glomeruli (also known as chronic transplant glomerulopathy). Infiltration of lymphocytes, plasma cells and eosinophils are noted in the renal interstitium.
- **Graft-versus-Host disease (GVHD):** It occurs when immunologically competent cells or their precursors are transplanted into immunologically crippled patients and transferred cells recognize alloantigens in the host. It occurs most commonly after allogenic bone marrow transplant. Immunocompetent T cells present in the donor marrow recognize the recipient's HLA antigen as foreign antigen and reacts against them. Both CD4+ and CD8+ T cells recognize and attract host tissues.
- **Acute GVHD:** This is characterized by an erythematous maculopapular rash; persistent diarrhoea or anorexia, or both. Also, there is liver disease with increased serum levels of bilirubin, alanine and aspartate aminotransferase and alkaline phosphatase. It occurs within first 3 months post-transplant.
- **Chronic GVHD:** It develops after 3 months post-transplant. Chronic GVHD resembles an autoimmune disease with malar rash, arthritis, sicca syndrome, obliterative bronchiolitis and cholestasis. They are susceptible to significant infections, particularly cytomegalo virus. They should receive prophylactic trimethoprim-sulphamethazole.
- **ANA (antinuclear antibody):** Seen in different autoimmune diseases.
- **Anti-double stranded DNA:** SLE (40–60%).
- **Anti-histone:** Drug- induced SLE.

- **Anti-Sm:** SLE (20–30%)
- **Anti centromere:** Limited Scleroderma (CREST)
- **Jo-1:** Inflammatory myopathy (also known as Histidyl-t-RNA synthetase)
- **SS-A (Ro):** Sjogren syndrome (70–95%), neonatal SLE with congenital heart-block
- **SS-B (La):** Sjogren syndrome (60–90%), neonatal SLE with congenital heart-block
- **Anti-DNA topoisomerase:** Diffuse scleroderma (Scl-70)
- **Renal changes in SLE (WHO classification):**
  a. *Class I*: Minimal change or no change (< 5% of cases)
  b. *Class II*: Mesangial lupus glomerulonephritis (0–25%)
  c. *Class III*: Focal proliferative glomerulonephritis (20–35%)
  d. *Class IV*: Diffuse proliferative glomerulonephritis (35–60%)
  e. *Class V*: Membranous glomerulonephritis (10–15%)
  f. *Class VI*: Advanced sclerotic glomerulonephritis (35–60%).
- **Antinuclear antibody staining pattern corresponding antigens:**
  a. *Homogeneous or diffuse nuclear staining*: Chromatin, histones
  b. *Rim or peripheral staining*: Double stranded DNA
  c. *Speckled pattern*: Antibody against Sm (Smith) antigen which is extractable (non-DNA) nuclear antigen, also against SS-A and SS-B reactive antigens. This is most common and least specific pattern.
  d. *Nucleolar pattern*: RNA (seen in systemic sclerosis)
  e. *Centromeric pattern*: Centromeres (seen in CREST syndrome)
- **CD4 T cell count and predisposition to infection:**
  a. CD4 T cell count >200 cells/mm^3: TB
  b. CD4 T cell count <200 cell/mm^3: *P.jiroveci*
  c. CD4 T cell count <100 cell/mm^3: *Cryptococcus*
  d. CD4 T cell count <50 cell/mm^3: CMV, MAC, IRIS (Immune reconstitution inflammatory syndrome in AIDS).
- **Amyloid:** It is a pathologic proteinaceous substance, deposited in the extracellular space in various tissues and organs of the body in a wide variety of clinical settings.
- **Type of Amyloid Protein:** (Major fibril protein) deposited in different diseases:
  a. Primary amyloidosis (multiple myeloma and other plasma cell dyscrasia): AL
  b. Secondary amyloidosis (rheumatoid arthritis, TB): AA
  c. Chronic renal failure: Aβ2
  d. Alzheimer's disease: Aβ
  e. Familial Mediterranean fever: AA
  f. Familial amyloidotic neuropathies: ATTR (abnormal or mutant ATTR)
  g. Systemic senile amyloidosis: ATTR (normal ATTR)
  h. Type 2 diabetes: AIAPP
  i. Isolated atrial amyloidosis: AANF.
- **Diagnosis of amyloidosis:**
  a. H&E stain: Amorphous eosinophilic extracellular substance
  b. Congo red stain: Pink or red color to tissue deposits
  c. Congo red stain with polarizing microscopy: Apple green birefringence
  d. Thioflavin T&S: (fluorescent stain): Yellow color under UV light
  e. Electron microscopy: Nonbranching fibrils of indefinite length and a diameter of approximately 7.5–10 nm.
  f. X-ray crystallography and Infrared spectroscopy: Characteristic cross β-plated sheet conformation.

NEOPLASIA

- **Neoplasia:** A neoplasm is an abnormal mass of tissue, the growth of which exceeds and is uncoordinated with that of the normal tissues and persists in the same excessive manner even after cessation of the stimuli which evoke the change (Defined by RA Willis, eminent British Oncologist in 1962).

The process of formation of neoplasm is called neoplasia.

So, neoplasm is new, uncontrolled growth of cells that is not under physiologic control. A "tumor" or "mass lesion" is simply a "growth" or "enlargement" which may not be neoplastic (such as granuloma). The term cancer implies malignancy, but **neoplasms** can be subclassified as either benign or malignant.

- **Hamartoma:** Disorganized but benign-appearing masses composed of cells indigenous to the particular site. For example, pulmonary chondroid hamartoma contains islands of disorganized, but histologically normal cartilage, bronchi and vessels.
- **Choriostoma:** This is a congenital anomaly which is better described as a heterotropic rest of cells. For example, a small nodule of well-developed and normally organized pancreatic substance may be found in the submucosa of the stomach, duodenum, or small intestine.
- **Differentiation:** It refers to the extent to which neoplastic parenchyma cells resemble the corresponding normal parenchymal cells, both morphologically and functionally; lack of differentiation is called **anaplasia**.
- **Pleomorphism:** Variation in size and shape of both the cells and the nuclei. Thus, cells within the same tumor are not uniform but range from large cells, many times larger than their neighbors, to extremely small and primitive appearing.
- **Hyperchromasia:** Increased nuclear material (chromatin) or DNA which is responsible for dark staining of the cells.
- **N:C ratio:** Nuclear-cytoplasmic ratio is normally 1:4 to 1:6 but may approach 1:1 in anaplastic cells (in neoplasm or tumor).
- **Atypical mitosis:** Normal mitosis is bipolar. But when the mitotic figures become bizarre and sometimes producing tripolar, quadripolar or multipolar spindles, these are called atypical mitoses.
- **Tumor giant cells:** Another feature of anaplasia. Some neoplastic cells possessing only a single huge polymorphic nucleus and others having two or more large, hyperchromatic nuclei.
- **Metaplasia:** Reversible change in which one differentiated cell type (epithelial or mesenchymal) is replaced by another cell type.
- **Dysplasia:** A change having loss in the uniformity of the individual cells and loss architectural orientation. Dysplastic changes are often found adjacent to foci of invasive carcinoma. Dysplasia literally means disordered growth. Is/are the
- **Anaplasia:** An absence of differentiation (extent to which neoplastic cells resemble normal cell both morphologically and functionally).
- **Metastasis:** It is the most reliable features of a malignant tumor, characterized by the spread of the tumor to other parts because of penetration into blood vessels, lymphatics and body cavities. The major exceptions are most malignant neoplasms of the glial cells in the central nervous system, called gliomas, and basal cell carcinoma (rodent ulcer) of the skin. Both are locally invasive forms of cancer, but they rarely metastasize.
- **Local invasion:** It is the second most reliable feature that differentiates from malignant from benign tumors. The malignant tumors show invasion, infiltration and destruction of the surrounding tissue.
- **Sentinel lymph node:** It is defined as the first lymph node or group of nodes draining a cancer. It is postulated that sentinel lymph node(s) is/are the target organs primarily reached by metastasizing cancer cells from the tumor. Sentinel lymph node biopsy (also known as sentinel node procedure) is used in the staging of certain types of cancer to see if

they have spread to any lymph node. It is useful for breast cancer, malignant melanoma, colon cancer and vulval cancer.

- **Skip metastasis:** Local lymph nodes, however may be bypassed, known as skip metastasis. This is because of venous-lymphatic anastomoses or because inflammation or radiation has obliterated lymphatic channels.
- **Warburg effect:** or aerobic glycolysis is the shifting of glucose metabolism by the cancer cells from the efficient mitochondria to glycolysis. It is seen because tumor cells have M2 isoform of pyruvate kinase enzyme. So, Warburg effect is a phenomenon predominantly observed in cancer cells wherein cells ferment glucose to lactic acid using glycolysis even in the presence of oxygen. Otto Warburg observed this effect in 1926 and postulated it to be the fundamental cause of cancer.
- **Hallmarks of cancer:**
  - i. Self sufficiency in growth signals: Due to oncogene activation
  - ii. Insensitivity to growth-inhibitory signals
  - iii. Evasion of apoptosis
  - iv. Limitless replicative potential
  - v. Development of sustained angiogenesis
  - vi. Ability to invade and metastasize
  - vii. Aerobic glycolysis (Warburg effect)
- **Proto-oncogenes:** Unmutated counterparts of oncogenes found normally in cell. Functions of protooncogenes are cell growth, inhibition of apoptosis and nuclear transcription. Chromosomal translocation is the commonest cause of proto-oncogenes.
- **Oncogenes:** Mutated or over expressed version of proto-oncogene that function autonomously. Oncogenes have no dependence on normal growth promoting signals and growth factors. Proto-oncogenes can be activated to oncogene by translocation and growth factors. Proto-oncogenes can be activated to oncogene by translocation (most common in hematologic malignancies), amplification and point mutation.
- **Oncoproteins:** Proteins encoded by oncogenes which promote cell growth in absence of growth promoting signals.

Proto-oncogenes (normal genes required for cell proliferation and differentiation)

↓

Oncogenes (genes promoting autoimmune cell growth in cancer cells)

↓

Oncoproteins (proteins lacking regulatory control and responsible for promoting cell growth)

- **RAS Oncogene:** The RAS genes, of which there are three in the human genome (H-RAS, K-RAS, N-RAS) where discovered initially in transforming retroviruses. Point mutation of RAS family genes is the single most common abnormality of proto-oncogenes in human tumors. Approximately 15–20% of all human tumors contain mutated versions of RAS proteins.
- **MYC oncogene:** The MYC proto-oncogene is expressed in virtually all eukaryotic cells. In contrast to the regulated expression of MYC during normal cell proliferation, persistent expression, and in some cases overexpression, of the MYC protein are commonly found in tumors.
  - a. C-MYC: Burkitt's lymphoma
  - b. L-MYC: Small cell carcinoma
  - c. N-MYC: Neuroblastoma.
- **Loss of heterozygosity (LOH):** Retinoblastoma develops when both the normal alleles of retinoblastoma gene (present on chromosome 13q14) are inactivated or altered. In familial cases of retinoblastoma, children are born with one normal and one defective copy of Rb gene. These children are called heterozygous at Rb locus because one allele of the gene is normal while the other is a mutant. So, till the time there is heterozygosity for the Rb gene, the cell behaviour is not affected and there is no chance of cancer development.

But when there is a mutation affecting the second allele, the chances of cancer increase. This means that the cell loses heterozygosity for the normal Rb gene (called as loss of heterozygosity).

- **P53 (guardian of the genome):** The p53 gene is located on chromosome 17p13.1, and it is the most common target for genetic alteration in human tumors. The official name of the gene is TP53 and the protein is p5 (for the sake of simplicity, both are referred to as "p53"). Little over 50% of human tumor contain mutations in this gene. Homozygous loss of p53 occurs in virtually every type of cancer, including carcinomas of the lung, colon, and breast (three leading cause of cancer deaths). In most cases, the inactivating mutations affect both p53 alleles and are acquired in somatic cells (not inherited in the germ line). The p53 gene is a tumor suppressor gene codes for 53kDa nuclear phosphoprotein. The non-mutant p53 gene is called as the 'wild type' of p53 gene.
- **APC (tumor suppressor gene):** It is also called gate-keeper of colonic neoplasia. It is component of Wnt signalling pathway. It is located in the cytosol of cells and controls cell fate, adhesion and cell polarity during embryonic development. It also controls oncogenic effects of β-catenin, so prevents carcinomas. Somatic mutation of APC gene causes carcinoma of stomach, colon, pancreas and melanoma. Inherited mutation causes familial adenomatous polyposis coli/colon cancer.
- **Micro RNA (miRNA):** These are small non-coding, ssRNA, approx. 22 nucleotides in length. They mediate sequence-specific inhibition of messenger RNA (mRNA) translation through the action of the RNA-induced silencing complex (RISC). They can either cause target mRNA cleavage or repress its translocation. *Examples*:
  a. Mir 34: It is activated by p53 gene. With its activation, p53 gene is able to repress the function of other genes.
  b. Mir-200: Promote epithelial-mesenchymal transitions, invasiveness and metastasis
  c. Mir-155: It upregulates genes that promote proliferation (Myc) and cause lymphoma.
- **Chromothripsis:** The word 'chromothripsis' literally means 'chromosome shattering'. Chromosomes that under chromothripsis first fragment into many pieces and then get stitched back together in a random order by DNA repair processes, most likely non-homologous end joining. This generates a highly rearranged chromosome (massive genomic rearrangement) from a single catastrophic event. It is known to be involved in both cancer and congenital diseases. It opposes the conventional theory that cancer is the gradual acquisition of genomic rearrangements and somatic mutations over time.
  The first evidence of chromothripsis came from whole-genome sequencing of CLL patients.
  Chromothripsis has been found in a range (3–25%) of other cancer types, such as neuroblastoma, medulloblastoma, bone cancers, multiple myeloma, and lung, renal, and thyroid cancers.
- **Genes promoting metastasis:** Ezrin (in rhabdomyosarcoma, and osteosarcoma)
- **Genes inhibiting metastasis:** NM23, KAI-1 (prostate cancer) and Ki 55 (malignant melanoma).
- **Metastatic oncogenes:** SNAIL, TWIST
- **Suppress metastasis of breast cancer:** Mir-335, mir-126
- **Promotes metastasis of breast cancer:** Mir 10^b
- **Smallest clinically detectable mass:** 1 g = 10^9 cells
- **Maximum mass compatible with life:** 1 kg = 10^{12} cells
- **Sarcoma causing lymph node metastasis:** Alveolar rhabdomyosarcoma (particularly solid variant), angiosarcoma, epithelioid sarcoma and synovial sarcoma.

- **Carcinoma causing haematogenous spread:**
  a. Renal cell carcinoma: Through renal vein
  b. Hepatocellular carcinoma (carcinoma of liver): Penetrate portal and hepatic radicals to grow within them (intravenous spread).
  c. Choriocarcinoma of testis (also other NSGCT or nonseminomatous germ cell tumor): Early hematogenous spread to lungs (most common site), liver, brain and other visceral sites.
- **Tumour lysis syndrome:** It is often seen with Burkitt's lymphoma, ALL, CLL, and arely solid tumors. It is caused by destruction of a large number of rapidly proliferating neolplastic cells. The biochemical features are:
  a. *Hyperuricemia*: Due to increased turnover of nucleic acids
  b. *Hyperkalemia*: Due to release of the most abundant intracellular cation potassium.
  c. *Hyperphosphatemia*: Due to release of intracellular phosphate
  d. *Hypocalcemia*: Due to complexing of calcium with the elevated phosphate
  e. *Lactic acidosis*
  f. *Hyperuricemia*: It can cause uric acid precipitation in the kidney causing acute renal failure.

MBBS Curriculum in Pathology and Question Papers

- MBBS Curriculum in Pathology
- West Bengal University of Health Sciences (WBUHS) 2023 and 2022 Question Papers

MBBS CURRICULUM IN PATHOLOGY

GOAL

The broad goal of the teaching of undergraduate student in Pathology is to provide the students with a comprehensive knowledge of the pathologic basis of disease, in order to enable him/her to achieve complete understanding of the natural course, clinical manifestations, complications and sequel of disease.

OBJECTIVES

1. Knowledge

At the end of the course, the student should be able to:

- Describe the structure and ultra-structure of a pathologically altered cell, mechanisms of cell degeneration, cell death and repair and be able to correlate structural and functional alterations.
- Explain the pathophysiologic processes which govern the maintenance of homeostasis, mechanisms of their disturbance and the morphological and clinical manifestations associated with it.
- Describe the mechanisms and morphologic patterns to tissue response to injury so that she/he can appreciate the pathophysiology of disease processes and their clinical manifestations.
- Correlate normal and altered morphology (gross and microscopic) of different organ systems in common diseases to the extent needed for understanding of disease processes and their clinical significance.

2. Skills

At the end of the course, the student should be able to:

- Describe the rationale and principles of commonly followed technical procedures of the diagnostic laboratory tests and interpretation of the results.
- Perform the simple bed-side tests on blood, urine and other biological fluid samples.
- Draw a rational scheme of investigations aimed at diagnosing and managing the cases of common disorders.
- Understand biochemical/physiological disturbances that occur as a result of disease in collaboration with pre-clinical departments.

3. Integration

At the end of training, he/she should be able to integrate the causes of disease and relationship of different etiological factors (social, economic and environmental) that contribute to the natural history of diseases most prevalent in India.

Course Contents

General Consideration:

The curriculum/course content shall include the topics in following categories: Up to 70% of the content as a whole and chapter-wise should be from MUST KNOW category; 20–25% should be from DESIRABLE TO KNOW category; and remainder 5% should be from NICE TO KNOW category. Accordingly, the THEORY LECTURES and FINAL (SUMMATIVE) ASSESSMENT should be as per the above.

The CHAPTER WISE course contents as per the category are as follows:

The topics for PRACTICAL (Pr) will be covered as a lecture during 1st hour of the Practicals followed by demonstration of gross specimens, microscopic slides, OSPE charts, instruments, or clinic pathological discussion (pertaining to the topic) to be covered in next 2 hours (Total duration of practical 3 hours, twice weekly). The goal should be to maintain the temporal correlation between the theory topics and the corresponding practical.

A. GENERAL PATHOLOGY:

1. CELL INJURY:

- **MUST KNOW:** Causes and mechanism of ischemic, toxic, free-radical/reperfusion induced injury; pathogenesis and pathology of reversible and irreversible cell injury; hyaline and fatty change (Pr). Necrosis: compare and contrast between different morphological patterns and their clinical correlation; gangrene (dry and weight) (Pr); compare and contrast between necrosis and apoptosis; mechanism of apoptosis and their clinical implications, compare and contrast between dystrophic and metastatic calcification; pigment deposition such as melanin, bilirubin, hemosiderin and anthracotic pigments **(Pr)**.
- **DESIRABLE TO KNOW:** Necroptosis.
- **NICE TO KNOW:** Cellular ageing, telomeres
- **Pr: Practical topics**

2. INFLAMMATION AND REPAIR:

- **MUST KNOW:** Features and causes; vascular events, cellular events in acute inflammation; cells and mediators of inflammation; morphological variant and outcome (ulcer, granulation tissue) (Pr) of acute inflammation; chronic inflammation (Pr): causes, types, non-specific and granulomatous (Pr) with examples; cutaneous wound healing and repair by primary and secondary union and factors modifying them; fracture healing.
- **DESIRABLE TO KNOW:** Growth factors, scar formation, keloid.
- **NICE TO KNOW:** Cell cycle and stem cells.
- **Pr: Practical topics**

3. HEMODYNAMIC DISTURBANCES:

- **MUST KNOW:** Pathogenesis and types of edema (transudate *vs* exudate); hyperemia vs congestion; chronic venous congestion (Pr): Lung (with heart failure cells), Liver (Nutmeg liver) and Spleen (Gamna–Gandy bodies); normal hemostasis, Virchow triad, coagulation cascade; thrombosis; infarct (Pr): red vs pale; embolism: formation, types and fate, effect on tissues; Shock: pathogenesis, types and organ specific changes.
- **DESIRABLE TO KNOW:** Rare causes of thrombophilia (antiphospholipid antibody syndrome, Factor V Leiden mutations, etc.)
- **Pr: Practical topics**

4. GROWTH DISTURBANCE AND NEOPLASIA:

- **MUST KNOW: Cellular adaptation (Pr):** Atrophy, hypertrophy, hyperplasia, metaplasia, dysplasia and intraepithelial neoplasia including carcinoma *in situ*, premalignant conditions. Neoplasia: Causes, classification, histogenesis and molecular basis, biological behaviour, benign versus malignant (Pr), nomenclature. Malignant neoplasms: Grade and stage, metastasis and invasion. Carcinogenesis: Environmental carcinogens, viral, chemical, occupational, hereditary. Gross and microscopic features, clinical correlation, mode of spread and prognosis of common benign and malignant tumors **(Pr)**.

- **DESIRABLE TO KNOW:** Laboratory diagnosis of cancer, Tumor markers, Para neoplastic syndromes.
- **NICE TO KNOW:** Newer diagnostic tool in cancer: immunohistochemistry, flow cytometry, karyotyping.
- **Pr: Practical topics, Soft tissue tumours of both benign/malignant (compare and contrast).**

5. IMMUNOLOGY:

- **MUST KNOW:** Immune system: organization (central and peripheral organs), cells, molecules and regulation; T and B cell receptor; Human leukocyte antigen/MHC; mechanism of different hypersensitivity reactions with examples; central and peripheral tolerance; autoimmune diseases: both organs specific and systemic with specific examples like SLE; Amyloidosis: classification, morphology (Pr), diagnosis:
- **DESIRABLE TO KNOW:** Immunology of Sjögren syndrome, Hashimoto thyroiditis, pathology of transplant rejection, graft versus host reaction.
- **Pr: Practical topics**
- **Redundant topic:** Immune deficiency: primary and secondary, tumor-host interaction, tumor immunology.

6. GENETIC DISORDERS:

- **MUST KNOW:** Basic concepts of genetic disorders (mutations, autosomal dominant, recessive, X-linked disorders) and some common examples. Down syndrome, Turner syndrome and Klinefelter syndrome.
- **DESIRABLE TO KNOW: Karyotyping**
- **NICE TO KNOW: Pedigree chart analysis**
- **Practical topics: None**
- **Redundant topic: All other** rare genetic disorders, storage disorders, mutation analysis, molecular diagnosis, etc.

7. INFECTIOUS DISEASE:

- **MUST KNOW:** Tuberculosis, Leprosy and HIV/AIDS to be included with horizontal integration with microbiology.
- **DESIRABLE TO KNOW (Pr):** Actinomyosis, mycetoma, rhinosporidiosis, hydatid disease, molluscum contagiosum; parasitic diseases: Malaria, filaria, amoebiasis
- **Pr: Practical topics**
- **Redundant topic:** All other bacterial, viral disease, Leishmania, Parasitic disease, etc.

8. INFANCY AND CHILDHOOD:

- **DESIRABLE TO KNOW:** Cystic fibrosis, Tumors: Neuroblastoma, Wilms' tumor, sacrococcygeal teratoma.
- **Redundant topic:** Nutritional disorders—Protein-energy malnutrition, vitamin deficiency.

9. MISCELLANEOUS DISORDERS (for student symposium):

- Occupational and environmental pathology.
- Alcohol and health
- Smoking and its effect
- Obesity and its relation with disease
- Diet and its relation to cancer and atherosclerosis
- Nutritional disorders: Protein energy malnutrition, vitamin deficiency.

B. HEMATOPATHOLOGY:

- **MUST KNOW:** Constituents of blood and bone marrow, regulation of hematopoiesis. **Anemia (MODULE) (Pr) (OSPE charts):** Classification and clinical features, Laboratory approach. Nutritional anemia: Iron deficiency, Vitamin B12 and Folate deficiency. Hemolytic Anemia: Classification and Laboratory diagnosis. Thalassemia, Haemoglobinopathies like Sickle cell anemia, Hereditary Spherocytosis. Aplastic Anemia, Pancytopenia. Leukemoid reaction, Leukemia (Pr) (OSPE): Acute and Chronic-classification (myeloid and lymphoid) and diagnosis. Multiple myeloma.
- **DESIRABLE TO KNOW:** G6PD deficiency, Acquired hemolytic anemia: **PNH**, Leukoerythroblastic blood picture, Autoimmune hemolytic anemia, hemolytic disease of newborn, MDS, Approach to a bleeding child, ITP, Coagulation disorders like Hemophilia, Von Willebrand Disease, DIC.
- **NICE TO KNOW: Flow cytometry in leukemia, rare thrombophilic states-APLA syndrome.**
- **Practical topics:** Blood transfusion practice: Grouping, Cross matching, Donor selection, and Component therapy, Rational use of blood transfusion, adverse reactions and transmissible infections.

C. SYSTEMIC PATHOLOGY:

1. CARDIOVASCULAR PATHOLOGY:

- **MUST KNOW:** Rheumatic heart disease, and Infective endocarditis, **Vegetation in heart**
- Hypertension, Pathogenesis, pathology and morphology of atherosclerosis and ischemic heart disease (acute myocardial infarction) **(Pr)**
- **DESIRABLE TO KNOW:** Vasculitis (Classification and selected entities), aneurysms, pericarditis
- **NICE TO KNOW:** Cyanotic and acyanotic heart disease (VSD, Fallot tetralogy)
- **Pr: Practical topics**
- **Redundant topic:** Cardiomyopathies, cardiac tumours, and others.

2. RESPIRATORY PATHOLOGY:

- **MUST KNOW:** Structure of bronchial tree and alveoli, defense mechanism, normal and altered lung function, concept of obstructive and restrictive lung disease, Pneumonia (lobar vs bronchopneumonia) (Pr), Lung abscess. Chronic obstructive pulmonary disease: Emphysema, Chronic bronchitis, Bronchial asthma, Bronchiectasis (Pr). Lung tumors (Pr): aetiopathogenesis and types (including newer prognostic and therapeutic markers).
- **NICE TO KNOW:** Mesothelioma, Interstitial lung disease, Hyaline Membrane Disease and ARDS.
- **Pr: Practical topics**
- **Redundant topic: Pulmonary hypertension**

3. HEAD and NECK and GASTROINTESTINAL PATHOLOGY:

- **MUST KNOW:** Oral pathology: Leukoplakia, Premalignant conditions and carcinoma. Salivary gland pathology: Common benign and malignant tumors (pleomorphic adenoma, Warthin tumor, Mucoepidermoid carcinoma, Adenoid cystic carcinoma) (Pr). Barrett esophagus. Gastritis-types, *H. pylori vs.* autoimmune gastritis. Benign vs malignant gastric ulcer (Pr), Tumors of stomach: carcinoma (Pr), MALT lymphoma. Inflammatory diseases of intestine: Typhoid vs Tubercular ulcer, Amoebic colitis, Ulcerative colitis (Pr) *vs* Crohn's disease, Appendicitis (Pr). Intestinal tumors: Polyps (Pr), adenoma-carcinoma sequence.
- **DESIRABLE TO KNOW:** Coeliac disease, GIST, Carcinoid
- **NICE TO KNOW: Hirschsprung disease**
- **Pr: Practical topics**
- **Redundant topic: Nasopharyngeal carcinoma, Laryngeal lesion, Ischemic bowel disease.**

4. LIVER AND BILIARY PATHOLOGY:

- **MUST KNOW:** Jaundice: types, etiopathogenesis **(Pr/OSPE)**, and differential diagnosis Viral Hepatitis: Acute and Chronic, Cirrhosis: Etiology, classification, Post necrotic, alcoholic, metabolic (Wilson), Morphology, complications. Alcoholic liver disease, NAFLD. Gallbladder diseases (Pr): Cholecystitis, cholelithiasis, carcinoma. Tumors of liver: hepatocellular carcinoma, metastasis.
- **DESIRABLE TO KNOW: LFT, Portal hypertension, Liver failure**
- **NICE TO KNOW: Neonatal cholestasis, biliary atresia,** Molecular classification of hepatic adenomas, carcinomas.
- **Pr: Practical topics**
- **Redundant topic: Vascular disease of liver, acute fatty liver of pregnancy,** Pancreatitis and Pancreatic tumors.

5. LYMPHORETICULAR PATHOLOGY:

- **MUST KNOW:** Lymphadenopathy-Causes, Lymphoma: Hodgkin and non-Hodgkin-classification scheme and morphology of selected lymphomas, Diseases of spleen-splenomegaly, hypersplenism
- **Pr: Practical topics**
- **Redundant topic:** Rare causes of lymphadenopathy, rare lymphomas.

6. URINARY TRACT PATHOLOGY:

- **MUST KNOW:** Structure and function of normal glomerulus, glomerular response to injury, Nephritic vs Nephrotic syndrome **(OSPE)**, Glomerulonephritis: Acute poststreptococcal/post infectious, Crescentic/RPGN, Nephrotic Syndrome (MCD, MGN, MPGN, and FSGS), diabetic nephropathy, chronic renal failure, polycystic kidney disease (Pr), Urinary tract infection and Pyelonephritis, Obstructive uropathy, Hydronephrosis, Nephrolithiasis. Renal tumors: Renal cell carcinoma (Pr), Benign hyperplasia of prostate, carcinoma prostate **(Pr)**.
- **DESIRABLE TO KNOW:** Acute tubular necrosis, benign and malignant nephrosclerosis, Urinary bladder: cystitis, urothelial carcinoma
- **NICE TO KNOW:** Gleason scoring for carcinoma prostate
- **Pr: Practical topics:** Renal function tests, Urinalysis

7. REPRODUCTIVE SYSTEM PATHOLOGY:

- **MUST KNOW:** Diseases of cervix: Cervical carcinoma (Pr), PAP stain, Screening and diagnosis (CIN). Hormonal influences and histology of different phases of Endometrium. Endometrial hyperplasia and carcinoma (Pr), Smooth muscle tumor (Pr), Endometriosis/ adenomyosis (Pr). Hydatidiform mole (Complete vs partial) (Pr) and Choriocarcinoma, Ovarian tumors (Pr). Diseases of breast-fibrocystic disease, Fibroadenoma, Breast Carcinoma, Phylloides tumor, Tumors of testis.
- **DESIRABLE TO KNOW:** Molecular basis of endometrial carcinoma
- **NICE TO KNOW:** Uncommon ovarian and testicular tumors, DUB
- **REDUNDANT:** Pelvic inflammatory disease, Valval and vaginal diseases, Genital tuberculosis. Paget disease of vulva. Semen analysis and investigation of infertility.
- **Pr: Practical topics**

8. MUSCULOSKELETAL PATHOLOGY:

- **MUST KNOW:** Osteomyelitis-Acute, chronic, tuberculous. Tumors: Classification, Osteosarcoma (Pr), Chondrosarcoma (Pr), Giant cell tumor (Pr), Ewing's sarcoma.
- **DESIRABLE TO KNOW: Rheumatoid arthritis (Pannus), Gout, Paget disease of bone,** Osteoporosis, Osteoarthritis.
- **NICE TO KNOW:** Rickets, Osteomalacia
- **REDUNDANT:** Tuberculous. Jaw-Ameloblastoma.
- **Pr: Practical topics**

9. ENDOCRINE PATHOLOGY:

- **MUST KNOW:** Non-neoplastic lesions of thyroid: Colloid goiter (Pr), Autoimmune thyroiditis (Hashimoto thyroiditis (Pr), thyrotoxicosis/Grave disease), tumors of thyroid (papillary, follicular, and medullary) **(Pr)**.
- **DESIRABLE TO KNOW: MEN syndrome, pheochromocytoma**
- **NICE TO KNOW:** Pituitary hyperfunction tumors, Hyperparathyroidism
- Pr: Practical topics.

10. NEUROPATHOLOGY:

- **MUST KNOW:** CSF and its disturbance, inflammatory disorders: Meningitis (Pyogenic, Tubercular, Viral, Others) with CSF charts (Pr) and Brain abscess. CNS tumors: Astrocytoma and Meningioma (Pr): classification
- **NICE TO KNOW:** Cerebrovascular accident, hemorrhage, aneurysm, Oligodendroglioma, ependymoma
- **REDUNDANT TOPIC:** Neurodegenerative/demyelinating disorder, muscular dystrophy, neuropathies
- **Pr: Practical topics**

11. SKIN TUMORS:

- **Squamous cell carcinoma, basal cell carcinoma, malignant melanoma (Pr)**
- Molecular mechanism of melanoma pathogenesis **(NICE TO KNOW)**
- **Pr: Practical topics**

PRACTICAL SKILLS

Acquisition of Skills:

The students should be able to:

- Acquire knowledge to collect, store and transport materials for various pathological tests including histopathology, cytopathology, hematopathology, blood bank and clinical pathology in a proper manner.
- Describe accurately and arrive at a logical diagnosis of common macroscopic findings in a pathological specimen such as pneumonia, cirrhosis, gangrene, etc.
- Specimens (gross appearance) such as pneumonia, cirrhosis, gangrene, etc.
- Interpret and arrive at a conclusive diagnosis in the microscopic analysis of common diseases like tuberculosis, carcinoma, acute inflammation, etc.
- Perform with accuracy and reliability various commonly performed hematological Procedures such as hemoglobin estimation, peripheral smear staining and reporting. At the same time, they will acquire knowledge on recent techniques of automation during their visit to lab.
- Calculate red cell indices and interpret the significance as well as common hematological abnormalities (microcytic hypochromic anemia, megaloblastic /macrocytic anemia/ pancytopenia) in CBC charts.
- Perform independently complete examination of urine and detect abnormal findings and interpret the results. They should also have an exposure to diagnostic kits available for urine tests.
- Perform independently grouping of blood.
- Aware of the procedure for common tests like ESR, PCV, vacutainers, bone marrow examination, semen analysis and interpret abnormal findings.
- Interpret abnormal laboratory (biochemical, hematological and serological) values of common diseases.
- Adopt universal precautions for self-protection and patient safety.

Practicals

1. Up to 15 hours (maximum) will be devoted to practical skills pertaining to hematology, clinical pathology, and blood banking as mentioned below:
   - Perform a complete urine examination and detect abnormalities and correlate clinically.
   - Perform with accuracy and reliability various hematological procedures such as Hemoglobin estimation, peripheral smear staining and reporting and blood grouping.
   - Observing or performing under guidance tests like ESR, PCV, bone marrow examination, and interpret abnormal findings.
2. *Remainderl 30–135 hours* of the entire practical shall be devoted to Identify and interpret gross and microscopic feature of pathological specimens and slides (as mentioned as **Pr** in course contents). This will also include discussion of case studies based on the real case scenario and appropriate laboratory findings of patients along with gross and microscopic findings wherever applicable to learn clinic pathological correlation (OSPE charts).
3. *Up to 3 hours each (total 12 hours) may be devoted for REVISION PURPOSE before formative and final/summative assessment.*

WEST BENGAL UNIVERSITY OF HEALTH SCIENCES (WBUHS) 2023 AND 2022 QUESTION PAPERS

The West Bengal University of Health Sciences
MBBS 2nd Professional Examination (New Regulation) March–April 2023

Subject: Pathology **Full Marks: 100**
Paper: I **Time: 3 hours**

Attempt all questions. The figures in the margin indicate full marks.

1. a. A 4-year-old boy was presented to paediatric OPD with growth retardation, prominence of cheek bones, pallor and splenomegaly. Peripheral blood smear shows marked anisocytosis, poikilocytosis, microcytosis, hypochromia along with target cells and fragmented red cells. The Hb level is 6 gm/dL. (1 + 4 + 4 + 6)
   i. What is your provisional diagnosis?
   ii. How do you classify this condition in this young age?
   iii. How will you proceed to confirm your diagnosis?
   iv. How will you explain the development of various clinical and laboratory features in this patient?

   b. A 30-year-old male met with roads traffic accident and had massive hemorrhage. The patient was pale, pulse was rapid and thread skin was cold and clammy. (2 + 3 + 10)
   i. What is the provisional diagnosis?
   ii. Classify the condition.
   iii. What are the different stages of the condition and their respective pathophysiology.

2. Answer the following: (3 × 10)
   a. Discuss wound healing by first and second intention.
   b. Describe the pathogenesis and staining characteristics of amyloid.
   c. Describe the pathogenesis of metastasis.

3. Write short notes on: (2 × 5)
   a. Role of AETCOM in an intravenous blood drawing session of an adolescent girl.
   b. Reactive Oxygen Species.

4. Explain the following statements: (5 × 4)
   a. Transfusion of blood component is more rational than whole blood transfusion.
   b. Leukaemia and leukemoid reactions are different.
   c. Tumor markers aid in diagnosis of malignancy.
   d. Inborn errors of metabolism usually follow autosomal recessive mode of inheritance.
   e. Reticulocyte count is helpful in differentiating types of anemia.

5. Choose the correct option for each of the following: (10 × 1)

i. Auer rods are derived from:

a. RNA
b. DNA
c. Primary granules
d. Secondary granules

ii. All are types of tissue macrophages except:

a. Littoral cell
b. Hoffbauer cell
c. Osteoclast
d. Osteoblast

iii. Leukocyte alkaline phosphatase (LAP) score is elevated in;

a. AML
b. CML
c. Myeloid metaplasia
d. Myeloid leukaemoid reaction

iv. Parvovirus B19 infection is often associated with:

a. Polycythemia Vera
b. Anaemia of chronic inflammation
c. Aplastic anemia due to bone marrow failure (hypocellularity)
d. Pure red cell aplasia.

v. Which of the following diseases is due to mutation of mitochondrial gene?

a. Leber hereditary optic neuropathy
b. Prader Willi syndrome
c. Angelman syndrome
d. Familial mental retardation

vi. A 40-year-old woman has had chronic congestive heart failure for the past 3 years. In the past 2 months, she developed a productive cough of rust colored sputum. A sputum cytology specimen now shows numerous hemosiderin laden macrophages. Which of the following subcellular structures in these macrophages is most important for the accumulation of this pigment?

a. Chromosome
b. Endoplasmic reticulum
c. Golgi apparatus
d. Lysosome

vii. Normal M:E ratio is:

a. 1:1
b. 3:1
c. 5:1
d. 10:1

viii. Which of the following CD markers is NOT primarily B-cell associated?

a. CD8
b. CD20
c. CD19
d. CD23

ix. Leprosy bacilli are:

a. Not acid fast
b. As acid fast as tubercle bacilli
c. Less acid fast
d. More acid fast compared to tubercle bacilli.

x. Classical markers for Hodgkin's disease are:

a. CD15 and CD20
b. CD15 and CD22
c. CD15 and CD30
d CD20 and CD30

The West Bengal University of Health Sciences
MBBS 2nd Professional Examination (New Regulation) March–April 2023

Subject: Pathology **Full Marks: 100**
Paper: II **Time: 3 hours**

Attempt all questions. The figures in the margin indicate full marks.

1. a. A 6-year-old boy developed puffiness of face, oliguria and mild hypertension two weeks after an attack of sore throat. (2 + 5 + 5 + 3)
 i. What is the provisional diagnosis?
 ii. What is the pathogenesis of the condition?
 iii. What laboratory investigations to be done to confirm the diagnosis?
 iv. Mention the fates of this condition.

b. A 65-year-old male smoker developed cough, occasional hemoptysis and marked weight loss in 4–6 weeks. Chest X-ray shows an opacity in right upper lobe. On examination one moderately enlarged, firm lymph node was found over the neck. (1 + 5 + 6 + 3)
 i. What may be the provisional diagnosis?
 ii. How will you proceed for a quick confirmation of your suspicion?
 iii. How will you classify this condition histologically?
 iv. What may be the complications in this case?

2. Answer the following: (3 × 10)
 a. Describe the pathogenesis of carcinoma of cervix.
 b. Describe the pathogenesis of peptic ulcer.
 c. Discuss the pathogenesis of nodular hyperplasia of prostate.

3. Write short notes on: (2 × 5)
 a. Leiomyoma of uterus.
 b. Pleomorphic salivary adenoma.

4. Explain the following statements: (5 × 4)
 a. Crohn's disease and ulcerative colitis have macroscopic and microscopic differences.
 b. Phyllodes tumor of breast is not always benign in behaviour.
 c. Alcoholism is not always a pre-requisite for cirrhosis.
 d. Diagnostic features of carcinoid tumour are specific
 e. Sequestrum leads to involucrum formation.

5. Choose the correct option for each of the following: (10 × 1)
 i. The cardinal features of Tetralogy of Fallot include all of the followings except:
  a. Atrial septal defect
  b. Ventricular septal defect

c. Obstruction to right ventricular outflow tract
d. Right ventricular hypertrophy.

ii. Which of the following statements is true for renal cell carcinoma:
a. It is not related to cigarette smoking.
b. Clear cell type of RCC is usually hereditary.
c. Most likely arise from glomerular epithelial cells.
d. Its characteristic tendency is to invade the renal vein.

iii. In Rheumatoid Arthritis, bone resorption is contributed by which cytokine?
a. IFN-gumma b. IL-17
c. RANKL d. TNF

iv. Modified macrophages of brain are:
a. Schwann cell b. Microglia
c. Astrocytes d. Ganglion

v. Emphysema associated most with alpha I antitrypsin deficiency is:
a. Panacinar b. Centriacinar
c. Distal acinar d. Irregular

vi. Long standing cases of Crohn's disease may develop the following complications except:
a. Malabsorption b. Toxic megacolon
c. Fistula formation d. Stricture formation

vii. Arias Stella reaction occurs in:
a. Ectopic tubal gestation only b. All ectopic gestations
c. Uterine gestation d. Uterine as well as ectopic gestation

viii. Astrocytoma occurring in children is commonly:
a. Fibrillary b. Pilocytic
c. Anaplastic d. Glioblastoma muttiforme

ix. Krukenberg's tumour may have all primary tumours listed below except:
a. Breast b. Stomach
c. Liver d. Pancreas

x. In an undescended testis, the following tumor develops most often:
a. Seminoma b. Teratoma
c. Choriocarcinoma d. Yolk sac tumor

The West Bengal University of Health Sciences
MBBS 2nd Professional Examination (New Regulation) May 2022

Subject: Pathology **Full Marks: 100**
Paper: I **Time: 3 hours**

Attempt all questions. The figures in the margin indicate full marks.

1. a. A 42-year-old male with H/o RTA presented with a lacerated injury of soft tissue of lower limbs without any fracture of bones. (2 + 5 + 3 + 5)
   i. What tissue will replace this devitalised injured tissue in the process of healing?
   ii. What are different stages of healing here?
   iii. What are the differences between healing by primary intention and by secondary intension?
   iv. Enumerate important complications of healing.

   b. A 30-year-old female presented with severe anaemia, weakness and dyspnoea. Blood examination showed: Hb as 6.0 g/dl and low MCV. (5 + 5 + 5)
   i. What is your provisional diagnosis?
   ii. What laboratory tests will you perform to confirm the diagnosis?
   iii. Discuss the causes and pathogenesis of this condition.

2. a. What is an infarct? Classify infarct and describe the factors that influence the development of an infact? (2 + 4 + 4)
   b. Define shock. Describe pathogenesis of hypovolemic shock. (2 + 8)
   c. What are conventional laboratory tests for thalassemia? (10)

3. Write short notes on following: (2 × 5)
   a. Idiopathic thrombocytopenic purpura.
   b. Role of AETCOM in medical teaching.

4. Explain the following statements: (5 × 4)
   a. Metaplasia is a double-edged sword.
   b. Sickle cell trait patient are resistant to falciparum malaria.
   c. Pre-transfusion screening of blood is mandatory.
   d. Causes of oedema are multifactorial.
   e. HPV is an oncogenic virus.

5. Choose the correct option for each of the following: (10 × 1)
   1. All, are true about chemokines except:
      a. Small protein (8–11 kD)
      b. Acts as chemoattractant
      c. Attracts monocytes
      d. Interferons are also included in this group

2. Naked granulomas are seen in:
   a. Wegener's granulomatosis
   b. Tuberculosis
   c. Syphilis
   d. Sarcoidosis
3. All are the effects of free radicals *except*:
   a. Lipid peroxidation
   b. Oxidative change in protein
   c. Breaks in DNA
   d. Synthesis of new protein
4. Karyorrhexis refers to:
   a. Cell membrane lysis
   b. Fading of cell nucleus
   c. Disintegration of cell nucleus
   d. Condensation of nucleus
5. The five stages of hemostasis are given below in random order. Put them in correct order (a) clot dissolution, (b) blood coagulation, (c) vessel spasm, (d) clot retraction, (v) formation of platelet plug:
   a. cabed
   b. acbde
   c. cebda
   d. ecdba
6. A malignant neoplasm is described as grade I on microscopic examination. What is best interpretation with this:
   a. Undifferentiated
   b. Moderately differentiated
   c. Well differentiated
   d. Poorly differentiated
7. Paraneoplastic syndrome is commonly seen with:
   a. Small cell carcinoma plug
   b. Colon adenocarcinoma
   c. Esophageal squamous cell carcinoma
   d. Retinoblastoma
8. Russel bodies are seen in:
   a. Plasma cells
   b. Myeloblast
   c. Lymphoblast
   d. Erythroblast
9. Autoimmune hemolytic anaemia is seen in:
   a. ALL
   b. AML
   c. CLL
   d. CML
10. All are features of apoptosis *except*:
    a. Cell size shrinkage
    b. Pyknosis of nucleus
    c. Cell membrane intact
    d. Presence of inflammatory cells

The West Bengal University of Health Sciences
MBBS 2nd Professional Examination (New Regulation) May 2022

Subject: Pathology **Full Marks: 100**
Paper: II **Time: 3 hours**

Attempt all questions. The figures in the margin indicate full marks.

1. a. A 46-year-old male presented with epigastric burning pain usually occurs 2–3 hrs after meal in day and is worse at midnight. (2 + 5 + 5 + 3)
   i. What is your provisional diagnosis?
   ii. Write about the risk factors and pathogenesis of this disorder.
   iii. Describe in short about the morphology of the disease.
   iv. Mention complications of the disease.

   b. A 55-year-old female presented with painless, hard fixed lump over breast. On examination, left axillary lymph nodes are palpable. (2 + 5 + 5 + 3)
   i. What is your provisional diagnosis?
   ii. Enumerate the risk factors of this disease.
   iii. Write about the classification of this disease
   iv. Describe the morphology of various types in short.

2. a. Write down the pathogenesis of cirrhosis of liver in a alcoholic patient. (10)
   b. Enumerate the histopathology of lung lesions in pneumococcal pneumonia. (10)
   c. What are the immunological mechanisms of glomerular injury? (10)

3. Write short notes on following: (2 × 5)
   a. Long-term complications of diabetes mellitus.
   b. Morphology of teratoma of ovary.

4. Explain the following statements: (5 × 4)
   a. Renal cell carcinoma can be associated with raised haematocrit.
   b. Explain how a colonic polyp can lead to colonic carcinom
   c. Ewing sarcoma and primitive neuroectodermal tumors are unified into a single category.
   d. Pulmonary tuberculosis in HIV infected persons is usually sputum negative.
   e. Dihydroxy testosterone plays a critical role in the pathogenesis of benign prostatic hyperplasia.

5. Choose the correct option for each of the following: (10 × 1)
   1. All are precursor lesions of lung carcinoma *except*:
      a. Squamous metaplasia
      b. Squamous dysplasia
      c. Atypical adenomatous hyperplasia
      d. Diffuse idiopathic pulmonary neuroendocrine cell hyperplasia

2. Majority of carcinoma of oropharynx harbors oncogenic variant of HPV; Particularly
   a. HPV-11
   b. HPV-16
   c. HPV-18
   d. HPV-21
3. Most characteristic finding of glomerulonephritis is
   a. Proteinuria
   b. Edema
   c. Oliguria
   d. Red cell casts in urine
4. All are the features of ulcerative colitis *except*:
   a. Pseudopolyps
   b. Ulcers
   c. Toxic megacolon
   d. Strictures
5. Which of the following is *not* a premalignant condition?
   a. Sessile serrated adenoma
   b. Hyperplastic polyp
   c. Juvenile polyposis syndrome
   d. Tubular adenoma
6. Renal transplant patients are prone to get infection with:
   a. Adenovirus
   b. EB virus
   c. Cytomegalovirus
   d. Coxsackievirus
7. Rosette's are found in:
   a. Neuroblastoma
   b. Liposarcoma
   c. Fibrosarcoma
   d. Leiomyoma
8. The tumour marker CA-125 is raised in which ovarian tumor:
   a. Papailary serous cystadeno carcinoma
   b. Malignant Brenner tumour
   c. Granulosa cell tumour
   d. Dysgerminoma
9. Tram track appearance is found in:
   a. IgA nephropathy
   b. Focal segmental glomerulosclerosis
   c. Membranoproliferative disease
   d. Good Pasture syndrome
10. Krukenberg tumour can be caused by all *except*:
    a. Colon carcinoma
    b. Carcinoma of breast
    c. Carcinoma of gallbladder
    d. Choriocarcinoma

Appendices

Appendix

I

Common Instruments in Pathology

HAEMATOLOGY INSTRUMENTS/ REAGENTS

Antisera (Antibody) for ABO and Rh Blood Grouping

- Blue-coloured vial: Antisera A
- Yellow-coloured vial: Antisera B
- Pink/red coloured vial: Antisera AB
- Colourless vial: Anti-D (Rh) grouping.

Uses

i. Antisera A, B, and AB for ABO blood grouping
ii. Anti-D for Rh grouping
iii. Both forward and reverse grouping can be done. Refer to Fig. 8.2A, page 95.

Bone Marrow Aspiration Needle

i. **Klima's needle:** In this needle, the adjustable guard is present along the length of the needle. This is more secure than the side guard present in Salah's BM aspiration needle. There is no side screw. Refer to Fig. 3.2B, page 36.
ii. **Salah's needle:** It has a guard which is fixed to the needle by a side screw. Refer to Fig. 3.1B, page 36.

Parts of BM aspiration needle:

- Trocar
- Cannula/stylet
- Adjustable guard or side guard.

Ideal bone marrow needle:

- Should be stout
- 7–8 cm in length
- Well-fitted stylet
- Edges well sharpened.

DLC Counter (Manual) for Differential Leukocyte Count (DLC)

Use: To determine the relative number (percentage, %) of each type of white blood cell presents in the blood.

Instrument: Made of steel with pressing keys and a knob at both ends. Refer to Fig. 2.11, page 23.

Graduated Pipette (1 ml)

Instrument: Glass pipette with etched marking of 0.1 each (Fig. AI.1).

Use: Dispensing required small volume of liquid.

Lancet (Blood Lancet)

Instrument: Similar to a small scalpel but with a double-edged blade or needle. It is made of metal having a sharp-pointed end with fixed depth. Blood lancet is generally disposable (Fig. AI.2).

Uses

i. To make punctures, such as a finger prick to collect capillary blood.

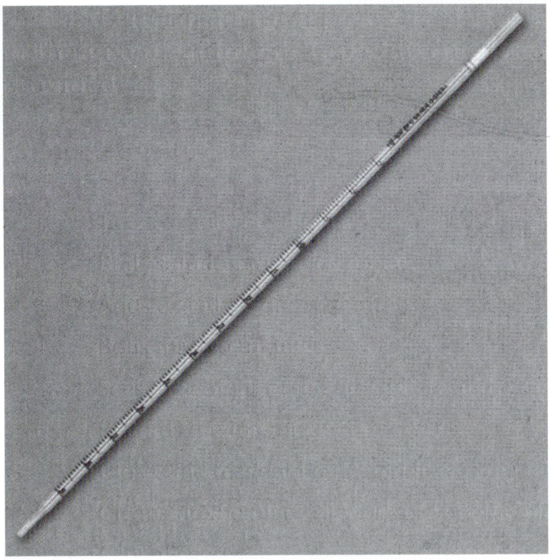

Fig. AI.1: Graduated pipette (1 ml)

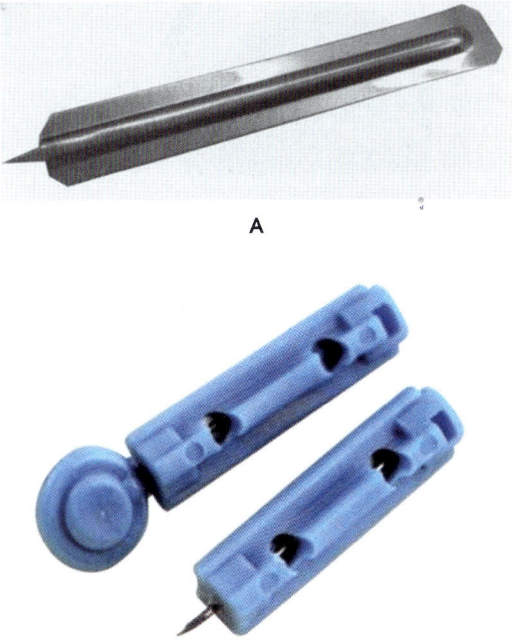

A

B

Fig. AI.2A and B: Blood lancet

ii. Also used to prick the skin in skin testing for allergies.

Neubauer (Improved) Counting Chamber or Haemocytometer

Hemo means blood; *Cyto* means cell; *Meter* means measurement/counter. Thus, it is an instrument used to count the blood cells.

Instrument: It is a thick crystal slide (made up of crystal glass). Generally, it measures 30 × 70 mm with a thickness of 4 mm. Two type: (i) Simple counting chamber (rarely used) which has one counting area in the central part, (ii) double chambers (commonly used) which have two counting areas that can be loaded independently. The depth is 0.1 mm in the double chambers, there is an H-shaped grove and on both sides two counting areas present.

Neubauer chamber's counting grid is 3 × 3 mm in size. The grid has 9 square divisions of width 1 mm. Refer to Fig. 4.3, page 49.

Uses

i. Usually used for counting blood cells (WBC, RBC or platelets)
ii. Sperm counts
iii. Cell count in body fluids.

Pasteur Pipette

Instrument: Also know as droppers or eye droppers. They are usually glass tubes tapered to a narrow point and fitted with a rubber bulb at the top. The combination of the Pasteur pipette and rubber bulb has also been referred to as a **teat pipette**. It has been named after French scientist Louis Pasteur. Pasteur pipette made of plastic is also available (Fig. AI.3).

Uses

i. Used for filling Wintrobe's tube with blood.

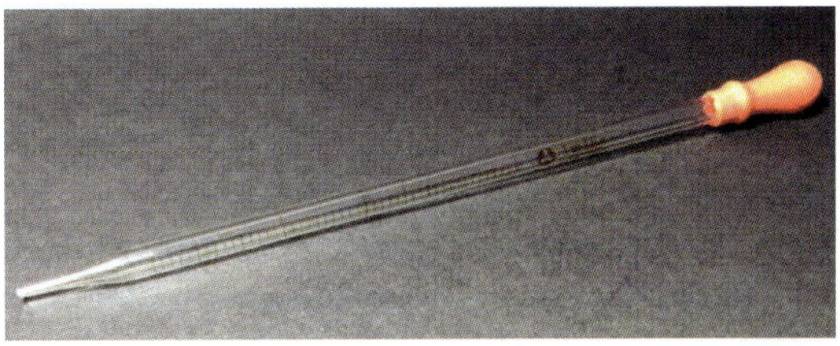

Fig. AI.3: Pasteur pipette

ii. Used to transfer small quantities of liquids or chemical solutions without exposing it to the external environment.

RBC Pipette

Refer to Chapter 4: Total Count of WBC, RBC and Platelets (Refer Fig. 4.8, page 51).

Sahli's Pipette, Haemoglobinometer Tube and Comparator Box

Refer to Chapter 6: Haemoglobin Estimation, Fig. 6.2, page 72).

Stopwatch

Instrument/device: It is a handled timepiece. Both manual and automatic versions are available. In manual timing, the clock is started and stopped by a person pressing a button. In automatic device, both starting and stopping are triggered automatically by sensors (Fig. AI.4).

Uses

i. Used to determine the timing of the end point of in tests for coagulation studies and haemostasis.
ii. Also used to record timings in sports (stop clock).

Thermometer for Water Bath

Instrument: Usually glass thermometer with precision (markings) (Fig. AI.5).

Use: For placing in water bath to take temperature recording.

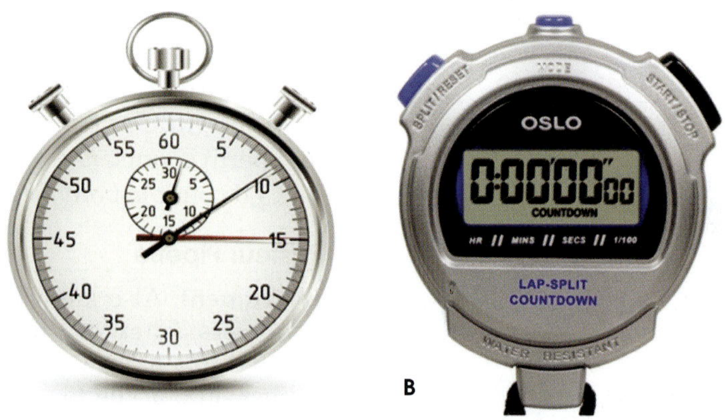

A B

Fig. AI.4A and B: (A) Manual stopwatch; (B) Automatic stopwatch

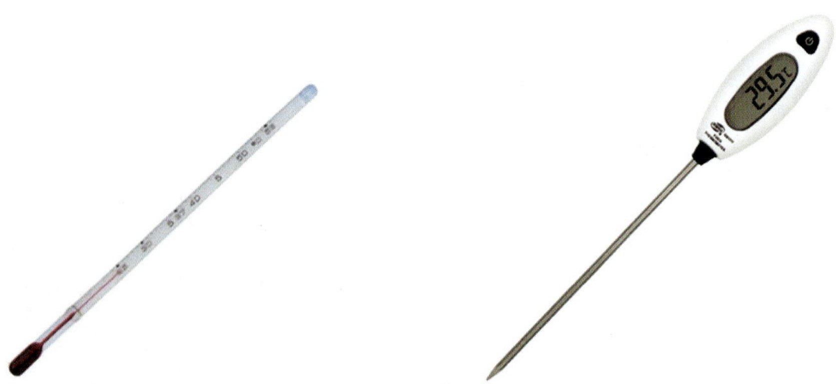

A Glass thermometer B Electric thermometer

Fig. AI.5A and B: Thermometer

Trephine Biopsy (Jamshidi Type) Needle

Instrument: Made of stainless steel with tapering end to reduce crush artifact. It has needle stilette and a guard. Refer to Fig. 3.3A, page 38.

Uses

i. To obtain bone marrow tissue. It is cylindrically shaped solid piece of bone marrow, 2 mm wide and 2 cm long (80 µl).
ii. Bone marrow tissue obtained is processed by paraffin embedding technique for microscopic examination.
iii. Can also be used for immunohistochemistry (IHC), flow cytometry (immunophenotyping) and PCR (polymerase chain reaction).

Vacutainers with Vacupuncture Needle

Schematic diagram of using vacutainer tube and vacutainer needle (Fig. AI.6).

Vacutainer needle + vacutainer holder + vacutainer tube (Fig. AI.7).

Refer to Chapter 1; Blood Collection and Anticoagulants (page 12).

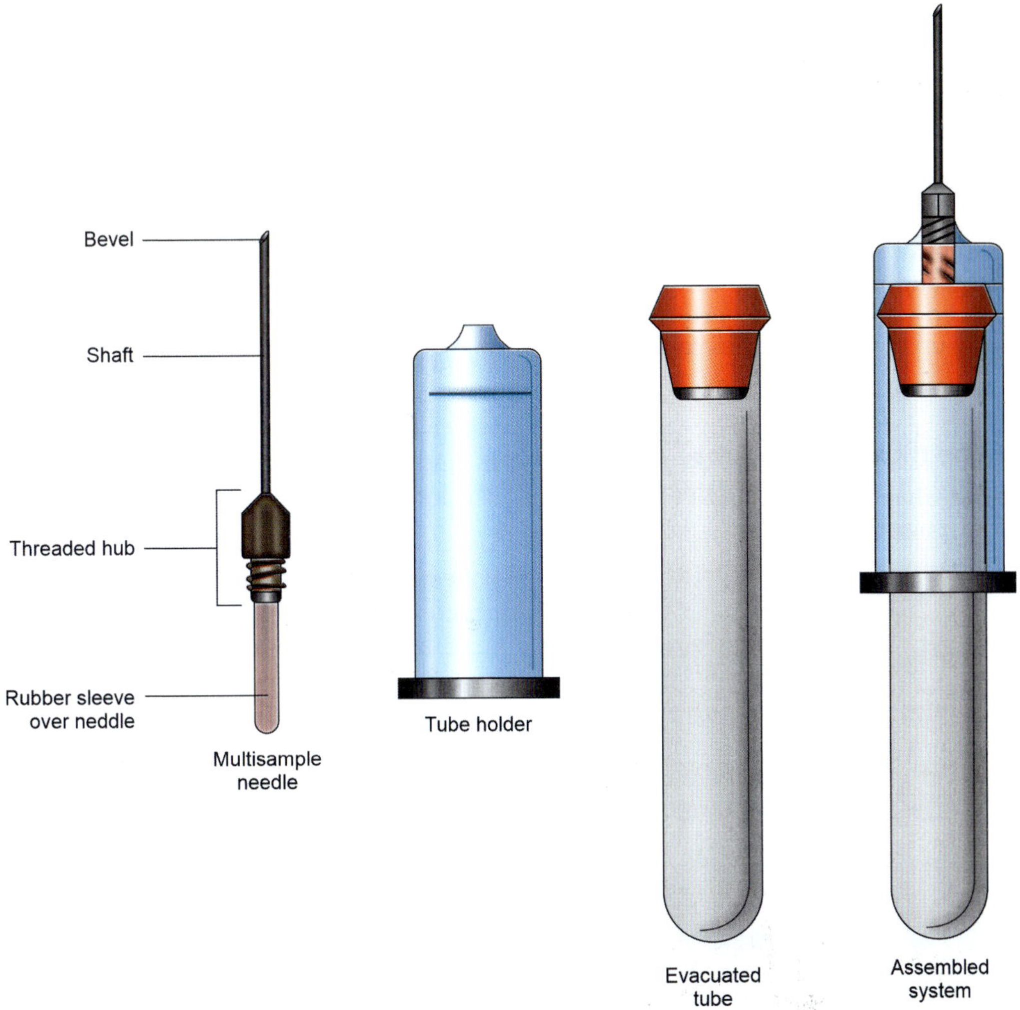

Fig. AI.6: Vacutainers with vacupuncture needle

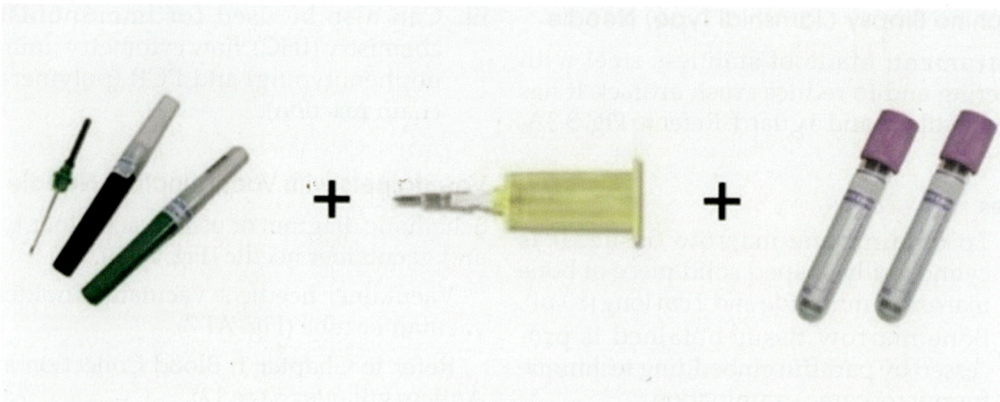

Fig. AI.7: Vacutainers system

Westergren's Pipette

Refer to Chapter 5; ESR and PCV, Fig. 5.1, page 58).

Westergren's Stand

Refer to Fig. 5.2, page 58.

Instrument: Made of stainless steel base with top support. Multiple ESR pipettes can be placed within it in a vertical position. Usually up to 6 ESR pipettes can be placed.

Use: To record ESR in Westegren method.

Wintrobe (Haematocrit) Tube

Refer to Chapter 5; ESR and PCV (Refer to Fig. 5.6, page 65).

Wintrobe's Stand (Fig. AI.8)

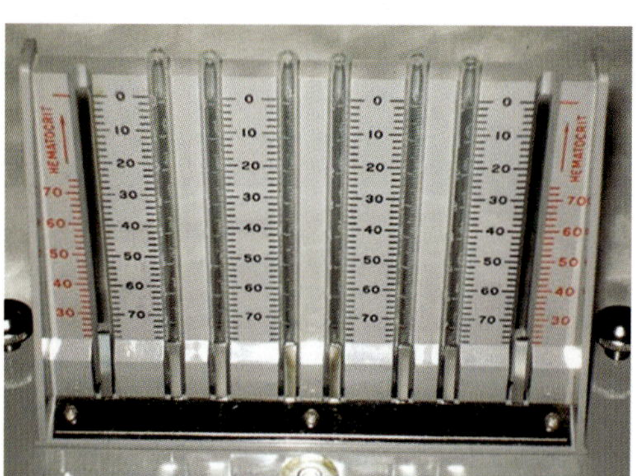

Fig. AI.8: Wintrobe's stand

Instrument: Made of good quality metal (stainless steel) and coated with enamel. Usually 2–8 Wintrobe's tubes can be placed.

Use: To record ESR in Wintrobe's method.

CLINICAL PATHOLOGY INSTRUMENTS/ REAGENTS

Dipstick for Urine

Reagent strip: A standard urine test strip may comprise up to 10 different chemical reagents which react (change color) when immersed in, and then removed from, a urine sample. The test is read after 30–120 seconds.

Use: To determine pathological changes in patient's urine in standard urinalysis (proteins, glucose, ketone, haemoglobin, bilirubin, urobilinogen, acetone, leukocyte, pH and specific gravity) (Refer Fig. 12.7, page 180).

Esbach's Albuminometer (Fig. AI.9)

Refer to Chapter 12; Urine Examination (pages 171 and 175).

Lumbar Puncture Needle

It is a sterile long slender needle with a stilette. It is about 10 cm long and has a bore of 1–1.5 mm.

Refer to Chapter 11; LP Needle, CSF and Body Fluids Fig. 11.1 (page 151).

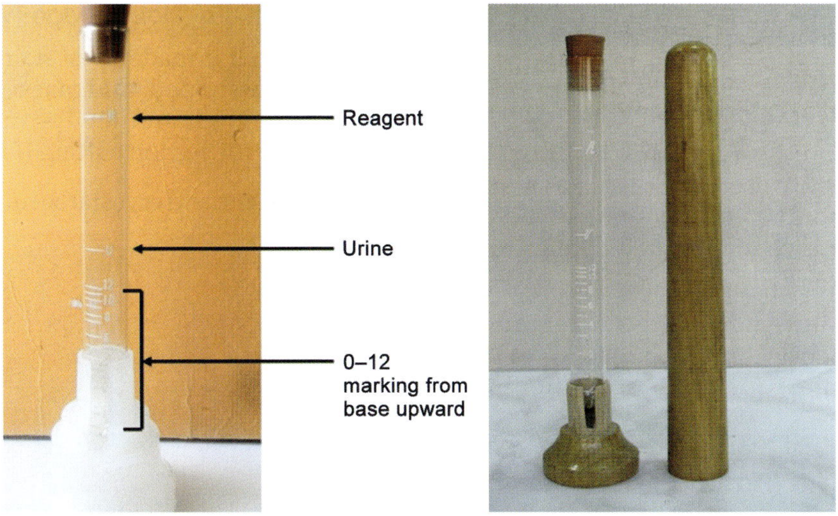

Fig. AI.9: Esbach's albuminometer

Urinometer (Hydrometer) (Fig. AI.10)

Refer to Chapter 12; Urine Examination (page 168).

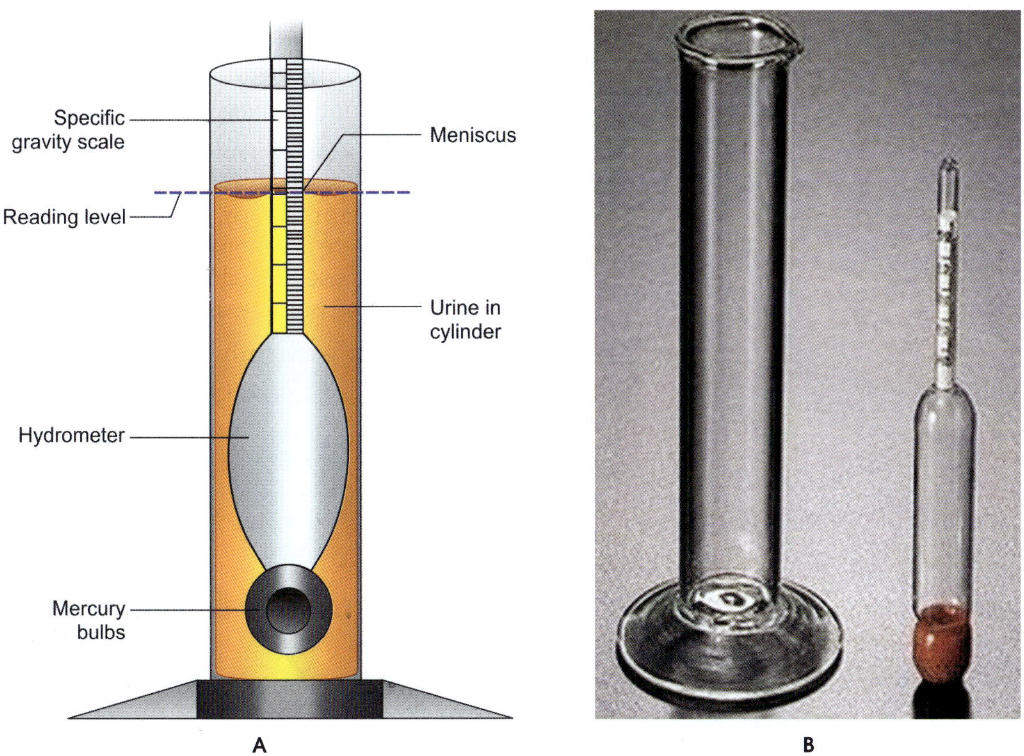

Fig. AI.10A and B: Urinometer (hydrometer)

HISTOPATHOLOGY

Block Moulds (Leuckhart's (L) Mould Method)

Description: L-shaped heavy brass. Two such pieces are used and placed as required to make paraffin block. It is named after Leuckhart invention in 1881. Refer to Fig. 13.3A, page 201.

Use: Tissue embedding. After adding fixative, biopsies are embedded in paraffin/wax for subsequent tissue sectioning in microtome.

Block Moulds (Plastic) or Cassettes

Description: Made of plastics and light weight. Refer to Fig. 13.4A, page 201.

Use: Same as metal block moulds.

Microtomy Blade (High and Low Profile)

Description: High profile disposable blades (Leica 818) are ultra-fine yet durable, the 80 mm long × 14 mm high × 0.35 mm thick blades, can make very thin sections. Low profile (Leica 819) disposable blades are 80 mm long, 8 mm high and 0.25 mm thick.

Both high and low profile blades are made of stainless steel (Fig. AI.11).

Use: Microtome and cryostat sectioning.

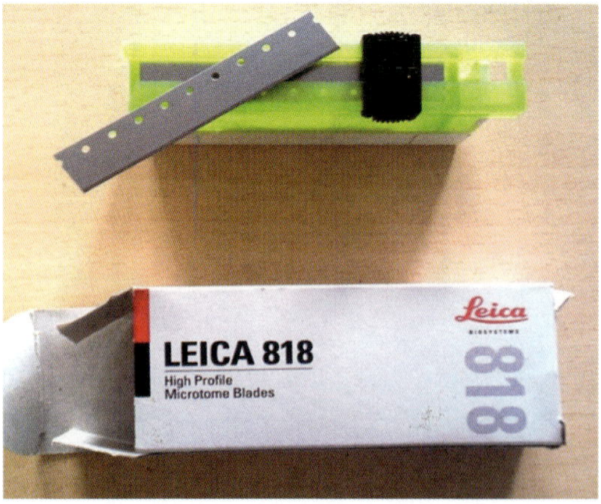

Fig. AI.11: Microtome blade (high profile)

Microtome Knife (Plain Wedge Type)

Description: It is made up of stainless steel. It is wedge-shaped and uses in rotary microtome. High and low profile placed within knife for section cutting (Fig. AI.12).

Use: Microtome and cryostat section cutting.

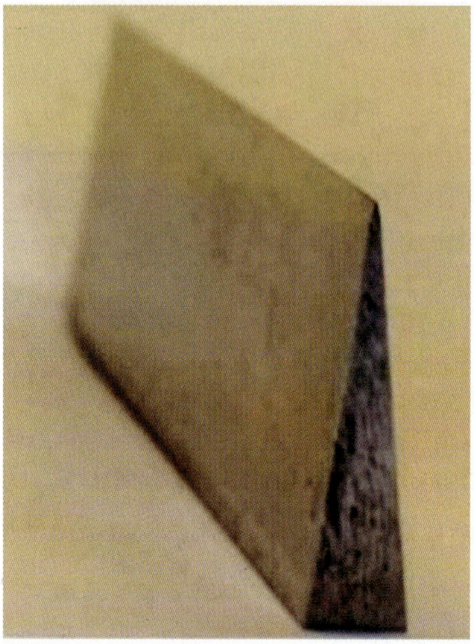

Fig. AI.12: Microtome knife

Tissue Capsule (Stainless Steel) Cassette

Description: This capsule is autoclavable, made of stainless steel, and resistant to most of the common laboratory acids and chemicals. There are many holes embedded on its lid and base to facilitate the fluid flow in it. It has secure positive snap cap (Fig. AI.13).

Use: Paraffin wax embedding for tissue processing.

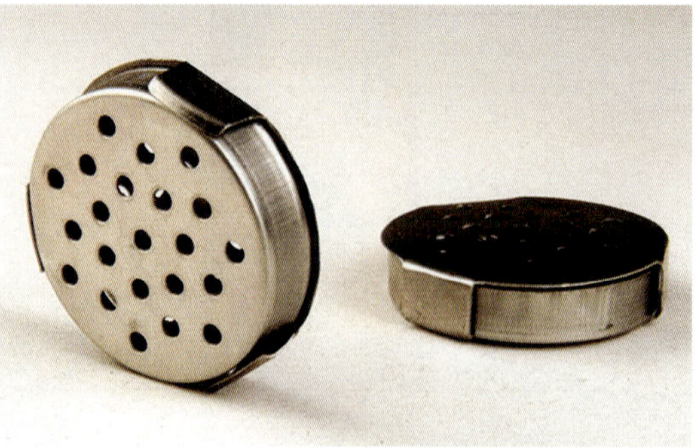

Fig. AI.13: Stainless steel cassette

CYTOPATHOLOGY

Ayre's Spatula

Description: It is a wooden spatula with U-shaped opening on one side and a flat surface on another. The broad end is for vaginal sample collection and the narrow end is for cervical sample collection.

Use: It is rotated 360° to collect cervical/ vaginal cells for Pap (Papanicolaou) staining. It is being replaced by cytobrush and Ayre's bury device/spatula. Refer to Fig. 16.5A, page 234.

Coplin Jar

Description: It is a covered glass (or plastic) vessel that is rectangular in cross section and grooved inside for holding microscope slides vertical during processing or staining. It can hold up to 10 slides of the size 1 × 3 inches (Fig. AI.14).

Use: For fixation of slides (alcohol), staining of smears or histologic sections.

Franzen Handle (Syringe Holder)

Description: Made up of stainless steel and can hold 10/20 ml syringe. It can produce a good negative pressure. The holder leaves one hand free to immobilize and to feel the target lesion. Other hand is used for aspiration (negative pressure).

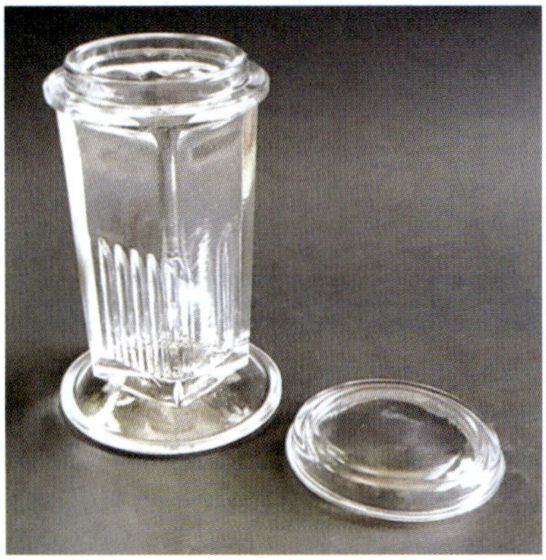

A

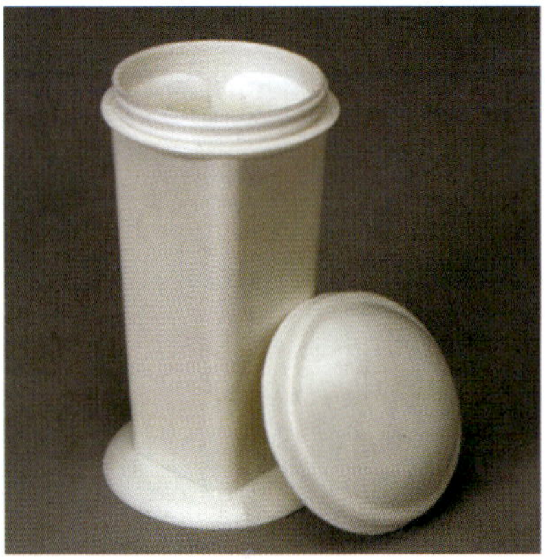

B

Fig. AI.14A and B: (A) Coplin jar (glass), (B) Coplin jar (plastic)

Use: To aspirate material during FNAC and making smears. Refer to Fig. 16.10, page 241.

Appendix

II

Reference Values (Range)

NORMAL REFERENCE VALUES IN HAEMATOLOGY

Parameters	Males	Females
• Haemoglobin (Hb)	13–18 g/dl	11–16 g/dl
• Haematocrit (PCV)	41–53 %	36–46 %
• ESR i. Westergren method	0–10 mm/1st hour	0–20 mm/1st hour
ii. Wintrobe method	0–7 mm/1st hour	0–14 mm/1st hour
• Mean corpuscular volume (MCV)	78–98 fl	78–98 fl
• Mean corpuscular haemoglobin (MCH)	28–32 pg	26–34 pg
• Mean corpuscular haemoglobin concentration (MCHC)	31–36 g/dl	31–36 g/dl
• Serum iron	80–180 μg/dl	30–160 μg/dl
• Total iron binding capacity (TIBC)	250–450 μg/dl	228–428 μg/dl
• Transferrin saturation	30–35 %	30–35%
• Serum ferritin	36–300 ng/ml (mean 90)	10–200 ng/ml (mean 18)
• Prothrombin time (PT)	11–14 seconds	11–14 seconds
• Activated partial thromboplastin time (APTT or PTTK)	35–45 seconds	35–45 seconds
• Haemoglobin A_1C	4–6 %	4–6%
• Serum fibrinogen	200–400 mg/dl	150–400 mg/dl
• RBC count	4.5–5.5 million/mm^3	3.8–5.2 million/mm^3
• WBC count or total leukocyte count (TLC)	4,000–11,000/mm^3 (4–11 × 10^9/L)	4,000–11,000/mm^3 (4–11 × 10^9/L)
• Platelet count	1,50,000–4,00,000/mm^3 (150–400 × 10^9/L)	1,50,000–4,00,000/mm^3 (150–400 × 10^9/L)
• Reticulocyte count (adult and children)	0.5–2.0 %	0.5–2.0%
• Reticulocyte count (infants)	2–6 %	2–6%
• Absolute eosinophil count	40–450 cells/mm^3	40–450 cells/mm^3

Differential Leukocytes Count (DLC)

• Neutrophils (polymorphs)	40–70% (2,00–7,500/mm^3 or µl)
• Lymphocytes	20–40% (1.500–4,00/mm^3 or µl)
• Monocytes	2–10% (200–800/mm^3 or µl)
• Eosinophils	1–6% (40–450/mm^3 or µl)
• Basophils	<1% (10–100/mm^3 or µl)

Critical Values in Haematology

Laboratory test values/findings	Risk/clinical significance
• Haemoglobin <7g/dl	• Myocardial ischaemia
• Haemoglobin >20 g/dl	• Hyperviscosity syndrome
• Total leukocyte count <2,000/mm^3	• Infections (especially when neutrophil) count falls below 500/mm^3)
• Total leukocyte count >50,000/mm^3	• Leukaemia, leukaemoid reaction
• Platelet count <40,000/mm^3	• Critical count, platelet/blood transfusion required
• Platelet count <20,000/mm^3	• Spontaneous bleeding
• Platelet count <10,000/mm^3	• Serious haemorrhage
• Platelet count <1,00,000/mm^3 (thrombocytopenia)	• Bleeding time increased
• Platelet count >10,00,000/mm^3 (thrombocytosis)	• Thrombosis
• Prothrombin time >30 seconds or >3 times control valve	• Bleeding
• Plasma fibrinogen <100 mg/dl	• Bleeding
• Activated partial thromboplastin time ≥75 seconds	• Bleeding
• D-dimer: Positive	• Disseminated intravascular coagulation (DIC)

Lipid Profile

Component	Reference value	
	Conventional	SI unit
• Total serum cholesterol		
i. Desirable for adults	<200 mg/dl	<5.17 mmol/L
ii. Borderline high	200–239/dl	5.17–6.18 mmol/L
iii. High and undesirable	>240 mg/dl	>6.21 mmol/L
• Triglycerides	<160 mg/dl	>1.55 mmol/L
• HDL cholesterol		
i. Low (undesirable)	<40 mg/dl	<1.03 mmol/L
ii. High, protective range	>60 mg/dl	1.55 mmol/L
• LDL cholesterol		
i. Desirable range	100–130 mg/dl	<3.34 mmol/L
ii. Borderline high	130–159 mg/dl	3.36–4.11 mmol/L
iii. High	160–189 mg/dl	4.11–4.20 mmol/L
iv. Very high	>190 mg/dl	>4.21 mmol/L

Clinical Chemistry

Component	Specimen	Reference value	
		Conventional units	SI units
• Alpha fetoprotein (AFP)	Serum	0–8.5 ng/ml	0–8.5 μg/L
• Aminotransferases (transaminases)			
i. Aspartate (AST, SGOT)	Serum	12–38 U/L	0.20–0.65 μkat/L
ii. Alanine (ALT, SGPT)	Serum	7–41 U/L	0.12–0.70 μkat/L
• Amylase	Serum	20–96 U/L	0.34–1.6 μkat/L
• Bilirubin	Serum		
i. Total		0.3–1.3 mg/dl	5.1–22 μmol/L
ii. Direct (conjugated)		0.1–0.4 mg/dl	1.7–6.8 μmol/L
iii. Indirect (unconjugated)		0.2–0.9 mg/dl	3.4–15.2 μmol/L
• Calcium (total)	Serum	8.7–10.2 mg/dl	2.2–2.6 mmol/L
• C-reactive proteins (CRP)	Serum	0.2–3.0 mg/L	0.2–3.0 mg/L
• Glucose (fasting)	Plasma		
i. Normal range		70–100 mg/dl	<5.6 mmol/L
ii. Impaired fasting glucose (IFG)		101–125 mg/dl	5.6–6.9 mmol/L
iii. Diabetes mellitus		>126 mg/dl	>7.0 mmol/L
• Glucose (2 hours postprandial or PP)	Plasma		
i. Normal		<140 mg/dl	<7.8 mmol/L
ii. Impaired glucose tolerance (IGT)		140–200 mg/dl	7.8–11.1 mmol/L
iii. Diabetes mellitus		>200 mg/dl	11.1 mmol/L
• Phosphatases	Serum		
i. Acid phosphatase		0–5.5 U/L	0.90 μkat/L
ii. Alkaline phosphatase		33–96 U/L	0.56–1.63 μkat/L
• Prostatic specific antigen (PSA)	Serum	0–4.0 ng/ml	0–4.0 μg/L
• Proteins (total)	Serum	6.7–8.6 g/dl	67–86 g/L
i. Albumin		3.5–5.5 g/dl	35–55 g/L
ii. Globulins		2.0–3.5 g/dl	20–35 g/L
iii. Albumin/globulin ratio		1.5–3:1	
• Troponins, cardiac (c Tn)			
i. Troponin I (c Tn I)	Serum	0–0.08 ng/ml	0–0.8 μg/L
ii. Troponin T (c Tn T)	Serum	0–01 ng/ml	0–0.1 μg/L
• Rheumatoid factor (RF)	Serum	<15 IU/ml	<15 KIU/L
• Blood urea nitrogen (BUN)	Blood	7–20 mg/dl	2.5–7.1 mmol/L
• Uric acid	Serum		
i. Males		3.1–7.0 mg/dl	0.18–0.41 μmol/L
ii. Females		2.5–5.6 mg/dl	0.15–0.33 μmol/L

Clinical Chemistry

Analyte	Reference value	
	Conventional	SI unit
• Sodium	136–146 mEq/L	136–146 mmol/L
• Potassium	3.5–5.0 mEq/L	3.5–5.0 mmol/L
• Chloride	95–107 mEq/L	95–107 mmol/l
• Urea	20–40 mg/dl	3.3–6.6 mmol/L
• Creatinine	0.6–1.2 mg/dl	53–106 μmol/L

Index